Physics of PET and SPECT Imaging

IMAGING IN MEDICAL DIAGNOSIS AND THERAPY

Series Editors: Andrew Karellas and Bruce R. Thomadsen

Published titles

Quality and Safety in Radiotherapy
Todd Pawlicki, Peter B. Dunscombe,
Arno J. Mundt, and Pierre Scalliet, Editors
ISBN: 978-1-4398-0436-0

Adaptive Radiation Therapy
X. Allen Li, Editor
ISBN: 978-1-4398-1634-9

Quantitative MRI in Cancer
Thomas E. Yankeelov, David R. Pickens,
and Ronald R. Price, Editors
ISBN: 978-1-4398-2057-5

Informatics in Medical Imaging
George C. Kagadis and Steve G. Langer, Editors
ISBN: 978-1-4398-3124-3

Adaptive Motion Compensation in Radiotherapy
Martin J. Murphy, Editor
ISBN: 978-1-4398-2193-0

Image-Guided Radiation Therapy
Daniel J. Bourland, Editor
ISBN: 978-1-4398-0273-1

Targeted Molecular Imaging
Michael J. Welch and William C. Eckelman,
Editors
ISBN: 978-1-4398-4195-0

Proton and Carbon Ion Therapy
C.-M. Charlie Ma and Tony Lomax, Editors
ISBN: 978-1-4398-1607-3

Comprehensive Brachytherapy:
Physical and Clinical Aspects
Jack Venselaar, Dimos Baltas, Peter J. Hoskin,
and Ali Soleimani-Meigooni, Editors
ISBN: 978-1-4398-4498-4

Physics of Mammographic Imaging
Mia K. Markey, Editor
ISBN: 978-1-4398-7544-5

Physics of Thermal Therapy:
Fundamentals and Clinical Applications
Eduardo Moros, Editor
ISBN: 978-1-4398-4890-6

Emerging Imaging Technologies in Medicine
Mark A. Anastasio and Patrick La Riviere, Editors
ISBN: 978-1-4398-8041-8

Cancer Nanotechnology: Principles and Applications in Radiation Oncology
Sang Hyun Cho and Sunil Krishnan, Editors
ISBN: 978-1-4398-7875-0

Monte Carlo Techniques in Radiation Therapy
Joao Seco and Frank Verhaegen, Editors
ISBN: 978-1-4665-0792-0

Image Processing in Radiation Therapy
Kristy Kay Brock, Editor
ISBN: 978-1-4398-3017-8

Informatics in Radiation Oncology
George Starkschall and R. Alfredo C. Siochi,
Editors
ISBN: 978-1-4398-2582-2

Cone Beam Computed Tomography
Chris C. Shaw, Editor
ISBN: 978-1-4398-4626-1

Tomosynthesis Imaging
Ingrid Reiser and Stephen Glick, Editors
ISBN: 978-1-4398-7870-5

Stereotactic Radiosurgery and Stereotactic Body Radiation Therapy
Stanley H. Benedict, David J. Schlesinger, Steven
J. Goetsch, and Brian D. Kavanagh, Editors
ISBN: 978-1-4398-4197-6

Computer-Aided Detection and Diagnosis in Medical Imaging
Qiang Li and Robert M. Nishikawa, Editors
ISBN: 978-1-4398-7176-8

IMAGING IN MEDICAL DIAGNOSIS AND THERAPY
Series Editors: Andrew Karellas and Bruce R. Thomadsen

Published titles

Physics of PET and SPECT Imaging

Edited by
Magnus Dahlbom, PhD
Department of Molecular and Medical Pharmacology
Division of Nuclear Medicine, David Geffen School of Medicine at UCLA

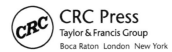

CRC Press
Taylor & Francis Group
Boca Raton London New York

CRC Press is an imprint of the
Taylor & Francis Group, an **informa** business

A TAYLOR & FRANCIS BOOK

CRC Press
Taylor & Francis Group
6000 Broken Sound Parkway NW, Suite 300
Boca Raton, FL 33487-2742

First issued in paperback 2020

ISBN-13: 978-1-4665-6013-0 (hbk)
ISBN-13: 978-0-367-78236-8 (pbk)

Lib ary of Congress Cataloging-in-Publication Data

Names: Dahlbom, Magnus, editor.
Title: Physics of PET and SPECT imaging / [edited by] Magnus Dahlbom.
Other titles: Imaging in medical diagnosis and therapy.
Description: Boca Raton, FL : CRC Press, Taylor & Francis Group, [2017] |
Series: Imaging in medical diagnosis and therapy
Identifiers: LCCN 2016033209| ISBN 9781466560130 (hardback ; alk. paper) |
ISBN 1466560134 (hardback ; alk. paper)
Subjects: LCSH: Tomography, Emission. | Single-photon emission computed tomography. | Imaging systems in medicine.
Classification: LCC RC78.7.T62 P55 2017 | DDC 616.07/575--dc23
LC record available at https://lccn.loc.gov/2016033209

To my family – my wife Maggie and my children Katarina, Kristian, Michele, and Vanessa for your constant support and encouragement, and infinite amount of love and patience.

Contents

Series preface   xi

Preface   xiii

Acknowledgment   xv

Editor   xvii

Contributors   xix

PART 1   BASICS   1

1 Principles of SPECT and PET imaging   3
   Magnus Dahlbom and Michael A. King

PART 2   TECHNOLOGY   41

2 Scintillators for PET and SPECT   43
   Charles L. Melcher and Lars Eriksson

3 Photodetectors   63
   Magnus Dahlbom

4 Acquisition electronics   91
   Thomas K. Lewellen

5 SPECT instrumentation   115
   Wei Chang, Michael Rozler, and Scott D. Metzler

6 PET instrumentation   163
   Andrew L. Goertzen and Jonathan D. Thiessen

PART 3   QUANTITATIVE IMAGING   193

7 Methodologies for quantitative SPECT   195
   Irène Buvat

8 Data corrections and quantitative PET   211
   Suleman Surti and Joshua Scheuermann

9 Image reconstruction for PET and SPECT   235
   Richard M. Leahy, Bing Bai, and Evren Asma

10 High-performance computing in emission tomography   259
    Guillem Pratx

11 Methods and applications of dynamic SPECT imaging   285
    Anna M. Celler, Troy H. Farncombe, Alvin Ihsani, Arkadiusz Sitek, and R. Glenn Wells

12 Dynamic PET imaging   321
    Sung-Cheng (Henry) Huang and Koon-Pong Wong

PART 4   MULTIMODALITY IMAGING   337

13 PET/CT   339
    Søren Holm, Osama Mawlawi, and Thomas Beyer

14 SPECT/CT   369
    Yothin Rakvongthai, Jinsong Ouyang, and Georges El Fakhri

15 PET/MRI   379
    Ciprian Catana

PART 5   PRECLINICAL IMAGING AND CLINICAL APPLICATIONS   411

16 Preclinical PET and SPECT   413
    Steven R. Meikle, Andre Z. Kyme, Peter Kench, Frederic Boisson, and Arvind Parmar

17 Clinical applications of PET/CT and SPECT/CT imaging   439
    *Johannes Czernin and Ora Israel, Ken Herrmann, Martin Barrio, David Nathanson, and
    Martin Allen-Auerbach*

Index   473

Series preface

Advances in the science and technology of medical imaging and radiation therapy are more profound and rapid than ever before, since their inception more than a century ago. Further, the disciplines are increasingly cross-linked as imaging methods become more widely used to plan, guide, monitor, and assess treatments in radiation therapy. Today, the technologies of medical imaging and radiation therapy are so complex and so computer driven that it is difficult for the persons (physicians and technologists) responsible for their clinical use to know exactly what is happening at the point of care, when a patient is being examined or treated. The persons best equipped to understand the technologies and their applications are medical physicists, and these individuals are assuming greater responsibilities in the clinical arena to ensure that what is intended for the patient is actually delivered in a safe and effective manner.

The growing responsibilities of medical physicists in the clinical arenas of medical imaging and radiation therapy are not without their challenges, however. Most medical physicists are knowledgeable in either radiation therapy or medical imaging, and expert in one or a small number of areas within their discipline. They sustain their expertise in these areas by reading scientific articles and attending scientific talks at meetings. In contrast, their responsibilities increasingly extend beyond their specific areas of expertise. To meet these responsibilities, medical physicists periodically must refresh their knowledge of advances in medical imaging or radiation therapy, and they must be prepared to function at the intersection of these two fields. How to accomplish these objectives is a challenge.

At the 2007 annual meeting of the American Association of Physicists in Medicine in Minneapolis, this challenge was the topic of conversation during a lunch hosted by Taylor & Francis Group and involving a group of senior medical physicists (Arthur L. Boyer, Joseph O. Deasy, C.-M. Charlie Ma, Todd A. Pawlicki, Ervin B. Podgorsak, Elke Reitzel, Anthony B. Wolbarst, and Ellen D. Yorke). The conclusion of this discussion was that a book series should be launched under the Taylor & Francis banner, with each volume in the series addressing a rapidly advancing area of medical imaging or radiation therapy of importance to medical physicists. The aim would be for each volume to provide medical physicists with the information needed to understand technologies driving a rapid advance and their applications to safe and effective delivery of patient care.

Each volume in the series is edited by one or more individuals with recognized expertise in the technological area encompassed by the book. The editors are responsible for selecting the authors of individual chapters and ensuring that the chapters are comprehensive and intelligible to someone without such expertise. The enthusiasm of volume editors and chapter authors has been gratifying and reinforces the conclusion of the Minneapolis luncheon that this series of books addresses a major need of medical physicists.

The Imaging in Medical Diagnosis and Therapy series would not have been possible without the encouragement and support of the series manager, Luna Han of Taylor & Francis. The editors and authors, and most of all I, are indebted to her steady guidance of the entire project.

William Hendee, Founding Series Editor
Rochester, Minnesota

Preface

The fields of positron emission tomography (PET) and single-photo emission computed tomography (SPECT) imaging are continuously developing. New developments in detector technologies have allowed a broad spectrum of new imaging possibilities. Much of this development comes from the discovery of new scintillator materials, improvements and innovation in photodetector development, and new innovative system designs and image reconstruction algorithms. All of these areas of development have allowed improved image quality, spatial resolution, and simultaneous multimodality imaging.

Although there are a few excellent textbooks on the subject of nuclear imaging, this book is intended as the first to focus on PET and SPECT instrumentation, reflecting the most recent developments, including the challenges of multimodality imaging.

The book is aimed at an audience of graduate students in biomedical physics and postdocs in molecular imaging and related fields. We also expect the book to be useful as a reference for other professionals involved in molecular imaging, in both academics and industry. One of my hopes in assembling it is to provide an advanced-level textbook that goes beyond the general concepts described in introductory textbooks.

The chapters are organized into five sections, starting with an introduction to the field from a researcher and clinician's perspective, and covering the basics of PET and SPECT physics. The second section addresses detector technology, starting with scintillators, photodetectors for use with scintillators, and solid-state detectors, in addition to a chapter that covers system electronics (e.g., digital pulse processing) and the use of advanced computing methods (e.g., use of the graphics processing unit for image reconstruction and processing). The third section turns to various aspects of producing quantitative images, such as techniques for image reconstruction, corrections to the data to produce quantitative images, and characterization and evaluation of images, as well as challenges of dynamic imaging in PET and SPECT. The fourth section covers instrumentation for multimodality imaging, which includes PET/CT, SPECT/CT, and PET/MR. The final section looks at specialized instrumentation used in preclinical imaging using PET and SPECT, with a final chapter on clinical applications.

Magnus Dahlbom

Acknowledgment

Foremost, I thank all the authors who have taken time out of their busy schedules to contribute with their knowledge and expertise to this book. I would like to thank Ms. Amber Hain for administrative support. Finally, I would like to give special thanks to Ms. Luna Han, Senior Publishing Editor at CRC Press for her help, guidance, and patience throughout this project.

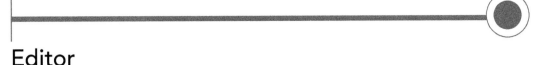

Editor

Magnus Dahlbom has been working in the field of nuclear medicine for close to 30 years. He earned his BSc in physics from the University of Stockholm in 1982. He earned his PhD from the University of California, Los Angeles (UCLA) in 1987. His PhD research was on high-resolution PET detectors and image processing. In 1989, he was part of the team that started the first clinical PET operation in the United States at UCLA. Around the same time, together with Drs. Edward J. Hoffman and Michael E. Phelps, he developed the whole-body PET imaging technique, which is currently used in more than 90% of all PET studies performed. His research interests are in PET and SPECT instrumentation and image processing. Since 1989, he has been the chief physicist at the Nuclear Medicine Services at UCLA, where he is responsible for all imaging instrumentation, including SPECT, SPECT/CT, and PET/CT systems. At UCLA, he is the faculty graduate advisor in the biomedical physics graduate program. He is teaching graduate-level courses on the basics of nuclear medicine imaging and instrumentation. Dr. Dahlbom has authored and coauthored more than 120 research papers and 11 book chapters on nuclear imaging instrumentation and processing. He was also coeditor of a PET/CT atlas. For the last 6 years, he has been serving as an editorial consultant to the editor in chief of the *Journal of Nuclear Medicine*.

Contributors

Martin Allen-Auerbach
Ahmanson Translational Imaging Division
David Geffen School of Medicine
University of California, Los Angeles
Los Angeles, California

Evren Asma
Toshiba Medical Research Institute USA, Inc.
(TMRU)
Vernon Hills, Illinois

Bing Bai
Toshiba America Medical Systems
Tustin, California

Martin Barrio
Ahmanson Translational Imaging Division
David Geffen School of Medicine
University of California, Los Angeles
Los Angeles, California

Thomas Beyer
QIMP Group Center for Medical Physics and
Biomedical Engineering
Medical University Vienna Vienna, Austria

Frederic Boisson
Australian Nuclear Science and Technology
Organisation (ANSTO)
Lucas Heights, New South Wales, Australia

Irène Buvat
Unité Imagerie Moléculaire In Vivo
Inserm/CEA/Université Paris Sud
Orsay, France

Ciprian Catana
Athinoula A. Martinos Center for Biomedical
Imaging
Charlestown, Massachusetts

Anna M. Celler
Department of Radiology
University of British Columbia
Vancouver, British Columbia, Canada

Wei Chang
Department of Diagnostic Radiology
Rush University Medical Center
Chicago, Illinois
(Now at Department of Radiology
University of Pennsylvania
Philadelphia, Pennsylvania)

Johannes Czernin
Ahmanson Translational Imaging Division
David Geffen School of Medicine
University of California, Los Angeles
Los Angeles, California

Magnus Dahlbom
Department of Molecular & Medical
Pharmacology
David Geffen School of Medicine
University of California, Los Angeles
Los Angeles, California

Georges El Fakhri
Gordon Center for Medical Imaging
Department of Radiology
Massachusetts General Hospital
and
Department of Radiology
Harvard Medical School
Boston, Massachusetts

Lars Eriksson
Molecular Imaging Siemens Medical Solutions
Knoxville, Tennessee

Troy H. Farncombe
Department of Nuclear Medicine
McMaster University
Hamilton, Ontario, Canada

Andrew L. Goertzen
Section of Nuclear Medicine
Health Sciences Centre
Department of Radiology
University of Manitoba
Winnipeg, Manitoba, Canada

Ken Herrmann
Department of Nuclear Medicine
Universitätsklinikum Würzburg
Würzburg, Germany

Søren Holm
Department of Clinical Physiology, Nuclear
Medicine & PET
University of Copenhagen
and Rigshospitalet
Copenhagen University Hospital
Copenhagen, Denmark

Sung-Cheng (Henry) Huang
Department of Molecular & Medical
Pharmacology
David Geffen School of Medicine
University of California, Los Angeles
Los Angeles, California

Alvin Ihsani
Massachusetts General Hospital
Harvard Medical School
Boston, Massachusetts

Ora Israel
Department of Nuclear Medicine
Rambam Health Care Campus and Rappaport
Faculty of Medicine
The Technion
Haifa, Israel

Peter Kench
Faculty of Health Sciences
The University of Sydney
Sydney, Australia

Michael A. King
Department of Radiology
University of Massachusetts Medical
School
Worcester, Massachusetts

Andre Z. Kyme
Brain and Mind Research Institute
The University of Sydney
Sydney, Australia

Richard M. Leahy
Signal and Image Processing Institute
Department of Electrical Engineering
University of Southern California
Los Angeles, California

Thomas K. Lewellen
Department of Radiology
University of Washington School of
Medicine
Seattle, Washington

Osama Mawlawi
Department of Imaging Physics
Division of Diagnostic Imaging
and Nuclear Medicine Physics Section
The University of Texas MD Anderson Cancer
Center
Houston, Texas

Steven R. Meikle
Faculty of Health Sciences
The University of Sydney
Sydney, Australia

Charles L. Melcher
Department of Materials Science and
Engineering
University of Tennessee
Knoxville, Tennessee

Scott D. Metzler
Department of Radiology
University of Pennsylvania
Philadelphia, Pennsylvania

David Nathanson
Ahmanson Translational Imaging Division
David Geffen School of Medicine
University of California, Los Angeles
Los Angeles, California

Jinsong Ouyang
Gordon Center for Medical Imaging
Department of Radiology
Massachusetts General Hospital
and Department of Radiology
Harvard Medical School
Boston, Massachusetts

Arvind Parmar
Australian Nuclear Science and Technology
Organisation (ANSTO)
Lucas Heights, New South Wales, Australia

Guillem Pratx
Radiation Biophysics Laboratory
Department of Radiation Oncology
Stanford University School of Medicine
Palo Alto, California

Yothin Rakvongthai
Department of Radiology
Faculty of Medicine
Chulalongkorn University
Bangkok, Thailand

Michael Rozler
Department of Diagnostic Radiology
Rush University Medical Center
Chicago, Illinois

Joshua Scheuermann
Department of Radiology Perelman School of Medicine
University of Pennsylvania
Philadelphia, Pennsylvania

Arkadiusz Sitek
Philips Research North America
Cambridge, Massachusetts

Suleman Surti
Physics & Instrumentation Group
Department of Radiology
University of Pennsylvania School of Medicine
Philadelphia, Pennsylvania

Jonathan D. Thiessen
Imaging Program
Lawson Health Research Institute
and Department of Medical
Biophysics
Western University
London, Ontario, Canada

R. Glenn Wells
Division of Cardiology
University of Ottawa Heart Institute
Department of Physics
Carleton University
Ottawa, Ontario, Canada

Koon-Pong Wong
Department of Molecular & Medical
Pharmacology
David Geffen School of Medicine
University of California, Los Angeles
Los Angeles, California

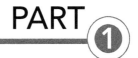
BASICS

1 Principles of SPECT and PET imaging   3
   Magnus Dahlbom and Michael A. King

Principles of SPECT and PET imaging

MAGNUS DAHLBOM AND MICHAEL A. KING

1.1	Introduction	4
1.2	Basic physics	4
	1.2.1 Units for mass and energy	4
	1.2.2 Stable and radioactive nuclides	5
	1.2.3 Six modes of radioactive decay	7
	1.2.4 Mathematics of radioactive decay	12
1.3	Interactions of radiation with matter	13
	1.3.1 Interactions of photons with matter	14
	1.3.2 Exponential attenuation of a beam of photons	16
1.4	Principles of photon detection	18
	1.4.1 Pulse height analysis	19
	1.4.2 Detection systems	21
	1.4.3 Scintillation detection	21
	1.4.4 Photodetectors	22
	1.4.4.1 Photomultiplier tube	22
	1.4.4.2 Solid-state photodetectors	23
	1.4.4.3 Solid-state detectors	24
1.5	Introduction to SPECT imaging	25
1.6	PET	28
	1.6.1 Basic principle	28
	1.6.2 Basic instrumentation design	30
	1.6.3 Coincidence detection	31
	1.6.4 Time resolution	31
	1.6.5 True coincidences	32
	1.6.6 Random coincidences	32
	1.6.7 Multiple events	33
	1.6.8 Scatter and attenuation	33
	1.6.9 Noise equivalent count rate (NECR)	34
	1.6.10 Time-of-flight PET	35

1.7   Image reconstruction   35
        1.7.1   Filtered backprojection   35
        1.7.2   Iterative reconstruction   36
1.8   Image analysis and evaluation   36
1.9   Summary   37
References   37

1.1 INTRODUCTION

Single-photon emission computed tomography (SPECT) and positron emission tomography (PET) are both well-established emission tomographic imaging methods used in clinical diagnosis and in research. Both are tomographic imaging methods that allow for *in vivo* studies of physiological processes by observing the distribution of the concentration of a radiotracer within the subject that is being studied. The radiotracers used are substances that are part of the normal physiological processes in the body, with the difference that they are labeled with a radionuclide that can be detected by external means. For instance, glucose metabolism can be studied by following the distribution of fluorodeoxy glucose labeled with ^{18}F (^{18}FDG), which emits a positron. The formation of skeletal tissue can be studied using methylene diphosphonate (MDP) labeled with ^{99m}Tc, which is a gamma emitter.

Both imaging modalities are used in numerous different applications. Clinically, the methods are used for primary diagnosis, staging of disease, and observing response to therapy. Both imaging methods are frequently used to study the efficacy of new drug treatments. Preclinical SPECT and PET are used in the development of new radiotracers where the new tracer is studied in animal models prior to human testing. Preclinical imaging is also being used to study the efficacy of new treatments in animal models prior to human trials. Preclinical imaging has become an important research tool to study and better understand the biology of certain diseases, such as cancers.

Emission tomography provides the ability to noninvasively *reconstruct* the three-dimensional (3-D) distribution of concentration of a radionuclide within an object. This is accomplished by acquiring information about the activity concentration along a large number of rays or line integrals through an object. Common for both SPECT and PET, external detector systems are utilized to detect photons that are emitted in the decay of the radionuclide. Although both SPECT and PET utilize the photon emission to localize the activity, the detection techniques and the requirements in terms of what radionuclides can be used are quite different. In this chapter, some of the basic and relevant physics to SPECT and PET are reviewed. This includes a summary of the various radioactive decay modes, photon interactions, and detection, and finally, an introduction and overview of the principles of SPECT and PET imaging.

1.2 BASIC PHYSICS

In this section, some of the basic concepts of atomic and nuclear physics are discussed. These concepts are important for the discussion of radioactive decay, interactions, and other relevant physical processes for nuclear imaging.

1.2.1 UNITS FOR MASS AND ENERGY

The units used in our everyday life for mass and energy are much too large and many times inconvenient for use in atomic and nuclear physics. Thus, we need to define units whose scale matches that of the material discussed in this book.

In classical physics, *mass* is defined as a body's resistance to acceleration. By Newton's second law, when a net force is applied to an object, it will undergo acceleration according to

$$\text{Force [newton]} = \text{mass [kg]} \times \text{acceleration [m/s}^2] \tag{1.1}$$

where the force is given in multiples of the derived unit newton (N), the mass of the object is in kilograms, and the resulting acceleration is given in meters per second squared. A kilogram is a huge amount of mass compared with that of nuclei and particles making up an atom. The unit of mass most convenient to use for these is the *universal mass unit* (umu). This is defined as 1/12 the mass of the carbon atom made up of six protons, six electrons, and six neutrons (^{12}C). This is approximately 1.7×10^{-27} kg. The universal mass unit has also been called the unified atomic mass unit and dalton. It replaced the older atomic mass unit (amu), which was based on the oxygen atom with eight protons, eight electrons, and eight neutrons (^{16}O).

Macroscopically, energy can be defined as the ability to do work. The unit of energy is the derived unit joule. Mechanically, it is the energy expended when a force of 1 N is applied to move an object 1 m. Electrically, 1 J of energy is expended when a coulomb (C) of charge is moved through a potential difference of 1 V. A coulomb is 6.25×10^{18} times charge on an electron. Thus, the charge on one electron is 1.6×10^{-19} C. If a single electron is moved through a potential difference of 1 V, this is equal to 1.6×10^{-19} J. Using this, the *electron volt* (eV) is defined as 1.6×10^{-19} J, and this is the unit of energy that is commonly used in atomic and nuclear physics. As a reminder, 1 keV = 1,000 eV or 10^3 eV and 1 MeV = 1,000,000 eV or 10^6 eV.

Mass and energy are related by the equation

$$E = mc^2 \tag{1.2}$$

where E is energy in joules, m is mass in kilograms, and c is the speed of light in a vacuum (~3×10^8 m/s). Using Equation 1.2 and the definitions for the universal mass unit and electron volt, 1 umu of matter equals 931.5 MeV of energy. For example, the mass of an electron is 0.000549 amu, which is equivalent to an energy of 0.511 MeV or 511 keV. This conversion of mass to energy is, for instance, very important in PET.

1.2.2 STABLE AND RADIOACTIVE NUCLIDES

Prior to discussing the various modes by which nuclei can transform or decay toward more stable configurations, we briefly define some terms that will be made use of in that discussion. Nuclei are made up of positively charged protons, and neutrons, which have no net charge. The mass of the neutron is slightly larger than that of the protons. If we do not want to differentiate between these two particles, we call them *nucleons*. A *nuclide* is a particular combination of nucleons. A *radionuclide* is a nuclide that naturally emits radiation. The notation used to denote a given nuclide is $^A_Z X$, where A is the *atomic mass number* or number of nucleons, Z is atomic mass number or number of protons, and X is the symbol of chemical element (defined by Z). Examples of nuclides of interest in PET and SPECT are $^{18}_9$F, $^{99}_{43}$Tc, and $^{201}_{81}$Tl.

The nuclides can be grouped into families, which share some common attributes. *Isotopes* are nuclides that have same the Z or same number of *protons*. Examples are $^1_1$H, $^2_1$H, and $^3_1$H, which are the three known isotopes of hydrogen. *Isobars* are nuclides that have the same atomic mass number of A or the same number of nucleons. $^{99}_{42}$Mo and $^{99}_{43}$Tc are examples of isobars. Isobars are very important, as three of the modes of radioactive decay we discuss occur between isobars. That is, they are isobaric modes of decay. *Isotones* are nuclides that have the same number of *neutrons*. $^3_1$H and $^4_2$He are examples of isotones.

Just like the electrons bound to the nucleus, the nucleons bound within the nucleus can exist in different energy states. *Isomers* are different *energy* states of the same nuclide. That is, isomers are when one or more of the nucleons are bound differently (in different energy states) between the two. $^{99}_{43}$Tc and $^{99*}_{43}$Tc are two isomers of $^{99}_{43}$Tc. The first is the ground state, and the second is an *excited* state, as indicated by the asterisk (*). If the excited state has a half-life longer than >~10^{-12} s, then we will call this a *metastable* state. $^{99m}_{43}$Tc is the metastable state of $^{99}_{43}$Tc, which is commonly used in nuclear imaging.

Stable nuclides are ones that do not naturally transform themselves and emit radiation in the process (configuration with greatest binding energy). There are approximately 275 known stable nuclides. Figure 1.1 shows a representation of where the stable nuclides would be as the curved line on a plot of the number of

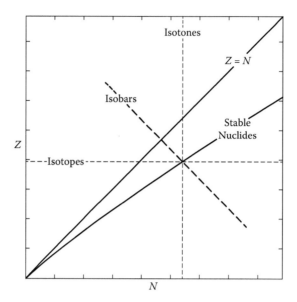

Figure 1.1 Representation of where the stable nuclides would be, as the curved line, on a plot of the number of protons versus number of neutrons. The solid diagonal line is an indication of nuclides, which have an equal number of protons and neutrons ($Z = N$).

protons versus number of neutrons. The solid diagonal line is an indication of nuclides, which have an equal number of protons and neutrons ($Z = N$). Note that at first, the stable nuclides lay along this line, but then the line curves so that eventually stable nuclides have approximately 1.5 times more neutrons than protons. The horizontal dashed line indicates where members of the same isotopic family would occur. Similarly, the vertical dashed line indicates where members of the same isotone family would occur and the 45° dashed diagonal line where members of the same isobar family would occur. To either side of this curve and extending beyond where it ends are the locations where the approximately 2200 known unstable or radioactive nuclides would be plotted. These nuclides, which naturally emit radiation in the process of transforming, are also call *radionuclides*.

Typically, the plot in Figure 1.1 is of the number of neutrons versus the number of protons, so that the plot for stable nuclides would curve upward instead of to the side. It has been plotted oppositely here to serve as an introduction to the chart of the nuclides. The chart of the nuclides is a plot of all of the known nuclides with selected properties, such as modes of decay, indicated within the box representing them. Figure 1.2 shows a version generated from data obtained from the Brookhaven National Laboratory (BNL) [1], in which color is used to indicate the mode of decay, with black being the stable nuclides.

In determining if it is possible for a radionuclide to undergo a decay to become another radionuclide, there are a number of conservation laws that need to be obeyed. Here, we consider only three of them. The first is the conservation of the *mass number* (A). The second is the conservation of the *total charge*. The third is the conservation of *mass and energy*. In the latter, we make use of matter being able to be converted to energy or energy to mass according to Equation 1.2. This leads to our being able to calculate the energy released (Q) in megaelectron volts during a potential decay as

$$Q\,[\text{MeV}] = \big(\text{Total Mass before decay [umu]} - \text{Total Mass after decay [umu]}\big) \times 931.5\,\text{MeV/umu} \qquad (1.3)$$

where 931.5 MeV/umu is the conversion between mass and energy given earlier. If Q is positive, then energy given off during decay is energetically favorable. If Q is negative, then energy has to be supplied for the decay to be feasible according to the conservation of mass and energy.

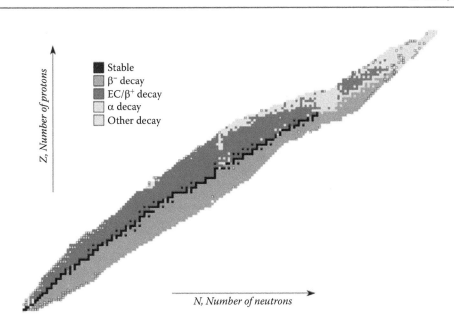

Figure 1.2 Chart of nuclides. Black squares indicate stable nuclides. Yellow squares indicate radionuclide decaying by alpha decay. Pink squares indicate radionuclides decaying by negatron or β⁻ decay. Blue squares indicate radionuclides decaying by either positron β⁺ decay or EC. White squares indicate other decay paths (e.g., spontaneous fission). (Chart generated from data from the National Nuclear Data Center, Brookhaven National Laboratory, Upton, NY, 2016.)

As an example, let us consider whether $^{12}_{6}C$ can decay by emitting a neutron, that is, whether the following transformation can take place:

$$^{12}_{6}C \rightarrow {}^{11}_{6}C + {}^{1}_{0}n + Q$$

Using Equation 1.3, we have the following:

$$Q\,[MeV] = \left(mass\,{}^{12}_{6}C - \left(mass\,{}^{11}_{6}C + mass\,{}^{1}_{0}n \right) \right) \times 931.5\,MeV/umu$$

There are many published sources of atomic masses, and many of these are available over the web. The one used in this discussion is the *Radiological Health Handbook* (RHH) published in 1970 by the U.S. Department of Health, Education, and Welfare [2]. Using the masses from the RHH [2], we obtain

$$Q = \left(12.00000\,umu - \left(11.011432\,umu + 1.008665\,umu \right) \times 931.5\,MeV/umu \right)$$

$$= -18.7\,MeV$$

Thus, the emission of a neutron does not occur without input of 18.7 MeV of energy. In fact, $^{12}_{6}C$ is a stable nuclide, which does not naturally undergo any of the six modes of decay that will be discussed in the next section.

1.2.3 Six modes of radioactive decay

The first mode of decay is *alpha* (α) *decay*. Alpha decay predominantly occurs when large nuclides decrease their mass through the emission of a $^{4}_{2}He$ nucleus (the alpha particle) to achieve greater binding energy per nucleon for the remaining nucleons. The $^4_2$He is the combination of nucleons emitted because it has the greatest binding energy per nucleon of any of the small combinations of nucleons. All the nuclides shown in yellow in Figure 1.2 will undergo alpha decay. The equation for alpha decay is given as

$$^A_Z P \rightarrow {}^{A-4}_{Z-2}D + {}^4_2He \tag{1.4}$$

where P is the parent nuclide and D is the daughter. Figure 1.3a shows how the P and D radionuclides would be related on the chart of the nuclides (i.e., P turns into D by loss of two protons and two neutrons with the emission of the alpha particle).

$^{226}_{88}$Ra is a naturally occurring radionuclide that is present due to it being a member of a decay chain starting with $^{238}_{92}$U, which has a half-life of 4.5×10^9 years. It undergoes alpha decay as shown in the following:

$$^{226}_{88}Ra \rightarrow {}^{222}_{86}Rn + {}^4_2He$$

The daughter $^{222}_{86}$Rn is a gas and seeps into cellars where it and its daughters make a significant contribution to the background equivalent dose to the U.S. population.

The energy level diagram for the decay of $^{226}_{88}$Ra is shown in Figure 1.3b. In these diagrams, moving farther down is going to a state of greater binding energy per nucleon, to the left is a decrease in the atomic number (Z), and to the right is an increase in the atomic number. Notice that two possible alpha decays are shown for $^{226}_{88}$Ra. One is to the ground state and the other is to an exited state. An isomeric transition (IT) between the excited state and the ground state is also indicated.

The energy release (Q) for this decay using the masses of the parent, daughter, and alpha from RHH [2] is 4.86 MeV. This energy is shared as kinetic energy between the daughter and alpha as dictated by the conservation of momentum. This explains why the energy for the alpha decay to the ground state in Figure 1.3b is listed as only 4.78 MeV. For alpha decay to occur, Q has to be not only positive, but also greater than ~3.9 MeV. This threshold energy is needed for the alpha to be able to break free from the daughter. In general, the larger Q is, the shorter the half-life once the threshold Q has been reached.

The second mode of decay is *beta* (β^-) *decay*, which is sometimes also called negatron decay to distinguish it from positron decay, which is discussed next. It is the first of three isobaric decay modes. Being an isobaric decay mode, the parent and daughter will both be members of the same isobaric family of nuclides. That is, they have the same number of nucleons and differ in the number of these that are protons versus the number that are neutrons.

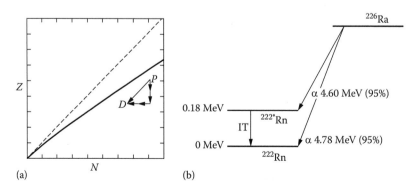

Figure 1.3 (a) Schematic of how the parent (*P*) and daughter (*D*) radionuclides would be related as positioned on the chart of the nuclides for alpha decay. (b) Energy level diagram for decay of ^{226}Ra. (Adapted from U.S. Bureau of Radiological Health Public Health Service, Radiological Health Handbook, U.S. Department of Health, Education, and Welfare, Washington, DC, 1970.)

Beta decay is basically the turning of a neutron into a proton with the emission of the beta particle and an antineutrino. The beta particle is an electron, which is created at the moment of emission. In fact, outside of the nucleus neutrons are not stable and undergo beta decay to protons ($_1^1H$ nuclei). This is energetically possible, as the mass of the neutron is larger than that of the proton, so that the energy release for this decay is 0.782 MeV, which is equal to the maximum kinetic energy of the emitted beta. The equation for beta decay is

$$_Z^A P \rightarrow \,_{Z+1}^A D + \,_{-1}^0 e + \bar{v} \tag{1.5}$$

where $_{-1}^0 e$ is the β^- particle or the negatron, and $\bar{v}$ is the antineutrino. Beta decay occurs below the line of stability on the chart of the nuclides. As shown in Figure 1.4a, it is how parent nuclides in this region transform to come closer to the line of stability by moving upward along the isobaric line for the family of isobars of which it is a member. In the BNL chart of nuclides in Figure 1.2, all of the nuclide positions shown in pink undergo beta negatron decay.

An example of beta decay of importance in nuclear imaging is that of $_{42}^{99}Mo$ to $_{43}^{99m}Tc$, since $_{43}^{99m}Tc$ is the most frequently employed radionuclide in SPECT imaging. This decay is given as

$$_{42}^{99} Mo \rightarrow \,_{43}^{99m} Tc + \,_{-1}^0 e + \bar{v}$$

The importance of it stems from it taking place inside generators used to produce $_{43}^{99m}Tc$ for clinical imaging. The transformation takes place with a 66 h half-life. $_{42}^{99}Mo$ is chemically bound to a column in the generator. $_{43}^{99m}Tc$, which has different chemical properties, is eluted from the column when sterile saline is drawn through it by a container with a vacuum initially in it.

The decay of $_{42}^{99}Mo$ is quite complex, as illustrated in Figure 1.4b. It can occur with the emission of any one of multiple different energy beta particles to a number of excited states of $_{43}^{99}Tc$. None of these states are the ground state. Following the beta decays, there are prompt ITs to other excited states, the metastable state, and the ground state. Immediately after beta decay, 86% of the time the transitions result in ^{99}Tc being in its 6 h half-life metastable state and 14% in the ground state. The decay of the metastable state is discussed subsequently in this section.

As mentioned above, the maximum kinetic energy of the beta particle is equal to the energy of release. This is true in general so long as the transition goes to the ground state of the daughter. However, it has been determined experimentally that the average energy given to the beta particle can vary from essentially 0 up to this maximum value. This distribution of values was one of the reasons that the existence of the antineutrino was postulated, so that it could carry away the remaining portion of the available energy.

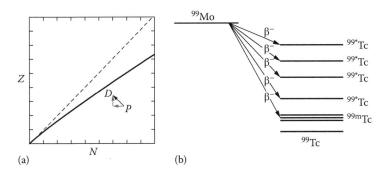

Figure 1.4 (a) Schematic of how the parent (P) and daughter (D) radionuclides would be related as positioned on the chart of the nuclides for beta decay. (b) Energy level diagram for the decay of ^{99}Mo. (Adapted from U.S. Bureau of Radiological Health Public Health Service, *Radiological Health Handbook*, U.S. Department of Health, Education, and Welfare, Washington, DC, 1970.)

The third mode of decay is *positron decay* (β⁺), which is the second of the isobaric decay modes to be discussed. Simplistically, it is the conversion of a proton into a neutron by the emission of a positive electron (the positron) and a neutrino. Neutrons are larger in mass than protons, so this takes place inside of a nucleus, where this conversion leads to the daughter nuclide having its nucleons even more tightly bound (i.e., there is an increase in the binding energy). The equation for positron decay is

$$\substack{A\\Z}P \rightarrow \substack{A\\Z-1}D + \substack{0\\+1}e + v \tag{1.6}$$

where $\substack{0\\+1}e$ is the positron (β⁺), and v is the neutrino. Nuclides rich in protons compared with the isobaric configuration(s) with largest binding energy occur above the line of stability in the chart of the nuclides. Thus, in positron decay the parent nuclide transforms down along the isobaric line to the daughter, as shown in Figure 1.5a. In the chart of the nuclides in Figure 1.2, the locations in blue all undergo positron decay.

An important example of positron decay is that of $\substack{18\\9}F$ to $\substack{18\\8}O$ according to

$$\substack{18\\9}F \rightarrow \substack{18\\8}O + \substack{0\\+1}e + v$$

This transition occurs with a 109.8 min half-life. That plus the chemical properties of fluorine make $\substack{18\\9}F$ the most commonly employed radionuclide for PET.

As in beta decay, the maximum energy given to the β⁺ is that predicted by the calculation of Q (assuming the transition is to the ground state of the daughter). However, in positron decay the parent has to be at least two times the rest mass energy equivalent of the electron or 1.022 MeV *larger* in mass than the daughter for decay to occur. Thus, the calculated Q for the decay of $\substack{18\\9}F$ is 0.635 MeV, as indicated in Figure 1.5b, which provides the energy level diagram for the decay of $\substack{18\\9}F$. Note that instead of being a straight diagonal line from the parent to the daughter, positron decay is indicated as first dropping straight down and then going diagonally off to the left. Positron decay is typically drawn in this way to indicate the requirement that it needs the equivalent decrease in mass of 1.022 MeV below the parent before it can occur. Note also that two modes of decay are indicated in this figure. The second mode is *electron capture* (EC or ε), which is the next mode to be discussed and, in many cases, an alternative or competing decay path to positron decay.

Once emitted, the positrons lose the kinetic energy they were given primarily through collisions with the electrons of atoms of the medium they travel through. Since positrons are the antiparticle to that of the electron, when all of their kinetic energy is gone, they will combine with an electron of the medium. In this process, they both *annihilate* with the emission of two 0.511 MeV photons at essentially 180° to each other. The energy for the two photons of 0.511 MeV comes from the conversion of the mass of the positron and electron into energy in the form of electromagnetic radiation. The emission of two equal energy photons at

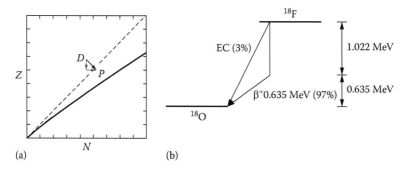

Figure 1.5 (a) Schematic of how the parent (*P*) and daughter (*D*) radionuclides would be related as positioned on the chart of the nuclides for positron decay and EC. (b) Energy level diagram for the decay of ¹⁸F. (Adapted from U.S. Bureau of Radiological Health Public Health Service, *Radiological Health Handbook*, U.S. Department of Health, Education, and Welfare, Washington, DC, 1970.)

~180° to each other is dictated by the conservation of momentum, provided that the electron–positron pair is at rest at the time of annihilation.

The fourth mode of decay is that of EC. It is the third and final isobaric mode of decay. It occurs when one of the orbital electrons of the atom enters the nucleus and combines with a proton to convert it into a neutron. It also can occur for nuclides above the line of stability on the chart of nuclides, as shown in Figure 1.5a, and thus is an alternative to positron decay in many cases. The locations where it can occur are also shown in blue on the chart of the nuclides (Figure 1.2). EC is also called K-capture if the orbital electron is from the K-shell, and L-capture if it is from the L-shell. When one does the analysis to determine the value of Q for EC, it is determined that EC can occur so long as the mass of the parent is larger than that of the daughter nuclide. Since there is no need for the margin of 1.022 MeV as required for positron decay, EC can occur for transitions not energetically possible for positron decay. The equation for EC is

$$_{Z}^{A}P - _{-1}^{0}e \rightarrow _{Z-1}^{A}D + \nu \tag{1.7}$$

In this case, the neutrino carries away all of the energy of release so long as the daughter goes to the ground state.

Some radionuclides that undergo EC can be used in SPECT imaging. This is because sometimes the decay is to an excited state of the daughter and the transition to the ground state leads to the emission of a photon, which can be used in imaging. Also, the loss of an orbital electron when it combines with the proton results in a vacancy in the electron binding structure. When this vacancy is filled by a less tightly bound electron, the difference in binding energy of the two states results in the emission of either a *characteristic radiation photon* or an *Auger* electron. The characteristic radiation photon is so named because its energy characterizes the change in binding energy of the electron, and thus the element it comes from. If the characteristic radiation is high enough in energy, it is called an x-ray, has a chance of escaping the body, and can thus be used in imaging. The Auger electron is another orbital electron of the atom to which the energy is transferred, so it can be freed from the atom.

An important example of a radionuclide used in SPECT that undergoes decay via EC is that of $_{81}^{201}$Tl. $_{81}^{201}$Tl chloride is used in cardiac perfusion imaging where a single injection during stress can be used to assess the coronary distribution of blood flow under high demand and delayed imaging can be used to assess redistribution. $_{81}^{201}$Tl undergoes decay according to

$$_{81}^{201}\text{Tl} + _{-1}^{0}e \rightarrow _{81}^{201}\text{Hg} + \nu + \text{x-rays} + \gamma\text{-rays}$$

where the γ-rays are emitted with ~10% abundance from de-excitation of the excited states of $_{81}^{201}$Hg. The characteristic x-rays are emitted about 88% of the time and are the primary photons used in imaging. The Q for this decay is 0.423 MeV by EC but –0.599 MeV via positron decay; thus, it solely occurs via EC.

The fifth and sixth modes of decay are forms of IT. That is, they occur when an excited nuclide de-excites to the ground state or a state closer to the ground state. These transitions can occur promptly as part of the decay to the daughter, or they can be delayed when the excited state is *metastable*. The equation for IT transitions is given as

$$_{Z}^{A*}P \rightarrow _{Z}^{A^{"*"}}P + \gamma \text{ and/or IC} \tag{1.8}$$

where the * in the resultant nuclide is because this could be the ground state, another excited state that will undergo a prompt transition, or a metastable state. Note that the identity of the resultant nuclide is the same as before the transition. Metastable states are indicated on the chart of the nuclides by dividing the entries in the box providing data for the nuclide into portions, one for each metastable state and the ground state.

The first mode of IT and fifth mode to be discussed is that of *gamma* (γ) *ray* emission. It is similar to that of the emission of a characteristic photon in that the γ-ray's energy is defined by the difference in energy

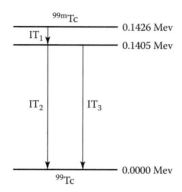

Figure 1.6 ITs from the metastable to the ground state of ^{99}Tc.

between the two energy states. Note the difference between x-rays and γ-rays is their origins. Characteristic x-rays are produced when electrons de-excite, and γ-rays when nucleons de-excite.

The second mode of IT and sixth mode to be discussed is that of *internal conversion* (IC). This happens when one of the orbital electrons of the atom enters the nucleus, receives the energy it de-excites, and leaves the atom with this energy minus its own binding energy. Given that this process results in the creation of a vacancy in the electron energy levels, characteristic radiation and Auger electrons are also associated with this process.

The determination of whether a given IT transition will be by γ or IC is random. However, the probability of occurrence of these depends of the properties of the given transition and have been tabulated for the radionuclides of clinical interest by the Medical Internal Radiation Dosimetry (MIRD) committee of the Society of Nuclear Medicine and Molecular Imaging (SNMMI) [3].

An important example of IT is that of the decay of $^{99m}_{43}$Tc to $^{99}_{43}$Tc. The energy level diagram for this decay adapted from [3] is shown in Figure 1.6. Note that IT_1 occurs ~99% of the time and goes by M or N shell IC with no γ. IT_2 goes ~88% of the time by emission of a 0.1405 MeV γ-ray, which is the photon used in medical imaging. The rest of the time it goes by IC for various energy shell electrons. Finally, IT_3 goes ~1% of the time primarily by IC electron emission.

There is another mode of IT, which occurs only when the transition energy is greater than 1.022 MeV. This is internal pair production. In this transition, instead of IC or γ-ray emission, an electron and a positron are emitted carrying away as kinetic energy the residual energy over 1.022 MeV needed to create this pair of particles. This is a low-probability event. However, because of the high sensitivity of PET imaging of the pair of photons emitted when positrons annihilate, PET of the internal γ-ray transitions when ^{90}Y undergoes β⁻ has been proposed as an alternative to SPECT imaging of the bremsstrahlung x-rays produced by the slowing of the β⁻ in the material [4].

1.2.4 Mathematics of radioactive decay

If dN represents the number of nuclei decaying during a very short period of time dt, then that number is just the negative (as these dN decrease the original number) of the number of nuclei at any point in time $N(t)$ times a constant λ called the decay constant. The equation governing the decay in the number of nuclei can then be written as

$$\frac{dN}{dt} = \lambda N(t) \tag{1.9}$$

Note that λ is the instantaneous fractional rate of decay and has units of time⁻¹. λ just depends on what radionuclide is decaying and not on factors such as temperature or pressure. The solution of this first-order differential equation is

$$N(t) = N_0 e^{-\lambda t} \tag{1.10}$$

where N_0 is the number of nuclei at $t = 0$.

In nuclear medicine, it is not the number of nuclei that is of interest, but rather the rate at which these nuclei are decaying. That is because this rate is related to the rate at which photons are being emitted, which is important to know when trying to judge the number of photons that will be acquired during imaging (as well as the radiation dose to the patient). The number of radioactive nuclei undergoing transformation per unit time ($-dN/dt$) is termed the *activity*. The negative is there because dN is a negative number, as stated before. By Equations 1.9 and 1.10, we can write

$$A(t) = -\frac{dN}{dt} = \lambda N(t) = A_0 e^{-\lambda t} \tag{1.11}$$

where A_o ($= N_o \lambda$) is the activity at t_0. Note that A depends on both N and λ. Thus, even if one has the same number of atoms for two different radionuclides, you will have different activities for them, as their λ values will be different.

There are two units employed with activity. The traditional unit is the *curie* (Ci) and was originally defined as the number of disintegrations in a gram of freshly isolated ^{226}Ra. Since the actual number of disintegrations per seconds of a gram of ^{226}Ra changed with improved counting methods, 1 Ci was defined as 3.7×10^{10} disintegrations per second (dps). Similarly, a millicurie will undergo 3.7×10^7 dps and a microcurie will undergo 3.7×10^4 dps. The curie is still commonly used in nuclear medicine clinics when discussing activities, especially in the United States. However, the International System of Units (SI) of activity, which is the *bequerel* (Bq), has replaced the curie in scientific communications. One bequerel is defined as 1 dps.

The decay constant is not what is tabulated for radionuclides. Instead, the *half-life* ($T_{1/2}$) is tabulated. The half-life is the time over which the activity (or the number of nuclei) decreases by a factor of 2 to 1/2 the original amount. Thus, in two half-lives it will decrease to ¼, and in three half-lives to 1/8. Using Equation 1.10, the following relationship between the decay constant and the half-life can be derived:

$$T_{1/2} = \frac{\ln 2}{\lambda} \approx \frac{0.693}{\lambda} \tag{1.12}$$

which provides the relationship between the two parameters for the rate of decay of a radionuclide. As an example, if $\lambda = 0.1155$ h^{-1}, then one will determine $T_{1/2} = 0.693/0.1155$ h^{-1} = 6.0 h, which is the $T_{1/2}$ for ^{99m}Tc. Using Equation 1.12 for the relationship between $T_{1/2}$ and λ, and that $2 = e^{\ln 2}$, Equation 1.11 can be written as

$$A(t) = A_o e^{-\lambda t} = A_o e^{\ln 2t/T_{1/2}} = A_o 2^{-t/T_{1/2}} \tag{1.13}$$

The last form is the one that one uses mentally when doing calculations in terms of multiples of $T_{1/2}$. It can also be used to give a ballpark estimate when time is not a multiple to $T_{1/2}$ and a calculator is not available.

1.3 INTERACTIONS OF RADIATION WITH MATTER

The radiations emitted in radioactive decays can be divided into ionizing and nonionizing based on whether a single particle or photon has enough energy to remove an electron from an atom. The distinction is important in terms of the potential for biological effects. The lethal dose for 50% of individuals irradiated in 30 days (LD$_{50/30}$) for humans is approximately 4 Gy (absorption of 4 J/kg) when ionizing radiation is delivered acutely and whole body. With some approximations, one can determine this would ionize 1 in 10^8 atoms and raise the body temperature 0.001°C. If delivered by nonionizing radiation, there would just be the temperature change. Nonionizing radiation will not be discussed further in this chapter, as it is not employed in SPECT and PET.

Ionizing radiation can be divided into *directly* and *nondirectly* ionizing types of radiation. Directly ionizing radiation consists of charged particles that were given kinetic energy during radioactive decays (α, β^-, β^+, etc.). These interact with the orbital electrons and protons in the nuclei of the material through which they are passing through the coulomb force. They do not have to actually physically "hit" electrons or nuclei to interact with them and thereby pass energy to them. They thus continually lose kinetic energy. Indirectly ionizing radiation consists of photons and particles with no net charge, such as neutrons, and they do not interact via the coulomb interaction. However, once they do interact with atoms, they can liberate charged particles, primarily secondary electrons. These secondary radiations will distribute the kinetic energy they are given to the medium in the same way that the primary radiations do for directly ionizing radiation. Thus, in the following the interactions of directly ionizing radiation are discussed, followed by a discussion of those of x- and γ-rays.

Most of the energy deposited by charged particles is through *collisional* losses. Collisions can be elastic where the total kinetic energy is conserved. But in most cases, the electrons and protons with which the radiation interacts are bound in atoms so that collisions will result is an *excitation* of these to a higher energy state, or an *ionization* whereby they are removed from being bound within the atom. In either case, the interactions are inelastic because some of the kinetic energy of the radiation is used to overcome part or all of the binding energy. Also, since nuclear binding energies are generally much greater than that of electrons, most of these interactions occur with the electrons, as opposed to protons, within nuclei. Ultimately, most of this energy ends up as heat.

Charged particles can also lose energy by the emission of a photon when they are slowed primarily through interacting with nuclei. This is called *bremsstrahlung*. The probability of bremsstrahlung emission is proportional to the inverse square of the mass of the particle. It is thus much lower for alpha particles than electrons. The emission probability is also proportional to the atomic number (Z) of the nuclei and the kinetic energy of the particle. Bremsstrahlung is, for instance, the major source of x-ray production in x-ray tubes where accelerated electrons strike a metal target typically made of tungsten ($Z = 74$).

1.3.1 INTERACTIONS OF PHOTONS WITH MATTER

There are five interactions by which photons of a high enough energy to be considered ionizing radiation interact with matter. Of these, only two are of major importance in nuclear medicine. We will discuss the five in the order in which they dominate the interactions taking place as the photon energy increases.

The first is *classical scattering*, so titled because it can be explained completely by classical physics. It is also call coherent or Rayleigh scattering. In this interaction, the photon interacts with the atom as a whole [5]. As a result of the interaction, the photon undergoes a change in direction with negligible energy loss to the atom. The scattering angle (ϕ) is small and increasingly biased in the forward direction as the initial energy of the photon (E_i) increases. The probability of classical scattering increases with atomic number (Z) of the atom and decreases with energy. It contributes only a small fraction of the interactions taking place in patients at the energies of interest in SPECT and PET imaging.

The second photon interaction is *photoelectric effect*. It is the first one of great importance in nuclear medicine. The photoelectric effect is schematically depicted in Figure 1.7. In this interaction, a photon is absorbed by a bound electron providing it all of its incident energy (E_i) [5]. This energy is used to overcome the binding energy of the electron (E_b), and the remainder (E_e) is carried away as kinetic energy by the electron, which is called a *photoelectron*. For this interaction to occur, the incident photon energy must be greater than the binding energy of the electron, or $E_i > E_b$. Thus, there is a threshold dependence on the individual electron binding energy for occurrence of the photoelectric effect. As soon as this threshold is reached, the photoelectric effect becomes the dominant mode of interaction for photons of that energy, replacing classical scattering. This results in a sudden increase in the probability of photon interaction as a function of energy, or an *absorption edge*. Beyond the threshold, the probability of interaction increases as the cube of the atomic number of the atoms of the material ($\sim Z^3$), and decreases with the cube of the energy ($\sim E^{-3}$). Thus, a doubling of the atomic number would increase the probability by a factor of ~ 8, and a doubling of the energy of the photon would decrease the probability by ~8. This dual dependence leads to the photoelectric effect remaining the dominant mode of interaction up to an energy of ~28 keV in the soft tissue of the body ($Z = 7.4$), ~48 keV in bone ($Z = 13.8$), ~250 keV in NaI ($Z = 50$), and ~500 keV in lead ($Z = 82$). The photoelectric effect thus plays a part in the absorbed dose from photon irradiation in body, providing contrast for bone and contrast agents in radiology, creation of the photopeak in scintillation detectors for use in imaging, and the usage of lead in collimators.

The third mode of interaction, and second of the two most important modes in SPECT and PET, is *Compton scattering*. During Compton scattering, the photon interacts with a loosely bound orbital electron (one whose binding energy is very small in comparison with that of the photon). This interaction is schematically depicted in Figure 1.8. The initial energy of the photon (E_i) is divided between that given to the *Compton electron* (E_e) (this now includes the electron binding energy) and that carried away by the scattered photon (E_s) [5]. The electron recoils at an angle φ relative to the original direction of the photon, which varies between 0° and 90°. The scattered photon travels at an angle θ, which can vary between 0° and 180°. Scattering at 180° is called *backscattering*. The relationship between the energy of the incident and scattered photons as a function of θ is [5]

$$E_s = \frac{E_i}{1 + \frac{E_i}{m_o c^2}\left(1 - \cos\theta\right)} \tag{1.14}$$

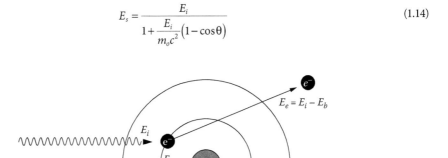

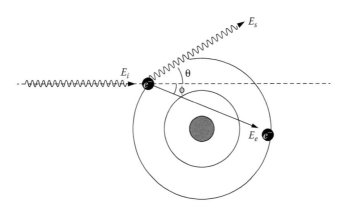

Figure 1.7 Depiction of photoelectric interaction. A photon comes in from the left, is absorbed by a K-shell electron, and provides enough energy to free the electron from the atom.

Figure 1.8 Depiction of Compton scattering. A photon comes in from the left; interacts with a loosely bound electron, freeing it from the atom; and is scattered at a lower energy to travel in a different direction.

where $m_o c^2$ is the rest mass energy of the electron, which is, as mentioned earlier, 511 keV.

The equation for the energy of the backscattered photon as a function of E_i can be derived by using a value of 180° as the scattering angle in Equation 1.14:

$$E_s = \frac{E_i}{1 + 2\dfrac{E_i}{m_o c^2}} \tag{1.15}$$

As per Equation 1.15, the energy of the backscattered photon starts very close to E_i for low-energy photons, reaches 90 keV for the 140 keV photons, and becomes 255 keV as E_i approaches infinity.

The probability of the Compton interaction does not directly depend on Z. Instead, it depends on *the number of electrons per gram*, or *electron density*, which depends on the ratio of Z to the atomic mass number (A) [5]. Recall that $A = Z + N$, where N is the number of neutrons. Small nuclides typically have near the same number of neutrons as protons. However, as the size of the nuclide increases, it becomes favorable to have more neutrons than protons to retain stability in the nucleus. Thus, as Z increases, the number of electrons per grams decreases slowly and the probability of the Compton interaction per gram thus also decreases slowly. The probability of Compton interaction decreases slowly with energy in comparison with the photoelectric effect. Because of this, Compton scattering becomes the dominant mode of interaction after the photoelectric falls below it in probability as photon energy increases. Also, due to this reduction in scattered photon energy with increasing angle of scattering, one can use energy windowing to include only a portion of the Compton scattered photons near the energy of E_i when imaging. This can significantly decrease but not eliminate the scattered photons imaged. Still, approximately 50% of the photons imaged are scattered for the energy window covering K x-rays of ^{201}Tl [6], and 25% for ^{99m}Tc [7].

The fourth mode of interaction is pair production. In this interaction, a photon interacting primarily with the nucleus can be converted into a pair of particles. To conserve charge, the particles are oppositely charged and thus are an electron and its antiparticle, the positron. In order for this interaction to occur, the photon must have sufficient energy to create these two particles, or 1.022 MeV (two times the 0.511 MeV rest mass energy of the electron). Any energy above this is carried away as kinetic energy, equally shared by the electron and the positron. The probability of pair production is thus zero until photon energies of 1.022 MeV, and unlike the other interactions, it increases with energy thereafter, eventually dominating Compton scattering at high photon energies. However, 1.022 MeV is much higher than the energy of the photon energies currently employed in radionuclide imaging. Pair production is therefore an interaction that is not observed in SPECT and PET.

The fifth mode of decay is *photodisintegration*. This occurs when photons interact with nucleons inside of the nucleus and results in the ejection of one or more nucleons. Since nuclear binding energies are much larger than the energy of photons employed in SPECT and PET, this interaction is not observed in SPECT and PET imaging.

1.3.2 EXPONENTIAL ATTENUATION OF A BEAM OF PHOTONS

When a beam of photons traverses a material, some of the photons will pass through the material without interacting. These *transmitted* photons are unaltered in energy or direction. Other photons will undergo one of the modes of interaction discussed in the preceding section, resulting in *attenuation* or a reduction in the intensity of the beam. As illustrated in Figure 1.9, the amount of attenuation that takes place depends on four factors. The first three are properties of the material, and the fourth is a property of the photons within the beam. The first factor, which impacts the relative amount of attenuation, is the *thickness* of the material (x in centimeters). When the thickness increases, so does the amount of attenuation, as the photons have to travel through more of the material. The second factor is the *density* (ρ in grams per cubic centimeter). This acts similarly to an increase in thickness, as an increase in density just compresses more of the material into the same distance. The third property of the material is the *atomic number* (Z). Generally, as Z increases, attenuation increases, but it also depends on what is the dominant mode of interaction in the material at the energy of the photons. For example, as mentioned when we discussed the interactions, the probability of Compton scattering does not depend directly on Z. Instead, it depends on the number of electrons per gram, which decreases slowly with Z. Thus, if Compton scattering is the dominate mode of interaction, a small increase in Z can cause a small decrease in attenuation on a per gram basis. Of course, a large change in Z could result in photoelectric effect becoming the dominant mode of interaction and attenuation then increasing. The fourth factor is the *energy* of the photons. Generally, as the energy of the photons increases, the attenuation decreases, but again, not always. For example, if the current energy is not sufficient to eject K-shell electrons via the photoelectric effect, then an increase in energy results in the K-shell electrons being able to be ejected. Then this increase in energy would lead to an increased relative amount of attenuation, as one would have gone from below to above a photoelectric absorption edge.

If the original intensity of the beam of photons is I_0, then the intensity I of the beam of photons after passing through a thickness x of some material is given as

$$I(x) = I_0 e^{-\mu(\rho, Z, E)x} \tag{1.16}$$

where $\mu(\rho, Z, E)$ is the *linear attenuation coefficient*, which is a function of the density (ρ) and atomic number of the material (Z), and energy E of the photons (Figure 1.9). The linear attenuation coefficient is the probability of attenuation per unit thickness, based on a very thin layer of material. The unit μ is usually given in cm^{-1}. The linear attenuation coefficient is the sum of the coefficients for the five individual interactions in the material for the given energy of photons. Since it depends on three factors, one does not find it tabulated. Instead, it is the *mass attenuation coefficient* (μ_m), whose units are square centimeters per gram, that is usually found. The mass attenuation coefficient is obtained from μ by dividing μ by ρ (i.e., $\mu_m = \mu/\rho$). It thus depends only on the materials atomic number and the energy of the photons. The linear attenuation coefficient can be obtained from the mass attenuation coefficient by

$$\mu = \rho\mu_m \tag{1.17}$$

Two-dimensional tables of μ_m can be found in the RHH [2], the text by Cherry et al. [5], and on the web at a URL of the National Institute of Standards and Technology (NIST) (http://www.nist.gov/pml/data/xraycoef/index.cfm). Since μ_m values for only selected energy values are tabulated, interpolation of some form is used to obtain values in between. Values for mixtures of materials not in the tables can be obtained as the sum of the individual elemental μ_m values, each multiplied by its fraction by weight [5]. When using tabulated values, one should be careful to note what interactions are included. For example, the table of μ_m values in [5] does not include classical scattering. Also, interpolation and the calculation of μ_m values for mixtures can be problematic near photoelectric absorption edges. NIST also supports the program XCOM for the calculation of values for user-specified photon energies and materials at http://www.nist.gov/pml/data/xcom/index.cfm.

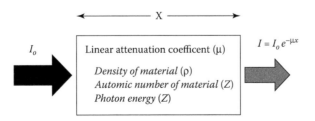

Figure 1.9 Depiction of the change in the intensity of a beam of photons passing through an absorber of thickness x and attenuation coefficient μ. The intensity of the primary photons will be reduced exponentially. The linear attenuation coefficient μ is dependent on the density of the material, the atomic number of the material, and the energy of the photons.

Just like in radioactive decay, where two alternative quantities are employed to quantify the decay rate characteristics for a radionuclide (λ and $T_{1/2}$), in attenuation there are two alternative quantities that are employed to characterize the attenuation properties of a material to a given energy beam of photons (μ and HVT). The *half-value thickness* (HVT) or *half-value layer* (HVL) is the thickness of the material required to reduce the beam of photons to one-half its initial intensity. Just like in Equation 1.12, in radioactive decay the relationship between μ and HVT is

$$HVT = \frac{\ln 2}{\mu} \approx \frac{0.693}{\mu} \tag{1.18}$$

Another value that is frequently useful is the tenth-value thickness (TVT). The TVT is the thickness of the material needed to reduce the intensity by a factor of 10. Unlike radioactive decay, it is μ and not HVT that is typically tabulated. Note that under the attenuation conditions discussed thus far, TVT = 3.3 HVT. This can be useful in estimating the attenuation without use of a calculator. Making use of the relationship between μ and HVT, Equation 1.16 can be rewritten as

$$I(x) = I_0 e^{-\mu x} = I_0 e^{-\ln 2 \, x / \text{HVT}} = I_0 2^{-x/\text{HVT}} \tag{1.19}$$

The last form is handy to use if x is a multiple of HVT.

Equation 1.16 is accurate only for a *monoenergetic* beam of photons, which is when all the photons have the same energy. If multiple energy photons are in the beam, then a separate μ should be employed for each. Equation 1.16 is also accurate only under the *good-geometry attenuation* or *narrow-beam* condition that as soon as a photon undergoes any interaction, it is no longer counted as a member of the beam [5]. Attenuation coefficients measured subject to these conditions are the good-geometry or narrow-beam attenuation coefficients. Compton scattered photons, even though they are reduced in energy, are not necessarily excluded from being counted due to the finite width of the energy windows used because of the limited ability to distinguish different energy photons (finite energy resolution) of our imaging systems. Thus, Equation 1.16 has to be modified to match the *broad-beam attenuation*, which actually occurs in emission imaging. This is done by the inclusion of the buildup factor B, which is dependent on both μ and x. The result is [5]

$$I(x) = I_0 B(\mu, x) e^{-\mu(\rho, Z, E)x} \tag{1.20}$$

Numerically, the buildup factor is the ratio of the sum of the transmitted and scatter photons to the transmitted photons only, or the relative increase in counts due to the inclusion of scattered photons. It thus depends on variables such as location in the attenuator, geometry and composition of the attenuator, energy of the photon, energy resolution of the imaging system, and energy window used in imaging.

1.4 PRINCIPLES OF PHOTON DETECTION

In both SPECT and PET, the radiation emitted from the imaged object is measured with external radiation detectors. The purpose of the detector system is to analyze the properties of the photons emitted, primarily the energy and the direction of emission. In the detector, a photon will undergo an interaction and deposit all or part of its energy in the detector volume. The energy deposited in the detector will produce a signal such as a burst of light in a scintillation crystal or electron–hole pairs in a solid-state detector. This signal is collected and is converted to an electrical signal that is fed into the processing electronics, which will be used to determine the energy of the event. The determination of the energy is necessary to decide whether the photon has traveled directly from the location of the radioactive decay to the detector (i.e., a primary photon) or has scattered prior to reaching the detector as the result of a photon interaction (e.g., Compton interaction). Since a scattered photon has changed direction, it has lost the directional emission information, originally carried by the primary photon, and these scattered photons should be rejected. Since a Compton interaction always results in a loss in photon energy, any detected photon with an energy lower than the primary photon energy is in general considered to be a scattered photon. Thus, to differentiate primary photons from scattered photons, the energy of each detected photon needs to be determined and examined.

In order for the detector to efficiently discriminate scattered photons from primary photons, the *energy resolution* of the detector should be as high as possible. Energy resolution refers to the uncertainty or variability in the observed signal from a detector when irradiated with monoenergetic photons. This variability is the result of statistical variations in the production of the signal, and for a given system, there are several contributing factors to this. For instance, in a scintillation detector system, there are statistical variations in the number of light photons in the scintillator following a photon interaction. In addition, there are statistical variations in the number of photoelectrons produced in the photodetector and variations in the multiplication factor of the photodetector.

In both SPECT and PET, the image quality and noise properties of the reconstructed image are dependent on the number of recorded primary photons or events. The efficiency of the detection system should therefore be as high as possible, and as many of the photons hitting the detector absorbed and recorded. The detection system should also be able to process each detected event fast to minimize dead-time losses at high detection rates.

In PET, where two annihilation photons originating from the same decay are used to localize the activity, it is also important for the detector system to have a high time resolution. This will increase the likelihood that two detected photons originated from the same annihilation event. The finite time resolution of PET detectors is primarily caused by statistical uncertainties in how fast the detectors respond following a photon interaction in the detector volume. When a pair of detectors are simultaneously struck by a pair of photons, the signals produced in each detector should ideally also be simultaneous. Due to statistical uncertainties, there is an inherent delay in when the signal is produced. There are several factors that contribute to the time resolution, including the rise and decay constant of the light in a scintillator, the amount of conversion efficiency of photon energy to scintillation light, and the mobility of electron–hole pairs in a solid-state detector.

In order to localize the photon emission and reconstruct the 3-D distribution of the isotope, it is also necessary to determine where the photon was detected and the direction of emission. The position of the detected photon is usually approximated by the location of the detector in space. Since the detector is made up of a volume of detector material, there is an uncertainty in the actual location of the physical extent of the detector. This is usually referred to as the spatial resolution of the detector. Some detector systems are designed as area or volume detectors, where the detector readout system determines the location where the photon was absorbed in the detector. The uncertainty in the positioning of the event in these detector systems adds to the uncertainty in the spatial resolution.

How the direction of the emitted photons is determined differs between the two imaging modalities and is discussed in more detail in later sections. In SPECT, the direction is determined by lead collimation, whereas in PET, the orientation is determined by electronic means.

All detector systems rely on photon interactions in the detector material to determine the energy of the photon. Compton and photoelectric interactions are the two dominant interaction types of the photons in the energy interval used in SPECT and PET (~70–511 keV). In both types of interactions, some or all of the photon's energy is transferred as kinetic energy to an electron, which will produce ionizations and excitations in the detector volume. It is the effect of both of these processes that is involved in generating the detector signal.

1.4.1 PULSE HEIGHT ANALYSIS

Radiation detectors can be operated in either current mode or pulse mode. In current mode, the interaction rate in the detector is so high that it is not possible to distinguish one interaction from another. What is measured in the detector is a factor related to the time average of the deposited energy in the detector. This is the detection mode used by the detector system in computed tomography (CT), where the photon flux generated by the x-ray tube is so high.

In pulse mode, the time between interactions is sufficiently long to allow recording of each interaction in the detector. This allows the electronics to integrate the signal produced in the detector, and measure how much energy was deposited and whether the event should be accepted or rejected. Since the height of the pulse produced by the detector is proportional to the energy deposition, the process of examining each pulse is usually referred to as pulse height analysis or spectroscopy.

If a detector is irradiated with monoenergetic photons and the pulse heights of the signals generated in the detector are histogrammed, a pulse height spectrum is generated. Since the pulse height spectrum shows the distribution of energy depositions in the detector, it is also called an energy spectrum. Based on the features of the energy spectrum, it is possible to make a decision on what pulses carry useful information for imaging and what pulses should be rejected. A typical pulse height spectrum from a scintillation detector is shown in Figure 1.10 when irradiated with 140 keV photons. It has a large peak, which represents full energy depositions in the detector, primarily from photoelectric interactions. This peak is usually referred to as the photopeak, and the centroid represents the energy of the photons the detector was irradiated with. The *photopeak* has a finite width or spread around the center, although the photons the detector was irradiated with were monoenergetic. This widening is the result of the statistical variation in the production of signal carriers in the detector. The amount of widening is characteristic of the detector material and is referred to as the *energy resolution*. The amount of widening depends on the detector material, but also on the photon energy.

At lower energies below the photopeak, there are energy depositions that are produced by Compton interactions in the detector where only a fraction of the photon energy is deposited on the detector. This region of the spectrum is usually referred to as the Compton distribution. In an ideal detector, with perfect energy resolution there would be a distinct separation of the photopeak and the Compton distribution. However, because of the energy resolution, the two interaction distributions blend into each other.

The energy depositions or events that fall under the photopeak are in general considered good events that should be kept to make up the final image. Since these events are close to the photon energy that is emitted, it is a high likelihood that these events have traveled straight from the radioactive decay to the detector without interacting and deflected along its path. Any photon that has interacted prior to reaching the detector will have an energy lower than the primary photon energy. These photons are referred to as scattered photons or events. In the energy spectrum, these photons will fall anywhere below the photopeak and will be mixed in with the Compton distribution. This is illustrated in the right spectrum of Figure 1.10, which was generated by placing the source behind 10 cm of scattering material. Compared with the left spectrum, the number of

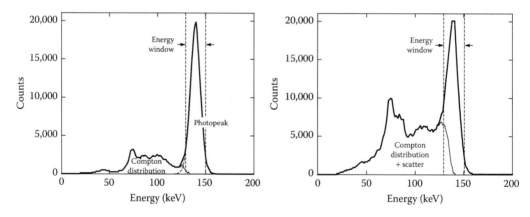

Figure 1.10 Examples of energy spectra of 140 keV photon measured with NaI (Tl) detector. The spectrum to the left was measured with the source in air. The spectrum is characterized by a large photopeak and the Compton distribution. The photopeak represents all full energy absorptions in the detector of the 140 keV photons. The Compton distribution represents partial energy absorptions in the detector (i.e., Compton interactions in the detector). Due to the finite energy resolution, there is a spillover of Compton events into the energy window defined by the photopeak. In the absence of scatter, there is only a minimal amount of spillover. The spectrum to the right was acquired with the source placed behind 10 cm of scattering material, which results in an increase of detected low-energy, scattered events. In this case, there is a larger amount of scattered events that spill over into the energy window.

low-energy events is substantially higher. In the interaction, these scattered photons have lost the original emission direction and should therefore be rejected. To separate the primary or unscattered events from scattered events, energy discrimination can be used. In energy discrimination, only events within a certain energy range or *energy window* are accepted. Any detector interaction outside this range will be rejected. The energy window should ideally be set wide enough to enclose the entire photopeak. Because of the finite energy resolution, some of the scattered events will blend in with the photopeak, as shown in Figure 1.10. If the energy window is set around the entire photopeak, a substantial amount of scatter will be accepted. How much scatter will be accepted depends on several factors, including primary photon energy, energy resolution, and size of the scattering medium [8]. To reduce the amount of detected scatter, the energy window is typically set as a percent width around the photopeak, which will minimize the amount of detected scatter with an acceptable loss in detected unscattered events (e.g., events in the tails of the photopeak).

For instance, imaging with 140 keV photons with a 15% energy window means that energy depositions in the detector ranging from 129.5 to 150.5 keV are accepted. Assuming the energy resolution of the detector is 9% full width at half maximum (FWHM), this energy window will still accept 95% of the events in the photopeak.

1.4.2 Detection systems

There are three main categories of radiation detectors: gas detectors, scintillation detectors, and solid-state detectors. Due to the poor detection efficiency at the energies of interest in SPECT and PET, gas detectors are rarely used, although there are some examples of systems that use gas detectors [9–11]. Scintillation detection systems are the most widely used type of detector system in both SPECT and PET and are discussed in subsequent sections and also in Chapter 2. Solid-state detectors have in recent years shown to be a promising detector technology, especially at the lower energies used in SPECT imaging. The use of these detectors is still somewhat limited and will only be briefly discussed in this chapter.

1.4.3 Scintillation detection

The most common detector for photon detection is a scintillation crystal coupled to a photodetector. A scintillation crystal is a material that has the ability to emit visible light photons following the interaction of a photon with an electron in the crystal lattice. The scintillation process is a property of certain materials that are grown into a crystalline solid [12].

When a photon interacts in the scintillator, a high energetic electron is produced that could be either a photoelectron or a Compton electron. The high energetic electron will produce excitations of electrons in the scintillation crystal lattice. These electrons will eventually de-excite back to the ground state, and in a scintillator, one of several possible de-excitation pathways is through the emission of a light photon. The number of light photons produced following the interaction is approximately proportional to the total amount of energy the photon deposited in the crystal in the photon interaction (i.e., the amount of energy transferred to the photo- or Compton electron).

The emission of the light photons following an interaction is not instantaneous but will instead typically follow a functional shape that has a very sharp initial rise time, followed by an exponential decaying tail with a *decay time constant* that is specific to the scintillator material. This time constant can vary between a few nanoseconds for some of the fastest scintillators to 1–2 μs for some of the slower scintillators. The decay time constant of the scintillation detector will affect how fast the detector can count. If the time constant is long, it will take some time before the detector is ready to accept another interaction. This is typically on the order of three to four times the decay time constant. If another pulse arrives within this time interval, this is referred to as pulse pileup [13], and this typically leads to a distortion of the signal and will in the end provide incorrect information regarding the amount of energy that was deposited in the detector interaction.

The light emitted from the scintillator is converted into an electrical signal by coupling the crystal to a photodetector, such as a photomultiplier tube (PMT) (see Section 1.4.4). The output from the photodetector allows analysis of the signal by the subsequent electronics to obtain energy and timing information from the detected event.

For scintillators used in SPECT and PET imaging, there are certain properties of the scintillator material that make it a suitable detector material. For both modalities, it is necessary to efficiently stop the photons in a small detector volume, preferably in one single interaction. This will maximize detection efficiency and also minimize losses in spatial resolution due to photon scatter in the detector. The detector should therefore have an effective Z such that photoelectric interaction is the dominant or most likely interaction type. At 140 keV (gamma emission from ^{99m}Tc), photoelectric interaction is the dominant interaction type for $Z > 31$. At 511 keV (annihilation radiation), photoelectric interaction is dominant for $Z > 79$. In addition, the detector should also have a high density since this increases the likelihood of capturing any secondary photons from a Compton interaction close to the initial interaction site (i.e., Compton photons captured in a subsequent photoelectric interaction). It should be mentioned that primary photons that undergo Compton interactions in the detector are good events and could be used in the image formation. However, since only a fraction of the photon energy is deposited in the detector, these events are in most imaging systems rejected, since they are indistinguishable from scattered photons originating from Compton interactions in the object that is being imaged.

The light yield of the scintillator is another factor that is of importance in the selection of suitable scintillators for use in SPECT and PET imaging. The *light yield* (i.e., number of scintillation photons per absorbed energy) will primarily affect the energy resolution of the detector. The more light that is produced, the better the energy resolution, which in turn will improve the detector's ability to distinguish primary photons from scattered radiation. The light yield depends on the scintillator material, and for a bright scintillator such as NaI (Tl), the light yield is 38,000 photons/MeV, with an average scintillation photon energy around 3 eV (13). This translates to an absolute energy conversion efficiency of 11.3%. For bismuth germanate (BGO), which is a less bright scintillation, the light yield is 8200 photons/MeV, with an average scintillation photon energy around 2.6 eV. In this case, the conversion efficiency is only 2.1%. On the other hand, BGO has a very high effective Z and density and is therefore very useful for detection of high energetic photons, including annihilation radiation.

The light yield also affects how accurately one can position the interaction within the detector volume. The most common detector system used in SPECT imaging is the scintillation camera, which consists of a large NaI (Tl) monolithic scintillation crystal coupled to an array of PMTs. The position of each event in the crystal is determined by a center of mass calculation using the signal from the array of PMTs. Just like the energy resolution, the spatial resolution of the scintillation camera is primarily determined by the amount of light produced in the photon interaction. The more light produced in the scintillator, the better the spatial resolution.

Although PET systems use a somewhat different detector technology (see Chapter 6), the spatial resolution and event positioning in PET detector modules are also highly dependent on the light yield of the scintillator.

The decay time constant of the scintillator light emission should be short enough to prevent pulse pileup at high event rates. The photon flux a detector uses in SPECT is typically fairly low, which permits the use of fairly slow scintillators with decay constants on the order of 2–300 ns. For instance, the decay constant of NaI (Tl) is 230 ns. Due to the higher photon flux in PET imaging, faster scintillators are required with a decay constant on the order 20–50 ns. LSO:Ce used in many modern PET systems has a decay constant of 40 ns.

1.4.4 Photodetectors

Once the light has been produced in the scintillation detector, the optical signal needs to be collected and converted to an electrical signal, which can be analyzed by the processing electronics. This is accomplished by coupling a photodetector to the scintillator. Ideally, the photodetector should also provide some amplification in the conversion process, since the amount of light produced by each photon interaction in the scintillator detector is extremely low. There are two main groups of photodetectors used in conjunction with scintillator detectors: PMTs and solid-state detectors.

1.4.4.1 PHOTOMULTIPLIER TUBE

The PMT is a vacuum tube with a photocathode and an anode [14]. Between the cathode and anode is an electron acceleration structure, consisting of a series of dynodes. To accelerate electrons between the dynodes, high voltage is applied between the cathode and anode, which is distributed across the series of dynodes.

When a scintillator is coupled to the photocathode of the PMT, the scintillator light photons will pass through the glass envelope, be absorbed in the photocathode, and produce photoelectrons in the process. Some of the photoelectrons will migrate to the surface of the photocathode and escape. The ratio of the number of emitted photoelectrons off the photocathode to the number of incoming scintillation light photons is usually referred to as the quantum efficiency (QE). In order to minimized signal losses, it is important that the QE be as high as possible, ideally 100%. However, for most photoemissive materials used in PMTs, the QE is on the order of 20%–30% in the range of wavelengths emitted from most scintillators. The QE is therefore a significant source of signal loss that affects both the energy resolution and the spatial resolution of the detector.

The voltage between the photocathode and the first dynode will accelerate the photoelectrons toward the first dynode. The voltage applied between the photocathode and the first dynode should be such that the electron gains enough energy to produce secondary electron emission in the dynode. Some of these secondary electrons will reach the surface of the first dynode and then be accelerated toward the second dynode. These electrons in turn will gain enough energy to produce secondary electrons in the second dynode. This process will continue along the whole dynode structure, and the total charge will be collected at the anode. The result is an amplification of the signal on the order of 10^6–10^7, in which the properties of the emitted scintillator light are to a great extent preserved, such as the rise and decay times. This signal from the PMT is then processed by subsequent electronics to determine energy and timing information.

The main advantage of the PMT is that it is a very stable and proven technology and is fast enough for most nuclear imaging situations. However, the PMTs are bulky due to the need for a glass envelope that withstands the vacuum and also contains the dynode structure. This imposes some restrictions on how the PMT technology can be used in the design of high-resolution imaging systems. The electron optics and the electron transport and amplification of the dynode chain of the PMT are also very sensitive to magnetic fields. In most applications, the sensitivity to an external magnetic field is not an issue. Shielding against weak magnetic fields, such as the earth's magnetic field, is accomplished with mu-metal shielding. However, in the presence of a strong magnetic field, the PMT is nonfunctional, which prevents its use in hybrid systems such as PET/MRI systems.

1.4.4.2 SOLID-STATE PHOTODETECTORS

Solid-state photodetectors for use with scintillators are typically of two kinds. There are the conventional silicon photodiode or the PIN diode, which provides no signal gain [15], and the avalanche photodiode (APD), which provides an internal signal gain [16]. Common for both types is that the light from the scintillator produces electron–hole pairs in the detector volume. By applying a voltage across the device, the electron–hole pairs are collected, and the collected charge is proportional to the amount of light that was emitted from the scintillator. Compared with PMTs, the QE is much higher for the solid-state detectors and is typically greater than 80% [13]. Another advantage of the solid-state devices is that they are more compact than PMTs. Smaller and more compact imaging devices can therefore be built with the silicon photodetectors. Solid-state detectors are also, in contrast to PMTs, insensitive to external magnetic fields. These devices are therefore currently the only option for photodetectors to be used in MRI-compatible scintillator-based nuclear imaging devices.

Since the PIN device does not provide any internal gain and also produces a significant amount of noise when used at room temperature, the signal-to-noise ratio (SNR) of the generated signal tends to be fairly poor when used for photon counting. This limitation can be overcome with specialized low-noise electronics and cooling of the devices [17]. Despite some of the challenges of the PIN diodes, there are examples of successful radionuclide imaging devices using this technology [17,18].

The APD is another type of solid-state detector that, in contrast to the PIN diode, provides an internal amplification of the signal. This is accomplished by producing a region within the diode where the electrical field is high enough to accelerate the charge carriers enough to create further ionizations and produce more electron–hole pairs. The result is the onset of an internal avalanche or multiplication, which results in an amplification of the signal. The APD is operated below the breakdown voltage, where the collected signal is still proportional to the amount of light that was produced in the scintillator. The gain of the APD results in a signal with better SNR properties than the PIN diode. However, the gain in the APD is only on the order of 10^2–10^3, which is fairly nominal in comparison with a PMT. Furthermore, the timing properties are worse for

APDs than PMTs, primarily due to the slower rise time of the signal from the APD. This prevents its use in systems where very fast timing is required, such as in time-of-flight (TOF) PET. The signal gain in an APD is also very sensitive to both voltage and temperature variations. APDs therefore need to be operated with very stable high-voltage supplies and in a highly regulated temperature environment.

In recent years, a special type of APD has been introduced, which is referred to as a silicon photomultiplier (SiPM), solid-state photomultiplier (SSPM), or multipixel photon counter (MMPC) [19]. These devices are all based on the same principle as the APD; however, the field strength within the diode is high enough to set off a self-sustained electron multiplication that is eventually quenched, by either passive or active means. This behavior is analogous to that of the electron multiplication observed in Geiger–Müller gas detectors. When operated in this so-called Geiger mode, the amplitude of the signal is constant and independent of the number of absorbed light photons. To make a device that is useful as a photon detector, the area of the detector is divided into hundreds or thousands of smaller microcells. Each one of these cells will produce a signal of equal amplitude when hit by one or more light photons. The sum of the signals from all of the individual cells is then approximately proportional to the number of scintillation photons absorbed by the photodetector.

The SiPM signal is only linear with the scintillator light if the number of microcells is much greater than the number of emitted light photons, which reduces the probability that more than one scintillation photon is absorbed in each cell. However, due to the finite number of microcells in the device, there is always a probability of multiple photon hits in the same cell, especially when the number of cells is not much larger than the number of emitted light photons. This results in a nonlinear energy response of the device; however, it has been shown that this can be calibrated and corrected for [20].

The SiPM combines many of the best properties of the APD and PMT. Like the APD, it is very compact, rugged, and light; has a high QE; is insensitive to magnetic fields; and has a signal gain similar to that of a PMT. The SiPM typically operates at only a few tenths of volts. They are also very fast and can provide timing resolution with fast scintillators on the order of a few hundred picoseconds, which makes it possible to use them in TOF PET [21].

1.4.4.3 SOLID-STATE DETECTORS

Solid-state detectors can also be used for direct detection of the γ-rays. When used as direct-detection detectors, they operate in a manner similar to that of the conventional ionization chamber. Analogous to the electron–ion pairs produced in an ionization chamber from a high energetic Compton or photoelectron, a large number of electron–hole pairs are produced in a semiconductor detector. These are the charge carriers that are collected to produce a signal that would represent the total amount of energy that was deposited in the detector in the photon interaction. The energy required to produce an electron–hole pair depends on the material, but is 3–5 eV for most practical detectors. Due to the low energy to produce an electron–hole pair in a semiconductor, a large number of signal carriers are produced from a single photon interaction. The large number of signal carries produced following a photon absorption results in a signal with excellent energy resolution. This is in contrast to a scintillation detector, described earlier, where energy resolution is limited by the number of photoelectrons produced at the photocathode in the PMT.

The most common materials used as direct-detection semiconductor detectors are silicon (Si), germanium (Ge), cadmium telluride (CdTe), and cadmium zinc telluride (CZT) [22,23]. Due to the low Z of Si [14] and Ge [24] and the need for cooling, these materials are not practical as detector materials for nuclear imaging applications. CdTe and CZT, on the other hand, both have an effective Z, similar to that of NaI, which makes them potential candidates for detector materials for low-energy photons in single-photon imaging applications. The excellent energy resolution of the solid-state detectors allows for more effective rejection of scatter than conventional scintillation camera-based imaging systems. A drawback of the solid-state detector technology is that the detector material is relatively expensive to manufacture. The systems that have been manufactured using this technology have therefore been limited to relatively small and compact organ-specific systems, such as systems designed for cardiac imaging [25,26].

Due the low effective Z and low detection efficiency of CdTe and CZT at 511 keV, this material is not expected to replace the scintillation detector in PET systems. However, several groups have investigated the possibility of using solid-state detectors in PET [27,28].

CdTe and CZT are like the solid-state photodetectors insensitive to magnetic fields. These detector materials can therefore be used in hybrid SPECT/MRI systems [29,30].

1.5 INTRODUCTION TO SPECT IMAGING

Tomography provides the ability to re-create or *reconstruct* 3-D distributions from information collected along ray or line integrals through the object from many directions. In emission tomography, the information acquired is related to the concentration of activity at each point along the ray as altered by attenuation, the inclusion of scattered photons, and other degradations. It takes two points or one point plus a direction to determine the path of a ray. In PET, which is discussed in Section 1.6, the ray is determined as the path between the pair of detectors detecting the pair of photons emitted at approximately 180° to each other when the positron annihilates. On the other hand, in SPECT only a single photon is employed in the detection. Thus, in addition to knowledge of where the photon was detected, information is required on along what path the detected photon traveled to reach the detector. This is provided by the use of collimators to restrict access to the detector such that photons traveling only along prescribed paths can reach it. Unlike the lenses used in optical imaging, which "bend" photons to bring them into focus on the detector, the collimators employing SPECT are designed to preferentially absorb photons not traveling along desired paths. This reduces the number of photons that reach the detector by a factor 10^3–10^4, but is essential in imaging, as illustrated in Figure 1.11. In this figure are shown the collection of line integrals imaged by the detector at a single position, which is called a *projection*.

In most commercial SPECT systems, the collimator, detector, and electronics that form the image are all included in a single unit, or the *camera head*. A schematic of a camera head is shown in Figure 1.12. The x- or γ-rays are emitted from the patient in a direction such that they can pass through the channels between the septa of the collimator and impinge upon the crystal of the scintillation detector. The septa are typically made of some lead alloy, which is highly absorbing for the x- or γ-rays. If the rays interact in the detector, the light emitted is in proportion to the deposited energy. This light then shines on the array of PMTs, each with its own preamp. The signal output by the preamps is then analyzed to determine the X and Y location of the interaction in the scintillation detector. A signal proportional to the total energy (Z) is also formed for use in deciding whether the detected photon's deposited energy falls within the range of values (window) for inclusion in the image.

To accomplish acquisition of the projections, general-purpose SPECT systems consist of a number of components, as illustrated in Figure 1.13. The first is an imaging table upon which the patient lies down supine, with his or her arms positioned over his or her head or at his or her side, depending on the clinical procedure. Typically, after the patient is in position on the table, the table is translated into the bore of the system to position the desired anatomy within the field of view (FOV) of the camera heads. A catcher on the opposite side of the gantry is frequently used to diminish the downward deflection of the table when the patient is on it.

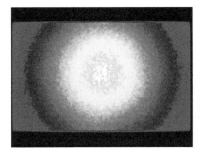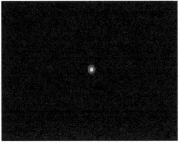

Figure 1.11 Images of a point source 10 cm from the camera head acquired without (left) and with (right) a collimator in place. Note that without the collimator, the intensity of the photons emitted by the point source falls off according to the inverse-square law with distance. With the collimator in place, an image of the point source is obtained.

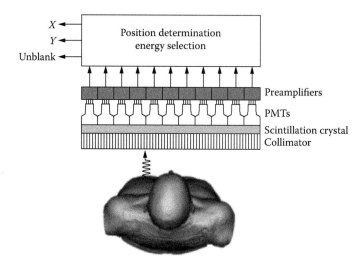

Figure 1.12 Schematic of major components of a gamma camera. Photons emitted from the patient will hit the collimator. If the direction of the photons aligns with the detector channels, they will reach the scintillation crystal. When the photons interact in the scintillation crystal, a light flash is produced. This light is collected by the array of PMTs. The signals from the PMTs will be processed by the electronics to determine the energy and the position of the photon interaction. If the energy of the interaction falls within the energy window, the event is saved and histogrammed into an image matrix.

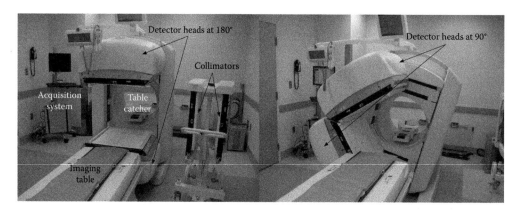

Figure 1.13 Modern two-headed SPECT system shown in two different configurations of the detector heads (180° to the left and 90° to the right).

The second component is one or more camera heads, each equipped with its own collimator. Two camera heads is the most common number currently; however, systems with one, three, or more heads are available. As shown in Figure 1.13, with two heads, the heads can usually be positioned opposed to each other (180°) for general SPECT imaging (left), and at 90° to each other for cardiac imaging (right). Attached to the front of the camera heads are the collimators. The collimators have contact sensors, which can halt movement of the system to avoid injury to patients. A mechanism is provided for exchanging collimators to enable the usage of collimators designed for different purposes. As illustrated on the left in Figure 1.13, the currently unused collimators are typically stored on carts so as to enable their being moved out of the way.

The third component is the gantry to which the heads are mounted. The heads can be moved closer to or away from the mechanical *center of rotation* (COR) to maximize spatial resolution by staying close to the surface of the patient without contacting him or her. The gantry rotates the heads about the COR to the series of angular increments necessary for reconstruction. The rotation can be *"step and shoot,"* in which acquisition only occurs when the heads are at the series of angular increments and not during rotation.

This eliminates angular motion during acquisition, but results in lost time while the camera rotates, during which patient imaging could have been performed. Alternatively, a *continuous* acquisition of projection data can occur, during which individual projection images are acquired while the camera is constantly moving. This maximizes the utilization of photon collection during acquisition, as there is no lost time stepping from one angle to the next. It does, however, introduce some uncertainty in the projection angle the data is acquired at. So long as the rotation during acquisition of a projection is small (~3° or less), this is usually not a problem.

The fourth component of SPECT systems is the acquisition system. This comes with a vender-supplied graphical user interface (GUI) to move the imaging table, camera heads, and gantry as needed to accomplish the acquisition of the projection set.

As mentioned above, the collimators mounted on the camera heads can be exchanged to adapt the system to different imaging needs. There are four basic collimator designs, and adaptations of each of these to the energy of the photons employed in imaging and the desired sensitivity and spatial resolution trade-off. The most common type of collimator employed in SPECT is the *parallel-hole collimator*, shown schematically in Figure 1.12. Figure 1.14 shows the front surface of an actual collimator. The thickness of the septa, septal length, and diameter of the hole can be varied to adapt parallel-hole collimators for usage with different energy photons. Collimators such as the one shown in Figure 1.14 designed for usage in imaging ^{99m}Tc and ^{201}Tl (photons of 150 keV or less) are called *low-energy* (LE) collimators. *Medium-energy* (ME) collimators are designed for usage with radionuclides such as ^{67}Ga and ^{111}In (~300 keV or less). Finally, *high-energy* (HE) collimators are designed for usage with radionuclides such as ^{131}I and ^{18}F (~500 keV or less). The trade-off between spatial resolution and sensitivity is usually given by the name, as ultra-high-resolution (UHR); high-resolution (HR); general-all-purpose (GAP), which can also be called medium-sensitivity (MS); or high-sensitivity (HS) collimator. These two naming conventions are combined when specifying a collimator, for example, the low-energy high-resolution (LEHR) collimator of Figure 1.14.

Other types of collimators include *pinhole*, which employs a single hole to view the object; *converging*, which employs holes whose rays converge to a single focal point (the fan-beam variant converges to a focal line) in front of the collimator; and *diverging*, which has holes that view a region of increasing size as one moves away from the face of the collimator. An important fact to remember is that the *spatial resolution of all collimator types gets worse with distance from the collimator face*. The rate, however, is dependent on the collimator type. Also, the variation in sensitivity to a point source with distance from the face is constant for parallel-hole collimators, increases for converging collimators up to the focal distance, and decreases for pinhole and divergent collimators.

An important aspect of SPECT (and all medical imaging) is that one should be sure the imaging system is operating properly before employing it clinically. This is the domain of *quality control* (QC), and information on how this relates to nuclear imaging can be found in the publications of Sokole [31], Zanzonico [32], and Case and Bateman [24].

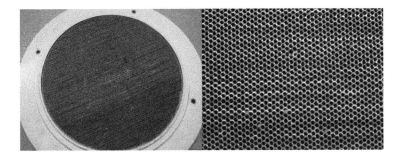

Figure 1.14 At the left is shown a LEHR parallel-hole collimator with the protective covering removed so that the collimator core is visible. This collimator was used in the 1980s on a mobile gamma camera. At the right is shown a close-up of the front face of the core made up of hexagonal-shaped channels (holes) formed by thin lead alloy septa.

1.6 PET

1.6.1 BASIC PRINCIPLE

In PET, only isotopes that decay through the emission of a positron are used, and it is the unique properties of this class of isotopes that are utilized to localize the radionuclide. When the positron is produced in the decay, it will be ejected with some kinetic energy from the nucleus (Figure 1.15). The energy of the positron depends primarily on the amount of energy available in the decays, and this energy is also shared between the positron, the neutrino, and the daughter nucleus. This means that the positron can be emitted with an energy anywhere from close to zero to the maximum available energy (E_{max}). The energy distribution of the emitted positrons is not uniform but is fairly symmetrical around half of the E_{max}. In the case of the decay of ^{18}F to ^{18}O, positrons are emitted at a maximum energy of 633 keV and with an average energy of about 310 keV.

Once ejected from the nucleus, the positron will travel some distance in the surrounding medium, as illustrated in Figure 1.15. The positron will lose its kinetic energy through inelastic collision with atomic electrons and will eventually reach thermal energies. The positive charge of the positron will attract it to an electron and form a hydrogen-like state known as *positronium*. Since the positron is the antiparticle of the electron, the positronium is very instable and will rapidly annihilate (the mean life of positronium is on the order of ~10^{-10} s). In order to conserve energy and momentum, two 511 keV photons (total rest mass energy of the electron–positron pair) are emitted in opposite directions (provided the net momentum of the electron–positron pair is zero). If the net momentum of the positron–electron pair is greater than zero at the time of annihilation, then the angle between the two 511 keV annihilation photons will deviate slightly from 180° [33].

The fact that the two simultaneously emitted photons have an energy of 511 keV and these two photons are emitted approximately 180° apart is what is utilized in PET to localize the radionuclide in a PET scanner. If the two 511 keV annihilation photons are registered by a pair of detectors within a narrow time window of a few nanoseconds, then it is assumed that somewhere along the line connecting the two detectors, an annihilation occurred that is also assumed to be the approximate location of the radioactive decay. This detection technique is commonly referred to as coincidence detection and originates from the work of Walther Bothe in the mid-1920s [34]; it has been used extensively in the studies of nuclear physics and cosmic radiation. Since this detection technique does not require any collimation and only relies on the detector electronics to determine the orientation of the emitted photons, it is sometimes referred to as electronic collimation.

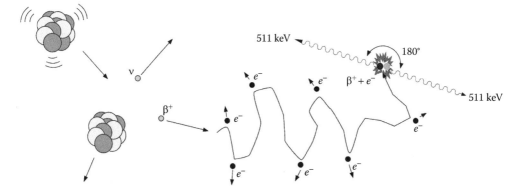

Figure 1.15 Illustration of the basic principle of PET. Nuclides with an excess of protons will decay through the emission of a positron (β^+). In the decay, a stable daughter nuclide is produced and a neutrino in addition to the positron. The positron will be emitted in the medium with some kinetic energy and interact with electrons and produce excitations and ionizations in the process. Eventually, the positron will have lost most of its energy and be attracted to an electron. This electron–positron pair will rapidly annihilate, and in the process, two 511 keV photons are emitted approximately 180° apart. The well-defined energy of the emitted photons, and that they are emitted back to back, is what is utilized in a PET system. If two photons are simultaneously detected, then it is assumed that a radioactive decay occurred somewhere along the line connecting the two detectors.

In a complete PET system, a large number of detectors are arranged around the object to be imaged. The most common configuration is to place the detector elements in a circular arrangement (Figure 1.16), where the diameter is large enough to accommodate the object to be imaged. For a typical clinical PET system, the diameter of the detector ring is typically around 80 cm. Several of these detector rings are placed next to each other to extend the axial FOV and increase detection efficiency. Each detector is designed to efficiently absorb and detect 511 keV annihilation photons. Since there are no collimators in front of the detectors to restrict the view of the detector elements, each detector element could potentially register coincidences between itself and any other detector element in the system. The result is a significantly higher detection efficiency in the system compared with a collimator-based SPECT system. The open geometry allows for the collection of a complete data set needed for image reconstruction without the need of any movements of the detectors. This allows the system to collect rapidly changing dynamic processes.

The line connecting a pair of detectors in a PET system is usually referred to as the line of response (LOR). When a pair of detectors records a coincidence, it is assumed that the direction of the emitted photon pairs is the same as the orientation of the LOR. However, this is only true if the photons are exactly 180° apart (i.e., the positron–electron pair is at rest at the time of annihilation). As mentioned earlier, if the positron–electron pair has some residual momentum, the emission angle of the photon pair will deviate from 180°. This deviation from 180° is on the order of 0.5° and is one of the factors that limits the spatial resolution in PET. This effect is sometimes referred to as photon noncollinearity, and the effect on the spatial resolution depends on

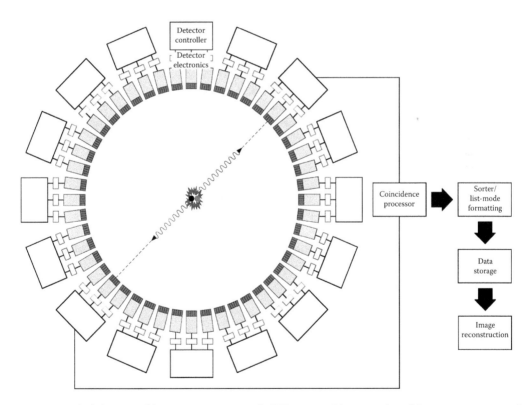

Figure 1.16 Block diagram of the main components of a PET scanner. A large number of detectors are arranged around the object to be imaged. Each detector module is connected to its own electronics. When a detector is struck by a photon, the signal is processed by the detector electronics. If the signal is a valid event (e.g., the energy falls within the energy window), it is passed on to the detector electronics, which will take the signals from a group of detectors and pass the position and timing information to the coincidence processor. The coincidence processor will determine if two detector modules registered two events within the predefined time window. If this is the case, the event will be saved and passed to the sorter system, where the event is saved in a sinogram or formatted for list-mode storage. The event is finally stored on disk. When the acquisition is finished, the data is reconstructed.

the system diameter. For a whole-body system, the contribution from the photon noncollinearity is close to 2 mm, whereas for a small-diameter preclinical system, this effect is a small fraction of a millimeter.

Since the detectors have some physical extent, the LOR is better described as a narrow tube instead of a line. The physical extent of the detector or the width of this narrow tube is one factor that limits the spatial resolution in PET. The geometric line spread function (LSF) at the midpoint between a pair of detectors will have a triangular shape with an FWHM equal to half the detector width [35]. At any off-center position, the LFS will take on a trapezoidal shape and the FWHM will widen.

Another approximation in PET is that it is assumed that the LOR aligns with the location of the radioactive decay. What the system is actually measuring is the location of the annihilation, which may occur at some distance away from the actual radioactive decay since the positron travels some distance before it annihilates. The range of the positron is dependent on the energy transferred to the positron in the decay, which in turn is isotope specific. For instance, the maximum energy transferred to a positron in the decay of ^{18}F is 635 keV, which corresponds to a range of 2 mm in tissue. The corresponding values in the decay of ^{15}O are 1.72 MeV and 8 mm. Thus, the spatial resolution is expected to be slightly worse for a study using ^{15}O as the radionuclide compared with ^{18}F.

During an acquisition, a large number of coincidences are recorded along a large number of LORs of different spatial locations and orientations. The number of recorded coincidences for each LOR will be proportional to the total or projected activity along the LOR. These projections of activity along the LORs then form a data set that can be used to reconstruct the 3-D distribution of the positron-emitting isotope within the object. Image reconstruction is discussed in more detail in Chapter 9.

1.6.2 BASIC INSTRUMENTATION DESIGN

Figure 1.17 illustrates the basic components of a PET scanner. The most basic system consists of a set of detectors arranged around the object to be imaged. The most common geometry is a circular arrangement of the detectors, but other geometries exist, such as square, hexagon, and octagon. Each detector module usually consists of an array scintillation detector coupled to a photodetector readout. The scintillation material used in PET should have a high effective atomic number and high density. These two factors will maximize the probability that the 511 keV photon deposits all of its energy in a single interaction (i.e., photoelectric interaction) in a small detector volume. This will in turn result in a high detection efficiency and also reduce resolution losses due to photon scatter in the scintillator.

The most common photodetector used in PET is the PMT. In the first generation of PET systems, each scintillator was coupled to its own PMT. As the scintillation detector elements were made smaller to improve

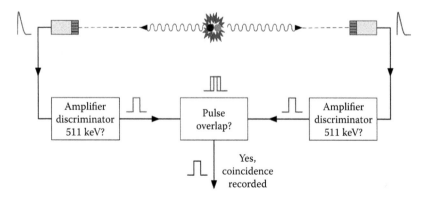

Figure 1.17 Schematic of a coincidence circuit. When a pair of detectors are struck by annihilation radiation produced from the same annihilation of a positron–electron pair, both detectors will generate a pulse that is fed into an amplifier and pulse height discriminator. The signal will be amplified and analyzed to determine whether the energy corresponds to 511 keV annihilation photon or not. If this is the case, a logic pulse is generated. These logic pulses are fed into a coincidence circuit, which looks for overlapping pulses from two inputs. If two pulses overlap, a coincidence is detected and the event is registered.

spatial resolution, it was no longer possible to continue with this detector design due to both the cost of the number of readout channels necessary and the space requirement of the PMTs. Current PET systems use a detector technology commonly referred to as block detectors [36,37], where an array of scintillator elements is coupled to a smaller array of PMTs, typically four. A light guide is placed between the scintillator array and the PMTs. This light guide directs the light produced in the scintillator elements in such a way that each element produces a unique signal pattern in the four PMTs. This allows for accurate detector element identification, and block detectors with up to 169 detector elements (13 × 13) coupled to only four PMTs have been constructed [38], providing a reduction in necessary readout channels of more than 40 compared with scintillators individually coupled to a PMT.

The outputs from the detector modules are then fed into a processing unit or detector controller that determines which detector element within the module was hit by a 511 keV photon, how much energy was deposited, and timing information when the interaction occurred. This information is then fed into a coincidence processor, which receives information from all detectors in the system. The coincidence processor determines if two detectors were registering an event within a predetermined time period (i.e., the coincidence time window). If this is the case, a coincidence has been recorded and information about the two detectors and the time the event occurred are saved. PET detector design and the overall system design are discussed in more detail in Chapter 6.

1.6.3 Coincidence detection

To register a valid event in PET, the two annihilation photons have to be detected in two separate detector elements within a narrow time window, typically on the order of a few nanoseconds. The simplest coincidence detection circuit consists of a pair of detectors placed on opposite sides of a positron-emitting source and is illustrated in Figure 1.17. Both detectors are connected to the necessary amplifiers, pulse shapers, pulse height analyzers (PHAs), and power supplies. The energy discriminators of the PHAs are set to only detect 511 keV photons, which usually means that events within a specific energy range will be accepted. This energy range or window depends on the energy resolution and the absorption properties of the detector. When an annihilation photon is fully absorbed in the detector, the PHA will generate a square or logic pulse with a fixed height and a width τ. The output from the two PHAs is then fed into a coincidence circuit, which will sense if there is an overlap of two pulses from the two inputs. If there is an overlap, a coincidence has been recorded and the coincidence circuit will in turn generate a logic pulse that is registered by a counter to record the event.

In a full PET system with more than 30,000 detector elements and more than 10^8 possible coincidence combinations, there are no dedicated coincidence circuits between each possible detector pair combination. Instead, detectors are grouped together and a significant amount of multiplexing takes place to determine which detector pair triggered the coincidence. Furthermore, the analog coincidence method described above has in modern PET systems been replaced by digital techniques, but still serves as an illustration of the principles of the coincidence method.

1.6.4 Time resolution

Ideally, if two annihilation photons are emitted from a source at the midpoint between the two detectors, the two PHAs should simultaneously generate the two logic pulses, and these should overlap without any time shift. However, all detection systems have an inherent slowness or delay before the detector signal is produced. This results in a finite temporal uncertainty within which coincidences can be determined. This is referred to as the time resolution of the system. There are a number of factors that contribute to the time resolution, and these factors depend greatly on the design of the detector system. For a scintillation detector system, the primary contributor to the loss of time resolution is the stochastic process of producing the signal following a photon interaction in the detector. After the absorption of the annihilation radiation, a discrete number of light photons are generated in the scintillator. Only a fraction of these will reach the photodetector and generate the signal carriers that will finally produce the signal that is analyzed by the subsequent processing electronics. In a PMT, the signal carriers are the photoelectrons emitted from the photocathode. Due to the quantum nature of the signal (i.e., a discrete number of photoelectrons), there will be a variance in the number of signal carriers when observing a large number of detected events. This will also result in a random time delay in when the first few photoelectrons will be emitted from the photocathode in the PMT. Since the arrival of these initial photoelectrons is used as a time stamp or time-pickoff to determine the coincidences, this random time delay or time jitter will affect how accurately in time a coincidence can be determined. The magnitude of the time delay depends primarily on how much light is produced in the scintillation detector for each photon absorption, at what rate the scintillation light is emitted, or the decay constant of the scintillation emission light, and how many photoelectrons are required to trigger the discriminator [39]. In general, the more light produced per absorption, the faster the first scintillation light photons will be produced, and the shorter the time constant of the light emission, the faster the scintillation photons will be produced, which will result in less time jitter.

In addition to the properties of the scintillation crystal, noise and signal degradation in the photodetectors and the subsequent pulse processing electronics are additional factors that contribute to time delay and signal degradation. For a given detector system, there is therefore a measurable time resolution. For older PET systems using BGO detectors, this time resolution was on the order of 6–10 ns [40]. Systems using the fastest scintillators that are practical for use in PET have a time resolution on the order of 375–525 ps [41–43]. Because of this inherent slowness of the detector system, it is necessary to give the logic pulses from the PHAs a finite width to ensure the pulses generated from an annihilation event overlap and the coincidence is recorded. Using a width of τ would ensure that all events separated by $\leq 2\tau$ are registered. The value of τ is usually set as wide as the time resolution of the detector pair.

1.6.5 TRUE COINCIDENCES

When two photons emitted from the same annihilation event are detected by a pair of detectors and generate a coincidence, then a true event has been recorded. These are the types of events that ideally only should be recorded by the detection system. However, there are additional types of coincidences that are recorded by the system that typically will have an adverse effect on the data.

1.6.6 RANDOM COINCIDENCES

The need to set a time window of finite width to ensure that most of the true coincidences are recorded allows for the possibility of detecting random coincidences. Random coincidences originate from two separate annihilations, where the orientation of the emitted annihilation photons is such that only one photon from each annihilation is detected. Since the coincidence is produced by two unrelated annihilations, these types of events do not provide any useful information about the activity distribution and should therefore be rejected. The random coincidences are unfortunately indistinguishable from the true coincidences, and the recorded coincidence is therefore a mix of the two event types. The random events tend to add a fairly uniform background to the true events, and if not corrected for, this background will reduce image contrast and compromise quantification.

It can be shown that the rate of detected random events between a pair of detectors is given by

$$R_{\text{Random}} = 2\tau R_1 R_2 \tag{1.21}$$

where 2τ is the coincidence time window, and R_1 and R_2 are the individual or singles count rates in detectors 1 and 2, respectively. Since the singles rates R_1 and R_2 are directly proportional to the activity in the FOV, the random rate is then proportional to the square of the activity in the FOV. Thus, if the activity is doubled, then the random rate will increase by a factor of four. The random rate is also directly proportional to the width of the coincidence window and can therefore be reduced by narrowing the time window. Since the coincidence window is dictated by the time resolution of the detector systems, the time window can typically not be reduced below the time resolution of the system without causing a loss in detection efficiency.

In order to maintain image contrast and quantitative accuracy of the reconstructed images, the collected coincidences along each LOR have to be corrected for the random coincidences. Since the measured coincidences are a mix of true and random coincidences, these coincidences are sometimes referred to as prompt coincidences. As the random coincidences are indistinguishable from the true coincidences, the random events cannot be rejected event by event. Instead, the number of registered random events has to be estimated. One method is to measure the singles count rates (R_1 and R_2) in the individual detectors, and knowing the width of the coincidence time window (τ), the random rate is then estimated using Equation 1.21. Other approaches for estimating the random rate are discussed in Chapter 8.

When correcting the prompt event for the presence of random events, additional statistical noise from the estimate of the random event is added to the net true events. The amount of noise added depends on the level of random event rate, but the random rate should in general be kept as low as possible, and should never exceed the net true count rate. Ideally, the net true count rate should increase linearly with injected activity in the FOV. Since the random count rate increases with the square of the activity, together with the noise degrading effect, there is a point where the amount of random events exceeds the net true rate. This point depends on several factors, including the properties of the scanner, the activity distribution, and the scatter environment. For any given imaging situation, the count rate behavior has to be characterized and the "optimal" activity level has to be determined [44].

1.6.7 MULTIPLE EVENTS

Multiple events are coincidences between three or more detected photons. These events may contain a true coincidence and a single unrelated photon, or be triggered by three unrelated photons. Because of the ambiguity of how to assign these events to a specific LOR, these events are rejected. Although these events do not directly increase noise, they indirectly increase noise due to the loss of events or dead time. The multiple event rate tends to increase to the third power of the activity level [45].

1.6.8 SCATTER AND ATTENUATION

As the annihilation photons travel through matter, there is a chance that the photons will undergo an interaction. At 511 keV, the most likely interaction type in most tissue types is Compton interaction, although some photoelectric interactions occur in bone due to the higher effective Z. As discussed earlier, in the Compton interaction, some of the photon energy is transferred to a loosely bound electron, and the remaining energy will appear as a scattered photon. The scattered photon energy will follow the Klein–Nishina probability distribution, but at 511 keV the scattered photons have a tendency to have forward direction with fairly small energy loss in the interaction (i.e., the energy of the scattered photon is only slightly lower than the original 511 keV photon check numbers). The consequences of the interaction are two. First, the intensity of true coincidences along a specific LOR is reduced or attenuated. Second, the scattered photons that are produced in the interaction will have a high probability of being detected due to the small energy loss, and therefore have a high likelihood of being accepted by the energy discriminator. Since one or both of the photons have changed direction, the event will be assigned to the incorrect LOR. If scattered events are not corrected for, the result in the final image is a loss in contrast [46–48].

If the loss of events along a LOR is not corrected for, the resulting image will have a distortion of the activity distribution, where the activity concentration in the center of the object will be underestimated. The amount of attenuation along a specific LOR depends on the total attenuation along the LOR. Consider the object in Figure 1.18, which has a uniform attenuation coefficient. If a point source is located at an unknown depth x in the object, and the total thickness of the object is D, then the probability that photon 1 will escape is

$$p_1 = e^{-\mu x} \tag{1.22}$$

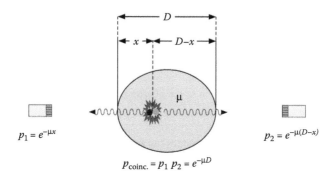

Figure 1.18 Illustration of attenuation in PET. If an annihilation occurs at an unknown depth x in a medium of uniform attenuation μ of thickness D, then the probability that the two annihilation photons will escape can be calculated. The probability that photon 1 will escape is $p_1 = e^{-\mu x}$, and the probability that photon 2 will escape is $p_2 = e^{-\mu(D-x)}$. The probability that both photons will escape is the product p_1 and p_2: $p_{coin} = p_1 p_2 = e^{-\mu(D-x)} e^{-\mu x} = e^{-\mu D}$. This probability for escape is the factor that the measured number of coincidences will be reduced by. In order to produce an image free of artifacts, the number of coincidences along every LOR has to be corrected by the inverse of this factor, i.e., $e^{\mu D}$, where D has to be estimated for each LOR.

The probability that the second photon will escape is similarly

$$p_2 = e^{-\mu(D-x)} \tag{1.23}$$

The probability that both photons will be detected is then

$$p_2 p_2 = e^{-\mu x} e^{-\mu(D-x)} = e^{-\mu D} \tag{1.24}$$

Thus, the amount of attenuation is independent of the location along the LOR of the source, and the amount of attenuation is only dependent on the total attenuation along the LOR. It can also be shown that this is true for a distributed source. If the attenuation is not uniform, the attenuation factor (μD) is replaced with a line integral of the attenuation coefficients along the LOR.

1.6.9 Noise equivalent count rate (NECR)

The correction of the total or prompt coincidence count rate for random and scattered coincidences adds noise to the net true coincidence count rate. The magnitude of the noise increase depends on several factors including activity in the FOV, count rates, and the scatter environment. In a low scatter situation and at low count rates, where the random count rate is expected to be low, the noise increase should be minimal. On the other hand, if the scatter and the randoms rates are high, then the noise contamination can be substantial. The noise equivalent count rate (NECR) is a metric used to describe this increase in noise due to the randoms and scatter corrections applied to the total coincidence count rate. The NECR is defined as [49]

$$\text{NECR} = \frac{T^2}{T + S + kR}$$

where T is the true count rate, S is the scatter count rate, R is the randoms or randoms count rate, and k is either 1 or 2, depending on how the randoms are estimated (i.e., 1 for estimation from singles and 2 from delayed coincidence measurement; see Chapter 8).

The NECR is the equivalent count rate that has the same level of statistical noise in the absence of scatter and random coincidences as the corrected net true count rate and is always less than the net true count rate. It has been shown that the NECR is proportional to the square of the noise in the reconstructed images [50]. This metric is frequently used to compare the performance of PET systems. Since both the scatter and random coincidences depend on the source distribution, these comparisons are only meaningful under highly standardized imaging conditions.

1.6.10 TIME-OF-FLIGHT PET

In the discussion of measuring coincidences, the difference in time of arrival of the two photons has been ignored. However, there is a measurable difference is arrival time of the two photons. If this time difference can accurately be measured, then the location of the annihilation can also be accurately determined. From classical mechanics, it can be shown that the location (x) of the annihilation along the line connecting the detector pair is

$$x = \frac{c\Delta t}{2} \tag{1.25}$$

where c is the speed of light and Δt is the difference in time of arrival of the two photons, and the origin (i.e., $x = 0$) is at the midpoint between the detector pairs. If ideal detectors existed (i.e., detectors with no timing uncertainty), then there would be no need for image reconstruction (see below). However, current detector technology only provides a timing resolution of a few hundred picoseconds, which translates to positioning uncertainty of a few centimeters. The TOF information can still be used in the image reconstruction to reduce image noise. It has been shown by Budinger [51] that the amount of reduction in noise is related to both the time resolution of the detection system and the distribution of the activity. If $SNR_{non\text{-}TOF}$ is the SNR of an object with a diameter D, reconstructed without TOF information, then the SNR of the object is

$$SNR_{TOF} \cong \sqrt{\frac{D}{\Delta x}}SNR_{non-TOF} = \sqrt{\frac{2D}{c\Delta t}}SNR_{non-TOF} \tag{1.26}$$

From this equation, it can be seen that the amount of reduction of noise is directly proportional to the time resolution and inversely proportional to the diameter of the imaged object. Based on this equation, larger objects would benefit more from using TOF in the measurements, rather than smear objects. This has also been shown in measurements on systems that allow TOF measurements [52].

1.7 IMAGE RECONSTRUCTION

The data collected in a SPECT and PET study is a collection of projections acquired at different angles. Each projection represents the total activity along a line in the object that is being imaged, viewed at a specific angle. If adequately sampled around the object, these projections or line integrals contain all the necessary information to reconstruct the 3-D activity distribution. There are a number of approaches for image reconstruction; these are described in detail in Chapter 9 of this book, but are briefly described here.

1.7.1 FILTERED BACKPROJECTION

The most commonly used analytical image reconstruction method is filtered backprojection (FBP) [53]. In FBP, the projection data is backprojected onto the image matrix at each angle. The backprojection operation will result in an image that resembles the true activity distribution, but with degraded resolution, lowered contrast, and the relative quantification lost.

These effects of backprojection can be described mathematically and can be reversed by applying a filter to the projection data prior to the operation. This filtering step will restore the resolution that would otherwise occur if the projections were simply backprojected and preserve the relative quantification between structures in the image.

Although the filter reverses the image degrading effects of backprojection, it also amplifies high-frequency noise (e.g., statistical noise). Since most SPECT and PET studies contain relatively high levels of statistical noise due to limited counting statistics, it is always necessary to apply a smoothing filter, which attenuates the high-frequency noise. Since the high spatial frequencies carry the information to visualize small objects and edges, this filtering will also result in a loss in resolution and ability to visualize and accurately quantify small objects. The amount of smoothing that is necessary to apply to the data depends on the level of statistical noise, which in turn depends on how many counts were acquired during the study. Furthermore, the level of smoothing also depends on what level of noise the observer finds acceptable in order to identify objects of a certain size of contrast in the image (i.e., contrast resolution). Images reconstructed with FBP from data acquired under clinical conditions will typically always have a significantly lower spatial resolution than the intrinsic resolution of the imaging system.

1.7.2 ITERATIVE RECONSTRUCTION

The second class of image reconstruction method used in both SPECT and PET imaging is the iterative reconstruction algorithms. These algorithms have to a great extent replaced the traditional FBP in both imaging modalities. The main reason for this is the improved image quality that can be achieved using iterative image reconstruction, especially in terms of improved SNR.

The basic principle for iterative reconstruction is to reconstruct an image that through a series of iterations best represents the data acquired by the imaging system. The iterative process starts with an initial estimate of the image, which is many times a uniform distribution. The next step is to sum up the image intensities along the same LORs as the scanner would acquire the data. This process is usually referred to as forward projection (i.e., the opposite of the backprojection operation described in Section 1.7.1). The forward projected data is then compared with the measured projection data. The difference between the measured and the forward projected data is then used to make adjustments to the previous image estimate along the measured LORs (e.g., a backprojection operation). This process is then repeated until the difference between the forward projected and measured data sets is minimized (i.e., convergence is reached).

One of the many advantages of the iterative reconstruction algorithms is that they attempt to arrive at an image or activity distribution that most likely would have created the measured projection data, taking into account both the effects of counting statistics and the physics of the measurements (e.g., scatter, normalization, and detector resolution) [54,55]. The drawback of the iterative reconstruction algorithms is that they are very computationally expensive, especially if the system model is very detailed. In contrast to FBP, where one backprojection is required, iterative reconstruction algorithms may require a large number of iterations before convergence is reached. A number of methods have therefore been developed to accelerate the reconstruction. One of the most commonly used acceleration techniques is the ordered subsets [56].

With increasingly powerful computers and the use of graphics processing units (GPUs) for image reconstruction (see Chapter 10), images reconstructed with sophisticated iterative algorithms are used routinely in clinical practice.

1.8 IMAGE ANALYSIS AND EVALUATION

Once the images have been reconstructed, they will be analyzed and interpreted. In clinical imaging, the images are evaluated many times qualitatively. This means that the physicians evaluate the images visually and look for abnormalities in the distribution of the radiotracer. For a given radiotracer, there is a normal distribution of the tracer. The abnormal uptake could, for instance, be a regional increase or decrease in tracer uptake in an organ. An increase in the uptake of ^{18}FDG, which reflects the glucose metabolism, could be an indication of a highly metabolic tumor. A decrease in the uptake of a flow tracer in the myocardium could be an indication of a partial blockage of the coronary arteries. Visual interpretation of the images is the most common method of image interpretation.

Both SPECT and PET have the ability to produce quantitative images, where the pixel values in the image represent the actual activity concentration in bequerels per milliliter. This requires a number of corrections to be applied to the raw data, either before, during, or after image reconstruction. How this is accomplished is discussed in more detail in Chapters 7 and 8. Producing images that are quantitative allows the possibility of better quantification of the uptake in a suspected lesion. Having quantitative images is a requirement in order to calculate the standardized uptake value (SUV) [57,58], which is a common index to characterize the uptake in lesions. The SUV is frequently used to differentiate malignant from benign tumors [59] and to evaluate the tumor response to therapy [60]. The SUV is a very attractive method for quantification due to its computational and methodological simplicity. All that is needed is accurate knowledge of the injected activity, time of injection, weight of the subject, and time of the acquisition. The SUV is, however, sensitive to a number of parameters, such as uptake time, body mass and fat content, glucose levels, spatial resolution, and image noise [61].

More sophisticated methods for quantitative imaging involve dynamic imaging. The acquired image data is then used together with pharmacokinetic models of the uptake and metabolism of the radiotracer to estimate rate constants. These methods for quantification are more complex and labor-intensive. Thus, they are typically not used routinely clinically. However, these methods are extensively used in research studies. Quantitative imaging is discussed in greater detail in Chapters 11 and 12.

1.9 SUMMARY

This chapter has presented an overview of the physics behind SPECT and PET imaging. Radioisotopes are used to produce the energetic photons used to localize the injected traces with external detectors. In both SPECT and PET imaging, the direction of the emission of the photons along a line in space is necessary to localize the radiotracer within the object that is being imaged. In SPECT, this is accomplished with large-area detectors with lead collimators. In PET, the back-to-back emission of annihilation photons when an electron–positron pair annihilates is used to determine the direction of the photon emission. By collecting a large number of these photon events by the detector at different angles and positions around the imaged object, the 3-D distribution of the radiotracer can be reconstructed. In clinical imaging, the images can be interpreted by a physician to determine whether the uptake is normal. Scientists can use the images to achieve a better understanding of the behavior of a radiotracer under development.

In this book, the various aspects of SPECT and PET imaging are discussed in detail in the subsequent chapters. Scintillation detectors and photodetectors are discussed in Chapters 2 and 3, respectively. Chapter 4 includes a discussion on the electronics used for these detector systems. Chapters 5 and 6 describe full SPECT and PET system design. How to produce images that are quantitative in SPECT and PET is covered in Chapters 7 and 8, respectively. Image reconstruction techniques are described in Chapter 9, and the developments in the use of GPUs for image reconstruction and data processing are discussed in Chapter 10. Dynamic imaging where a time series of images is acquired to extract kinetic information of the radio tracer and organ function is covered in Chapters 11 and 12. Multimodality imaging where SPECT and PET instrumentation are combined with CT is covered in Chapters 13 and 14. PET and MRI are discussed in Chapter 15. The applications of the two imaging modalities are covered in the final two chapters: preclinical applications are discussed in Chapter 16 and clinical applications are presented in Chapter 17.

REFERENCES

1. National Nuclear Data Center, Brookhaven National Laboratory, 2016, Upton, NY.
2. U.S. Bureau of Radiological Health Public Health Service. 1970. *Radiological Health Handbook*. U.S. Department of Health, Education, and Welfare, Washington, DC.

3. Weber, D. A., and L. T. Dillman. 1989. *MIRD—Radionuclide Data and Decay Schemes*. Society of Nuclear Medicine, New York.

4. Gates, V. L., A. A. H. Esmail, K. Marshall, S. Spies, and R. Salem. 2011. Internal pair production of 90Y permits hepatic localization of microspheres using routine PET: Proof of concept. *J Nucl Med* 52:72–76.

5. Cherry, S. R., J. A. Sorenson, and M. E. Phelps. 2012. *Physics in Nuclear Medicine*. Elsevier/Saunders, Philadelphia.

6. Hademenos, G. J., M. A. King, M. Ljungberg, I. G. Zubal, and C. R. Harrell. 1993. A scatter correction method for Tl-201 images—A Monte-Carlo investigation. *IEEE Trans Nucl Sci* 40:1179–1186.

7. Devries, D. J., and M. A. King. 1994. Window selection for dual photopeak window scatter correction in Tc-99m imaging. *IEEE Trans Nucl Sci* 41:2771–2778.

8. Jaszczak, R. J., K. L. Greer, C. E. Floyd Jr., C. C. Harris, and R. E. Coleman. 1984. Improved SPECT quantification using compensation for scattered photons. *J Nucl Med* 25:893–900.

9. Jeavons, A., D. Townsend, M. Wensveen, R. Magnanini, P. Frey, and A. Donath. 1985. The development of the HIDAC positron camera. *Eur J Nucl Med* 11:A40–A40.

10. Jeavons, A. P., R. A. Chandler, and C. A. R. Dettmar. 1999. A 3D HIDAC-PET camera with sub-millimetre resolution for imaging small animals. *IEEE Trans Nucl Sci* 46:468–473.

11. Lacy, J. L., C. S. Martin, and L. P. Armendarez. 2001. High sensitivity, low cost PET using lead-walled straw detectors. *Nucl Instrum Methods A* 471:88–93.

12. Birks, J. B. 1964. *The Theory and Practice of Scintillation Counting*. Pergamon Press, Oxford.

13. Knoll, G. F. 2010. *Radiation Detection and Measurements*. John Wiley & Sons, Hoboken, NJ.

14. Zworykin, V. K., G. A. Morton, and L. Malter. 1936. The secondary emission multiplier—A new electronic device. *Proc IRE* 24:351–375.

15. Suffert, M. 1992. Silicon photodiode readout of scintillators and associated electronics. *Nucl Instrum Methods A* 322:523–528.

16. McIntyre, R. J. 1966. Multiplication noise in uniform avalanche diodes. *IEEE Trans Electron Devices* 13:164–168.

17. Gruber, G. J., W. S. Choong, W. W. Moses, S. E. Derenzo, S. E. Holland, M. Pedrali-Noy, B. Krieger, E. Mandelli, G. Meddeler, and N. W. Wang. 2002. A compact 64-pixel CsI(Tl)/Si PIN photodiode imaging module with IC readout. *IEEE Trans Nucl Sci* 49:147–152.

18. Kindem, J., C. Y. Bai, and R. Conwell. 2010. CsI(Tl)/PIN solid state detectors for combined high resolution SPECT and CT imaging. In *2010 IEEE Nuclear Science Symposium Conference Record (NSS/MIC)*, pp. 1987–1990. Institute of Electrical and Electronics Engineers, Piscataway, NJ.

19. Dolgoshein, B., V. Balagura, P. Buzhan, M. Danilov, L. Filatov, E. Garutti, M. Groll, et al. 2006. Status report on silicon photomultiplier development and its applications. *Nucl Instrum Methods A* 563:368–376.

20. Stewart, A. G., V. Saveliev, S. J. Bellis, D. J. Herbert, P. J. Hughes, and J. C. Jackson. 2008. Performance of 1-mm(2) silicon photomultiplier. *IEEE J Quantum Electron* 44:157–164.

21. Buzhan, P., B. Dolgoshein, E. Garutti, M. Groll, A. Karakash, V. Kaphn, V. Kantserov, et al. 2006. Timing by silicon photomultiplier: A possible application for TOF measurements. *Nucl Instrum Methods A* 567:353–355.

22. Schlesinger, T. E., J. E. Toney, H. Yoon, E. Y. Lee, B. A. Brunett, L. Franks, and R. B. James. 2001. Cadmium zinc telluride and its use as a nuclear radiation detector material. *Mater Sci Eng R* 32:103–189.

23. Zanio, K., H. Montano, and F. Krajenbrink. 1975. Cadmium telluride x-ray spectrometer. *Appl Phys Lett* 27:159–160.

24. Case, J. A., and T. M. Bateman. 2013. Taking the perfect nuclear image: Quality control, acquisition, and processing techniques for cardiac SPECT, PET, and hybrid imaging. *J Nucl Cardiol* 20:891–907.

25. Bocher, M., I. M. Blevis, L. Tsukerman, Y. Shrem, G. Kovalski, and L. Volokh. 2010. A fast cardiac gamma camera with dynamic SPECT capabilities: Design, system validation and future potential. *Eur J Nucl Med Mol Imaging* 37:1887–1902.

26. Erlandsson, K., K. Kacperski, D. van Gramberg, and B. F. Hutton. 2009. Performance evaluation of D-SPECT: A novel SPECT system for nuclear cardiology. *Phys Med Biol* 54:2635–2649.

27. Pratx, G., and C. S. Levin. 2007. Accurately positioning events in a high-resolution PET system that uses 3D CZT detectors. In *2007 IEEE Nuclear Science Symposium Conference Record (NSS/MIC)*, vols. 1–11, pp. 2660–2664. Institute of Electrical and Electronics Engineers, Piscataway, NJ.

28. Yin, Y. Z., S. Komarov, H. Y. Wu, T. Y. Song, Q. A. Li, A. Garson, K. Lee, G. Simburger, P. Dowkontt, H. Krawczynski, and Y. C. Tai. 2009. Characterization of highly pixelated CZT detectors for sub-millimeter PET imaging. In *2009 IEEE Nuclear Science Symposium Conference Record (NSS/MIC)*, vols. 1–5, pp. 2411–2414. Institute of Electrical and Electronics Engineers, Piscataway, NJ.

29. Meng, L. J., J. W. Tan, and G. Fu. 2007. Design study of an MRI compatible ultra-high resolution SPECT for in vivo mice brain imaging. In *2007 IEEE Nuclear Science Symposium Conference Record (NSS/MIC)*, vols. 1–11, pp. 2956–2960. Institute of Electrical and Electronics Engineers, Piscataway, NJ.

30. Hamamura, M. J., S. Ha, W. W. Roeck, L. T. Muftuler, D. J. Wagenaar, D. Meier, B. E. Patt, and O. Nalcioglu. 2010. Development of an MR-compatible SPECT system (MRSPECT) for simultaneous data acquisition. *Phys Med Biol* 55:1563–1575.

31. Busemann-Sokole, E., and International Atomic Energy Agency. 2003. *IAEA Quality Control Atlas for Scintillation Camera Systems*. International Atomic Energy Agency, Vienna.

32. Zanzonico, P. 2008. Routine quality control of clinical nuclear medicine instrumentation: A brief review. *J Nucl Med* 49:1114–1131.

33. DeBenedetti, S., C. E. Cowan, W. R. Konneker, and H. Primakoff. 1950. On the angular distribution of two-photon annihilation radiation. *Phys Rev* 77:205–212.

34. Bothe, W. 1955. Coincidence method. *Science* 122:861–863.

35. Hoffman, E. J., S.-C. Huang, and M. E. Phelps. 1979. Quantitation in positron emission computed tomography. I. Effect of object size. *J Comput Assist Tomogr* 3:299–308.

36. Casey, M. E., and R. Nutt. 1986. A multicrystal two dimensional BGO detector system for positron emission tomography. *IEEE Trans Nucl Sci* 33:460–463.

37. Dahlbom, M., and E. J. Hoffman. 1988. An evaluation of a two-dimensional array detector for high-resolution PET. *IEEE Trans Med Imaging* 7:264–272.

38. Brambilla, M., C. Secco, M. Dominietto, R. Matheoud, G. Sacchetti, and E. Inglese. 2005. Performance characteristics obtained for a new 3-dimensional lutetium oxyorthosilicate-based whole-body PET/CT scanner with the National Electrical Manufacturers Association NU 2-2001 standard. *J Nucl Med* 46:2083–2091.

39. Post, R. F., and L. I. Schiff. 1950. Statistical limitations on the resolving time of a scintillation counter. *Phys Rev* 80:1113.

40. Moses, W. W. 2003. Time of flight in PET revisited. *IEEE Trans Nucl Sci* 50:1325–1330.

41. Jakoby, B. W., Y. Bercier, M. Conti, M. E. Casey, B. Bendriem, and D. W. Townsend. 2011. Physical and clinical performance of the mCT time-of-flight PET/CT scanner. *Phys Med Biol* 56:2375–2389.

42. Daube-Witherspoon, M. E., S. Surti, A. Perkins, C. C. M. Kyba, R. Wiener, M. E. Werner, R. Kulp, and J. S. Karp. 2010. The imaging performance of a LaBr3-based PET scanner. *Phys Med Biol* 55:45–64.

43. Bettinardi, V., L. Presotto, E. Rapisarda, M. Picchio, L. Gianolli, and M. C. Gilardi. 2011. Physical performance of the new hybrid PET/CT Discovery-690. *Med Phys* 38:5394–5411.

44. Watson, C. C., M. E. Casey, B. Bendriem, J. P. Carney, D. W. Townsend, S. Eberl, S. Meikle, and F. P. Difilippo. 2005. Optimizing injected dose in clinical PET by accurately modeling the counting-rate response functions specific to individual patient scans. *J Nucl Med* 46:1825–1834.

45. Germano, G., and E. J. Hoffman. 1988. Investigation of count rate and deadtime characteristics of a high resolution PET system. *J Comput Assist Tomogr* 12:836–846.

46. Levin, C. S., M. Dahlbom, and E. J. Hoffman. 1995. A Monte Carlo correction for the effect of Compton scattering in 3-D PET brain imaging. *IEEE Trans Nucl Sci* 42:1181–1185.

47. Ollinger, J. M. 1995. Detector efficiency and Compton scatter in fully 3D PET. *IEEE Trans Nucl Sci* 42:1168–1173.

48. Watson, C. C., D. Newport, M. E. Casey, R. A. DeKemp, R. S. Beanlands, and M. Schmand. 1997. Evaluation of simulation-based scatter correction for 3-D PET cardiac imaging. *IEEE Trans Nucl Sci* 44:90–97.

49. Strother, S. C., Casey, M. E., and Hoffman, E. J. 1990. Measuring PET scanner sensitivity: Relating countrates to image signal-to-noise ratios using noise equivalent counts. *IEEE Trans Nucl Sci* NS-37(2): 783–788.

50. Dahlbom, M., Schiepers, C., and Czernin, J. 2005. Comparison of noise equivalent count rates and image noise. *IEEE Trans Nucl Sci* 52(5): 1386–1390.

51. Budinger, T. F. 1983. Time-of-flight positron emission tomography: Status relative to conventional PET. *J Nucl Med* 24:73–78.

52. Karp, J. S., S. Surti, M. E. Daube-Witherspoon, and G. Muehllehner. 2008. Benefit of time-of-flight in PET: Experimental and clinical results. *J Nucl Med* 49:462–470.

53. Brooks, R. A., and G. Di Chiro. 1976. Principles of computer assisted tomography (CAT) in radiographic and radioisotopic imaging. *Phys Med Biol* 21:689–732.

54. Lange, K., and R. Carson. 1984. EM reconstruction algorithms for emission and transmission tomography. *J Comput Assist Tomogr* 8:306–316.

55. Shepp, L. A., and Y. Vardi. 1982. Maximum likelihood reconstruction for emission tomography. *IEEE Trans Med Imaging* MI-1:113–122.

56. Hudson, H. M., and R. S. Larkin. 1994. Accelerated image reconstruction using ordered subsets of projection data. *IEEE Trans Med Imaging* 13:601–609.

57. Zasadny, K. R., and R. L. Wahl. 1993. Standardized uptake values of normal tissues at PET with 2-[fluorine-18]-fluoro-2-deoxy-D-glucose: Variations with body weight and a method for correction. *Radiology* 189:847–850.

58. Huang, S. C. 2000. Anatomy of SUV. Standardized uptake value. *Nucl Med Biol* 27:643–646.

59. Griffeth, L. K., F. Dehdashti, A. H. McGuire, D. J. McGuire, D. J. Perry, S. M. Moerlein, and B. A. Siegel. 1992. PET evaluation of soft-tissue masses with fluorine-18 fluoro-2-deoxy-D-glucose. *Radiology* 182:185–194.

60. Romer, W., A. R. Hanauske, S. Ziegler, R. Thodtmann, W. Weber, C. Fuchs, W. Enne, M. Herz, C. Nerl, M. Garbrecht, and M. Schwaiger. 1998. Positron emission tomography in non-Hodgkin's lymphoma: Assessment of chemotherapy with fluorodeoxyglucose. *Blood* 91:4464–4471.

61. Keyes, J. W., Jr. 1995. SUV: Standard uptake or silly useless value? *J Nucl Med* 36:1836–1839.

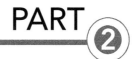
TECHNOLOGY

2 Scintillators for PET and SPECT   43
   Charles L. Melcher and Lars Eriksson
3 Photodetectors   63
   Magnus Dahlbom
4 Acquisition electronics   91
   Thomas K. Lewellen
5 SPECT instrumentation   115
   Wei Chang, Michael Rozler, and Scott D. Metzler
6 PET instrumentation   163
   Andrew L. Goertzen and Jonathan D. Thiessen

Scintillators for PET and SPECT

CHARLES L. MELCHER AND LARS ERIKSSON

2.1	Introduction	43
2.2	The scintillation process	44
2.3	Properties of commercial scintillators	46
2.4	Scintillators used in PET	48
2.5	Properties of scintillators for PET	48
2.6	Timing with scintillation detectors and TOF PET possibilities	51
	2.6.1 Photomultiplier tube–based detectors	51
	2.6.2 Silicon photomultiplier–based detectors	53
	2.6.3 Comparison of time resolution data obtained with PMTs and SiPMs	54
2.7	SPECT	55
2.8	Scintillator choices	55
2.9	Current SPECT systems	57
2.10	Small-Animal SPECT	57
2.11	New trends in SPECT imaging	57
2.12	Future research directions	58
	References	58

2.1 INTRODUCTION

A scintillator is a material with the ability to absorb ionizing radiation, such as x-rays or gamma rays, and to convert a fraction of the absorbed energy into visible or ultraviolet (UV) photons. The conversion process typically takes place on a timescale of nanoseconds to microseconds, thus producing a brief pulse of photons corresponding to each gamma ray or x-ray that interacts with the scintillator material [1]. The light pulse, the intensity of which is approximately proportional to the energy deposited in the scintillator, is sensed by a photodetector and converted into an electrical signal.

Scintillators may be liquid or solid, organic or inorganic, crystalline, polycrystalline, or glass. Organic liquid and plastic scintillators often are used for detection of charged particles and neutrons. For the detection of energetic photons, such as the gamma rays used in PET and SPECT, inorganic single-crystal scintillators are most often used because of their generally higher density and higher atomic number, which lead to better detection efficiency.

In PET, inorganic scintillator crystals are used to record pairs of gamma rays produced by the annihilation of positrons emitted by injected radionuclide tracers. The most common detector geometry comprises multiple rings of block detectors that are either partially or fully pixelated [2,3]. Typically, a 2×2 photosensor array is used to read out an array of scintillator elements with as many as 169 crystals. The ultimate performance of the camera is strongly tied to both the physical and scintillation properties of the crystals. For this reason, researchers have investigated virtually all known scintillator crystals for possible use in PET and SPECT [4]. Despite this massive research effort, only a few different scintillators have been found that have a suitable combination of characteristics, and only three (thallium-doped sodium iodide [NaI:Tl], bismuth germanate [BGO], and cerium-doped lutetium oxyorthosilicate [LSO:Ce]) have found widespread use [5]. A few others, namely, barium fluoride (BaF$_2$), cesium fluoride (CsF), cerium-doped gadolinium oxyorthosilicate (GSO:Ce), and most recently, cerium-doped lanthanum bromide (LaBr$_3$), have been used in experimental systems. Cerium-doped yttrium-lutetium aluminate (LuAP) has been used in some small-animal PET scanners. A few commercial systems have been built based on GSO.

In SPECT, large scintillator plates are used to image single-photon-emitting radionuclides. Thallium-doped sodium iodide is almost universally used. SPECT instrumentation is closely tied to the development of NaI:Tl, which began with Hofstadter's initial work in 1948 [6], and to Anger's invention of the scintillation camera [7]. The spatial resolution of an Anger camera is determined partly by a parallel-hole collimator located in front of the scintillator plate and partly by the principle of Anger logic, in which the interaction point of a gamma ray with the scintillator point is determined by an algorithm that weights the light intensity detected by several photomultiplier tubes (PMTs). SPECT uses one or more detector heads to obtain the views necessary for image reconstruction. Either one gamma camera is rotated through 360°, or up to three heads looking at different views of the object are rotated in order to have a full set of views for a three-dimensional reconstruction. Good energy resolution is important to ensure that the detected single photon is not a scattered photon. For a review of SPECT imaging and instrumentation, see Chapters 5 and 7 in this book or Peterson and Furenlid [8].

2.2 THE SCINTILLATION PROCESS

Efficient detection of gamma rays and x-rays by scintillators requires compositions that are optimized in several ways. Good detection efficiency requires high density and high effective atomic number to maximize the cross sections for photoelectric absorption, Compton scattering, and pair production. Luminescence centers should exhibit high quantum efficiency for good light output and electric dipole–allowed radiative transitions for short decay times and, consequently, high-count-rate capability in high-flux scenarios such as active interrogation. The host material band gap should be small in order to minimize the energy required for the production of electron–hole (e–h) pairs, but must be larger than the activator's energy transition from the excited state to the ground state. Low defect concentrations are needed for fast and complete energy transfer from the matrix to the luminescence centers. Minimal absorption of the emitted light is necessary for good light collection by the photosensor, and an index of refraction near 1.5 is preferred in order to minimize internal reflections. Chemical inertness and mechanical strength facilitate cost-effective detector processing and high detector reliability and lifetime.

Since the ability to theoretically predict the detailed energy conversion characteristics of specific scintillator compositions is limited, most scintillator development has proceeded on a largely empirical basis. However, as scintillator performance in general continues to improve, it becomes increasingly important to understand the fundamental mechanisms that determine the maximum performance of specific scintillator compositions. Better understanding of the roles of defects and the development of crystal growth processes that minimize their formation are crucial to achieving high-resolution scintillation detectors for gamma ray spectroscopy.

The mechanism of scintillation can be characterized as a sequence of three major steps: (1) the creation of primary electrons and holes via ionization of the matrix material, the subsequent creation of numerous secondary excitations, and thermalization to create unbound e–h pairs and bound pairs (excitons); (2) the migration of e–h pairs to luminescence (activation) centers; and (3) the emission of the luminescent center itself [9,10]. The first step, ionization, is an intrinsic property of the material that is mainly related to the band gap and is not significantly affected by defects, impurities, or crystal growth conditions. Robbins [9] showed that the ionization efficiency, that is, the number of e–h pairs created per unit of absorbed gamma ray energy, can be calculated from the fundamental physical properties of the scintillator crystal, including the band gap, the high-frequency and static dielectric constants, and the optical longitudinal photon energy. For some scintillator materials, these parameters are well known, and consequently, the ionization efficiency can be calculated with reasonable confidence. For some newer scintillators, however, some of the parameters are not known precisely, thus resulting in a significant uncertainty in the calculated efficiency. A rule of thumb is that the average energy to create an e–h pair is approximately 1.5–2.0 E_g (E_g = band gap energy) for ionic crystals and 3–4 E_g for covalently bonded crystals. Due to electron–electron relaxation, the energy of an electron (or hole) eventually falls below the threshold to create further ionization, and it then thermalizes via electron–phonon interactions. In this way, up to approximately 75% of electron energy may be "lost" to nonradiative processes. The second step, energy migration, may be strongly affected by defects. It is generally understood that shallow charge traps affect the rate at which the energy is transferred to the excited states of luminescent centers due to the temporary trapping and subsequent detrapping of migrating excitons or unbound e–h pairs. Deeper traps can create delayed excitation and emission from luminescence centers known as afterglow. The third step, luminescence emission, is often characterized in terms of its quantum efficiency, that is, the ratio of the radiative transition rate to the total (radiative + nonradiative) transition rate. Nonradiative emission may become more likely due to elevated temperature or defects in close proximity to the luminescent center.

The steps of the scintillation mechanism occur on a wide range of timescales. In the case of photoelectric absorption of the incoming gamma ray, typically an electron is ejected from the K-shell of an atom with an energy equal to the incoming gamma ray energy minus the K-shell energy. The atom with the K-shell hole relaxes either by generating an Auger electron or through a series of radiative steps through the outer shells. Both the primary electron and the Auger electron relax via electron–electron interactions on a timescale of 1–100 fs, which is similar to the timescale of radiative relaxation of a K-shell hole. The result of this step is a large number of conduction band electrons, valence band holes, and core and valence band excitons. As mentioned above, the next step, thermalization, involves electron–phonon interactions in which electrons move to the bottom of the conduction band and holes move to the top of the valence band, thus producing e–h pairs with energy equal to the band gap. This process occurs on a timescale of roughly 1–10 ps. The time for e–h migration to luminescence centers varies widely according to the distance between centers, as well as the number and depth of traps created by crystalline defects and impurities. Times as long as 1–10 ns are not uncommon. The timescale of the final step, luminescence emission, ranges from <1 ns to >1 ms. Many useful scintillators utilize the 5d–4f transition with a characteristic time constant of 20–70 ns (e.g., Ce^{3+}), or the $4f^65d$–4f transition with a characteristic time constant of approximately 1 μs (e.g., Eu^{2+}).

From the timescales noted above, it is apparent that the observed emission time of a scintillator is dominated by the migration time of excitons and e–h pairs and the excited state lifetime of the luminescence center. In a perfect defect-free scintillation crystal with a single type of luminescence center with a single radiative transition, the excited state of the luminescence centers would be populated in ≪100 ps and emission would decay exponentially with a time constant corresponding to the lifetime of the excited state of the center. In addition, the scintillation efficiency or "light yield" would be predictable on the basis of the band gap and the quantum efficiency of the luminescence center, and light yield would be proportional to excitation energy, thus producing energy resolution that is limited only by the variance in the number of emitted photons. However, the light yield is often lower than expected, the scintillation decay is often slower than the radiative lifetime of the luminescence center, and the light yield is often not proportional to the absorbed gamma ray energy. It is generally understood that light yield and decay time are related in some way to energy migration (although the details are not always fully understood), and nonproportionality may be related as well.

Comparison of the scintillation decay time of a scintillator to the radiative lifetime of the luminescence center is a straightforward technique for revealing the existence of imperfect energy migration. The scintillation decay is typically measured using the time-correlated single-photon counting technique using standard laboratory electronics that have been readily available for decades. Measurement of the radiative lifetime of the luminescence center, however, requires a nanosecond or faster pulsed light source whose energy matches the transition energy of the center. Earlier measurements of this type were performed at synchrotrons, and the technique was therefore applied to a limited number of materials. Later, pulsed nitrogen lasers provided pulsed excitation, but only for cases in which the center's excitation overlapped the laser's fixed wavelength (337 nm). Today, nanosecond pulsed light-emitting diodes (LEDs) and faster pulsed lasers are available with a large variety of wavelengths, thus facilitating lifetime studies of a variety of luminescence centers.

2.3 PROPERTIES OF COMMERCIAL SCINTILLATORS

The ideal scintillator for PET would have a combination of several physical and scintillation properties (Table 2.1). A high detection efficiency for the gamma rays of interest requires both high atomic number for a large photoelectric cross section and high density for a large Compton scattering cross section. These are the two main interactions through which 511 keV gamma rays interact with the scintillator crystals. For good coincidence timing and high-count-rate capability, a short decay constant is required. In other words, the pulse of scintillation photons must be as brief as possible. A high light output allows a large number of crystal elements to be coupled to a single photodetector, and good energy resolution allows a clear identification of full energy events. The transmission of the scintillation light pulses into the photodetector is best when the refractive index of the scintillator material is similar to that of the entrance window and coupling material, usually near 1.5. In some materials, color centers may be easily produced by ionizing radiation, thus impeding the transmission of the scintillation light through the scintillator itself. Therefore, a resistance to this effect, known as radiation hardness, is desirable. Some scintillators are hygroscopic; that is, they readily absorb water from the atmosphere and therefore require special packaging to hermetically seal them. Nonhygroscopic materials have an advantage in that simpler packaging may be used. Mechanical ruggedness is desirable because it makes fabrication of small crystals easier. Because a PET scanner may use 5,000–12,000 cc of scintillator crystals, the growth of large volumes of crystals at a reasonable cost must be feasible.

The ideal scintillator for SPECT would have many of the same attributes as a PET scintillator, but with a different priority (Table 2.2). Because SPECT detectors are typically large single-crystal plates, the ability to grow very large-size crystals is a requirement. High light output is necessary since the light spreads out over a large area and is measured by several PMTs. Timing is not an issue because only single gamma rays are measured and the count rate is low. Good energy resolution is desirable. Density and effective atomic number are important, but less so than in PET due to the lower energies encountered in SPECT.

Because the truly ideal scintillator for PET and SPECT has not yet been discovered, one must look at the characteristics of materials that do exist and choose the one best suited to the application. Table 2.3 shows the physical properties of the seven scintillators that have been used in PET so far, listed in order of decreasing density. Both BGO and LSO:Ce have excellent physical properties. They have a high density and atomic number, which results in efficient detection of gamma rays, and are also rugged and nonhygroscopic, which

Table 2.1 Properties of the ideal scintillator for PET

Crystal property	Purpose
High density	High-gamma-ray detection efficiency
High atomic number	High-gamma-ray detection efficiency
Short decay time	Good coincidence timing
High light output	Large ratio of crystals to readout channels
Good energy resolution/good proportionality	Identification of full energy events
Appropriate emission wavelength	Match to photosensor
Transparent at emission wavelength	Efficient light transport
Appropriate index of refraction	Minimal reflection at sensor window
Radiation hardness	Stable performance
Rugged	Easier fabrication of small pixels
Nonhygroscopic	Simplifies packaging
Cost-effective growth	Reasonable cost

Table 2.2 Properties of the ideal scintillator for SPECT

Performance criteria	Scintillator properties
Anger logic readout	High light output
Continuous crystal plate	Large-scale crystal growth
High density	High-gamma-ray detection efficiency
High atomic number	High-gamma-ray detection efficiency
Appropriate emission wavelength	Match to photosensor
Appropriate index of refraction	Minimal reflection at sensor window
Low cost	Rapid and high yield growth

Table 2.3 Physical properties of some common scintillator crystals

Crystal	Density (g/cm^3)	Effective atomic number	Hygroscopic?	Rugged?
NaI:Tl	3.67	51	Yes	No
BGO ($Bi_4Ge_3O_{12}$)	7.12	75	No	Yes
GSO (Gd_2SiO_5:Ce)	6.71	59	No	No (cleaves)
BaF_2	4.88	53	No	Yes
CsF	4.64	53	Very	No
LSO (Lu_2SiO_5:Ce)	7.40	65	No	Yes
$LaBr_3$:Ce	5.06	47	Very	No

Table 2.4 Scintillation and optical properties of some common scintillators

Crystal	Primary decay constant (ns)	Secondary decay constant (ns)	Emission intensity (photons/MeV)	Emission wavelength (nm)	Index of refraction
NaI:Tl	230	10,000	38,000	410	1.85
BGO ($Bi_4Ge_3O_{12}$)	300	None	8,200	480	2.15
GSO (Gd_2SiO_5:Ce)	60[a]	600[a]	15,000	430	1.85
BaF_2	0.8	600	4,000	220	1.48
CsF	4	None	1,500	390	1.49
LSO (Lu_2SiO_5:Ce)	42	None	35,000	420	1.82
$LaBr_3$:Ce	16[a]	None	65,000	360	2.30[a]

[a] Varies with Ce concentration.

allows relatively simple detector fabrication. GSO is also a good candidate, except that it cleaves easily, which makes detector fabrication more difficult.

Table 2.4 shows the scintillation and optical properties of the seven PET scintillators, listed in order of increasing decay constant. BaF_2 has the shortest decay constant by far: 0.8 ns. Unfortunately, the emission is weak and located in the far UV at 220 nm, which requires PMTs with more expensive quartz windows. It also has a long secondary component of 600 ns. CsF has a very short decay constant of 4 ns, but its intensity is so weak that this scintillator is seldom used. LSO:Ce has the best combination of a short decay constant, 40 ns, and high emission intensity. In addition, it has no secondary decay component.

NaI:Tl is essentially the only scintillator used in SPECT, and its properties are found in Tables 2.3 and 2.4.

2.4 SCINTILLATORS USED IN PET

NaI:Tl was discovered in 1948 by Hofstadter [6]. It quickly became the scintillator of choice for radiation detection because of its high light output, that is, efficient conversion of deposited gamma ray energy to scintillation photons. The large light pulses are easily processed by conventional pulse shaping electronics. The main disadvantage of NaI:Tl is its low detection efficiency for gamma rays above 200 keV, as a result of low density and moderately low atomic number. At the energies typically used in SPECT (140 keV), the detection efficiency of NaI:Tl is satisfactory, and it is used almost exclusively in that application. However, for higher energy applications, such as PET (511 keV), NaI:Tl has been replaced, for the most part, by materials with higher density and atomic number. An additional disadvantage of NaI:Tl is that it is highly hygroscopic. As a result, a great deal of effort has gone into the development of hermetic packaging to protect the material from moisture in the atmosphere.

BGO emerged in the early 1970s, with initial studies reported by Weber and Monchamp [11]. Although the light output of BGO is only about 15% of that of NaI:Tl, its dramatically higher detection efficiency, as a result of density almost twice that of NaI:Tl, as well as a much higher atomic number, has made it a very popular choice for the detection of radiation above a few 100 keV. PET is the major ongoing application of BGO crystals today, despite the fact that their relatively long decay constant of 300 ns limits coincidence timing resolution and may result in high system dead-time losses.

Scintillators with short decay constants offer the possibility of time-of-flight (TOF) PET, in which opposing detectors measure the difference in the arrival times of a pair of gamma rays. In this way, the location of the positron event can be localized along the line connecting the two detectors. In the 1980s, two fast scintillators, CsF and BaF_2, were investigated. CsF has very low light output and is very hygroscopic and, consequently, has seen relative little use despite its short decay constant of 4 ns. BaF_2 has an even faster decay of less than 1 ns and a similar light output, but is nonhygroscopic. Therefore, in the early 1980s it was used in several PET scanners [12] for TOF PET. However, because of its relatively low density and atomic number, it eventually gave way to BGO.

One way to increase the spatial resolution of a tomograph is to couple multiple scintillator crystals with different decay constants to a single photodetector. Pulse shape discrimination is used to identify the crystal element of interaction. GSO has been used in conjunction with BGO and LSO in this way for a high-resolution tomograph [13,14]. A tomographic design using GSO exclusively has also been reported [15]. Fabrication of GSO detectors requires great care, because the crystals cleave easily. Thus, special techniques are needed to avoid cracking the crystal elements during cutting.

LSO:Ce offers one of the best combinations of properties for PET of the scintillators available today [16,17]. It has high density and a high atomic number for good gamma ray detection efficiency, a short decay constant for good coincidence timing, and high light output that allows for the use of many small elements per PMT. In addition, it is mechanically rugged and nonhygroscopic, thus allowing relatively simple fabrication of detectors. LSO:Ce has a low level of natural radioactivity as a result of the presence of ^{176}Lu, but the counting rate from this isotope is a small fraction of the typical counting rates from the injected tracers; thus, it is not a significant problem for PET. LSO:Ce has been used in a high-resolution brain tomograph [18], high-resolution animal tomographs [19], combined PET/MRI detectors [20], and combined PET/SPECT cameras [21,22]. Large-scale commercial production of LSO:Ce was realized around 2000 [23].

2.5 PROPERTIES OF SCINTILLATORS FOR PET

Despite the investigation of virtually every known scintillator for possible use in PET, only three have seen widespread use so far, NaI:Tl, BGO, and LSO:Ce. An experimental TOF PET system exists, based on $LaBr_3$, and a few commercial systems based on GSO:Ce have been offered. In this section, the properties of the first three important scintillators are compared in more detail.

One of the most important properties of a scintillator for PET is gamma ray detection efficiency. Because of the desire to shorten scan times and maintain low tracer activity, the crystals must detect as many of the gamma rays emitted as possible. This is the primary reason for the popularity of BGO. Gamma rays with an energy of 511 keV interact with solid matter primarily through two phenomena, the photoelectric effect and the Compton effect. In the photoelectric effect, the gamma ray is absorbed by an atom that ejects an electron (photoelectron) and also produces either characteristic x-rays or Auger electrons. The end result is that the full energy of the gamma ray is absorbed. In Compton scattering, the gamma ray loses a fraction of its energy to an electron through scattering. The energy of the electron is likely to be absorbed in the crystal, whereas the scattered gamma ray may or may not be absorbed. The distribution of energy between the electron and the gamma ray is determined by the scattering angle.

The detection efficiency of a detector may be characterized by the fraction of incident gamma rays that are partially or fully absorbed by it. For a detector of thickness x, exposed to a monoenergetic beam of gamma rays, the initial gamma ray intensity, I_o, is attenuated according to

$$I(E) = I_o(E)e^{-\mu x}$$

where:

 I is the intensity of gamma rays passing through the detector without interacting at all
 μ is the linear attenuation coefficient

The gamma rays that do interact in the detector by depositing either their full or partial energy are given by

$$A = 1 - e^{-\mu x}$$

Thus, it is clear that the fraction of incident gamma rays that are partially or fully absorbed is determined by the linear attenuation coefficient (for an idealized geometry). Figure 2.1 compares the linear attenuation coefficients for NaI:Tl, BGO, and LSO:Ce. From these data, the advantages of BGO and LSO:Ce over NaI:Tl are clear. At 511 keV, $\mu = 0.96$ cm^{-1} for BGO and $\mu = 0.87$ for LSO:Ce, whereas for NaI:Tl, μ is only 0.35 cm^{-1}. Consequently, to achieve similar efficiency, NaI:Tl detectors must be more than twice as thick compared with BGO and LSO:Ce detectors.

In most PET scanners, the emission of the scintillation crystals is converted to electrical signals by PMTs. To produce the largest signal, the scintillation emission should be as intense as possible, and the wavelength of the emission should match the wavelength of maximum photomultiplier sensitivity. Because bialkali photomultipliers with glass entrance windows, the most commonly used type, have a maximum sensitivity near

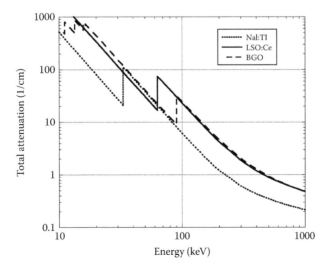

Figure 2.1 Total attenuation for energetic photons.

400 nm, it is advantageous for the scintillator to have its emission maximum near this wavelength. Both NaI:Tl and LSO:Ce have intense emissions that peak near that wavelength, whereas BGO has a much weaker and longer wavelength emission (480 nm) (Figure 2.2). The intensity of the scintillation emission strongly affects the number of crystal elements that can be coupled to a single PMT or, stated another way, strongly affects the ratio of scintillation elements to electronic channels. With BGO, block detectors today use up to 16 crystal elements per PMT, whereas LSO:Ce detectors use up to 42 crystal elements per PMT (the Siemens mCT block has 169 LSO pixels viewed by four PMTs). Thus, LSO:Ce makes possible significant cost savings as a result of the reduced number of photomultipliers and associated electronics per detector element.

In PET, the decay constant of the scintillation emission is very important, because singles count rates are typically very high, and coincidence resolving time (CRT) should be as small as possible to reject unwanted random events. A short scintillation decay constant is a benefit in both instances. Figure 2.3 compares the scintillation decay of NaI:Tl, BGO, and LSO:Ce. BGO has the longest decay, 300 ns. The primary decay

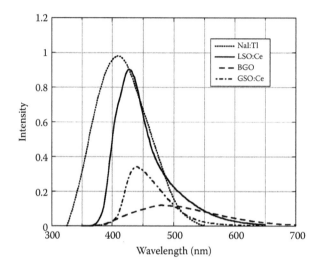

Figure 2.2 Comparison of emission spectra.

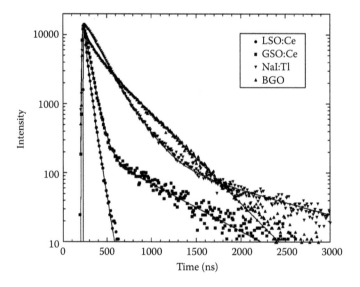

Figure 2.3 Comparison of scintillation time profiles.

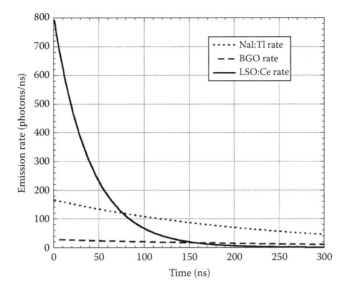

Figure 2.4 Comparison of photoemission rates.

constant of NaI:Tl is somewhat shorter, 230 ns, but an additional secondary decay of several microseconds is also present. The decay constant of LSO:Ce is several times shorter, 40 ns, and no secondary component is present.

Because the quality of a PET image is strongly dependent on the CRT of the detectors, a figure of merit that has been used for PET scintillators is the number of photons emitted per nanosecond. In this way, both the overall intensity of the emission and the duration of the pulse are accounted for in one parameter. Figure 2.4 compares the photons emitted per nanosecond for NaI:Tl, BGO, and LSO:Ce. LSO:Ce has a large advantage over BGO in this respect, because LSO:Ce's emission is both intense and fast, whereas BGO's emission is much weaker and slower. LSO:Ce is also better than NaI:Tl in this respect, because although NaI:Tl's emission is stronger than LSO:Ce, the decay constant is more than five times longer.

In view of the increasing interest in TOF PET, a more detailed description of timing with scintillators is given below.

2.6 TIMING WITH SCINTILLATION DETECTORS AND TOF PET POSSIBILITIES

2.6.1 PHOTOMULTIPLIER TUBE–BASED DETECTORS

In a scintillator, the detection process starts when the initial gamma radiation is absorbed and converted into thermalized electrons and holes. The next step is the migration of some fraction of the e–h pairs to luminescence centers, followed by the emission of photons. The rise time (τ_R) of the scintillation pulse is primarily determined by the migration process, while the decay time (τ_D) and the emission wavelength are characteristics of the luminescent ions. The light output (N_{ph}) is determined by the number of e–h pairs created, the efficiency of e–h migration, and the radiative efficiency of the luminescence centers. The photosensor converts N_{ph} to N_{phe} (number of photoelectrons) with a quantum efficiency that is characteristic of the sensor. In this section, the photosensor is assumed to be a PMT. The signal produced by the scintillator–PMT combination can then be characterized by

$$I = \text{const} \times \left[e^{-t/\tau_D} - e^{-t/\tau_R} \right]$$

The Hyman theory of time resolution of scintillation detectors was originally developed for plastic scintillators [24] and subsequently used by Moszyński and colleagues [25,26] to predict time resolution of plastic scintillators coupled to PMTs. More recently, Moszyński and colleagues have successfully used the theory to predict time resolution of inorganic scintillation detectors such as LSO:Ce [27,28]. Using the Hyman theory, the standard deviation of the time resolution of the scintillation detector (δ_τ) is given by

$$\delta_\tau = H(\tau_R, \tau_D, h, \mathrm{PMT}(\sigma)) \times r \times \tau_D / \sqrt{N_{phe}}$$

where the Hyman function H depends on the rise time, the decay time, the triggering fraction h of the anode pulse, the PMT gain and timing characteristics (time jitter of PMT defined by its standard deviation σ and the single-photon electron response with a standard deviation σ), and the gain dispersion of the PMT electron multiplier, defined by r. N_{phe} represents the number of photoelectrons produced in the PMT.

For a given σ/τ_D ratio, the Hyman function can be reduced to a simple function of h, and therefore the Hyman function can be represented by a family of functions $H(h)$, each of them identified by the ratio σ/τ_D. Each curve has a minimum reached for the optimal setting of the discriminator threshold h, thus giving the best time resolution.

As an example, we can apply the Hyman theory to an LSO:Ce scintillator, evaluated by Conti et al. [29]. In this case, a 5 mm LSO:Ce cube codoped with 0.1% Ca has a 37 ns decay time and photoelectron number of $N_{phe} = 4020$. Using the Hyman graphs shown in Figure 8 in [27], a simple interpolation between the minima for the $\sigma/\tau_D = 1/24$ curve and the $\sigma/\tau_D = 1/48$ curve shows the minimum of the Hyman function for a 37 ns decay time to be $H \approx 0.12$. The dispersion constant of $r = 1.03$ is taken from [27]. The standard deviation, δ_τ, for the time resolution is given by

$$\delta_\tau = 0.12 \times 1.03 \times 37,000 / \sqrt{4,020}$$

This implies that the best time resolution (full width at half maximum [FWHM]) of the LSO:Ce detector cube with XP2020Q PMT is expected to be

$$\Delta T = 2.35 \times 72 = 170 \ \mathrm{ps}$$

The actual timing resolution measured by Conti et al. [29] for this configuration was 165 ps, in good agreement with the Hyman theory prediction. It is notable that LSO:Ce has a fast rise time, so the time resolution is predominantly controlled by the decay time and the number of photoelectrons created. In fact, if the Hyman function can be expressed as a family of curves identified by σ/τ_D, experimental studies have shown that $H(\tau_D)$ is a weak function of $1/\tau_D$, of the type $H = \mathrm{const} \times \tau_D^{-\alpha}$ with $\alpha \approx 0.5$. Szczesniak et al. [28] observed that by plotting $\Delta T \times \sqrt{N_{phe}}$ as a function of $\sqrt{\tau_D}$ for a series of different scintillators, all measured on a XP20D0 PMT, a linear relationship was found between $H(\tau_D)$ and $\sqrt{\tau_D}$. This implies that the time resolution for a scintillation detector is proportional to the square root of the decay time over the number of photoelectrons or

$$\Delta T \propto = \sqrt{\tau_D / N_{phe}}$$

This expression has been shown to be an accurate prediction for scintillators with a negligible rise time by Glodo et al. [30] for LaBr$_3$ with increased Ce doping. The time resolution prediction in the above equation was used by Conti et al. [29] to classify different scintillators into a TOF figure of merit. For the chosen pixel dimension (2 cm thickness), the LSO:Ce scintillator was the best choice. However, if the LaBr$_3$ thickness is extended to 3 cm, this scintillator may have a figure of merit close to LSO:Ce.

2.6.2 SILICON PHOTOMULTIPLIER–BASED DETECTORS

In recent years, a new photosensor concept, the silicon photomultiplier (SiPM), has been developed. This is a photodetector consisting of an array of avalanche photodiode (APD) microcells working in Geiger mode. SiPMs are insensitive to magnetic fields and have a high gain and a fast response time. Some of the advantages can be summarized as follows:

- Excellent single photoelectron response
- Compactness
- Insensitivity to magnetic fields
- Low operation voltage (~100 V) and high gain (10^5–10^6)
- No damage when exposed to light under bias

There are, however, some limitations that have to be considered.

- A high dark count rate
- A high sensitivity to temperature variations
- Signal response is not linear in light exposure
- Cross talk between the cells may complicate the interpretation of the response
- After-pulses are generated

In a SiPM, the hundreds or thousands of Geiger-mode APDs are connected and operated in parallel, thus constituting an efficient proportional light sensor. The microcells are all identical, with dimensions generally from 25 to 100 μm, and each cell operates as an independent photon counter in Geiger mode when the bias voltage is higher than the breakdown voltage. A photon that interacts with one of the cells creates free carriers that give rise to a Geiger-type discharge. Since every cell is connected to the bias voltage via individual resistors, this discharge is quenched when the voltage of the cell drops below the breakdown voltage. After a short recovery time, the cell is once again ready to detect the next photon. The signal from a cell always has the same shape and amplitude, and so the cell can be seen as a binary device. The nonlinearity of the SiPM signal is related to the limited number of microcells compared with the number of scintillation photons, but it may also be related to a mismatch between the SiPM dead time and the scintillator decay time.

An important question is how well we understand the relationship between the SiPM response and the light output from a scintillator, especially in view of the limitations listed above. There are a number of models that describe the operation of the SiPM via both analytical [31,32] and Monte Carlo simulation approaches [33,34]. Monte Carlo simulations can account for most SiPM phenomena and give a fairly accurate description of the SiPM response and its variance.

Since the discharge currents from the cells are added on a common load resistor, the output signal from a SiPM is the sum of the signals from all the cells firing at the same time, and the photon detection efficiency is defined as

$$PDE = QE \times f \times p_a$$

where:

QE is the quantum efficiency at the emission wavelength

f is a fill factor, the ratio of the area occupied by the cells to the total device area

p_a is the probability for a Geiger breakdown, a function of the bias voltage, and the breakdown voltage

For a Hamamatsu MPPC S-10362-33-050C device, the PDE is ~50%, which is significantly higher than the quantum efficiency of commonly used PMTs such as XP2020Q, which may be ~25%–30%.

2.6.3 COMPARISON OF TIME RESOLUTION DATA OBTAINED WITH PMTS AND SiPMS

Timing results for LSO:Ce scintillators coupled to PMTs and SiPMs are shown in Tables 2.5 and 2.6. Assuming that LSO:Ce has an intrinsic timing resolution, it seems that the SiPM results are possibly closer to this limiting value. Seifert et al. [32] reported a CRT of 138 ps obtained with two detector assemblies consisting of $3 \times 3 \times 5$ mm^3 LYSO:Ce crystals mounted on MPPC-S10362-33-050C SiPMs. This implies an unfolded (one-detector) LSO:Ce-SiPM detector resolution of less than 100 ps. The best unfolded PMT–LSO:Ce detector value is very close to Seifert et al.'s LSO:Ce data [32], around 100 ps for an H6610 PMT (Hamamatsu) coupled to a 6 mm LSO:Ce cube [35]. These results appear to be very close to the limiting intrinsic timing resolution for LSO:Ce, although even smaller crystal dimensions may be needed to avoid contributions from the length of the light paths. In Table 2.6, we have listed the results of Yeom et al. [36] using a $3 \times 3 \times 5$ mm^3 LSO:Ce crystal. They have, however, an additional measurement for a $2 \times 2 \times 3$ mm^3 crystal with a result of 125 ps.

Seifert et al. also measured a $3 \times 3 \times 5$ mm^3 LaBr$_3$ scintillator (5% Ce) using the same SiPM and obtained a CRT of 95 or 67 ps unfolded. LaBr$_3$ is a very interesting scintillator for TOF PET applications since it has a very short decay time [32] of ~15 ns. On the other hand, it is less dense than LSO:Ce. Since the TOF gain can be assumed to be proportional to 1/CRT [29], the TOF gain related to a PET system would be 10.5 for LaBr$_3$ and 7 for LSO. For crystals of the same dimensions ($4 \times 4 \times 20$ mm^3), the detection efficiency of LSO:Ce is four times higher than that for LaBr$_3$. Using longer crystals for LaBr$_3$ (30 mm) and shorter crystals for LSO:Ce (20 mm) in order to compensate for the density difference, the detection efficiency of LSO:Ce detectors would still be more than a factor of two higher than that of LaBr$_3$. By combining both stopping power and TOF gain, LSO:Ce still seems to be the best TOF PET scintillator [29] for architectures based on either PMTs or SiPMs.

Table 2.5 PMT-LSO:Ce timing

References	LSO:Ce dimensions (mm^3)	N$_{phe}$ for 511 keV	LSO:Ce decay time (ns)	PMT used	CRT (ps)	Unfolded time resolution (ps)
Szczesniak et al. [62]	10*10*5	3300	46.2	XP3060	283	200
Szczesniak et al. [62]	10*10*5	4100	46.2	XP20D0	235	166
Szczesniak et al. [62]	10*10*5	2800	46.2	R5320	245	173
Conti et al. [29]	5*5*5	4010	37	XP2020Q	233	165
Eriksson et al. [35]	6*6*6	4050	33	H6610	141	100

Table 2.6 SiPM LSO:Ce timing

References	LSO:Ce dimension (mm^3)	N$_{phe}$ for 511 keV	LSO:Ce decay time (ns)	SiPM used	CRT (ps)	Unfolded time resolution (ps)
Seifert et al. [32]	3*3*5	3,300	43.8	S10362-33-050C	138	98
Gundacker et al. [63]	2*2*5	16,000 (N$_{ph}$/MeV)	40	S10931-050P	142	100
Yeom et al. [36]	3*3*5	n/a	n/a	S10362-33-050C	147	104
Yeom et al. [36]	2*2*3	n/a	n/a	S10362-33-050C	125	88

n/a, not available.

2.7 SPECT

The origin of the SPECT technique can be traced back to the pioneering work of David Kuhl and Roy Edwards during the late 1950s to early 1960s. Both longitudinal and transaxial tomography were investigated, and they were the first investigators to describe a true transaxial approach for emission tomography [37,38]. They used NaI:Tl scintillation detectors, and the gamma rays emitted by the source distributions entered the detectors via collimated holes. The detectors were rotated and translated to collect the information necessary for a back-projection reconstruction. To speed up the process, two or more detectors could be used. The Mark III was brought into use in 1965 and was able to determine, for example, the cerebral blood volume by using red blood cells labeled with Tc^{99m}. Around 1976, the final version, Mark IV, consisted of 32 collimated detectors. For measuring the attenuation, they used a collimated radioactive source behind the body and a collimated detector in front of the body that were operated in a manner similar to that of x-ray computed tomography (CT).

A second starting point for single-photon imaging dates back to the work of Hal Anger and the invention of the Anger camera, or gamma camera [7]. With Anger cameras, the translation steps are no longer necessary; only the rotational part is. The Anger camera consists of a NaI:Tl plate with a thickness appropriate for detecting the single photon energy used, usually between 6 and 10 mm for the 140 keV gamma ray from Tc^{99m}. The scintillator response is read out by an array of PMTs. The light from each scintillation event spreads out and generates signals in several PMTs. The relative intensities of the PMTs are used to determine the location of the scintillation event on the scintillator plate. The direction of each gamma ray impinging on the scintillator plate is defined by the collimator, usually a parallel-hole array. The activity distribution is shown on a two-dimensional display. For whole-body SPECT situations, the basic Anger concept with a large scintillator area has prevailed, while for smaller gamma cameras, pixel-based approaches are preferred to give a more uniform response.

Paul Harper and colleagues at the University of Chicago were the first investigators to explore the use of an Anger camera for transaxial tomography [39]. In 1968, Gerd Muehllehner investigated a transaxial tomographic approach using a rotatable chair placed in front of a stationary camera [40]. The concept of a rotatable chair was used quite a few times, for example, in the 1970s by Thomas Budinger and Grant Gullberg [41] and by Stig Larsson [42]. Ron Jaszczak and colleagues worked on a dual Anger camera system, the Searle dual gamma camera whole-body SPECT system [43]. In Europe during the late 1970s, Stig Larsson at Karolinska University in Stockholm was evaluating a prototype rotating-camera SPECT system [42].

The objective of SPECT, like PET, is to determine the tissue activity distribution of the injected tracer. For this, we need a full set of projections, with sufficient angular sampling. If the projections are determined sequentially, we can assume that the activity distribution is fairly static during the data acquisition. If the different projections are taken with rotating detectors, we also need to accurately determine the center of rotation. Since the detectors are rotated, the response of the detectors must be insensitive to orientation and position. The PMTs are typically shielded with mu-metal, since the electron multiplication in the PMT may be affected by variations of the earth magnetic field as discussed by Stig Larsson [42]. The final steps are the corrections of tissue attenuation and the image reconstruction itself. Early on, filtered backprojection approaches were used, but nowadays iterative reconstructions are routinely employed.

2.8 SCINTILLATOR CHOICES

Instrumentation for SPECT imaging mostly uses gamma cameras based on NaI:Tl scintillators. The ROST method [44], for example, can be used to grow extremely large single crystals, up to 500 kg, and the Bridgman growth is also used to produce large single crystals from which scintillator plates are cut. The typical detector geometry is a parallel-hole lead or tungsten collimator located on the patient side of the scintillator plate with an array of PMTs optically coupled to the opposite side of the plate. The scintillator plate is approximately 40 × 50 cm in area and 6–10 mm thick, although plates up to 25 mm with a grooved surface have been used. The collimator is used to define the direction of gamma rays incident on the plate, and Anger logic is used to determine the interaction points of gamma rays with the scintillator plate. The use of Anger logic results in dead space near edges. Pixilation of the scintillator and one-to-one coupling of pixels to photosensors can be used to avoid this problem and is important in small-field-of-view (organ-specific) cameras and some small-animal SPECT systems. Pixilation can also provide better spatial resolution, but comes with added cost and complexity.

CsI:Tl has detection efficiency similar to that of NaI:Tl, but the emission wavelength is significantly longer, 540 nm versus 420 nm, and therefore better suited to photodiode light detection. It also has a longer decay time of approximately 1 μs, although this is usually not an issue due to the low count rate typical in SPECT. Its lower hygroscopicity relaxes packaging requirements. It is used by Digirad in the Cardius camera. CsI:Na is similar but with a shorter wavelength more suitable for PMTs; it is used in the LinoView small-animal SPECT camera. Scintillator choices for SPECT are summarized in Table 2.7.

New scintillators with more light and faster time response have been considered for SPECT, such as $LaBr_3$ and $LaCl_3$. The intrinsic spatial resolution for a given scintillator is governed by its light output and the light readout technique. The use of Anger logic with NaI:Tl scintillators results in ~4 mm resolution, whereas ~2.5 mm resolution can be achieved with $LaBr_3$:Ce. The energy resolution establishes part of the scatter discrimination. For NaI:Tl, the Tc^{99m} 140 keV energy resolution is around 9%, and for $LaBr_3$:Ce, it is around 6%. The improved energy resolution from 9% to 6% would allow the Compton scatter background to be reduced from 35% to as low as 25% [45]. However, implementation of $LaBr_3$:Ce has been hindered by high cost and more demanding packaging due to higher hygroscopicity. Also, the current state of the art of $LaBr_3$:Ce crystal growth is not sufficient to produce single-crystal plates of the size used for SPECT. Therefore, pixelated $LaBr_3$:Ce is the only choice.

Microcolumnar crystal arrays of CsI:Tl have been developed for x-ray detection. In this case, the detector layers are needle like crystals that are grown together. Since the needles have small sizes and individually can channel light, the intrinsic spatial resolution is improved. The thickness, however, is limited, which practically means they are only used in low-energy gamma ray imaging and in x-ray applications [46,47].

Room temperature semiconductors have attractive possibilities for SPECT. The leading candidate is $Cd_{(1-x)}Zn_xTe$, or CZT, which has a detection efficiency similar to that of NaI(Tl) at 140 keV for the same-thickness material. The advantage of semiconductors is the fact that electrons and holes created by the ionization from gamma rays are collected directly at electrical contacts rather than requiring the conversion of scintillation light by a photosensor. In this way, energy resolution of ~4% can be achieved at 140 keV, which is better than any available scintillator. The improved energy resolution and the resulting ability to distinguish various radioisotopes from each other may offer the potential for new multi-isotope applications. In addition, CZT can be segmented into small pixels to provide excellent spatial resolution, although the count rate is limited by slow charge transport compared with the much faster photon transport in scintillators. At this point, the high cost, especially for thick crystals, limits the use of CZT to small-animal and organ-specific systems.

Table 2.7 Scintillator candidates for SPECT

Scintillator	Density (g/cm³)	Effective Z	Decay time (ns)	Emission wavelength (nm)	Light yield (% of NaI)	Energy resolution at 140 keV (%)
NaI:Tl	3.67	50	230	420	100	9
CsI:Tl[a]	4.5	54	800 (60%) 3400 (40%)	550	~150	11
CsI:Na	4.5	54	630	420	85	11
$LaBr_3$:Ce[a]	5.29	46.9	17 (100%) (5% Ce)	360	~150	6
$LaCl_3$:Ce	3.9	47.3	20	350	~125	6
$Cd_{(1-x)}Zn_xTe$	5.78	49.1	n/a	n/a	n/a	4

[a] Scintillation Materials Research Center data.
n/a, not available.

2.9 CURRENT SPECT SYSTEMS

The typical performance of a conventional SPECT system based on two rotating NaI:Tl detector heads is as follows. Each detector head has a field of view of 40×55 cm. The intrinsic spatial resolution is 4 mm FWHM, and the SPECT reconstructed resolution is around 1 cm. The energy resolution for 140 keV photons is ~9.5%. The planar count rate sensitivity per detector head, using the low-energy high-resolution collimator, is around 100 cps/MBq [48], or 0.01% [49].

SPECT imaging and the use of single-photon radionuclides have advantages not available with positron emitters. Compared with PET, SPECT imaging may provide a much longer timescale as a wide range of isotopes exist, with different half-lives to better adapt to tracer kinetic requirements. These include Tc^{99m}, I^{123}, and In^{111}. Since the SPECT tracers have different single photon energies, multiple tracers can be used simultaneously. The Tc^{99m} isotope has a half-life of 6 h, and In^{111} a half-life of 2.8 day. This implies that SPECT provides information for up to a week, instead of the few hours provided by F^{18} (110 min half-life), for molecular pathways with long turnover rates. The fact that more than one SPECT tracer can be used simultaneously in a study implies, in addition, that more than one molecular pathway may be monitored in one study, although this places additional demands on detector performance. For example, both blood flow and receptor kinetics can be measured in one study, as discussed by Meikle et al. [48].

SPECT/CT was first suggested by Hasegawa et al. [50], but the current implementation has mostly gained popularity from the existing PET/CT systems [51]. In the same way as for PET/CT, attenuation correction based on the CT attenuation maps is a significant improvement over the prior methods. As in PET/CT, the coregistration of the SPECT images with the CT provides anatomical landmarks. The CT information also provides highly accurate control of patient orientation. SPECT/CT of course has the same limitations as PET/CT, such as patient motion.

2.10 SMALL-ANIMAL SPECT

Preclinical imaging with SPECT has become a major research area over the last 10–15 years. The demand for *in vivo* imaging in the preclinical arena has grown rapidly with the development of animal models of human diseases, including transgenic mice [48,52]. Investigation of rodents and other small animals makes high resolution necessary, perhaps one order of magnitude higher than for clinical human studies. This requirement necessitates, in addition, high sensitivity to obtain images with sufficient statistics without long acquisition times and without delivering doses higher than required by the tracer principles.

To achieve high resolution in clinical SPECT systems, usually an assembly of high-resolution pinhole collimation detectors is used [53]. A major challenge for small-animal SPECT is still the detection efficiency, often ~ 0.1%.

2.11 NEW TRENDS IN SPECT IMAGING

SPECT and SPECT/CT have often been used for therapy and therapy planning. Perhaps radioiodine therapy is the best-known and performed procedure. But there are other well-established therapies, for example, inflammable joint disease and metastasized tumors. Liver tumors not possible to surgically cure can be efficiently treated with nuclear medicine techniques monitored by SPECT and SPECT/CT imaging. Recently, these techniques have been extended to include prostate cancer (PCa). New imaging agents like ^{99m}Tc-MIP-1404 bind to prostate-specific membrane antigen (PSMA), a protein found in PCa cells, and with SPECT imaging, the tumor sites may thus be visualized. PSMA is expressed in normal human prostate epithelium but is upregulated in PCa, including metastatic disease, thus being an attractive molecular target for the detection of primary and metastatic PCa.

The ^{99m}Tc-MIP-1404 ligand is a small molecule with a reasonably fast uptake in PSMA. If the uptake is high, this may indicate a fast-developing disease, thus giving an opportunity to differentiate aggressive from nonaggressive PCas. If a therapeutic tracer such as ^{177}Lu is bound to a PSMA-seeking ligand, a therapeutic tool may be created. Such a tool may find and potentially disable the cancer cells. ^{177}Lu bound to J591 has been tested in phase I and phase II trials and has been found to reduce PSA levels, thus indicating a therapeutic effect. Alternatively, ^{177}Lu can first be used as a PSMA identifier and then be used for therapy with much higher doses.

^{99m}Tc-MIP-1404 is rapidly cleared from the circulation with minimal urinary activity, but moderate (15%–20%) liver and kidney uptake. In men with metastatic PCa, ^{99m}Tc-MIP-1404 is rapidly localized to lesions in lymph nodes and bone on a 1 h timescale. SPECT/CT images demonstrated excellent lesion contrast. In most patients, more lesions were demonstrated with ^{99m}Tc-MIP-1404 than bone scan. In all subjects with a Gleason score over 7, ^{99m}Tc-MIP-1404 SPECT clearly identified the PCa sites confirmed by histopathology and PSMA staining.

^{177}Lu-J591 imaging was able to identify all known sites of disease in all treated subjects [54]. A subsequent phase II study demonstrated 94% tumor targeting [55]. ^{111}In-J591 imaging before ^{90}Y-J591 treatment revealed 89% of known bony lesions and the majority (69%) of soft tissue lesions [56]. In a few selected cases, J591 demonstrated lesions that were not apparent on the bone scan but were identified on MR or conventional imaging as the lesion progressed [57]. SPECT images have confirmed both osseous and soft tissue uptake. Currently, one of these compounds, ^{99m}Tc-MIP-1404, is under evaluation in an international phase II study of patients scheduled for radical prostatectomy with a high risk of lymph node involvement.

2.12 FUTURE RESEARCH DIRECTIONS

Researchers continue to actively investigate potential new scintillator materials, because a tomograph's performance depends so strongly on the characteristics of the detectors. Most of the effort has focused on high-density and high-atomic-number materials, as well as materials with potentially very short decay constants. Surveys of large numbers of candidates [58] have failed to identify any practical scintillators for PET. Recent research has therefore shifted toward computational efforts to model potential materials [59,60]. Hopefully, an improved understanding of the underlying physics of scintillation processes will lead to the ability to predict the characteristics of new scintillator materials without actually synthesizing them.

In addition to searching for new scintillator materials, investigators have combined known scintillators in novel ways, such as phoswich detectors, which combine two dissimilar scintillators in the same detector. For instance, layers of LSO:Ce and NaI:Tl have been combined to make a camera that provides both PET and SPECT capability [21]. The LSO:Ce layer is used for PET imaging, and the NaI:Tl layer is used for SPECT imaging. Similarly, researchers have constructed prototype detectors of LSO:Ce and YSO:Ce for the same purpose [61].

REFERENCES

1. P. A. Rodnyi, *Physical Processes in Inorganic Scintillators*, vol. 14, Boca Raton, FL: CRC Press, 1997.
2. M. Casey and R. Nutt, A multicrystal two dimensional BGO detector system for positron emission tomography, *IEEE Transactions on Nuclear Science*, vol. 33, pp. 460–463, 1986.
3. M. E. Casey, R. Nutt, and T. D. Douglas, Two dimensional photon counting position encoder system and process, U.S. Patent 4749863, 1988.
4. G. F. Knoll, *Radiation Detection and Measurement*, New York: Wiley, 2010.
5. C. L. Melcher, Scintillation crystals for PET, *Journal of Nuclear Medicine*, vol. 41, pp. 1051–1055, 2000.
6. R. Hofstadter, Alkali halide scintillation counters, *Physical Review*, vol. 74, p. 100, 1948.
7. H. O. Anger, Scintillation camera with multichannel collimators, *Journal of Nuclear Medicine*, vol. 5, pp. 515–531, 1964.
8. T. E. Peterson and L. R. Furenlid, SPECT detectors: The Anger camera and beyond, *Physics in Medicine and Biology*, vol. 56, p. R145, 2011.

9. D. Robbins, On predicting the maximum efficiency of phosphor systems excited by ionizing radiation, *Journal of the Electrochemical Society*, vol. 127, pp. 2694–2702, 1980.

10. A. Lempicki, A. Wojtowicz, and E. Berman, Fundamental limits of scintillator performance, *Nuclear Instruments and Methods in Physics Research Section A: Accelerators, Spectrometers, Detectors and Associated Equipment*, vol. 333, pp. 304–311, 1993.

11. M. J. Weber and R. R. Monchamp, Luminescence of Bi4Ge3O12: Spectral and decay properties, *Journal of Applied Physics*, vol. 44, pp. 5495–5499, 1973.

12. M. Yamamoto, D. C. Ficke, and M. M. Ter-Pogossian, Experimental assessment of the gain achieved by the utilization of time-of-flight information in a positron emission tomograph (Super PETT I), *IEEE Transactions on Medical Imaging*, vol. 1, pp. 187–192, 1982.

13. L. Eriksson, C. Bohm, M. Kesselberg, J. Litton, M. Bergstrom, and G. Blomquist, A high resolution positron camera, in *The Metabolism of the Human Brain Studied with Positron Emission Tomography*, ed. T. Greitz, D. H. Ingvar, and L. Widen, New York: Raven Press, 1985, pp. 33–46.

14. S. Holte, H. Ostertag, and M. Kesselberg, A preliminary evaluation of a dual crystal positron camera, *Journal of Computer Assisted Tomography*, vol. 11, pp. 691–697, 1987.

15. J. S. Karp, S. Surti, M. E. Daube-Witherspoon, R. Freifelder, C. A. Cardi, L.-E. Adam, et al., Performance of a brain PET camera based on anger-logic gadolinium oxyorthosilicate detectors, *Journal of Nuclear Medicine*, vol. 44, pp. 1340–1349, 2003.

16. C. L. Melcher and J. S. Schweitzer, Cerium-doped lutetium oxyorthosilicate: A fast, efficient new scintillator, *IEEE Transactions on Nuclear Science*, vol. 39, pp. 502–505, 1992.

17. C. L. Melcher and J. S. Schweitzer, A promising new scintillator: Cerium-doped lutetium oxyorthosilicate, *Nuclear Instruments and Methods in Physics Research Section A: Accelerators, Spectrometers, Detectors and Associated Equipment*, vol. 314, pp. 212–214, 1992.

18. M. Schmand, L. Eriksson, M. Casey, M. Andreaco, C. Melcher, K. Wienhard, et al., Performance results of a new DOI detector block for a high resolution PET-LSO research tomograph HRRT, *IEEE Transactions on Nuclear Science*, vol. 45, pp. 3000–3006, 1998.

19. A. F. Chatziioannou, S. R. Cherry, Y. Shao, R. W. Silverman, K. Meadors, T. H. Farquhar, et al., Performance evaluation of microPET: A high-resolution lutetium oxyorthosilicate PET scanner for animal imaging, *Journal of Nuclear Medicine*, vol. 40, p. 1164, 1999.

20. Y. Shao, S. Cherry, K. Farahani, R. Slates, R. Silverman, K. Meadors, et al., Development of a PET detector system compatible with MRI/NMR systems, *IEEE Transactions on Nuclear Science*, vol. 44, pp. 1167–1171, 1997.

21. M. Schmand, M. Dahlbom, L. Eriksson, M. Andreaco, M. Casey, K. Vagneur, et al., Performance of a LSO/NaI (Tl) phoswich detector for a combined PET/SPECT imaging system, *Journal of Nuclear Medicine*, vol. 29, p. 9P, 1998.

22. B. J. Pichler, T. Gremillion, V. Ermer, M. Schmand, B. Bendriem, M. Schwaiger, et al., Detector characterization and detector setup of a NaI-LSO PET/SPECT camera, *IEEE Transactions on Nuclear Science*, vol. 50, pp. 1420–1427, 2003.

23. C. L. Melcher, M. A. Spurrier, L. Eriksson, M. Eriksson, M. Schmand, G. Givens, et al., Advances in the scintillation performance of LSO: Ce single crystals, *IEEE Transactions on Nuclear Science*, vol. 50, pp. 762–766, 2003.

24. L. Hyman, Time resolution of photomultiplier systems, *Review of Scientific Instruments*, vol. 36, pp. 193–196, 1965.

25. B. Bengtson and M. Moszyński, Timing properties of scintillation counters, *Nuclear Instruments and Methods*, vol. 81, pp. 109–120, 1970.

26. J. Bialkowski, Z. Moroz, and M. Moszyński, Further study of timing properties of scintillation counters, *Nuclear Instruments and Methods*, vol. 117, pp. 221–226, 1974.

27. M. Moszyński, T. Ludziejewski, D. Wolski, W. Klamra, and V. Avdejchikov, Timing properties of GSO, LSO and other Ce doped scintillators, *Nuclear Instruments and Methods in Physics Research Section A: Accelerators, Spectrometers, Detectors and Associated Equipment*, vol. 372, pp. 51–58, 1996.

28. T. Szczesniak, M. Moszynski, A. Syntfeld-Kazuch, L. Swiderski, M. A. S. Koschan, and C. L. Melcher, Timing resolution and decay time of LSO crystals co-doped with calcium, *IEEE Transactions on Nuclear Science*, vol. 57, pp. 1329–1334, 2010.

29. M. Conti, L. Eriksson, H. Rothfuss, and C. L. Melcher, Comparison of fast scintillators with TOF PET potential, *IEEE Transactions on Nuclear Science*, vol. 56, pp. 926–933, 2009.

30. J. Glodo, W. Moses, W. Higgins, E. Van Loef, P. Wong, S. Derenzo, et al., Effects of Ce concentration on scintillation properties of LaBr$_3$: Ce, *IEEE Transactions on Nuclear Science*, vol. 52, pp. 1805–1808, 2005.

31. H. T. van Dam, S. Seifert, R. Vinke, D. Dendooven, H. Lohner, F. J. Beekman, et al., A comprehensive model of the response of silicon photomultipliers, *IEEE Transactions on Nuclear Science*, vol. 57, pp. 2254–2266, 2010.

32. S. Seifert, H. T. van Dam, R. Vinke, P. Dendooven, H. Lohner, F. J. Beekman, et al., A comprehensive model to predict the timing resolution of SiPM-based scintillation detectors: Theory and experimental validation, *IEEE Transactions on Nuclear Science*, vol. 59, pp. 190–204, 2012.

33. J. Pulko, F. Schneider, A. Velroyen, D. Renker, and S. Ziegler, A Monte-Carlo model of a SiPM coupled to a scintillating crystal, *Journal of Instrumentation*, vol. 7, p. P02009, 2012.

34. A. K. Jha, H. T. van Dam, M. A. Kupinski, and E. Clarkson, Simulating silicon photomultiplier response to scintillation light, *IEEE Transactions on Nuclear Science*, vol. 60, pp. 336–351, 2013.

35. L. Eriksson, S. Cho, M. Aykac, C. L. Melcher, M. Conti, M. Eriksson, and C. Michel, Comparison of count rate sensitivity performance for a LSO-TOF system with a Cherenkov radiation based PbF2-TOF system, in *IEEE Nuclear Science Symposium and Medical Imaging Conference*, Anaheim, CA, 2012, pp. 3108–3111.

36. J. Y. Yeom, R. Vinke, and C. S. Levin, Optimizing timing performance of silicon photomultiplier-based scintillation detectors, *Physics in Medicine and Biology*, vol. 58, p. 1207, 2013.

37. D. E. Kuhl and R. Q. Edwards, Image separation radioisotope scanning, *Radiology*, vol. 80, pp. 653–662, 1963.

38. D. E. Kuhl and R. Q. Edwards, Cylindrical and section radioisotope scanning of the liver and brain, *Radiology*, vol. 83, pp. 926–936, 1964.

39. P. V. Harper, R. M. Beck, D. E. Charleston, B. Brunsten, and K. A. Lathrop, Three dimensional mapping and display of radioisotope distributions, *Journal of Nuclear Medicine*, vol. 6, p. 332, 1965.

40. G. Muehllehner, Radioisotope imaging in three dimensions, *Journal of Nuclear Medicine*, vol. 9, p. 337, 1968.

41. T. F. Budinger and G. T. Gullberg, Three-dimensional reconstruction in nuclear medicine emission imaging, *IEEE Transactions on Nuclear Science*, vol. 21, pp. 2–19, 1974.

42. S. A. Larsson, Gamma camera emission tomography: Development and properties of a multi-sectional emission computed tomography system, *Acta Radiologica Supplementum*, vol. 363, p. 1, 1980.

43. R. J. Jaszczak, The early years of single photon emission computed tomography (SPECT): An anthology of selected reminiscences, *Physics in Medicine and Biology*, vol. 51, p. R99, 2006.

44. V. I. Goriletsky and S. K. Bondarenko, Production of preset quality large NaI(Tl) single crystals for detectors used in medical instrument building, *Materials Science and Engineering: A*, vol. A288, pp. 196–199, 2000.

45. W. W. Moses and K. S. Shah, Potential for RbGd 2 Br 7:Ce, LaBr 3:Ce, LaBr 3:Ce, and LuI 3:Ce in nuclear medical imaging, *Nuclear Instruments and Methods in Physics Research Section A: Accelerators, Spectrometers, Detectors and Associated Equipment*, vol. 537, pp. 317–320, 2005.

46. V. Nagarkar, T. Gupta, S. Miller, Y. Klugerman, M. Squillante, and G. Entine, Structured CsI (Tl) scintillators for x-ray imaging applications, *IEEE Transactions on Nuclear Science*, vol. 45, pp. 492–496, 1998.

47. M. P. Tornai, C. N. Archer, A. G. Weisenberger, R. Wojcik, V. Popov, S. Majewski, et al., Investigation of microcolumnar scintillators on an optical fiber coupled compact imaging system, *IEEE Transactions on Nuclear Science*, vol. 48, pp. 637–644, 2001.

48. S. R. Meikle, P. Kench, M. Kassiou, and R. B. Banati, Small animal SPECT and its place in the matrix of molecular imaging technologies, *Physics in Medicine and Biology*, vol. 50, p. R45, 2005.

49. A. Rahmim and H. Zaidi, PET versus SPECT: Strengths, limitations and challenges, *Nuclear Medicine Communications*, vol. 29, pp. 193–207, 2008.

50. B. H. Hasegawa, K. Iwata, K. H. Wong, M. C. Wu, A. J. Da Silva, H. R. Tang, et al., Dual-modality imaging of function and physiology, *Academic Radiology*, vol. 9, pp. 1305–1321, 2002.

51. T. Beyer, D. W. Townsend, T. Brun, P. E. Kinahan, M. Charron, R. Roddy, et al., A combined PET/CT scanner for clinical oncology, *Journal of Nuclear Medicine*, vol. 41, pp. 1369–1379, 2000.

52. B. L. Franc, P. D. Acton, C. Mari, and B. H. Hasegawa, Small-animal SPECT and SPECT/CT: Important tools for preclinical investigation, *Journal of Nuclear Medicine*, vol. 49, pp. 1651–1663, 2008.

53. F. J. Beekman, F. van der Have, B. Vastenhouw, A. J. van der Linden, P. P. van Rijk, J. P. H. Burbach, et ßal., U-SPECT-I: A novel system for submillimeter-resolution tomography with radiolabeled molecules in mice, *Journal of Nuclear Medicine*, vol. 46, pp. 1194–1200, 2005.

54. N. H. Bander, M. I. Milowsky, D. M. Nanus, L. Kostakoglu, S. Vallabhajosula, and S. J. Goldsmith, Phase I trial of 177 lutetium-labeled J591, a monoclonal antibody to prostate-specific membrane antigen, in patients with androgen-independent prostate cancer, *Journal of Clinical Oncology*, vol. 23, pp. 4591–4601, 2005.

55. S. T. Tagawa, H. Beltran, S. Vallabhajosula, S. J. Goldsmith, J. Osborne, D. Matulich, et al., Anti-prostate-specific membrane antigen-based radioimmunotherapy for prostate cancer, *Cancer*, vol. 116, pp. 1075–1083, 2010.

56. M. I. Milowsky, D. M. Nanus, L. Kostakoglu, S. Vallabhajosula, S. J. Goldsmith, and N. H. Bander, Phase I trial of yttrium-90-labeled anti-prostate-specific membrane antigen monoclonal antibody J591 for androgen-independent prostate cancer, *Journal of Clinical Oncology*, vol. 22, pp. 2522–2531, 2004.

57. N. H. Bander, Technology insight: Monoclonal antibody imaging of prostate cancer, *Nature Clinical Practice Urology*, vol. 3, pp. 216–225, 2006.

58. S. E. Derenzo, W. Moses, J. Cahoon, R. Perera, and J. Litton, Prospects for new inorganic scintillators, *IEEE Transactions on Nuclear Science*, vol. 37, pp. 203–208, 1990.

59. J. Andriessen, P. Dorenbos, and C. Van Eijk, Calculation of energy levels of cerium in inorganic scintillator crystals, *MRS Proceedings*, vol. 348, pp. 355–365, 1994.

60. S. E. Derenzo, M. Klintenberg, and M. J. Weber, Ab-initio cluster calculations of hole formation and trapping in PbF{sub 2} and PbF{sub 4}, *IEEE Transactions on Nuclear Science*, vol. 46, pp. 1969–1973, 1999.

61. M. Dahlbom, L. MacDonald, M. Schmand, L. Eriksson, M. Andreaco, and C. Williams, A YSO/LSO phoswich array detector for single and coincidence photon imaging, *IEEE Transactions on Nuclear Science*, vol. 45, pp. 1128–1132, 1998.

62. T. Szczesniak, M. Moszynski, L. Swiderski, A. Nassalski, P. Lavoute, and M. Kapusta, Fast photomultipliers for TOF PET, in *Nuclear Science Symposium Conference Record, 2007 (NSS '07)*, Piscataway, NJ: IEEE, 2007, pp. 2651–2659.

63. S. Gundacker, E. Auffray, B. Frisch, T. Meyer, P. Jarron, and P. Lecoq, SiPM photodetectors for highest time resolution in PET, in *International Workshop on New Photon-Detectors*, Orsay, France, 2012.

Photodetectors

MAGNUS DAHLBOM

3.1	Introduction	64
3.2	Photomultipler tube	65
	3.2.1 Photocathode	66
	3.2.2 Electron multiplication	68
	3.2.3 Spatial uniformity	69
	3.2.4 Dark current	70
	3.2.5 Magnetic fields	70
	3.2.6 Time response	70
	3.2.7 Voltage divider	71
	3.2.8 Special PMT configurations	72
	3.2.8.1 Position-sensitive PMTs	72
	3.2.8.2 Hybrid PMTs	73
	3.2.8.3 Microchannel plate	75
3.3	Semiconductor detectors	75
	3.3.1 PIN photodiodes	76
	3.3.1.1 Noise	76
	3.3.2 Avalanche photodiodes	77
	3.3.2.1 Gain	78
	3.3.2.2 Noise	79
	3.3.2.3 Applications of APDs	80
	3.3.3 Silicon photomultiplier	80
	3.3.3.1 Basic operation	80
	3.3.3.2 Quenching	83
	3.3.3.3 Photodetection efficiency	83
	3.3.3.4 Linearity	84
	3.3.3.5 Noise and dark current	84
	3.3.3.6 Time resolution	85
	3.3.3.7 Digital silicon photomultiplier	85
	3.3.3.8 Applications	86
3.4	Summary	86
References		86

3.1 INTRODUCTION

The detector systems used almost exclusively in SPECT and PET systems are scintillation detector based. In these detector systems, the gamma rays emitted from the object that is being imaged will interact in the scintillation crystal. Depending on the interaction type, an energetic photoelectron or Compton electron is produced and set in motion, which will produce ionizations and excitations in the crystal. As the electrons de-excite back to the ground state, some of the transitions will result in the emission of light photons. The number of light photons emitted is proportional to the amount of energy that was transferred to the electron in the interaction. The purpose of a photodetector is to collect and absorb the scintillation photons and convert the light energy into an electrical signal that can be processed by the subsequent electronics to determine the energy and position of the interacting gamma ray.

The main challenge in scintillation detector systems is to detect and amplify the extremely low signal that is produced in the burst of light photons, each with an energy in the neighborhood of 3–4 eV. The number of photons that is produced in the interaction depends on the light yield of the scintillation crystal and the energy of the interacting gamma ray. NaI (Tl) is a scintillator that has a light yield of 38,000 photons/MeV [1]. Following a photoelectric interaction of a 140 keV photon in a NaI (Tl), approximately 5300 scintillation photons will be produced. These scintillation light photons are emitted isotropically in the crystal in following the interaction. Since the photodetector is only coupled to one face of the scintillator, it is necessary to place reflectors on the sides not coupled to the photodetector to prevent escape of the light. These reflectors are not perfect and will absorb some of the scintillation photons. To reduce reflections at the scintillator–photodetector interface, the scintillation crystal is usually coupled to the photodetector with some coupling material (e.g., optical grease), which might absorb some of the scintillation light photons. A mismatch in indexes of refraction of the scintillation crystal, coupling material, and photodetector may produce light losses due to internal trapping. All of these processes will result in only a fraction of the light photons actually reaching the photodetector. In a scintillation camera using a NaI (Tl), only about 50%–60% of the light will actually reach the photodetectors. Due to the low number of scintillation light photons that will escape the crystal, it is important that the photodetector absorbs as much of the light as possible, and preferably also has the ability to amplify the signal without adding any additional noise. It is also important that the temporal properties of the signal are preserved, including the rise and decay time of the signal.

When considering a photodetector for PET and SPECT, there are certain performance parameters that are of particular importance. In a scintillator-based SPECT system, each event needs to be accurately positioned within the scintillation crystal. In addition, the energy of each absorbed event needs to be determined. Both the accuracy and the precision of the energy determination depend on the how well the photodetector performs. The light collection, which will affect the signal amplitude and statistical variation in the signal output, is therefore of great importance. These characteristics are also of importance in PET, however; in PET, the timing properties of the signal are also of concern. The timing properties of the detector system are important since they are what allow the PET system to sort out and correlate what pairs of detected events originate from the same photon annihilation. How accurately a detector system can do this is referred to as the time resolution of the system. The time resolution of the scintillation detector system is primarily determined by the light emission characteristics of the scintillator material used. Some of the factors that affect this are the time it takes for the excited electrons to migrate to the activator sites in the crystal lattice, the decay constant of the scintillation light, and the scintillation light yield. The timing properties of the signal are usually characterized by the rise and decay time of the signal. The rise time is especially critical since this will determine how quickly the detector generates a signal following the absorption of a photon. As soon as the signal from the detector exceeds any predetermined threshold, defined by the inherent noise level of the detector, this will trigger the timing circuitry and define the point in time when the signal was generated. The faster the rise time, the faster this time stamp is generated and the better the time resolution of the system. This method of triggering is referred to as leading-edge timing and is a common and effective method for triggering. Any variability in when the time stamp is generated will introduce an uncertainty in time, which is sometimes referred to as time jitter or time slew, depending on the source of the inaccuracy [1]. There are several factors that affect the timing uncertainty, such as noise in the signal and the dynamic range of the signals, and the signal shape. A detailed discussion on the time-pickoff methods and timing uncertainties can be found in [1].

In PET, which relies on fast timing signals, it is of importance that the inherent signal properties of the scintillation light are preserved and not degraded when the light is converted to an electrical signal by the photodetector. In a non-time-of-flight (TOF) system, a time resolution of a few nanoseconds is necessary to accurately assign two detector signals to an annihilation event. If the photodetector adds a few hundred pico-seconds of uncertainty to the overall timing information, this may not be that critical. However, in TOF PET it is desirable to determine the difference in time of detection of a pair of photons as accurately as possible, preferably within a few hundred picoseconds. It is therefore important that the photon detector does not add uncertainty in the timing properties of the signal.

Another factor of consideration is the stability of the detector system. In order to maintain a consistent performance of the imaging system, it is important that the detector system and, in particular, the photode-tectors are stable. This will reduce the frequency with which the system has to be recalibrated.

There are two main classes of photodetectors utilized with scintillation crystals: photoemissive devices such as the photomultiplier tube (PMT) and semiconductor devices. Both of these groups are specialized devices with different operating characteristics that will be discussed in the following sections.

3.2 PHOTOMULTIPLER TUBE

The PMT is a very sensitive and fast device that is widely used as a photodetector in scintillator-based detec-tor systems. The PMT was developed in the 1930s to amplify signals from weak light sources. The PMT was later used in physics experiments together with fluorescence screens to detect alpha particles. This was first described in a classified report by Curran and Baker in 1944 [2]. Since this work was performed as part of the Manhattan project, it was withheld from publication until 1948 [3].

The PMT is still the most commonly used photodetector in scintillator-based SPECT and PET imaging systems. Figure 3.1 illustrates the basic elements of a PMT. The PMT consists of a photocathode, focusing

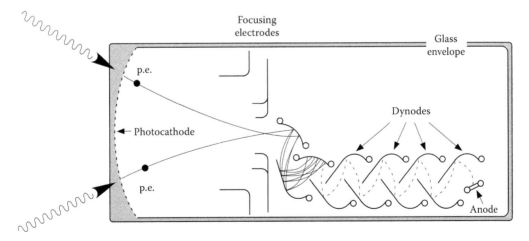

Figure 3.1 Schematic of a PMT. A light photon will eject a photoelectron (p.e.) from the photocathode. The focusing electrodes will guide the p.e. toward the first dynode. When the electron impinges on the first dynode, it will eject secondary electrons. These will be attracted to the second dynode. This process will be repeated down the series of dynodes. The result is a multiplication of the signal, which is collected at the anode.

electrodes, an electron multiplying structure, and an electron collector or anode, all contained within a sealed vacuum tube.

The transparent entrance window is a surface on the PMT to which the scintillator is coupled. The photocathode, which consists of a photoemissive surface, is located on the inside (i.e., the vacuum side) of the entrance window. When the scintillation photons are absorbed in the photocathode, photoelectrons are emitted into the vacuum. By the applying a voltage between the photocathode and the acceleration structure, an electric field is created. This electric field will, together with a series of focusing electrodes, guide the photoelectrons toward the multiplication structure. This consists of a series of electrodes or dynodes, where a potential is applied between each pair of dynodes. At each stage, the signal is amplified through secondary electron emission as the electrons impinge on each dynode. The end stage of the multiplication structure is the anode, where the multiplied electrons are collected and which is the readout stage of the PMT. Because of the electron multiplication structure, together with the inherent low-noise properties of the PMT, the signal-to-noise ratio (S/N) of the output signal is very high.

3.2.1 PHOTOCATHODE

The purpose of the photocathode is to absorb the scintillation light photons and subsequently emit photoelectrons that are collected and amplified by the dynode structure. There are two types of photocathodes used in PMTs: the transmission or semitransparent type and the reflection or opaque type. In the reflection-type photocathode, the scintillation light photons pass through the glass envelope of the PMT and are then fully absorbed in the photocathode. The photoelectrons are emitted in the opposite direction of the incident light, hence the name reflection-type photocathode. This type of photocathode is typically used in side-on PMTs.

The transmission-type photocathode is used in head-on or end-on PMTs, which is the type of PMT that is used in scintillator-based SPECT and PET systems. In the transmission type, the photocathode is located directly on the inner surface of the entrance window. In this case, the scintillation light photons pass through the glass envelope and are absorbed in the photocathode. The photocathode has to be thick enough to absorb the scintillation light, but also thin enough to allow escape of the photoelectrons to the surface to allow collection by the first dynode.

The conversion efficiency or sensitivity of the photocathode is typically characterized by the quantum efficiency (QE). The quantum efficiency (QE) is defined as

$$QE[\%] = 100 \times \frac{\text{number of emitted photoelectrons}}{\text{number of incident photons}} \tag{3.1}$$

The QE should ideally be as close as possible to 100%; however, most standard photocathodes do not have a QE greater than 20%–30% [4].

Another metric of the conversion efficiency of the photocathode is the radiant sensitivity, S. It is defined as current generated by the photoelectrons emitted from the photocathode divided by the incident radiant flux at a given wavelength, and is given in units of amperes per watts [5]. Commonly used is also the relative radiant sensitivity, where the maximum radiant sensitivity is normalized to 100%. The relationship between the QE and the radiant sensitivity S at a given wavelength λ (nm) is given by

$$QE[\%] = 100 \times \frac{1240}{\lambda} S \tag{3.2}$$

The QE and S of the photocathode have a strong dependency on the wavelength of the incident light, and this dependency is referred to as the spectral response (Figure 3.2). The spectral response is dependent on both the material used in the photocathode and the material of the entrance window. The cutoff of the spectral response at longer wavelengths depends on the photocathode material and is due to the fact that the energy transfer to the electron is not high enough to allow the electron to escape. At short wavelengths

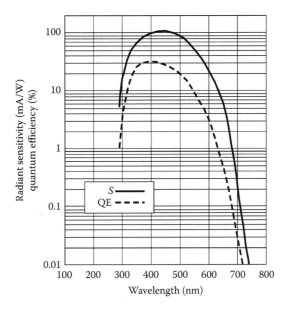

Figure 3.2 Spectral response. QE and radiant sensitivity (S) as a function of wavelength for a borosilicate PMT with a bialkali photocathode. At long wavelengths (>700 nm), the energy of the photons is not high enough to eject an electron. The cutoff at short wavelengths (<300 nm) is due to absorption in the glass envelope. Using UV transmitting glass, the transmission can be extended down to ~200 nm.

(i.e., ultraviolet [UV]), the cutoff is due to the absorption of the light in the entrance window. Borosilicate glass, which is the most commonly used window material, transmits light from the infrared region (IR) to 300–350 nm [1]. Using entrance windows of UV transmitting glass, quartz, or MgF_2, the transmission can be extended down to below 200 nm [1].

The photocathode is made of compound semiconductor consisting of alkali metals with a low work function. Some of the more common photocathodes materials are the bialkali (Sb-Rb-Cs and Sb-K-Cs) and multialkali (Na-K-Sb-Cs) photocathodes. The bialkali photocathodes have a spectral response from around 200 nm (UV region) to 600 nm (visible light). The multialkali photocathodes have a wider spectral response, from 200 to 850 nm (IR). Photocathodes made from GaAsP crystals activated with cesium have a narrower spectral response than the previously mentioned photocathode materials, but a QE close to 50% in the visible region [6]. PMTs with GaAsP photocathodes are more expensive to manufacture than standard bialkali PMTs. Recent optimization efforts in the manufacturing process of bialkali photocathodes have resulted in the production of PMTs with a maximum QE above 40% [6].

The spectral response of the photocathode should be matched with the emission spectrum from the scintillator in use. For instance, bialkali photocathodes have a peak QE at around 370 nm, which is fairly well matched to the emission spectrum of many scintillators used in nuclear imaging devices, such as NaI (Tl), lutetium oxyorthosilicate (LSO), and bismuth germanate (BGO).

The QE of the photocathode has a direct influence on the statistical variance of the signal in a scintillation detector system. The variance in the number of photoelectrons produced off the photocathode can be assumed to follow Poisson statistics. If, on average, N photoelectrons are produced after a gamma ray absorption in the scintillator, then the variance in the signal is also N and the standard deviation is $\sqrt{N}$. This variance in the signal also propagates into the multiplied signal. Even if the scintillator is irradiated with monoenergetic photons, there will be an observed variance in the measured signal, which is seen in the width of the photopeak in an energy spectrum where the measured full width at half maximum (FWHM) is proportional to $\sqrt{N}$. The effect of this variance is also observed in spatial resolution in scintillation cameras where the positioning of the events is determined by the signals collected by the PMTs. If the QE is improved, this should also increase the N, which should improve both energy resolution and spatial resolution of a gamma camera system.

3.2.2 Electron multiplication

The amplification of the signal in the PMT takes place in the multiplication structure. Once the photoelectrons have been emitted from the photocathode, they need to be guided toward the multiplication or dynode structure. Figure 3.3 show examples of dynode structures that are commonly used. An electric field produced by a voltage applied between the photocathode and the first dynode will, together with focusing electrodes, guide and accelerate the electrons toward the first dynode. When the photoelectrons strike the dynode, they will have gained enough kinetic energy to produce secondary electron emission. The dynode material and the applied voltage are selected such that the ratio of the number of emitted electrons to the number of incident electrons is greater than 1. This multiplication process continues between the dynodes, and the total charge produced in the process is collected at the final anode stage.

If a positive potential of 100 V is applied between the photocathode and the first dynode, a photoelectron will have gained a kinetic energy of approximately 100 eV as it strikes the dynode. This energy is enough for the electron to produce excitation of electrons to the conduction band in the dynode. Assuming a band gap of 2–3 eV of the dynode material, 30–50 excited electrons are produced by a single impinging electron. The directions of these secondary electrons are random, and only a few of these will therefore move toward the surface of the dynode. Although some of the electrons are moving toward the surface of the dynode, many of them will not have enough energy to reach the surface or to overcome the potential barrier at the surface and will therefore not be able to escape. As a result, only a small fraction of the initially excited electrons will escape the dynode surface to contribute to the secondary electron emission. The number of secondary electrons emitted not only is dependent on the properties of the dynode material, but also is sensitive to the applied voltage. If the potential difference between the photocathode and the dynode is reduced, a lower number of electrons are excited. On the other hand, a larger fraction of these will be produced at the surface, which will increase the probability for escape. Conversely, if the potential difference is increased, more electrons are excited, but at greater depths within the dynode, which will lower the probability of escape. Because of these counteracting effects, there is an optimal operating voltage that will maximize the secondary electron emission.

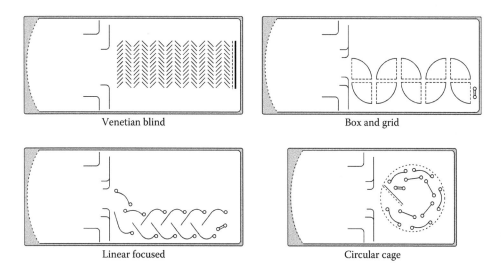

Venetian blind

Box and grid

Linear focused

Circular cage

Figure 3.3 Example of four commonly used different dynode structures in head-on PMTs. The *venetian blind* produces an *n* electric field that has very good collection efficiency of the photoelectrons. The foil structure of the dynodes makes it less sensitive to magnetic fields. The *box-and-grid* structure has very high collection efficiency of the photoelectrons, which results in good detection efficiency and uniformity. In the *linear focused*, the spread in electron trajectories is minimized, which results in low TTS. Using a *circular cage* structure results in a compact PMT, and it also has a fast response time.

The secondary electron emission ratio δ or dynode multiplication factor is given by

$$\delta = \frac{n_e}{n_i} \tag{3.3}$$

where:

n_i is the number of primary (incoming) electrons
n_e is the number of secondary (emitted) electrons

For a PMT with n dynode stages, the overall ideal gain or multiplication μ would be

$$\mu = \alpha \delta^n \tag{3.4}$$

where α is the probability that the photoelectron will have a trajectory such that it will impinge on the effective area of first dynode and produce secondary emissions that will result in further multiplication in the subsequent dynodes. This is commonly referred to as the collection efficiency. For a well-designed and properly adjusted PMT, α should be close to 1; however, if the voltage between the photocathode and the first dynode is low, then a drop in the collection efficiency may result.

For conventional dynode materials such as BeO, MgO, and Cs_3Sb, values for δ per stage are typically 4–6. For a PMT 10 stage (i.e., 10 dynodes) with a multiplication factor of 4 per stage, the overall gain would be $\sim 4^{10}$, or approximately 10^6. Thus, the PMT provides a very large amplification of the initially very weak incoming signal generated by the light from the scintillator.

The secondary electron emission ratio is dependent on the dynode material and the applied voltage:

$$\delta = kE^{\beta} \tag{3.5}$$

where:

k is a constant
E is the voltage between a pair of dynodes
β is the dynode material and structure-dependent coefficient, which has a value of 0.7–0.8

If V is the overall voltage applied between the cathode and the anode, then the gain can be written as

$$\mu = \delta^n = \left(kE^{\beta} \right)^n = \left[k \left(\frac{V}{n+1} \right)^{\beta} \right]^n = \frac{k^n}{(n+1)^{\beta n}} V^{\beta n} = KV^{\beta n} \tag{3.6}$$

Since PMTs typically have 8–14 stages, the gain is expected be proportional to $V^6 - V^{12}$. The strong dependency of the gain on the voltage requires that the high-voltage supply be extremely stable, since any small fluctuation in voltage would be magnified with a factor of 6–12 at the signal output.

3.2.3 SPATIAL UNIFORMITY

The uniformity of the PMT refers to the variation in signal output at the anode across the area of the photocathode and can be large in PMTs with a large-area photocathode. The uniformity depends primarily on how uniform the photocathode is, but also on the collection efficiency of the photoelectrons by the first dynode. The uniformity also has a dependency on wavelength and the applied voltage. As the incoming light shifts toward longer wavelengths, the uniformity becomes dependent on the surface conditions of the photocathode. If the applied bias is too low, then the electron collection efficiency between the dynodes may degrade, which in turn may affect the uniformity. In general, head-on tubes provide better uniformity than side-on tubes. The dynode structure used in the multiplication structure also affects the uniformity. For instance, the box-and-grid type and venetian blind-type provide better uniformity than the linear-focused type. A method to even out the effects of photocathode nonuniformities is to add a diffuser or light guide between the scintillator and the PMT. In scintillation cameras, the spatial resolution and positioning linearity are directly affected by the uniformity of the PMTs used. Thus, the uniformity of the PMTs is one of the most important parameters in the selection of the PMT used.

3.2.4 DARK CURRENT

Even when a biased PMT is placed in complete darkness, a small current can be measured at the anode. This current is typically referred to as the anode dark current and determines the lower limit of light detection. The dark current has a strong dependency on the applied voltage. There are several sources that contribute to the dark current where the main source is due to thermionic emission or electrons within the PMT. In particular, electron emissions from the photocathode are a significant contributor, since these will be multiplied by the dynode structure.

The current-caused thermionic electron emission from the photocathode is directly proportional to the area of the photocathode. The dark current from thermionic electron emissions can be reduced by cooling of the PMT. In general, the dark current is several orders of magnitude lower in comparison with the signal produced by the photoemission of the light produced by scintillators used in SPECT and PET.

3.2.5 MAGNETIC FIELDS

PMTs are very sensitive to magnet fields, which affects the electron collection and multiplication structure. Even a weak magnetic field such as the earth's can produce a degrading effect on the performance of the PMT. The magnetic field will perturb the trajectories of the electrons as they pass through the PMT structure, and the result is a loss in signal due to reduced electron collection. How much signal loss depends on the strength and orientation of the magnetic field and the construction of the PMT. The collection of the photoelectron by the first dynode is the stage of PMT that is most sensitive to magnetic fields. For instance, a PMT in which the trajectories of the electrons from the photocathode to the first dynode are long is more likely to be more adversely affected by a magnetic field than a tube where this path length is short.

By enclosing the PMT in a μ-metal shield that extends beyond the photocathode, the effects of weak magnetic fields can be reduced. In a SPECT system, where the detector head is rotating around the object that is being imaged, the orientation of the earth's magnetic field relative to the PMTs in the detector is not constant. The signal amplitude could therefore potentially vary depending on the orientation of the detector head, which was also observed on older SPECT systems [7,8]. In modern systems, this effect has been eliminated by the use of appropriate magnetic shielding around the PMTs.

3.2.6 TIME RESPONSE

The time response of the detector system is very critical in PET, especially in systems where the TOF information is collected. Any degradation of the timing properties of the signal in the detector chain should therefore be minimized. Although the PMT has a very fast time response, it may degrade the signal because of timing characteristics of the particular PMT design. This degradation is attributed to the difference in path lengths of the trajectories as the electrons travel from the point of emission of the photocathode to the first dynode. There are two components that describe the timing properties of a PMT: the electron transit time (TT) and transit time spread (TTS). The electron TT is the average time between the emission of the photoelectrons from the photocathode and the collection of the burst of electrons at the anode (Figure 3.4). The average TT depends on the design of the PMT and is on the order of 5–80 ns. The TT is not a degrading factor itself since it only introduces a fixed time delay. However, the TTS does effect the timing properties since this introduces an uncertainty in when the photoelectron emitted from the photocathode was generated and, in turn, when the photon was absorbed in the scintillator.

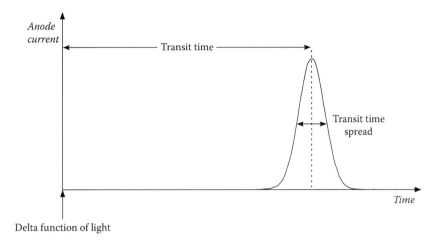

Figure 3.4 Illustration of TT and TTS. The TT is the average time between when the photoelectron is emitted from the photocathode and a current (i.e., multiplied signal) is measured at the anode. The TTS is spread in the TT in multiple measurements.

The time response is primarily dependent on the type of dynodes used, but also has a dependency on the applied voltage. PMTs using linear-focused or metal channel dynodes have the least amount of TTS, whereas tubes with box-and-grid and venetian blind dynodes have worse TTS performance. In addition to using a linear-focused dynode structure, fast PMTs use a spherical shape of the photocathode surface in order to minimize the difference in path lengths of photoelectrons emitted at the center compared with those emitted at the edge.

3.2.7 VOLTAGE DIVIDER

In order to accelerate the photoelectrons toward the multiplication structure, a bias voltage has to be applied between the photocathode and the subsequent dynodes. This bias should be high enough to provide good collection of the photoelectrons by the first dynode. Furthermore, the bias should provide enough acceleration of the electrons between the dynodes to produce adequate secondary electron multiplication. Since the signal carriers in the PMT are electrons, the potential of the first dynode with respect to the photocathode has to be positive in order to attract the electrons to the dynode. The succeeding dynodes have to be held at a positive potential with respect to the preceding dynode in order to move the multiplied electrons toward the anode.

The voltage distribution between the components in the PMT is provided by a high-voltage supply and a resistive voltage divider. The applied high voltage can either be positive (cathode grounding) or negative (anode grounding), as shown in Figure 3.5. In the case of positive high voltage, the photocathode is grounded, whereas the anode is at positive potential. When negative high voltage is applied, the photocathode is held at negative potential and the anode is grounded. Both configurations have pros and cons. When operating the PMT at positive direct current (dc) voltage, the anode is held at the same potential as the applied high voltage. In order to pass the multiplied signal from the anode, it has to be capacitively coupled to the processing electronics. However, this capacitive coupling may compromise the timing properties of the signal and may not be suitable where fast timing is necessary (e.g., TOF PET).

For fast timing application, a PMT is typically operated at negative high voltage where the anode is directly coupled to the processing electronics. In this case, the potential at the photocathode is at supplied negative voltage. If the glass envelope is in contact with grounded structures, the small conductivity of the glass may result in small currents flowing between the photocathode and the ground, which may lead to a degradation or damage to the PMT. This can be avoided by placing a μ-metal screen around the PMT and letting the screen have negative voltage.

The distribution of voltages between the photocathode and the dynodes is highly dependent on the application. Typically, a greater potential is applied between the photocathode and the first dynode in comparison

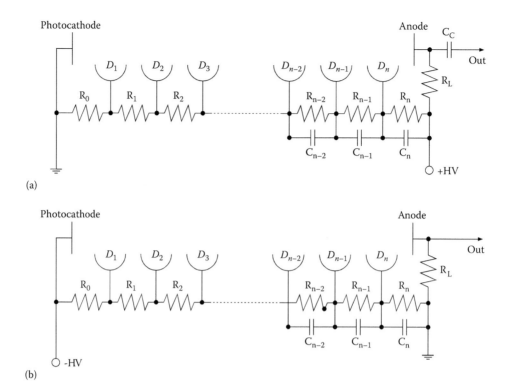

Figure 3.5 Voltage divider. Schematics of voltage divider circuits used to distribute the high voltage (HV) between the dynodes in a PMT. The resistors (R_i) between the dynodes ensure that the proper voltage is applied between each stage to allow the electron multiplication to take place. The capacitors (C_n) at the later stages ensure that the voltage is maintained, which could otherwise drop due to high currents at these stages. (a) Anode grounding. In this circuit, the photocathode is held at negative potential and the anode is at ground. (b) Cathode grounding. In this circuit, the photocathode is held at ground and the anode at positive potential. To protect the processing electronics, a coupling capacitor (C_C) has to be placed between the anode and the output. This capacitor may in some situations degrade the timing properties of the signal. In timing applications, such as TOF PET, anode grounding is used since the coupling capacitor can be eliminated.

with the succeeding dynode-to-dynode voltages. This ensures a high collection efficiency by the first dynode of the photoelectrons.

It is also common to connect capacitors in parallel with the resistors at the later stages of the PMT. The purpose of these so-called stabilizing capacitors is to prevent voltage drifts due to the high current flowing through the dynodes at the later multiplication stages. More detailed information regarding the design of voltage divider circuits can be found in [5].

3.2.8 SPECIAL PMT CONFIGURATIONS

3.2.8.1 POSITION-SENSITIVE PMTs

A conventional PMT does not provide any spatial information regarding where on the photocathode the scintillation photons were absorbed. Since the PMT is a fairly bulky device and there are restrictions on how small a PMT can be made due to the requirement that the photocathode and the multiplication structure have to be contained within a glass vacuum tube, it is difficult to construct high-resolution imaging devices where a large number of closely packed scintillation crystals are coupled to individual PMTs. In a conventional scintillation camera, this is resolved by coupling a large monolithic NaI scintillation crystal to an array of fairly large PMTs. Using Anger positioning logic [9] allows each event to be positioned to within 3 mm at 140 keV, which is in general adequate for most clinical SPECT applications.

In the block detectors used in PET, a similar but slightly different approach is used where an array composed of individual scintillation crystals is coupled to a smaller number of PMTs, typically four. Using the signal from the four PMTs and Anger-type positioning logic allows fairly accurate positioning of each event to within the dimensions of each crystal element [10,11]. This detector design works well where the detector elements are on the order of 4×4 mm^2 [12].

In high-resolution application where a resolution of better than 2 mm is needed, the Anger positioning readout is not adequate and a position-sensitive PMT (PS-PMT) is required.

Several types of PS-PMTs have been developed since these devices were first introduced in the 1980s. The main difference between these designs is the electron multiplication structure and the anode readout used.

The multichannel PMT (MC-PMT) consists of multiple distinct PMTs within the same vacuum enclosure, where multiple parallel dynode structures collect the photoelectrons from a common photocathode [13–15]. After multiplication in the individual dynode structures, the signal is read out at the anode, where each channel has its own separate anode. This design provides spatially separated signals with a minimal amount of electronic cross talk between channels. To reduce optical cross talk in the entrance window, one design used optical fibers to direct the scintillation light toward the photocathodes [16]. Although the spatial definition of events is excellent and the cross talk between channels is low in MC-PMTs, the main drawback is that the size of the active area of each channel is relatively large, which imposes limits on how small the crystal elements can be that are coupled to the PMT. Another drawback is that the active area of these PMTs tends to be relatively small, which results in a significant dead space.

In the grid-type dynode PMT, the dynodes are composed of layers of grid-type dynodes from which secondary electrons are emitted. To reduce spatial spread of the emitted electrons, a focusing mesh is added at each dynode layer. Despite the focusing mesh, there is a substantial spread on the order of 8–10 mm FWHM of electron cloud as it reaches the anode.

The focused mesh dynode structure reduces the problem of spatial spread of the electron cloud as the signal is multiplied. This structure is composed of multiple layers of small cusp-shaped dynodes. Between the dynode layers are guard plates with holes that help focus the secondary electron onto the next layer of dynodes.

The current generation of PS-PMTs uses metal channel–type dynodes together with a multianode readout (Figure 3.6). The metal channel dynode structure results in very low cross talk between channels. The reason for this is that the distance between each dynode stage is short, which means that there is less chance for electrons to spread laterally to adjacent channels. Instead, the multiplication cascade will flow directly toward the anode. Since electron trajectories between each multiplication stage are relatively short, the device is fairly compact. Another advantage of the short electron trajectories of the metal channel dynode structure is that they make it less sensitive to magnetic fields.

The anode structure used also differs between PS-PMTs designs. One common design in older PS-PMTs is the cross-wire readout scheme. In this design, the anode consists of two layers of parallel wires, where the wires in each layer are perpendicular to each other. The wires in each layer are read out by a charge division readout scheme, together with a center of gravity calculation to provide spatial information in each orthogonal direction. This readout scheme only requires that four signals have to be read out in these PMTs. Later generations of PS-PMTs use either cross-plates or multianodes for readout (Figure 3.6), where each anode is read out independently. This allows for more accurate positioning, although more electronic readout channels are required.

Although the most recent generation of PS-PMTs provides very high spatial resolution, together with low dead space, the cost of these devices limits their widespread use. A large imaging system for clinical use would most likely become prohibitively expensive if PS-PMTs were used as photodetectors. These PMTs are therefore used primarily in smaller, specialized high-resolution systems, such as preclinical imaging systems (Chapter 16).

3.2.8.2 HYBRID PMTs

The hybrid PMT (HPMT) combines a conventional PMT and a photodiode into one unit [17]. Like a conventional PMT, scintillation photons are absorbed in the photocathode from which photoelectrons are emitted.

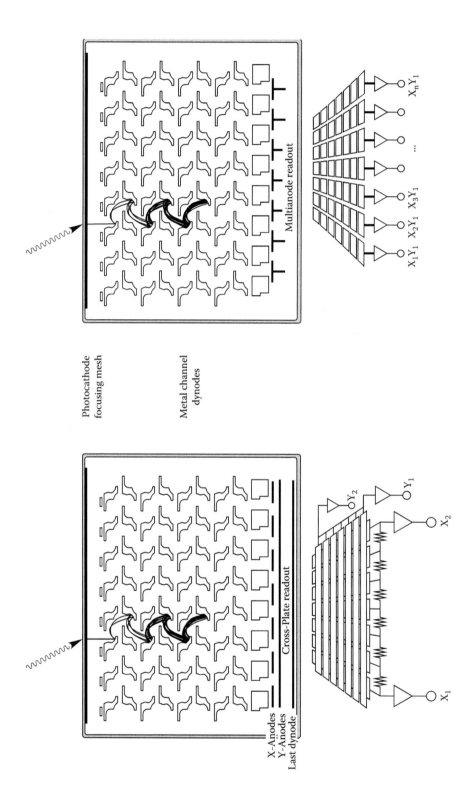

Photocathode
focusing mesh

Metal channel
dynodes

Multianode readout

X_1Y_1 X_2Y_1 X_3Y_1 ... X_nY_1

X-Anodes
Y-Anodes
Last dynode

Cross-Plate readout

X_1 X_2 Y_1 Y_2

Figure 3.6 PS-PMTs. Examples of the two readout schemes used in PS-PMTs. Left: In the cross-plate anode readout, a set of orthogonal plates are used to determine the position of the emitted photoelectron. After passing the dynode, the electrons will eventually hit the last dynode. At this stage, electrons will bounce back to and hit the X- and Y-anodes. Using a charge division readout scheme, the centroid of the electron cloud hitting the anodes can be calculated. Right: In the multianode readout, the multiplied signal from the dynodes is read out by an array of individual anodes. These will directly give the position of the event.

In the HPMT, the dynode structure has been replaced with a photodiode, which can be either a conventional PIN diode or an avalanche photodiode (APD) (Section 3.3.2). The photoelectrons are accelerated and focused toward the photodiode by a voltage on the order of 8 kV that is applied between the photocathode and the photodiode. The large voltage will accelerate the electrons enough to penetrate the photodiode and produce electron–hole pairs in the photodiode. In the single acceleration step, one photoelectron will produce approximately 1600 electron–hole pairs. If an APD is used as the photodiode, the signal will be further amplified, depending on the avalanche gain, which is typically on the order of 10–100. The overall gain of the HPD is thus on the order of 10^4–10^5, which is not as high as in a conventional PMT. However, the main advantage of the HPMT is that it has a very fast time response and low TTS. Since the distance between the photocathode and the photodiode is very short, it can also be made very compact. The short electron trajectory between the photocathode and the photodiode allows this device to be functional even in relatively strong magnetic fields.

Using a position-sensitive APD as the photodiode makes the HPMT position sensitive.

3.2.8.3 MICROCHANNEL PLATE

In a microchannel plate, the discrete dynode structure is replaced with a continuous channel where a voltage is applied between both ends [17]. Electrons entering a channel at an angle will hit the channel wall and produce secondary electron emissions. These will continue down the channel and produce further multiplication and eventually be collected by the anode located at the exit side of the plate. In the microchannel plate, thousands of small glass tubes (15–50 μm diameter) are fused together to form the multiplier structure. The main advantage of this device is that it is very fast, has low TTS, is compact, and is insensitive to magnetic fields. Since the multiplication occurs in discrete channels, there is no lateral spread in the multiplication process. This makes this structure suitable as a position-sensitive device, which can be accomplished by using a crosswire or multianode at the readout stage. The large dead space of the front face and high cost have prevented it from becoming feasible as a photodetector in PET and SPECT systems.

3.3 SEMICONDUCTOR DETECTORS

Semiconductor or solid-state detectors are another class of photodetectors that can be used as readout with scintillators. These photodetectors or photodiodes have several properties that make them very attractive as an alternative to conventional PMTs. The quantum efficiency of a photodiode is substantially higher than that of a conventional PMT. Unlike PMTs, the charge carriers do not have to escape a surface to contribute to the signal. The QE can therefore be as high as 80%, or even higher in photodiodes. The small dimensions of the device mean that the charge has to move over a relatively short distance, making the time response similar to that of PMTs. The small size of the device allows for the construction of very compact detector systems. Unlike most PMTs, these photodetectors are insensitive to magnetic fields, which currently makes them the only viable option for photodetectors for scintillator-based detector systems that are MRI compatible.

Semiconductor photodiodes utilize the electrical properties at the junction that is formed in silicon of different concentration levels of carrier types [18]. In n-type silicon, electrons are the majority carriers. This is produced by adding tracer amounts of pentavalent impurities such as phosphorus to the silicon, which is tetravalent when the crystal is grown. In p-type silicon, holes (i.e., electron vacancies) are the majority carriers. These holes are produced by adding tracer amounts of trivalent impurities such as boron to the silicon crystal. If the concentration of impurities is high, these materials are typically referred to as n^{++}- or p^{++}-type silicon, depending on the impurity type. On the other hand, if the impurity concentration is low, the material is referred to as n- or p-type materials. Sometimes, the notation ν- and π-type material is used to indicate a low concentration of n- and p-type impurities, respectively.

A p-n junction can be formed by ion implantation or diffusion of a p-type impurity, such as boron, into a substrate of n-type silicone. This will convert the n-type substrate to p-type in the region of the diffusion, and the p-n junction will be formed at the penetration depth of the implanted impurities. In the region of the junction, electrons in the n-type material will diffuse toward the p-type material. Conversely, the holes in the p-type material will diffuse in the opposite direction toward the n-type material. Due to the migration of electrons and holes in opposite directions, an electric field is produced across a region that is suppressed of free or loosely bound charge (i.e., electrons and holes). This region is referred to as the depletion region. Any charge that is generated in this region, for instance, by scintillation light, is quickly removed by the electrical field and produces a signal. Although this configuration could potentially work as a photodetector, the performance would be very poor. Due to the low field strength of the electric field of the unbiased junction, there is a high likelihood for trapping and recombination of the charge produced in the depletion region. In addition, the thickness of the depletion region is also very thin, which will affect the light absorption. To make the *p-n* junction work as a photodetector, a reversed bias has to be applied across the diode. This will ensure that the charge produced in the depletion region is efficiently collected by the electrodes. The bias will also increase the thickness of the depletion region, which will improve the absorption efficiency of the light.

Although a wide variety of semiconductor-based photodetectors have been developed, there are three kinds that are suitable to be used with scintillators. The first kind is the PIN photodiode, which does not provide any gain of the signal. The second kind is the APD, in which the signal is amplified. A third kind of semiconductor-based photodetector is the silicon photomultiplier (SiPM), which has evolved from the APD. Since its initial development, this device has received a lot of attention because it combines many of the best properties of a PMT and a semiconductor photodetector. These devices will be discussed in the next sections of this chapter.

3.3.1 PIN PHOTODIODES

A PIN (or p-i-n) diode is a photodiode with a lightly *n*-doped or intrinsic region at the *p-n* junction. A schematic of a typical PIN photodetector is illustrated in Figure 3.7. This structure allows for the depletion depth to about 100 μm when reversed biased. This results in an improved absorption efficiency of the impinging light, especially at longer wavelengths. In addition, the electronic noise is reduced due to a reduction in capacitance. The limit of the spectral response of a PIN diode at long wavelengths depends on the band gap energy of silicon, which is 1.12 eV. This corresponds to a wavelength of 1100 nm. At short wavelengths, the cutoff depends on the absorption properties of the material and the thickness of the diffusion layer (i.e., the entrance window). If the diffusion layer is too thick, most of the light will be absorbed there instead of in the depletion layer, resulting in a reduced QE. The cutoff at short wavelengths is around 320 nm for normal PIN photodiodes. In UV-enhanced photodiodes, the cutoff can be extended to below 200 nm. To protect the entrance window from mechanical damage and to allow efficient coupling of the scintillator, the photodiode is covered with glass or plastic resin coating. This allows light transmission down to about 300 nm. At shorter wavelengths, quartz windows should be used in order to avoid significant light absorption ion in the coating.

3.3.1.1 NOISE

Because of the small signal amplitude produced by the light from scintillators, together with the lack of internal gain of the PIN photodetector, noise is a major problem in these devices. This is a particular problem for large-area devices when operated in pulse mode.

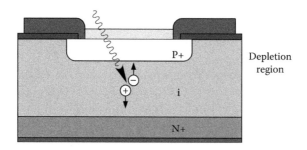

Figure 3.7 Schematic of the structure of a PIN photodiode. When light photons interact in the depletion region of the biased PIN diode, the electrons and holes produced will be collected by the anode and cathode, respectively. The photocurrent produced will not be amplified, and the gain of the PIN diode is therefore 1.

Noise in photodiodes consists of two components: series and parallel noise. The series noise increases with detector capacitance. Since the capacitance increases with the area of the device, devices greater than 1 cm^2 tend to produce excessive noise levels. The parallel noise is caused by variation in leakage current in the device. Leakage current tends to increase with the size of the device, which also prevents the use of large-area devices [19]. As the thickness of the device is increased, the capacitance of the diode will decrease, which reduces the series noise. However, the leakage current will increase as the thickness increases, which will increase the parallel noise. The typical thickness of photodiodes used for scintillator readout is typically 300–500 μm, which has been found to provide a good balance of acceptable levels of serial and parallel noise. Leakage current is also strongly dependent on temperature and can be reduced by cooling the photodiode.

In order to extract the best spectroscopic properties of the signal, long shaping time constants are used in the subsequent amplifying electronics, which makes it difficult to use PIN diodes in applications requiring fast timing (e.g., PET) [19].

Silicon devices are also sensitive to the incoming high-energy photons that are not absorbed in the scintillation detector. Since the energy of the incoming photons is significantly higher than the amount of energy absorbed in the detector as light photons, the signal from a direct-hit gamma is orders of magnitude higher. This is sometimes referred to as the nuclear countereffect. In order to minimize this, the photodiode should be kept as thin as possible. However, reducing the thickness will increase the capacitance, which will increase the serial noise.

Since the PIN device does not provide any internal gain and also produces a significant amount of noise when used at room temperature, the S/N of the generated signal tends to be fairly poor when used for photon counting. The lower limit of detection of the PIN photodetector is in the neighborhood of a few hundred light photons. This makes it extremely challenging to use these devices as photodetectors together with the scintillators and the gamma energies typically used in radionuclide imaging. This limitation can be overcome with specialized low-noise electronics and cooling of the devices [20]. Despite the challenges of using PIN diodes as a photodetector, there are examples of successful imaging devices using this technology [20,21].

3.3.2 AVALANCHE PHOTODIODES

The APD is a type of photodiode that, in contrast to the PIN diode, provides an internal amplification of the signal. This is accomplished by producing a more complex impurity concentration profile within the silicon substrate. When the bias is applied, a high electric field region is produced, which is high enough to accelerate the primary carriers enough to ionize bound carriers through impact ionizations. These secondary carriers can in turn ionize more carriers, and the result is the onset of an internal avalanche or multiplication, which amplifies the signal. The amplification of the signal alleviates some of the S/N problems seen in conventional photodiodes, as discussed in the previous section. The APD operates at significantly higher voltages than a conventional photodiode.

Since there are two kinds of carriers produced (electrons and holes) in the photodetector, both capable of producing secondary carriers, there is a positive feedback effect that could lead to breakdown, resulting in an infinite gain and also possibly damage. The amount of positive feedback is dependent on the relative impact ionization rates of the two carriers. It can be shown that to achieve high S/N, high finite gain, and wide bandwidth in an APD, the relative impact ionization rates between electrons and holes should be large. In addition, the device should be designed in such a way that the multiplication is initiated by the carrier with the higher ionization rate. In silicon, the impact ionization rate for electrons is one to two orders of magnitude higher than that of holes, which therefore makes it a suitable material for APDs [22].

A common APD design is the reach-through APD (Figure 3.8). In this device, regions in the depletion region are created: a drift region and a multiplication region. The two diffusions or ion implantations are adjusted such that when the bias is applied to the device, the depletion region of the diode reaches through to the low concentration π-region when the electric field at the junction is slightly less than required to cause avalanche breakdown. If additional voltage is applied, the depletion will rapidly extend out to the p^+ contact, whereas the electric field will only slowly increase. Since the ionization rates of the carriers increase exponentially with electric field, the main advantage of this device is a relatively slow variation in gain with applied

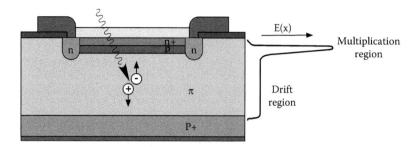

Figure 3.8 Schematic of the structure of a reach-through APD. When the bias is applied, drift and multiplication regions are created. The electrons produced after a photon interaction will drift toward the multiplication region where the signal is amplified.

bias; thus, the gain of this device will be less sensitive to voltage variations than some other APD designs. Another advantage of this device is a fast response time, high gain, and relatively low noise. The light enters through the p^+ contact, and the carriers are generated in the π-region. The electric field in this region is high enough to provide maximum carrier velocities, thus ensuring a fast response time. The thickness of the p^+ contact has to be adjusted to allow maximum transparency of the incoming light in combination with an antireflecting coating.

The reach-through structure allows for the construction of a fairly thick device, which increases the absorption efficiency. However, this has the drawback of increasing the nuclear effect (i.e., increased likelihood of direct absorption of gamma rays). Because of the energy deposition of a direct hit from a gamma ray, these events generate pulses of high amplitude. These pulses can, under most circumstances, be eliminated by energy discrimination.

3.3.2.1 GAIN

The multiplication factor or gain of an APD is an exponential function of the width of the multiplication region times the ionization rate of the electrons (α) and holes (β) and the location x within the multiplication region [19,22]:

$$M(x) = \frac{e^{-\int_x^w (\alpha-\beta)dx'}}{1-\int_0^w \alpha e^{-\int_{x'}^w (\alpha-\beta)dx'} dx'} \tag{3.7}$$

Since ionization rates α and β are dependent on the electric field, the gain has an exponential dependence on the applied bias. A simplified empirical expression of the gain M as a function of applied bias V is given by [23]

$$M(V) = \frac{1}{1-(V/V_b)^n} \tag{3.8}$$

where:
V_b is the breakdown voltage (i.e., voltage where a self-sustained avalanche occurs)
n is a material-dependent constant

The multiplication factor in practical APD is typically on the order of 50–200, which is fairly nominal in comparison with a PMT. It is possible to achieve higher gains by operating the APD at voltages close to the breakdown voltage. However, at these voltages, the gain is extremely sensitive to the applied voltage, which needs to be highly regulated in order to avoid instability in gain, and possibly breakdown. The gain of the APD also has a strong temperature dependency, where the gain is reduced by a few percent per increase in

Celsius degrees. The temperature therefore also has to be well regulated to avoid gain drifts. A temperature-induced gain drift can be compensated for by the adjustment of the bias voltage as the temperature changes (active gain control) [24].

3.3.2.2 NOISE

At low light levels, the APD is limited by the shot noise and the leakage current of the APD. Since the bulk leakage I_b current is multiplied, the total leakage current I_d is given by

$$I_d = I_s + I_b M \tag{3.9}$$

where:

I_s is the nonmultiplied surface current

Under constant voltage and stable conditions, the avalanche multiplication is initiated by an electron–hole pair that will, on average, produce a gain of the photocurrent of M. However, there is a significant fluctuation in the M between events. This fluctuation in M is referred to as the excess noise factor and is the main factor that adds noise to the signal in an APD. The excess noise factor, F, is given by [22]

$$F = \kappa M + \left(2 - \frac{1}{M}\right)(1 - \kappa) \tag{3.10}$$

$$\kappa = \beta / \alpha$$

where:

α is the ionization rates of electrons
β is the ionization rates of holes

Since the ionization rate for electrons is much higher than that of holes in silicon and typical gains are greater than 20, the expression for the excess noise factor can be approximated by

$$F \approx 2 + \kappa M \tag{3.11}$$

As can be seen from this equation, the excess gain factor is dependent on the gain and is at minimum 2. The total noise current for an APD under dark conditions (i.e., the photocurrent is zero) is given by

$$i_s^2 = 2q\left[I_b B M^2 F + I_s\right] \tag{3.12}$$

where:

q is the electron charge
B is the bandwidth

When the APD is coupled to a scintillator and operated at higher light levels, the noise current is given by

$$i_s^2 = 2q\left[\left(I_{ph} + I_b\right)B M^2 F + I_s\right] \tag{3.13}$$

I_{ph} is the photocurrent before multiplication. Since the excess noise factor F is dependent on the gain M, the noise current has a very strong dependence on the gain. Since the signal also increases with the gain, it is possible to find a gain at which the S/N is maximized. The S/N can be written as

$$\frac{S}{N} = \frac{I_{ph}^2 M^2}{2q\left[\left(I_{ph} + I_b\right)B M^2 F + I_s\right] + \dfrac{4kTB}{R_L}} \tag{3.14}$$

where the first and second terms in the denominator are the shot noise and the thermal noise, respectively, and k is Bolzmann's constant, T is the temperature in kelvin, and R_L is the load resistance. The thermal noise can be reduced by using a larger load resistance; however, this degrades the timing properties of the signal. For an APD, the signal can be multiplied without increasing the total noise until the shot noise reaches a level equal to the thermal noise.

3.3.2.3 APPLICATIONS OF APDS

APDs have for many years been suggested as a candidate to replace the PMTs in PET systems, especially in high-resolution systems where the size of the PMT is a limiting factor [25,26]. APDs were initially used in high-resolution preclinical PET systems [27,28] and have been primarily used in PET/MRI systems, where the magnetic field prevents the use of PMTs. APDs have been manufactured not only as single-element photodetectors, but also as monolithic arrays and position-sensitive devices [29,30]. These have been specifically designed for high-resolution preclinical PET systems. In terms of energy resolution, the performance of APDs is quite favorable compared with that of PMTs. Timing properties, however, are worse for APDs than PMTs, primarily due to the slower rise time of the signal from the APD. This prevents their use in systems where very fast timing is required, such as in TOF PET. As mentioned earlier, signal gain in an APD is also very sensitive to both voltage and temperature variations. APDs therefore need to be operated with very stable high-voltage supplies and in a highly regulated temperature environment, which adds cost to the design of the detector system [31–33].

3.3.3 SILICON PHOTOMULTIPLIER

The conventional mode of operation of the APD is to keep the applied voltage well below the breakdown voltage. The reason for this, as discussed in Section 3.3.2.3, is to maintain stability and avoid excessive noise. At this operating point, the APD will produce a linearly amplified signal of the photocurrent induced by the absorbed scintillation light.

If the applied voltage to the APD is further increased, the signal will start losing the linearity between the photocurrent and amplitude (Figure 3.9). Eventually, the APD will enter a mode that is referred to as Geiger mode, where the generation of signal carriers is self-sustained until the process is terminated or quenched [34]. In this mode of operation, the avalanche can be initiated by as little as a single electron–hole pair (i.e., one light photon) and the output signal is very high. However, the signal produced will have the same pulse height, independent of the number of electron–hole pairs produced by the absorbed light photons. When operated in Geiger mode, the APDs are referred to as single-photon APDs (SPADs) or Geiger APDs (G-APDs) [35]. G-APDs have been used in a variety of low-light detection applications, including single-molecule detection, luminescence microscopy, studies of fluorescent decays, and luminescence in physics, chemistry, and biology [36]. In addition to having a very high sensitivity, the G-APD is very fast and can provide timing resolution on the order of tens of picoseconds. It is also designed to be operated at much lower voltages than conventional APDs (tens of volts compared with hundreds). Since the G-APD does not provide any energy information, it is not useful as a photodetector for a scintillation crystal. On the other hand, a large array of small, independently operating G-APDs coupled to a single scintillation crystal can produce a signal that is proportional to the amount of light absorbed in the photodetector. If the number of elements or cells in the array is significantly greater than the number of light photons emitted from the scintillator, then there is a low likelihood that more than one light photon will be absorbed in each cell. Since each of the cells operates independently, each one absorbing a scintillation photon will produce a signal of approximately equal amplitude. By summation of all the signals from the individual cells, a signal that is proportional to the amount of light absorbed is produced. The summed signal should be proportional to the energy deposition in the scintillator. These multielement G-APDs are usually referred to as SiPM [37], solid-state photomultiplier (SSPM) [38], and multipixel photon counter (MMPC) [39].

3.3.3.1 BASIC OPERATION

The SiPM consists of a two-dimensional array of individual, independently operating APDs, all operating in Geiger mode (Figure 3.10). Each element in this array is usually referred to as a cell or μcell. The number of

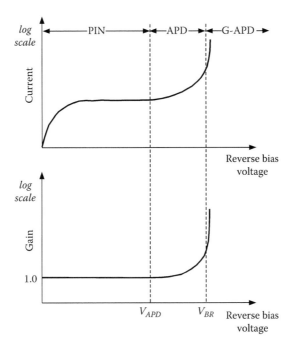

Figure 3.9 Current and gain dependency of applied bias in photodiodes. If the applied bias is too low, the electron and holes will recombine and result in a loss in signal. As the voltage is increased, all charge is collected (i.e., zero recombination). In this region, the gain is unity. When the voltage exceeds V_{Av}, the carriers can produce secondary ionizations and the current and gain increase. This is the operational region of APDs. If the voltage exceeds V_{Br}, a self-sustained avalanche is produced where the current and the gain will go toward infinity, unless the process is quenched. In the region, the diode operates as a G-APD. (Adapted from Dinu, N., in *Photodetectors*, ed. B. Nabet, Woodhead Publishing, Cambridge, UK, 2016, pp. 255–294.)

μcells in a single SiPM depends on the particular design and application but can be anywhere from 100 to 10,000 per mm². Currently, SiPMs are manufactured commercially in sizes from 1×1 to 6×6 mm².

The SiPM μcells are based on the reach-through structure used in conventional APD, which was discussed in Section 3.3.3. Each μcell consists of a *p-n* junction with dimensions on the order of 10–100 μm (Figure 3.10). When the reversed bias is applied, a very thin multiplication region (~1 μm) is created within the depletion layer. In order to operate the junction in Geiger mode, the electric field in the multiplication layer has to exceed $>3 \times 10^5$ V/cm. Since the multiplication layer is so thin, this can be accomplished by just applying only a few tenths of volts across the contacts. The SiPM is typically operated at a few volts above the breakdown voltage.

When an avalanche is triggered by a photon absorption in a μcell, the output pulse is proportional to the capacitance C of the μcell and the overvoltage (ΔV):

$$A \sim Q = C\Delta V = C\left(V_{bias} - V_{br}\right) \qquad (3.15)$$

where V_{bias} is the applied bias voltage and V_{br} is the breakdown voltage. Since the μcells are manufactured on the same substrate, the operational properties of each μcell should ideally be identical. All μcells in the SiPM should therefore produce pulses that are approximately equal in amplitude. In reality, there are nonuniformities in both gain and noise properties between the individual μcells. The typical gain of each μcell is in the range of 10^5-10^6, which is in the same order of magnitude as the gain observed in PMTs. The readout of the sum of the signals produced by the cells in SiPM is done through a common load resistor. Since each cell operates as a binary device, each producing a signal of equal amplitude, the summed signal is directly proportional to the number of triggered cells. As long as the number of cells is much larger than the number of

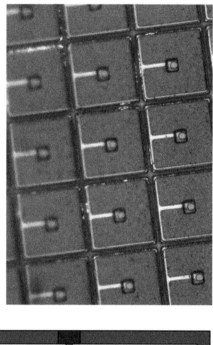

Top view

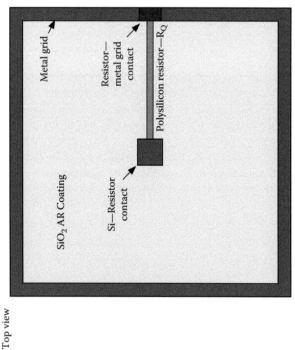

Side view

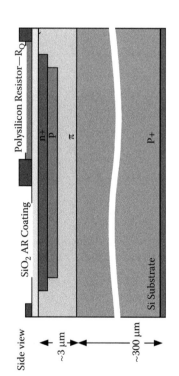

Figure 3.10 Left: Schematic of the structure of a passively quenched SiPM element. Similar to an APD, a *p-n* junction is created where the electrical field is high enough to initiate an avalanche. The integrated resistor (R_Q) serves as the quenching resistor to stop the avalanche. Right: Micrograph of a section of a SiPM showing the array of G-APD that makes up the device. (From Renker, D., and E. Lorenz, *J. Instrum*, 4, 2009. With permission)

incident photons, the signal amplitude will be proportional to the number of light photons that were absorbed in the cells.

The signal generation due to the breakdown process in the SiPM can be considered to be a three-step process: discharge, quenching, and recovery. The optical photons will initiate the avalanche and produce a *discharge*. The current flowing through the quenching resistor or the active quenching circuit will drop the bias below the breakdown voltage and *quench* the avalanche process. The final step is the *recovery*, where the bias is restored to the level prior to the onset of the avalanche. From the time of the onset of the avalanche until the restoration of the bias, the SiPM will be nonresponsive.

The gain of a SiPM has a very strong temperature dependency, which is primarily caused by the temperature dependency of V_{br}. Mazzillo et al. [40] measured that V_{br} in their device had a temperature coefficient of V_{br} of 30.6 mV/°C. If the V_{bias} is kept constant, the overvoltage ΔV will decrease, which will result in a decrease in gain. For stable operation, the temperature has to be controlled to within a fraction of a degree. Alternatively, the bias can be adjusted to compensate for the change in ΔV caused by the temperature change [41].

3.3.3.2 QUENCHING

Since the SiPM is operating in Geiger mode, the avalanche initiated by an electron–hole pair will be will be self-sustaining unless it is quenched. The quenching of the signal can be accomplished by either passive [42] or active [43] quenching. In passive quenching, a resistor is placed in series with each individual cell (Figure 3.10), which will lower the electrical field strength as the avalanche progresses. This will in turn prevent the formation of further signal carriers and eventually terminate the avalanche. How quickly the signal is quenched depends on the product of the resistance R_q of the quench resistor and the capacitance of the cell. This time depends primarily on the capacitance of the μcell and the resistance of the quenching resistor. Assuming that the recharge follows an exponential buildup, the bias would be restored to 95% of its initial value after 3τ and 99% after 5τ where τ is equal to $R_q C$. The recovery time will determine the count rate capability of the SiPM.

In many SiPM designs with passive quenching, polysilicon resistors are used for the quenching resistor. These resistors have a negative temperature coefficient, where the resistance increases by cooling, which will prolong the recovery time [44,45]. This dependency can be reduced by using thin metal film quenching resistors, which have a lower temperature coefficient [46].

In active quenching, the quenching resistor is replaced with a fast trigger and switching circuit [36]. This circuit senses the onset of the avalanche and drops the bias to below the breakdown voltage. After a predetermined hold-off time, the voltage is returned to the operational level. The advantage of active quenching is that the termination and restoration of the cell are faster than in passive quenching, which is limited by the time constants of the cell capacitance and the quenching resistor. However, active quenching circuitry adds complexity to the manufacturing of the SiPM.

3.3.3.3 PHOTODETECTION EFFICIENCY

The ability of a SiPM to detect a light signal depends on several factors, in addition to the QE defined for an APD or a PMT. This efficiency is usually referred to as the photodetection efficiency (PDE) and is defined as the product of three components:

$$PDE = QE \times f \times p_a \qquad (3.16)$$

where:

  QE   is the quantum efficiency
   f is the geometric fill factor
  p_a is the probability that an avalanche will be initiated by an electron–hole pair

Similarly to the PIN diodes and APDs, the QE of SiPM has a strong wavelength dependency, which depends on the light transmission through the contact layer and the absorption properties of the SiPM.

The fill factor is the ratio of the active area to the total area of the SiPM. This number is less than 1 since there will always be dead space between the μcells due to the presence of the necessary structures, such as electrical and optical isolation, quenching resistance, and metal grid connectors. These will all reduce the active area of the SiPM. In general, the smaller the μcells, the lower the fill factor since the dead space between cells tends to remain fairly constant while the cell size is reduced. Fill factors are typically in the range of 0.2–0.8.

Not all photon absorptions in a SiPM will result in the onset of an avalanche. Instead, there is a finite probability for this to occur, and the factor p_a accounts for this. This probability depends on where in the μcell the electron–hole pair was generated and the likelihood of electron–hole pair recombination. Increasing the overvoltage will reduce recombination and therefore increase the likelihood of initiating an avalanche. However, excessive overvoltage may lead to an increase in noise and after-pulsing (see Section 3.3.3.5). Values of p_a are in the range of 0.5–1.00 [47].

3.3.3.4 LINEARITY

As mentioned previously, a SiPM, the signal amplitude from an individual cell, is independent of the number of photons absorbed in the cell. The amplitude of the signal from the SiPM therefore only reflects the number of triggered μcells rather than the actual number of absorbed light photons. If the number of cells in the SiPM is much larger than the number of emitted light photons, then there is a very small likelihood that two or more photons would be absorbed in the same cell. However, if the number of cells is not much larger than the number of incident photons, then the probability for the absorption of two or more photons in the same μcell increases. This results in a nonlinearity between the signal amplitude and the number of absorbed light photons, which also limits the dynamic range of the SiPM. This nonlinearity not only depends on the ratio of absorbed light photons to the number of cells, but also has a dependence on the PDE. The relationship between the number of triggered cells, N_{trigger}, and the number of incident light photons, N_{photons}, can be described by [48]

$$N_{\text{trigger}} = N_{\text{cells}} \left(1 - e^{-\text{PDE} \frac{N_{\text{photons}}}{N_{\text{cells}}}} \right) \quad (3.17)$$

As long as the product of the PDE and N_{photons} is much smaller than N_{cells}, the device will have a linear behavior. Increasing the number of μcells in the SiPM will improve the linearity; however, this will reduce the fill factor and therefore also the PDE.

This nonlinearity also has a dependency on the applied voltage. Since the probability of triggering an avalanche, p_a, increases with the overvoltage, this will also increase the PDE (Equation 3.16). This in turn will increase the term in the exponent, which will worsen the nonlinearity [49].

When the SiPM is used as a photodetector together with a scintillator, this will result in nonlinear energy response of the detector system:

$$S \sim E\left(1 - e^{-kE}\right) \quad (3.18)$$

where E is the photon energy and k is the constant specific to the particular SiPM. The nonlinearity tends to shift and compress higher energies toward lower energies, which will degrade energy resolution and make absolute energy determination challenging [50,51]. However, it is possible to linearize the signal using Equation 3.18. This requires that the constant k is determined, which can be accomplished by a relatively straightforward calibration procedure [52]. This linearization procedure will become progressively less accurate as the signal reaches saturation levels. At energy levels where all μcells are triggered, the signal will entirely lose its relationship between energy and amplitude. It is therefore important that the SiPM used has the appropriate dynamic range for the scintillator and the energy interval of interest.

3.3.3.5 NOISE AND DARK CURRENT

Dark current in a SiPM includes pulses that are either uncorrelated or correlated to the primary avalanche event. These events are also referred to as primary and secondary dark pulses, respectively. Primary dark pulses are avalanches triggered by thermally generated carriers in the μcell. The dark pulse rate increases with the area of the device, overvoltage, and temperature, and is approximately 1 MHz/mm^2 at room temperature [53]. Recent design and manufacturing improvements have resulted in SiPMs with a significantly reduced dark pulse rate of around 100 kHz/mm^2 at room temperature [54]. By cooling of the device, thermally generated dark pulses are reduced.

Since most dark pulses have the amplitude of one photoelectron, increasing the triggering threshold above this level can reduce the dark pulse rate. By further increasing the threshold, the dark pulse rate is reduced by almost an order of magnitude for one additional photoelectron level [45]. Thermal noise is typically not a problem when using SiPMs with a scintillator since the number of μcells triggered by the absorbed light photons is well above the thermal noise level. Increasing the trigger level may, however, compromise the timing information in the signal and time resolution [55,56].

Secondary dark pulses are generated as a consequence of the primary avalanche events, which include after-pulse events and cross talk. During the primary avalanche event, there is a finite probability that some of the produced carriers will be captured in deep traps in the silicon [57]. Deep traps refer to energy levels in the middle of the band gap that are produced by defects or impurities in the silicon. Trapped carriers are eventually released with delay, depending on the lifetime properties of the trap involved. When the carrier is released, it can produce a secondary avalanche, which is referred to as an after-pulse. The after-pulses can occur during a period of several 100 ns following the primary avalanche and tend to prolong the recovery time. The number of trapped carriers is proportional to the number of carriers or charge produced in the avalanche. Since the charge is proportional to the overvoltage (Equation 3.14), after-pulsing increases with overvoltage. Cooling tends to increase the lifetime of the traps, which will prolong the after-pulsing, which in turn will extend the recovery time.

Cross talk is another contributing factor to the secondary pulses in a SiPM. This occurs when the primary avalanche triggers an avalanche in an adjacent cell. This secondary avalanche can be triggered by emission of photons produced by the primary avalanche. An avalanche breakdown event may produce three photons per 10^5 carriers with an energy greater than the band gap of silicon (1.14 eV) [58]. The photons can be absorbed in an adjacent cell and initiate a secondary avalanche. Cross talk can also be initiated by lateral diffusion of carriers to an adjacent cell if the absorption of the light photon occurs deep in the SiPM. Isolating the cells by adding metal-coated trenches between the μcells can reduce both sources of cross talk. This will, however, reduce the fill factor and the active area of the device and lower the PDE.

3.3.3.6 TIME RESOLUTION

The lower limit of the time resolution that can be achieved with a SiPM system is determined by time jitter that is caused by the time fluctuation when the signal from the SiPM is generated following the absorption of a light photon. This is analogous to the TTS observed in PMTs (Section 3.2.6). In a SiPM, this time jitter is caused by two main factors. First, there is a variation in the TT of the carries from the point of light photon absorption in the depletion layer to the high-field multiplication region. The field strength in this region is typically high enough that the carrier will reach the saturation velocity of 10 ps/μm. The contribution of this component depends on the thickness of the depletion region, where a thin depletion will provide less time jitter than a thick one. Second, there is a statistical variation in the buildup of the avalanche signal in the multiplication region from the initial carrier produced by the absorbed light photon. This factor is the main contributor to the time jitter in a SiPM. Additional factors contributing to the rise time of the pulse shape and timing resolution of the SiPM are the cell capacitance and μcell dimensions. Since larger μcells have a larger capacitance, these tend to be slower than devices with smaller μcells. The overall time jitter reported for SiPMs is 50–100 ps [59,60], which makes them as suitable as a photodetector in TOF PET systems. Several groups have reported on sub-100 ps coincidence time resolution of SiPMs with fast PET scintillators, such as LSO and LaBr$_3$ [61,62]. It should be mentioned that these measurements were performed under lab conditions and not in an actual full system configuration. Nevertheless, they show the excellent potential for the SiPM as a photodetector in PET.

3.3.3.7 DIGITAL SILICON PHOTOMULTIPLIER

An interesting property of the SiPM is that the signal from the device is inherently digital since each μcell acts as a binary switch. When a light photon is absorbed in a μcell, the cell will switch its state from 0 to 1. The total of all 1 states is then the total number of absorbed light photons. In a conventional analog SiPM, a summed pulse is generated that is analyzed in the conventional way using amplifiers, discriminators, and so on. In a digital SiPM (dSiPM), the SiPM is fully integrated with the analysis and logic circuitry in such a way that the output from the device is a digital representation of the signal amplitude and a time stamp when the event occurred [63–65]. In the implementation of a dSiPM by Philips, each μcell is integrated with its own active quench circuit. Furthermore, each μcell can be individually enabled or disabled in case of an excessive dark count rate, which should improve the S/N and minimize the time-degrading effects from the photodetector to the signal (e.g., time jitter). Using a pair of Philips dSiPMs coupled to $3 \times 3 \times 5$ mm^3 LYSO scintillators, a coincidence resolving time of close to 120 ps has been reported [66]. This value was achieved under very idealized laboratory conditions and is probably not likely to be achieved in a full system with larger scintillation detectors. Nevertheless, it illustrates the excellent timing information that can be achieved with the dSiPM.

3.3.3.8 APPLICATIONS

The SiPM has emerged as a very attractive and viable alternative to the conventional PMT in radioisotope imaging, in particular in PET and PET/MRI. SiPM has been used in several prototype PET systems, primarily MR-compatible preclinical systems [67–72], but also in clinical systems [73,74]. In the study by Krizsan et al. [72], the performances of two virtually identical systems were compared, where the only difference was the photodetector readout. They found that the imaging performance of a system using SiPM photodetectors was similar to that of a system using PS-PMTs. The only drawback of the SiPM system was that the tiling of individual SiPMs to create a large-area photodetector introduced some artifacts in the flood image.

Two of the major manufacturers of clinical PET systems are using SiPM as the photodetectors. General Electric (GE) is using SiPMs in its Signa PET/MR system, which allows simultaneous TOF PET and MR imaging and has a time resolution of better than 400 ps [74]. In the Philips Vereos PET–computed tomography (CT) system, dSiPMs are used [73]. This system also allows TOF imaging and has a time resolution of 325 ps. For comparison, the Siemens PET/CT system mCT, which uses conventional PMTs, has a time resolution of 527 ps [12]. The fact that SiPMs are used in commercial clinical PET systems is in indication that this technology might replace the PMTs as photodetectors, at least in high-performance PET systems, in the not too distant future. This technology is also very likely to be used in hybrid SPECT/MRI systems [75,76].

3.4 SUMMARY

In this chapter, the functionality of the main types of photodetectors used in PET and SPECT imaging systems has been presented. At the present time, PMTs are the technology used in most imaging systems. PMT is a mature, stable, and proven technology and provides the necessary performance in most imaging situations. However, PMTs have limitations that make their use in some applications suboptimal or not suitable at all. PMTs are fairly bulky devices and may therefore limit the spatial resolution that can be achieved. A severe limitation of the PMT is that it cannot be used in magnetic fields. Although innovative designs have overcome some of these limitations, these designs usually mean compromises, such as a loss in detection efficiency or S/N. Silicon photodetectors have for many years showed promise to be a replacement of the PMT in PET and SPECT imaging, but the performance and cost of conventional PIN diodes and APD have prevented them from becoming viable alternatives, especially in commercial systems. The improvements in the performance of the SiPM have shown that this technology might replace the PMTs as the photodetector in some system designs.

REFERENCES

1. Knoll, G. F. 2010. *Radiation Detection and Measurement.* Wiley, Hoboken, NJ.
2. Curran, S. C., and W. R. Baker. 1944. A photoelectric alpha particle detector. U.S. Atomic Energy Commission Report MDDC 1296. Technical Information Division, Oak Ridge Operations, Oak Ridge, TN.

3. Curran, S. C., and W. R. Baker. 1948. Photoelectric alpha-particle detector. *Rev Sci Instrum* 19:116.

4. Moses, W. W. 2009. Photodetectors for nuclear medical imaging. *Nucl Instrum Methods Phys Res A* 610:11–15.

5. Hamamatsu Photonics. 2007. *PMT Handbook*. Hamamatsu Photonics, Shizuoka, Japan.

6. Suyama, M., and K. Nakamura. 2009. Recent progress of photocathodes for PMTs. In *International Workshop on New Photon Detectors*, Matsumoto, Japan.

7. Larsson, S. A. 1980. Gamma camera emission tomography. *Acta Radiol Suppl* 363:1–75.

8. Rogers, W. L., N. H. Clinthorne, B. A. Harkness, K. F. Koral, and J. W. Keyes Jr. 1982. Field-flood requirements for emission computed tomography with an Anger camera. *J Nucl Med* 23:162–168.

9. Anger, H. O. 1958. Scintillation camera. *Rev Sci Instrum* 29:27–33.

10. Casey, M. E., and R. Nutt. 1986. A multicrystal two dimensional BGO detector system for positron emission tomography. *IEEE Trans Nucl Sci* 33:460–463.

11. Dahlbom, M., and E. J. Hoffman. 1988. An evaluation of a two-dimensional array detector for high-resolution PET. *IEEE Trans Med Imaging* 7:264–272.

12. Jakoby, B. W., Y. Bercier, M. Conti, M. E. Casey, B. Bendriem, and D. W. Townsend. 2011. Physical and clinical performance of the mCT time-of-flight PET/CT scanner. *Phys Med Biol* 56:2375–2389.

13. Engels, R., R. Reinartz, and J. Schelten. 1999. A new 64-channel area detector for neutrons and gamma rays. *IEEE Trans Nucl Sci* 46:869–872.

14. Roney, J. M., and C. J. Thompson. 1984. Detector identification with four BGO crystals on a dual PMT. *IEEE Trans Nucl Sci* 31:1022–1027.

15. Uchida, H., Y. Yamashita, T. Yamashita, and T. Hayashi. 1983. Advantageous use of new dual rectangular photomultiplier tube for positron-CT. *IEEE Trans Nucl Sci* 30:451–454.

16. Shao, Y. P., S. R. Cherry, S. Siegel, R. W. Silverman, and S. Majewski. 1996. Evaluation of multi-channel PMT's for readout of scintillator arrays. In *1995 IEEE Nuclear Science Symposium and Medical Imaging Conference Record*, vols. 1–3, pp. 1055–1059. IEEE, Piscataway, NJ.

17. Suyama, M. 2007. Latest status of PMTs and related sensors. In *International Workshop on New Photon-Detectors*, Kobe, Japan.

18. Sze, S. M., and K. K. Ng. 2007. *Physics of Semiconductor Devices*. Wiley-Interscience, Hoboken, NJ.

19. Pichler, B., and S. Ziegler. 2004. Photodetectors. In *Emission Tomography: The Fundamentals of SPECT and PET*, ed. M. Wernick and J. Aarsvold, pp. 255–267. Elsevier, San Diego.

20. Gruber, G. J., W. S. Choong, W. W. Moses, S. E. Derenzo, S. E. Holland, M. Pedrali-Noy, B. Krieger, E. Mandelli, G. Meddeler, and N. W. Wang. 2002. A compact 64-pixel CsI(Tl)/Si PIN photodiode imaging module with IC readout. *IEEE Trans Nucl Sci* 49:147–152.

21. Kindem, J., C. Y. Bai, and R. Conwell. 2010. CsI(Tl)/PIN solid state detectors for combined high resolution SPECT and CT imaging. In *2010 IEEE Nuclear Science Symposium Conference Record (NSS/MIC)*, pp. 1987–1990. IEEE, Piscataway, NJ.

22. Webb, P. P., R. J. McIntyre, and J. Conradi. 1974. Properties of avalanche photodiodes. *RCA Rev* 35:234–278.

23. Miller, S. L. 1955. Avalanche breakdown in germanium. *Phys Rev* 99:1234–1241.

24. Kataoka, J., R. Sato, T. Ikagawa, J. Kotoku, Y. Kuramoto, Y. Tsubuku, T. Saito, et al. 2006. An active gain-control system for avalanche photo-diodes under moderate temperature variations. *Nucl Instrum Methods Phys Res A* 564:300–307.

25. Lecomte, R., D. Schmitt, A. W. Lightstone, and R. J. McIntyre. 1985. Performance characteristics of BGO-silicon avalanche photodiode detectors for PET. *IEEE Trans Nucl Sci* 32:482–486.

26. Shah, K. S., R. Farrell, L. Cirignano, R. Grazioso, P. Bennett, S. R. Cherry, and Y. P. Shao. 1999. Planar APD arrays for high resolution PET. *Proc SPIE* 3770:104–111.

27. Lecomte, R., J. Cadorette, S. Rodrigue, D. Rouleau, and R. Yao. 1996. Performance of the Sherbrooke avalanche photodiode PET scanner: A new high resolution device for animal research. *J Nucl Med* 37:744–744.

28. Shao, Y., R. W. Silverman, R. Farrell, L. Cirignano, R. Grazioso, K. S. Shah, and S. R. Cherry. 1999. A compact high resolution PET detector using an APD array. *J Nucl Med* 40:75.

29. Shah, K. S., R. Grazioso, R. Farrell, J. Glodo, M. McClish, G. Entine, P. Dokhale, and S. R. Cherry. 2004. Position sensitive APDs for small animal PET imaging. *IEEE Trans Nucl Sci* 51:91–95.

30. Ziegler, S. I., B. J. Pichler, G. Boening, M. Rafecas, W. Pimpl, E. Lorenz, N. Schmitz, and M. Schwaiger. 2001. A prototype high-resolution animal positron tomograph with avalanche photodiode arrays and LSO crystals. *Eur J Nucl Med* 28:136–143.

31. Fontaine, R., F. Belanger, N. Viscogliosi, H. Semmaoui, M. A. Tetrault, J. B. Michaud, C. Pepin, J. Cadorette, and R. Lecomte. 2005. The architecture of LabPET (TM), a small animal APD-based digital PET scanner. In *IEEE Nuclear Science Symposium Conference Record*, vol. 5, pp. 2785–2789. IEEE, Piscataway, NJ.

32. Pichler, B. J., B. K. Swann, J. Rochelle, R. E. Nutt, S. R. Cherry, and S. B. Siegel. 2004. Lutetium oxyorthosilicate block detector readout by avalanche photodiode arrays for high resolution animal PET. *Phys Med Biol* 49:4305–4319.

33. Grazioso, R., N. Zhang, J. Corbeil, M. Schmand, R. Ladebeck, M. Vester, G. Schnur, W. Renz, and H. Fischer. 2006. APD-based PET detector for simultaneous PET/MR imaging. *Nucl Instrum Methods Phys Res A* 569:301–305.

34. Dautet, H., P. Deschamps, B. Dion, A. D. Macgregor, D. Macsween, R. J. Mcintyre, C. Trottier, and P. P. Webb. 1993. Photon-counting techniques with silicon avalanche photodiodes. *Appl Optics* 32:3894–3900.

35. Zappa, F., A. L. Lacaita, S. D. Cova, and P. Lovati. 1996. Solid-state single-photon detectors. *Opt Eng* 35:938–945.

36. Cova, S., M. Ghioni, A. Lacaita, C. Samori, and F. Zappa. 1996. Avalanche photodiodes and quenching circuits for single-photon detection. *Appl Optics* 35:1956–1976.

37. Buzhan, P., B. Dolgoshein, L. Filatov, A. Ilyin, V. Kantzerov, V. Kaplin, A. Karakash, et al. 2003. Silicon photomultiplier and its possible applications. *Nucl Instrum Methods Phys Res A* 504:48–52.

38. Stapels, C., W. G. Lawrence, J. Christian, M. R. Squillante, G. Entine, F. L. Augustine, P. Dokhale, and M. McClish. 2005. Solid-state photomultiplier in CMOS technology for gamma-ray detection and imaging applications. In *IEEE Nuclear Science Symposium Conference Record*, pp. 2775–2779. IEEE, Piscataway, NJ.

39. Yamamoto, K., K. Yamamura, K. Sato, S. Kamakura, T. Ota, H. Suzuki, and S. Ohsuka. 2007. Development of multi-pixel photon counter (MPPC). In *2007 IEEE Nuclear Science Symposium Conference Record*, vols. 1–11, pp. 1511–1515. IEEE, Piscataway, NJ.

40. Mazzillo, M., F. Nagy, D. Sanfilippo, G. Valvo, B. Carbone, A. Piana, P. G. Fallica, and S. Coffa. 2013. Silicon photomultipliers development at STMicroelectronics. *Proc SPIE* 8773.

41. Marrocchesi, P. S., M. G. Bagliesi, K. Batkov, G. Bigongiari, M. Y. Kim, T. Lomtadze, P. Maestro, F. Morsani, and R. Zei. 2009. Active control of the gain of a 3 mm × 3 mm silicon photomultiplier. *Nucl Instrum Methods Phys Res A* 602:391–395.

42. Brown, R. G. W., K. D. Ridley, and J. G. Rarity. 1986. Characterization of silicon avalanche photodiodes for photon-correlation measurements. 1. Passive quenching. *Appl Optics* 25:4122–4126.

43. Brown, R. G. W., R. Jones, J. G. Rarity, and K. D. Ridley. 1987. Characterization of silicon avalanche photodiodes for photon-correlation measurements. 2. Active quenching. *Appl Optics* 26:2383–2389.

44. Mazzillo, M., G. Condorelli, D. Sanfilippo, G. Valvo, B. Carbone, G. Fallica, S. Billotta, et al. 2009. Silicon photomultiplier technology at STMicroelectronics. *IEEE Trans Nucl Sci* 56:2434–2442.

45. Renker, D., and E. Lorenz. 2009. Advances in solid state photon detectors. *J Instrum* 4.

46. Nagano, T., K. Yamamoto, K. Sato, N. Hosokawa, A. Ishida, and T. Baba. 2011. Improvement of multi-pixel photon counter (MPPC). In *2011 IEEE Nuclear Science Symposium and Medical Imaging Conference (NSS/MIC)*, pp. 1657–1659. IEEE, Piscataway, NJ.

47. Piemonte, C. 2006. A new silicon photomultiplier structure for blue light detection. *Nucl Instrum Methods Phys Res A* 568:224–232.

48. Stewart, A. G., V. Saveliev, S. J. Bellis, D. J. Herbert, P. J. Hughes, and J. C. Jackson. 2008. Performance of 1-mm(2) silicon photomultiplier. *IEEE J Quantum Electron* 44:157–164.

49. Roncali, E., and S. R. Cherry. 2011. Application of silicon photomultipliers to positron emission tomography. *Ann Biomed Eng* 39:1358–1377.

50. Kolb, A., E. Lorenz, M. S. Judenhofer, D. Renker, K. Lankes, and B. J. Pichler. 2010. Evaluation of Geiger-mode APDs for PET block detector designs. *Phys Med Biol* 55:1815–1832.

51. Musienko, Y., E. Auffray, A. Fedorov, M. Korzhik, P. Lecoq, S. Reucroft, and J. Swain. 2008. SSPM readout of LSO, (Lu-Y)AP:Ce and PWO-II pixels for PET detector modules. *IEEE Trans Nucl Sci* 55:1352–1356.

52. Llosa, G., N. Belcari, M. G. Bisogni, G. Collazuol, S. Marcatili, P. Barrillon, C. de la Taille, et al. 2009. Energy, timing and position resolution studies with 16-pixel silicon photomultiplier matrices for small animal PET. *IEEE Trans Nucl Sci* 56:2586–2593.

53. Dolgoshein, B., V. Balagura, P. Buzhan, M. Danilov, L. Filatov, E. Garutti, M. Groll, et al. 2006. Status report on silicon photomultiplier development and its applications. *Nucl Instrum Methods Phys Res A* 563:368–376.

54. Acerbi, F., A. Ferri, G. Zappala, G. Paternoster, A. Picciotto, A. Gola, N. Zorzi, and C. Piemonte. 2015. NUV silicon photomultipliers with high detection efficiency and reduced delayed correlated-noise. *IEEE Trans Nucl Sci* 62:1318–1325.

55. Gatti, E., and V. Svelto. 1966. Review of theories and experiments of resolving time with scintillation counters. *Nucl Instrum Methods* 43:248–268.

56. Post, R. F., and L. I. Schiff. 1950. Statistical limitations on the resolving time of a scintillation counter. *Phys Rev* 80:1113–1113.

57. Cova, S., A. Lacaita, and G. Ripamonti. 1991. Trapping phenomena in avalanche photodiodes on nanosecond scale. *IEEE Electron Device Lett* 12:685–687.

58. Lacaita, A. L., F. Zappa, S. Bigliardi, and M. Manfredi. 1993. On the bremsstrahlung origin of hot-carrier-induced photons in silicon devices. *IEEE Trans Electron Dev* 40:577–582.

59. Acerbi, F., A. Ferri, A. Gola, M. Cazzanelli, L. Pavesi, N. Zorzi, and C. Piemonte. 2014. Characterization of single-photon time resolution: From single SPAD to silicon photomultiplier. *IEEE Trans Nucl Sci* 61:2678–2686.

60. Dinu, N. 2016. 8: Silicon photomultipliers (SiPM). In *Photodetectors*, ed. B. Nabet, pp. 255–294. Woodhead Publishing, Cambridge, UK.

61. Nemallapudi, M. V., S. Gundacker, P. Lecoq, E. Auffray, A. Ferri, A. Gola, and C. Piemonte. 2015. Sub-100 ps coincidence time resolution for positron emission tomography with LSO:Ce codoped with Ca. *Phys Med Biol* 60:4635–4649.

62. Schaart, D. R., S. Seifert, R. Vinke, H. T. van Dam, P. Dendooven, H. Lohner, and F. J. Beekman. 2010. LaBr(3):Ce and SiPMs for time-of-flight PET: Achieving 100 ps coincidence resolving time. *Phys Med Biol* 55:N179–N189.

63. Degenhardt, C., G. Prescher, T. Frach, A. Thon, R. de Gruyter, A. Schmitz, and R. Ballizany. 2009. The digital silicon photomultiplier: A novel sensor for the detection of scintillation light. In *2009 IEEE Nuclear Science Symposium Conference Record*, vols. 1–5, pp. 2383–2386. IEEE, Piscataway, NJ.

64. Frach, T., G. Prescher, C. Degenhardt, R. de Gruyter, A. Schmitz, and R. Ballizany. 2009. The digital silicon photomultiplier: Principle of operation and intrinsic detector performance. In *2009 IEEE Nuclear Science Symposium Conference Record*, vols. 1–5, pp. 1959–1965. IEEE, Piscataway, NJ.

65. Haemisch, Y., T. Frach, C. Degenhardt, and A. Thon. 2012. Fully digital arrays of silicon photomultipliers (dSiPM): A scalable alternative to vacuum photomultiplier tubes (PMT). *Phys Proc* 37:1546–1560.

66. van Dam, H. T., G. Borghi, S. Seifert, and D. R. Schaart. 2013. Sub-200 ps CRT in monolithic scintillator PET detectors using digital SiPM arrays and maximum likelihood interaction time estimation. *Phys Med Biol* 58:3243–3257.

67. Lerche, C. W., J. E. Mackewn, R. Ayres, B. Weissler, P. Gebhardt, T. Solf, B. Goldschmidt, et al. 2012. MR image quality and timing resolution of an analog SiPM based pre-clinical PET/MR insert. In *2012 IEEE Nuclear Science Symposium and Medical Imaging Conference Record (NSS/MIC)*, pp. 2802–2806. IEEE, Piscataway, NJ.

68. Mackewn, J. E., C. W. Lerche, B. Weissler, K. Sunassee, R. T. M. de Rosales, A. Phinikaridou, A. Salomon, et al. 2015. PET performance evaluation of a pre-clinical SiPM-based MR-compatible PET scanner. *IEEE Trans Nucl Sci* 62:784–790.

69. Llosa, G., C. Lacasta, N. Belcari, M. G. Bisogni, G. Collazuol, S. Marcatili, P. Barrillon, et al. 2009. Monolithic 64-channel SiPM matrices for small animal PET. In *2009 IEEE Nuclear Science Symposium Conference Record*, vols. 1–5, pp. 2658–2661. IEEE, Piscataway, NJ.

70. Thompson, C. J., A. L. Goertzen, P. Kozlowski, F. Retiere, G. Stortz, V. Sossi, and X. Z. Zhang. 2013. Measurement of energy and timing resolution of very highly pixellated LYSO crystal blocks with multiplexed SiPM readout for use in a small animal PET/MR insert. In *2013 IEEE Nuclear Science Symposium and Medical Imaging Conference (NSS/MIC)*, pp. 1–5. IEEE, Piscataway, NJ.

71. Dokhale, P., C. Stapels, J. Christian, Y. F. Yang, S. Cherry, W. Moses, and K. Shah. 2009. Performance measurements of a SSPM-LYSO-SSPM detector module for small animal positron emission tomography. In *2009 IEEE Nuclear Science Symposium Conference Record*, vols. 1–5, pp. 2809–2812. IEEE, Piscataway, NJ.

72. Krizsan, A. K., I. Lajtos, M. Dahlbom, F. Daver, M. Emri, S. A. Kis, G. Opposits, et al. 2015. A promising future: Comparable imaging capability of MRI-compatible silicon photomultiplier and conventional photosensor preclinical PET systems. *J Nucl Med* 56:1948–1953.

73. Miller, M., J. Zhang, K. Binzel, J. Griesmer, T. Laurence, M. Narayanan, D. Natarajamani, S. Wang, and M. Knopp. 2015. Characterization of the Vereos digital photon counting PET system. *J Nucl Med* 56:434.

74. Levin, C. S., S. H. Maramraju, M. M. Khalighi, T. W. Deller, G. Delso, and F. Jansen. 2016. Design features and mutual compatibility studies of the time-of-flight PET capable GE SIGNA PET/MR system. *IEEE Trans Med Imaging* 35:1907–1914.

75. Bouckaert, C., S. Vandenberghe, and R. Van Holen. 2014. Evaluation of a compact, high-resolution SPECT detector based on digital silicon photomultipliers. *Phys Med Biol* 59:7521–7539.

76. Georgiou, M., G. Borghi, S. V. Spirou, G. Loudos, and D. R. Schaart. 2014. First performance tests of a digital photon counter (DPC) array coupled to a CsI(TI) crystal matrix for potential use in SPECT. *Phys Med Biol* 59:2415–2430.

Acquisition electronics

THOMAS K. LEWELLEN

4.1 Basic goals of an acquisition system   91
4.2 Pulse integration and basic signal multiplexing   94
4.3 System topologies   97
4.4 Supporting software   103
4.5 Summary   112
References   113

4.1 BASIC GOALS OF AN ACQUISITION SYSTEM

As is evident in the chapters of this book, there are many different kinds of detector systems, and that leads to many different options in detector electronics. The role of the acquisition electronics system is to gather data from detector units and pass it to a host system for storage. This seemingly simple task presents many issues for a system designer to consider. Among them are (1) data rates and size, (2) physical space constraints, (3) power and heat issues, (4) scalability, (5) cost, and (6) special constraints (e.g., work in a magnetic field). In general, the data to be collected for each interaction in a system includes the amount of energy deposited in a detector or detector array, when the event occurred, and for imaging systems, some kind of spatial decoding of where the event occurred. For our purposes, we begin the exploration of acquisition electronics by defining two basic approaches to the design of such systems: (1) acquire all the "raw" data from the detectors (basic pulse information for each event) and (2) prequalify or process data before it is transferred to the host computer. The raw approach gives the image formation and data analysis tools maximum flexibility but can lead to very large data sets and very high data transfer rates. The prequalify approach generally uses various criteria to reject events not expected to be of interest and to preprocess some of the data to reduce the data bandwidth needed to transfer data to the host computer.

To further complicate the discussion, there are both analog and fully digital detectors. Analog detectors output a voltage or current pulse when an event occurs (Figure 4.1). The area under the pulse is related to the total amount of energy deposited in the detector element, and the shape of the pulse reflects both the scintillation process and any bandwidth-limiting components between the event location and the point the pulse is brought out of the detector for processing. A digital detector, for our purposes, is a device that reads out the event data directly into a digital format within the detector unit and does not provide any analog data to the acquisition electronics system (e.g., the Philips digital [Frach et al. 2009]). However, to date the vast majority of nuclear medicine imaging systems use analog detector modules, and that will be our focus. We mention some of the mode changes in acquisition electronics design for digital detectors later in this chapter. The topology selected for any detector system may be influenced by what a given laboratory or manufacturer has previously developed and can be adapted to the current design. If there are no major modifications required, adaptation of existing processing boards can be a major time and cost saver. However, we should also note that if a designer is faced with major modifications to existing boards and possible compromises in

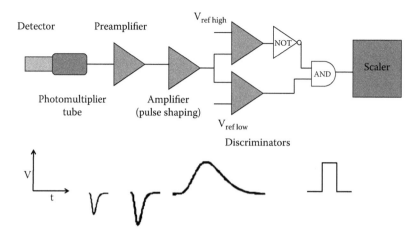

Figure 4.1 Classic single-channel pulse analyzer chain depicting the analog signal path from the detector through shaping and the subsequent processing by a pulse height analyzer (discriminator pair) that selects an energy range and counts (scaler) how many events fall within that energy range.

the desired data to be collected, then it may well be worth the significant cost and effort required to develop entirely new processing electronics. Undertaking such a design task is nontrivial, and such a decision should be undertaken carefully after a survey of available options in terms of commercial electronics offerings, possible collaborations with other universities or commercial vendors, and a realistic evaluation of the in-house capabilities to design and fabricate custom systems.

Figure 4.1 depicts the classic single-detector spectroscopy system based on a scintillation crystal and a photomultiplier tube (PMT). The idealized pulse processing is indicated for each stage at the bottom of the figure. For a more complete discussion of pulse processing and shaping techniques, we suggest a text such as the relevant chapters in Knoll (2010). For our purposes, it is sufficient to note that the pulse from the detector is normally characterized by a fast rise time and an exponential-like falloff as the signal is produced (in this example, light from the scintillator amplified by the PMT). After the detector, there may be a preamplifier—an amplifier that drives cables that may or may not actually amplify the signal. While most preamplifiers try to maintain the pulse shape, there is always some bandwidth limiting inherent in the devices, and the pulse shape may be altered. Then, in a classical analog system, the pulse is shaped—in this case, integrated and converted into a Gaussian-like pulse shape with a height proportional to the amount of energy that was deposited in the detector. In this example, a pair of comparators is used to define a pulse height region (window) for pulses that are to be counted. The comparator outputs results in a logic pulse that triggers a counter. The main point here is that the detector pulse is typically integrated and then either stored by the host computer (the raw mode) or preprocessed in some way (like applying an energy window—a window around the pulse heights we wish to accept).

In either raw or prequalify mode, we can list a series of common features that the acquisition system should provide. The first we have already mentioned—the integration of the detector signal so that the data we acquire represents all of the energy deposited in the detector. The integration can be done with a shaping amplifier or similar analog device, as indicated in Figure 4.1. An alternative that is used in many systems is to continuously digitize the pulse from the preamplifier (or even directly from the detector) and perform the pulse integration in a device such as a field-programmable gate array (FPGA) (Haselman et al. 2009a). In either case, the system designer has to consider count rate effects and how to correct for them. The two most common issues are pulse pileup and baseline shift. Figure 4.2 illustrates the pileup problem. To obtain the most accurate estimate of the amount of energy deposited in a detector, one would like to integrate the pulse until the tail reaches the baseline (as indicated by the 4τ arrow in the figure, where τ is the decay time of the scintillation light). But if a second event occurs in the same detector module within the integration period (second pulse sequence in Figure 4.2), then the integrated pulse will be distorted, providing what appears to be a single event with incorrect energy information. Pileup is the main cause of the loss of events as the count rate increases in an imaging system (the main component to the system dead time in a properly designed

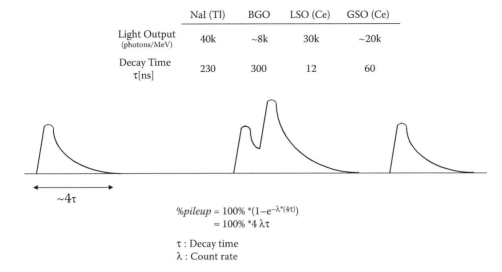

	NaI (Tl)	BGO	LSO (Ce)	GSO (Ce)
Light Output (photons/MeV)	40k	~8k	30k	~20k
Decay Time τ[ns]	230	300	12	60

$\sim\!4\tau$

$\%pileup = 100\% * (1 - e^{-\lambda * (4\tau)})$
$\approx 100\% * 4\,\lambda\tau$

τ : Decay time
λ : Count rate

Figure 4.2 Illustration of pulse pileup—two detector pulses overlap, resulting in a loss of counts when the pulses are integrated. The table at the top shows decay times (τ) of scintillators, and the equation determines the percent pileup as a function of count rate and decay time.

acquisition system). Figure 4.2 shows a basic estimate of pileup loss as a function of count rate and pulse decay time. One solution to reduce pileup loss is to shorten the integration period so that the system can detect two pulses. However, the second pulse of such a pair will still be distorted by the tail of the previous pulse (we get the correct number of pulses, but not all the correct energy information). To reduce such effects, the detector pulse shape can be changed with techniques such as clipping, where the pulse is inverted, delayed, and reflected back on itself to create a shorter pulse—but in the process also lose some of the accuracy of the measurement of how much energy was deposited in the detector (do not integrate all of the information in the original detector pulse). Another solution is to detect the pulses arriving and simply reject any pulses that pile up within the integration time window. This results in loss of data but solves the pulse distortion issue. For more sophisticated systems, several approaches to correct pileup have been developed, and we will illustrate one in more detail later in this chapter. Of course, if a system count rate is low enough, pileup is not a problem. But keep in mind the count rate you need to worry about is the raw detector count rate that is presented to whatever is doing the pulse integration—and it is the count rate before any qualification criteria are imposed. In a typical imaging system with an energy window qualification, the count rate to the pulse integration system can be much higher than the observed count rate after the energy window is applied.

A second common feature is a trigger system—some way to detect that a pulse has arrived. The trigger often records a time at which the event occurred, as well as providing a logic pulse signaling other parts of the electronics that an event is to be processed. There are a variety of methods for generating such a trigger. The simplest approach is a simple threshold detector that sends out a logic pulse if the detector signal goes above a low-level set point. Often, they have logic to not send out a pulse if the signal is too short (a noise spike) or, in some cases, too long (pileup). There are other options that are often used for fast timing applications where one desires to generate a trigger (and associated time stamp) consistently no matter what the size of the pulse is. The techniques include variations of constant fraction timing (Knoll 2010), crossover timing, and statistical approaches, such as fitting idealized pulse shapes to a fully digitized pulse (preserving the pulse shape for the estimation process). In a PET scanner, the acquisition system may include all the needed processing (analog or digital) to perform fast timing determination and impose timing windows on the coincidence data for dividing the events into prompts and randoms. The system may also only impose loose criteria on the timing to reduce the amount of data to be sent to the host and let the fine timing window(s) be applied during image reconstruction.

A third common feature is that of energy selection. Most systems impose energy-based criteria on qualifying an event to be processed. This can be done in the main acquisition electronics system or after the fact (if all the energy information is being saved) by the host computer. Such qualification can be as simple as applying a single energy window to the integrated signal to accept or reject it. But the process can become more demanding for some types of detectors that can generate more than one signal per event (e.g., detector systems designed to provide depth-of-interaction [DOI] data) or need to preserve more of the energy distribution information for subsequent processing by the image reconstruction algorithm. Even when more detailed energy information is being preserved for subsequent processing, the acquisition system may still impose a window criterion on a summation of all the signals for a single detected event to reject data that has no chance of being used in the image reconstruction process. For example, a PET scanner with DOI capability might impose a restriction that any event with a total energy deposition of less than 300 keV be rejected.

For imaging applications, the location of the event within the detector volume is needed. The different imaging systems, such as PET and SPECT, generally use different detector designs, and the decoding of the position information is often unique to the particular detector design. A system designer has to weigh the many issues we listed earlier to decide where to implement the position decoding algorithms. For example, it might be best to record the data event by event (list mode) and perform all of the position decoding during the image reconstruction process—resulting in large data files. Alternatively, the acquisition electronics can include such decoding in its basic design—as is often the case in single-photon imaging systems and essentially all non-time-of-flight PET scanners—and store the data in sinogram format.

We will revisit many of the above common features as we look more carefully at some of the typical designs for acquisition systems.

4.2 PULSE INTEGRATION AND BASIC SIGNAL MULTIPLEXING

We have already mentioned that pulse integration can be implemented in either analog or digital format. In the end, we need to digitize the pulses related to energy and position if the integration is done via analog components. We generally show nice smooth diagrams of what a detector pulse looks like. But reality is not that simple, and the pulses from the detector are generally noisy. Often, the detector pulse is smoothed (bandwidth limited) by design to reduce the noise—in particular if one is using direct digitizing of the pulse shape and wants to sample the shape accurately. Figure 4.3 illustrates such a case where the main detector pulse (the unfiltered pulse) has a great deal of noise that is smoothed with an appropriate analog filter and then digitized (in this case, at a 65 MHz sampling frequency). Note that such smoothing changes the pulse shape but does not change the pulse integral value. Even when a system designer uses a shaping amplifier for the integration, some degree of pulse smoothing is always present just due to cables and other passive components between the detector and the amplifier. The when the amplifier is used for pulse integration, the integration time is normally determined by selection of resistance and capacitance values in the analog pulse shaping or integration circuit. By changing these time constants, the integration time can be optimized for the type of detector pulse being processed. When analog integration is used, the typical system sends the integrated pulse to an analog-to-digital converter (ADC). In this configuration, the ADC is normally set up to digitize the height of the pulse from a shaping amplifier (an alternative is to shape but not integrate the pulse in the amplifier and then use the ADC to integrate the charge in pulse during a time interval defined by other external electronics—gating the signal to the ADC). If a designer decides to save cost and share one ADC between multiple detectors with analog integration, a sample-and-hold circuit is often placed between each amplifier and the ADC. This circuit stores the peak pulse height, and then each of the stored signals are routed to the ADC one at a time. This approach is no longer as common given the reduction in cost in ADCs and the preference of many designers to digitize the pulse directly and do the integration digitally. When doing the integration digitally, one must optimize the pulse bandwidth shaping (Figure 4.3) to the ADC sampling rate. The faster the sampling rate, the higher the cost and power and heat requirements. Thus, the system designer must understand all of the downstream pulse processing requirements to ensure that the sampled pulse has the necessary information. If the sampling rate is relatively slow, then the pulse must be smoothed enough so that the noise "spikes" do not produce biased results. As can be appreciated in the example in Figure 4.3, if the 65 MHz sampling rate were used with the unfiltered pulse,

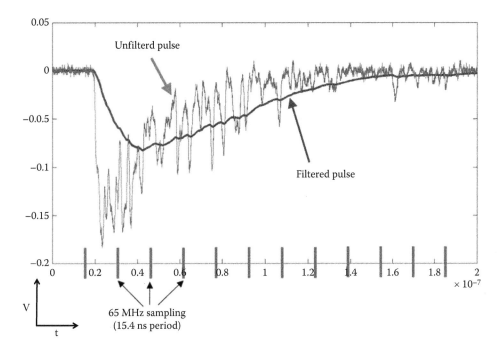

Figure 4.3 Example of one approach to digital sampling of a detector pulse. In this case, the analog pulse is first filtered to reduce noise and then sampled at a rate appropriate for the filtered pulse shape.

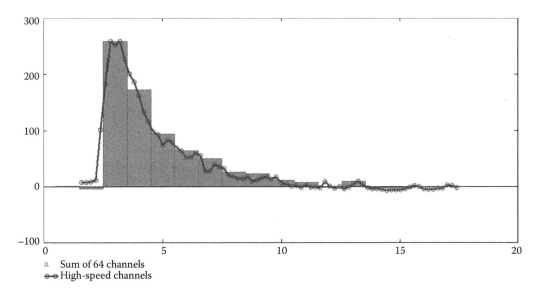

Figure 4.4 Comparison of slower and faster sampling of a pulse. For timing, the slow pulse sample does not sample the rise time of the pulse adequately for most timing applications. The faster sampling allows better timing estimation since it provides at least some samples on the rising edge of the pulse. For estimation of timing from digital sampling, the needed timing resolution will impact the minimum sampling rate required.

major errors would occur in the final pulse integration due to the peaks and valleys in the noise spectrum. By filtering the pulse, the ADC samples will be closer to the real pulse shape and accurate pulse integration will be achieved.

If timing is being done digitally, it may be necessary to use a higher digitizing rate for the signal being used to generate the timing information. Consider Figure 4.4, where data is plotted from a digitizing system connected to a 64-channel PMT. In this system, the 64 anodes are bandwidth limited to about 20 MHz and sampled at 60 MHz. At the same time, the common anode signal (common to all 64 channels and thus representing the total signal in the PMT) is digitized at a higher rate (in this example, at 300 MHz). If the sum of the 64 individual channels is compared with the high-speed channel, we should get essentially the same integrated values representing the total signal generated in the detector—and that is indeed the case in this example. However, when the signals are processed to determine a timing value (e.g., for a PET coincidence system), the signal digitized at 300 MHz preserves more of the leading edge of the detector pulse, and that leads to a much better estimation of when the pulse actually started with whatever timing algorithm is utilized (such as a fitted model pulse or a constant fraction estimator).

As we mentioned earlier, pulse pileup and baseline shifts are issues that impact both analog and digital integration schemes at higher count rates. Many analog shaping amplifiers include circuits to reduce baseline shift (Knoll 2010), but these circuits often have to be adjusted for a given detector and count rate range to get the best results. If one is using a digital integration scheme, there are several methods that can be implemented to sample the baseline between pulses and correct for changes in the baseline value. Typically, some averaging of many samples is used before adjusting the baseline (Haselman et al. 2010). Several pulse pileup correction schemes have also been developed for both analog pulse integration systems (Lewellen et al. 1990) and digital implementations (Haselman et al. 2010; Liu et al. 2007). Most of these schemes assume information is known about the correct pulse shape for a nonpileup event and then use various methods to recover the pulse, subtracting the tail effects from the previous pulse(s). We will provide a few more details of one such technique for a digital system in Section 4.4.

As mentioned above, if a designer wishes to minimize the number of ADCs in a system, some form of multiplexing or pulse summing may be utilized. An illustration of the sample-and-hold approach with the various held signals routed through an ADC is illustrated in Figure 4.5, where the basic front end organization of a General Electric Advance PET scanner is depicted. In this case, each detector block consists of four PMTs coupled to an array of crystals. The blocks were arranged such that the signals from six blocks were summed into X, Y, and Z (two position indices and one total energy value), along with timing data, and then held after the amplifier stages and multiplexed through a single bank of ADCs (one ADC for each of the signals). The advantage to this scheme is the reduction in the number of ADCs required and a reduction in the number of data channels to send to the host. Some of the disadvantages are that you still need to apply analog gain adjustments for each major element in the chain, and you can develop a nonuniform dead-time response in the multiplexing scheme if the block detector rates are mismatched or very high. A somewhat similar approach has been used for "classic" Anger gamma camera designs where the PMT signals were normally summed using a resistive network to produce an X, Y coordinate pair and a total energy signal. Those values are then digitized and sent to the host computer (Figure 4.6). The main advantage is the reduction of the number of signal channels (reducing between 35 and 70 PMT signals to just 3 signals). The main disadvantage is that the entire detector contributes to dead time since all of the PMTs are treated as one ensemble of signal sources. As acquisition systems have evolved, they have addressed the disadvantages of both the simple multiplexing and summing schemes we have just looked at.

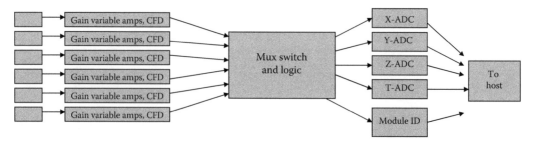

Figure 4.5 Example of multiplexing detector data into a set of ADCs as used in a General Electric Advance PET scanner. Each detector block (left) has four PMTs, and a group of six detector blocks are multiplexed into four ADCs to process events. CFD, constant fraction discriminator; Mux, multiplixer.

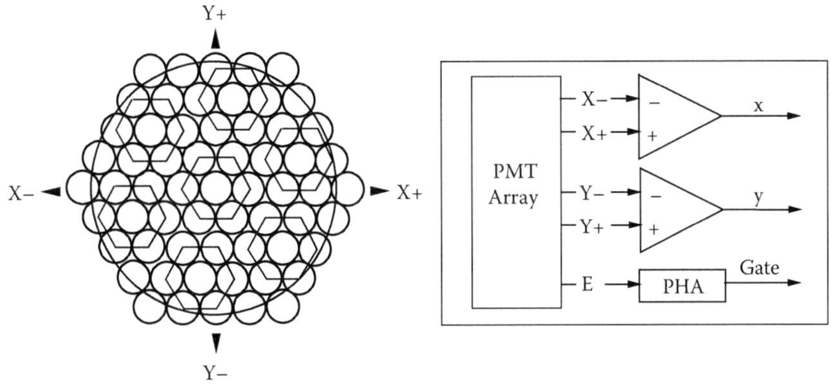

Figure 4.6 Another example of multiplexing of many PMTs into a smaller number of signals as used in the classic Anger camera. Each PMT (small circles in the left figure) is connected to three resistive summing circuits: X, Y (position) and E (energy for the pulse height analyzer [PHA]). This scheme is utilized in a similar way in modern detector systems, such as block detectors and multianode PMTs.

4.3 SYSTEM TOPOLOGIES

There are many topologies that have been adopted to link the detectors to the host computer(s). The design of a given topology generally takes into account the expected data rates at each step of the acquisition process and the cost of implementing a given system. A major consideration is the potential for data loss due to part of the acquisition chain not being able to handle the count rate. We have already discussed pulse pileup and noted that in a properly design system, it is the major contribution to dead time (data loss). Thus, as the system design is analyzed, the ideal goal should be to have all the stages past the integration step fast enough to not contribute to data loss. Of course, there are limitations in any real-world system and the designer must once again choose options based on the expected rates, what data loss might be acceptable (and correctable), and the limitations of existing hardware or the expected cost to develop new hardware. There is not one perfect solution, and there is considerable variety in the kinds of systems that have been developed.

Starting from the detector module, the first step in the acquisition system design is the processing of the detector signals. If it is an analog detector, this usually means implementing either integrating amplifiers or a set of free-running ADCs. Along with the pulse integration or digitization, there is usually some sort of event trigger circuit to alert the downstream electronics that an event has been detected. In the case of a PET system, this circuit also provides the timing information that will be needed to determine whether events are in coincidence. This data is then collected and any processing at the detector level is performed. As we have discussed, this can include position calculations, energy or timing qualifications, or other processing designed to reduce the amount of data to be passed on to the next stage of the acquisition system. At this stage of the processing, one normally finds a device such as an FPGA that does the main event processing. It is also common to find a dedicated local processor for control and command functions and assisting in sending data to the next stage of the acquisition system. These processors are often small single-board computers or, even more common in modern systems, a processor embedded in the FPGA. Such processors in the FPGA can be either hardware cores of common processors or soft processors built up from gates and memories in the FPGA. The soft processors are generally slower than the hardware core options, but offer the advantage of optimizing the processor configuration for the tasks to be performed. The final data is then packaged and sent on to the host processor. How these different stages are configured and interconnected is what we term the topology of the acquisition system.

In our laboratory, we like to refer to three basic categories of system topologies: (1) summing, (2) parallel, and (3) serial. In each case, one can define a variant, which we term layered, to reflect the insertion of data reduction or multiplexing processing in the chain before the data gets to the host system. Data reduction includes options such as applying energy windows early in the processing to reject events we are certain we do not want to process or computing position information before sending it on to the host. In this chapter, we use the term *multiplexing* to indicate that the data shares some common processing elements (such as a set of ADCs) that require the detector data to be sequenced in some manner through the common processing element, such as we have already shown in Figure 4.5, without loss of information other than possible dead-time issues if the data rate is greater than the common processing element bandwidth. One example of the summing approach (e.g., Figure 4.6) we have already mentioned. A more generic depiction of this approach is shown in Figure 4.7. While we have chosen to use the term *summing*, we can also refer to this approach as one form of data reduction, with the aim of reducing the amount of data to be transferred to the host for each event. The major advantage of such an approach is to reduce the needed bandwidth capability of the host to accept data and to make the data sets smaller. The primary disadvantage of a simple summing scheme is that some of the information from the detector array, such as pulse shape, can be lost.

The basic parallel approach is to take the data from each detector and pass it to the host on a very fast bus or large collection of parallel data ports. Let us consider some examples of a layered version of a parallel topology. One such scheme is diagramed in Figure 4.8—a simplified diagram of the kind of layering found in some

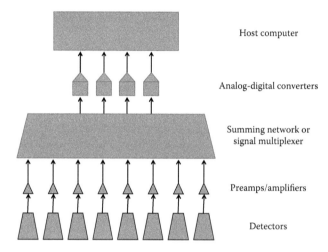

Figure 4.7 One of the possible acquisition topologies. In this example, the detector signals are summed (e.g., Figure 4.6) or multiplexed (e.g., Figure 4.5) and then the signals are digitized and passed on to a host computer.

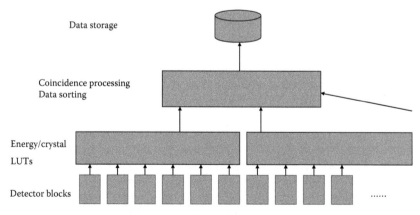

Figure 4.8 The use of summing or multiplexing can be generalized as depicted, where each detector feeds a set of electronics to process the basic data, much as shown in Figures 4.4 and 4.5. But the detectors are grouped so that there are parallel data paths from them to the host computer to find a balance between complexity and data rates. The goal is to reduce data rates at each layer, using fewer parallel channels to pass on the data to the next layer. This topology is sometimes termed layered parallel. In this example, the detector analog signals are digitized then routed to processing electronics to apply corrections for energy spectra differences between crystals and convert the detector analog data into discrete crystal addressed. Then the data is combined routed to electronics to apply coincidence and energy selection criteria and sort the data into sinograms for storage.

PET scanners. In this case, the detector block information is digitized (using either analog integration with ADCs or direct digitizing of the detector pulses) and passed to a processing unit. Usually, the detector bocks are grouped to several processing boards based on board capacities and data rate expectations. Continuing on with Figure 4.8, the middle layer does the position calculation (in this example, assigning an event to a crystal in a block detector) and applies energy windows to the data to reject events not of interest for the particular target applications of the scanner. The data is then passed to the next layer, where coincidence timing is done to determine if an event is a prompt or random. The data may also be binned into a convenient representation, such as a sinogram or list-mode data, and then passed on to a storage subsystem (what we normally term the host in this chapter). Another example of a layered parallel topology is the acquisition system used in ClearPET (Streun et al. 2002). For this system, the designers multiplexed four 64-channel PMT-based detectors to a single FPGA for event processing and then connected each of the several FPGA boards to the host computers using optical links.

Another approach to what we term parallel is to put each ADC on a very high-speed, multiple-bit data bus, such as the VME bus. Figure 4.9 shows a simplified diagram of such a system where each ADC occupies an address on the VME bus and can do direct memory writes (direct memory access [DMA]) of the data to the host computer memory (Bruyndonckx et al. 2001). One can argue this is not really a direct parallel scheme since there is a wide data bus to the host rather than several direct connections (one connection to the host per ADC). However, if the designer is careful to ensure that the data bus can handle the data rates, we still regard this as a parallel system in that a wide data bus of parallel bits is used to connect the ADCs to the host.

Another layered approach that has been used in various systems is to take advantage of the built-in high-speed serial communication capabilities found in most modern FPGAs. A general diagram of such a system is shown in Figure 4.10. Typically, the detector signals are processed by an FPGA (after either going through an analog integration system or, more commonly in recent years, using free-running ADCs to digitize the pulse train from the detector) and data is preprocessed as desired, which can include exchange of data between the FPGAs using their built-in serial communication channels. Such exchanges can include timing information that can be used to determine if events are in coincidence for a PET system or combing of data from different photosensors on a large crystal for determination of event position or any number of data reduction schemes.

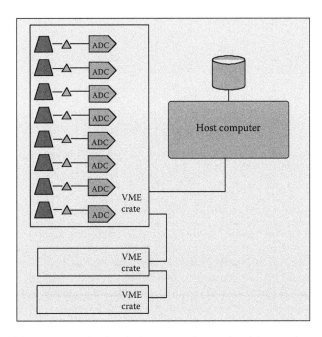

Figure 4.9 Fully parallel—one example. If each detector is digitized and then its data sent to the host computer without any summing or multiplexing, it is often termed a fully parallel topology. This figures shows one such example where the detector data is digitized and then sent to the host computer over a VME bus. Adapters for most host computers allow the VME bus to be an extension to the host I/O or memory bus. This topology is often used for detector testing but is also used in some PET systems (e.g., Bruyndonckx et al. 2001).

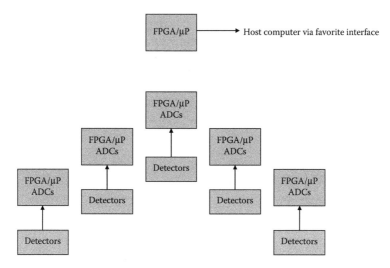

Figure 4.10 Another example of a layered topology where the detector signals are processed by local FPGAs and then the data is shared between the FPGAs using the device's built-in high-speed serial communications resources, with one of the FPGAs acting as the gateway to the host computer. For clarity, the high-speed serial links are not shown in the figure. This topology is sometimes called distributed parallel. High-speed serial communication built into the FPGAs is used to send data around. This allows coincidences to be determined locally by the FPGAs, which reduces the data rate to the host interface FPGA.

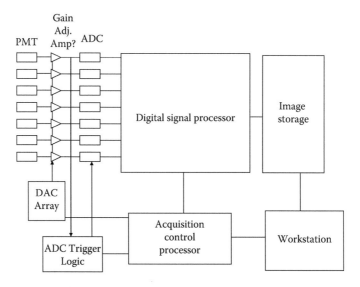

Figure 4.11 Generic diagram of the topology used in most modern scintillation cameras where each PMT is digitized and event position estimation, including corrections for spatial and energy linearity, as well as flood uniformity, is applied in processing logic in the detector head before being passed on to the host computer. Adj., adjustable.

The data that is determined to be of interest for the host computer can then be sent up to the host via multiple channels (such as the parallel optical links used in ClearPET) or via a single high-speed channel from a single node within the collection of FPGAs processing the detector data—as indicated in Figure 4.10. The concentration of data from the detector arrays into a single high-speed data path to a single host computer is a common trend in more recent acquisition system designs. In fact, most modern gamma cameras (single-photon imaging systems) use a topology similar to this approach in that each PMT is digitized and then processed by one or more devices, such as FPGAs. Corrections such as linearity, energy, and center of rotation are generally applied on the fly by the FPGAs and the data stored by a local processor. Figure 4.11 shows such a generic system where a single large crystal is viewed by an array of PMTs.

There are many options for how the acquisition electronics are connected to the host computer. We have already indicated options for parallel connections, including multiple parallel data ports, VME bus, and optical links (such as Glink). To that short list one can add the many variations of the PCI bus extenders—connecting the internal PCI bus found in just about all computers to external peripherals. There are other options, such as network switches that allow a number of acquisition nodes to be connected to a computer using Ethernet or fiber channel hardware. Another class of connection of the acquisition node to the host computer is that of the serial peripheral buses, such as USB and FireWire (or even custom Ethernet systems that do not use switches but point-to-point connections using Ethernet hardware). There are also new standards such as Thunderbolt that can either support some of the other standards (such as PCI Express, USB, and FireWire). As we consider these various options for any system, we need to once again consider data transfer rates, cost of development, and cost of construction. Part of the cost of development is to what extent we can use standard bus protocols to reduce the amount of development time (in terms of both hardware and software). Table 4.1 lists some of the many bus and communication options to connect acquisition node electronics together and to connect the system to the host computer. Some of the options, such as the standard PCI bus and the VME bus, are generally found inside of card rack systems (or crates) that have the bus on the backplane, along with power connections to allow the insertion of cards for the various functions desired. The cards can include standard commercial hardware such as single-board computers or arrays of devices such as FPGAs designed for general-purpose computing and control. More often than not, those systems found inside imaging systems that use one of these standard buses with many parallel data paths use the crates and perhaps some single-board computers or motion controllers, but implement the main acquisition functions on custom cards tailored to the specific scanner needs. The main reason for this approach is that the general-purpose cards often are not easily adaptable to the specific tasks needed for the scanner and result in

Table 4.1 List of some of the bus options for use in data acquisition systems

Bus technology	Rate	Rate
Ethernet (10BASE-X)	10 Mbit/s	1.25 MB/s
Fast Ethernet (100BASE-X)	100 Mbit/s	12.5 MB/s
10 Gigabit Ethernet (10B+GASE-X)	10 Gbit/s	1.25 GB/s
100 Gigabit Ethernet	100 Gbit/s	12.5 GB/s
FireWire 400 (IEEE 1394)	400 Mbit/s	50 MB/s
FireWire 800 (IEEE 1394b)	800 Mbit/s	98 MB/s
External PCI Express 2.0x1	4 Gbit/s	500 MB/s
External PCI Express 2.0x2	8 Gbit/s	1 GB/s
External PCI Express 2.0x4	16 Gbit/s	2 GB/s
External PCI Express 2.0x8	32 Gbit/s	4 GB/s
External PCI Express 2.0x16	64 Gbit/s	8 GB/s
GPIB/HPIB (IEEE 488)	64 Mbit/s	8 MB/s
Fiber Channel 1	1 Gbit/s	100 MB/s
Fiber Channel 4	4 Gbit/s	531 MB/s
USB 2.0 (full speed)	12 Mbit/s	1.5 MB/s
USB 3.0 (super speed)	5 Gbit/s	600 MB/s
eSATA (SATA 600)	6 Gbit/s	600 MB/s
Thunderbolt	10 Gbit/s × 2	781 MB/s × 2
HDMI 1.3	10.2 Gbit/s	1.275 GB/s
IEEE 802.11 n (wireless)	600 Mbit/s	75 MB/s
IEEE 802.11ac (wireless, maximum theoretical speed)	6.93 Gbit/s	850 MB/s
VME64	400 Mbit/s	40 MB/s
SPI bus (maximum)	100 Mbit/s	12.5 MB/s
HyperTransport (1 GHz, 16 pairs)	32 Gbit/s	4 GB/s
PCI Express 2.0 (× 16 links)	128 Gbit/s	16 Gb/s

having to use more cards and components than would be required with a custom card—making the system less compact and not as power efficient.

The trend is to use various forms of serial buses (e.g., Ethernet, Express PCIx1, USB, and FireWire) to interconnect the various major components of the acquisition system to each other and the host. Using bus systems that are used extensively in other commercial devices and desktop computers (e.g., USB and Ethernet) also allows the use of relatively low-cost components and the adaptation of standard software drivers and low-level application program interface (API) software provided by the various computer operating system vendors—for both the host and embedded processors or single-board computers that are generally included in the acquisition node electronics. Systems using Ethernet have generally taken one of two routes (Figure 4.12). One approach is the traditional direct connection of each node to a switch that is in turn connected to the host. An alternative that removes the switch and makes managing the system easier is to implement a point-to-point connection scheme where each node receives or generates data and passes it to the next node and eventually to the host computer. This approach requires more custom software work to be done in implementing the nodes, but the hardware parts are common and the many embedded processors and single-board computer options available to a designer make this a practical way to proceed. Such topologies are not limited to Ethernet but can also be implemented with some standard serial buses (e.g., FireWire) or by utilizing the point-to-point serial interconnection hardware found in many FPGAs and similar programmable devices that support standards ranging from SPI to Express PCIx1. For many research systems, the USB serial bus standard has been adopted due to a wide variety of inexpensive USB hardware available and the support of USB by all common computers. The downside of a USB approach is the necessity of using USB hub devices to connect the nodes to the host—it does not support a direct daisy chain serial bus connection, such as provided by FireWire or SPI. But the hubs are also inexpensive and can be either purchased or fabricated from standard parts. There are differences in these various bus options that include not only cost, but also efficiency. For example, the FireWire bus supports large data packets and has minimal overhead, but also can only support a maximum of 64 nodes. USB 2 can support up to 256 nodes, but has smaller maximum data packet sizes and more overhead for each transfer request—reducing the maximum data transfer rates. The newer USB 3 standard significantly increases the speed and maximum data packet sizes on the bus, but requires more wires in the interconnections than USB 2. When using standard serial bus protocols (e.g., FireWire and USB 2/3), most protocols allow definition of multiple logical devices in each node, as well as options on how the data is to be transmitted. For example, FireWire and USB support both asynchronous and isochronous transfers. When using isochronous transfers, each node is allocated fixed time segments to send data to the host. Used for a great deal of high-speed, continuous data streams like video, it can also be used for systems with only a few detectors (e.g., a dual-headed gamma camera). For more complicated systems, the

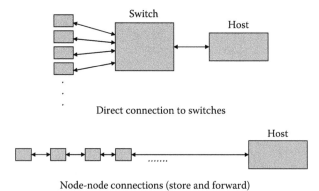

Figure 4.12 Examples of using Ethernet as the means to interconnect various components in the detector chain. The top figure illustrates the use of an Ethernet switch or hub to connect the detector units to the host. The bottom figure shows the use of the Ethernet hardware to connect the detector modules and the host on a single bus and let the detector modules process data and forward data of interest to the other modules and the host. This typically results in more complexity at each detector node (e.g., custom electronics and software) and does not allow the use of off-the-shelf hardware.

asynchronous mode is more appropriate since it allows the host to allocate time for each node to transfer data as needed. The use of multiple logical devices per node allows implementation of a command and control communication channel that is independent of the data channel. In such a system, the host usually sends a request to each node to see if they have data or need to report any errors or other conditions. If there is data, then the host issues a read command to the data channel and a block of data is sent to the host. In all cases, the bus protocol has error checking and send and receive acknowledgment logic built into the bus protocol so that any transmission errors can be trapped and new requests issued as needed. If there are other control functions needed, such as gantry motions, either an additional card can be added or one of the nodes can be configured with additional logical units to service such requirements.

The many serial bus options allow implementation of many different types of topologies. Probably the three most common are depicted in Figure 4.13. The *bus* topology refers to a serial bus where each node is connected to the serial bus and can communicate directly with the host computer or each other. The *tree* topology reflects using serial bus systems that require each node to only talk directly to the host computer, and even then through hubs such as used in USB systems. The *token pass* option is where we use serial links to connect nodes in a circular arrangement so that each node can create or forward data to the next. There is generally one node that determines when there is a collection of data that should be passed to the host computer. When using any kind of serial transfer scheme, it is important to define data structures and command and control protocols that minimize the bus overhead for each transfer. To get the maximum transfer rates, data generally needs to be packed into large data frames that use the maximum block transfer size the bus can support. In designs were each acquisition node transfers data directly to the host, that usually means that sequence of occurrence of events from each detector module is not maintained. The general solution is to include with each event a time tag matched to a master clock or other system-wide reference so that events can be sorted by time after the host receives data. In systems that use event-by-event gathering in a local computing node, the sequence can be preserved. But such system architectures then require more compute speed at the gathering node and often do not preserve all of the possible data information from the detectors. If data is being acquired in list mode, then the host system often does all of the data sorting and, in the case of PET, fine coincidence determination based on the time stamps in the data stream. Such options again point out the necessity of the acquisition system designer having a good understanding of how the data is to be utilized.

4.4 SUPPORTING SOFTWARE

If one is developing his or her own system or using a commercial system with various logic elements, there is always the issue of software tools and packages that support the tasks to be performed. One approach is to use a commercial software system that supports various kinds of commercial acquisition products. Examples include LabVIEW and MATLAB. Both of these programming environments support a variety of instruments connected with standard interfaces such as Ethernet or the general-purpose instrument bus (GPIB). There are tools within these environments to allow control of many standard cards found on commercial acquisition and control systems, such as devices from National Semiconductor, adapters for VME bus card cages, GPIB bus devices, and microtelecommunication computer crates and cards. There are also a large variety of analog and digital processing cards for VME and Fastbus systems, as well as more traditional standards used in my physics laboratories, such as the Nuclear Instrumentation Module (NIM) and Computer Automated Measurement and Control (CAMAC) standards. There are many companies making ADC cards and other general-purpose processing cards for these systems, and they have been used in many detection acquisition and control systems. They have not made a great impact in PET and SPECT imaging applications. Issues such as the physical space taken up by the card crates, the challenges of adapting general-purpose devices for imaging system-specific tasks, cost, and in some cases, speed of data acquisition have led most nuclear medicine imaging system commercial vendors and research laboratories to other solutions.

For prototyping detectors, the NIM, CAMAC, and VME modules are still used by many groups. There are some open-source software systems for acquiring data from such systems that have been developed by high-energy and nuclear physics groups that are adaptable for prototyping PET and SPECT detectors. For example,

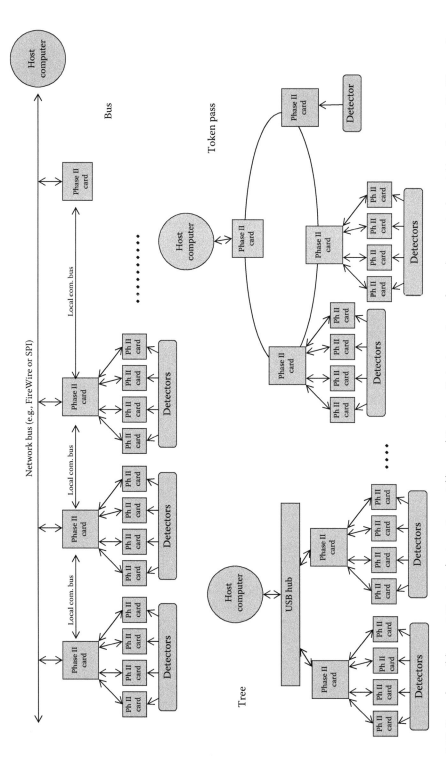

Figure 4.13 Several possible acquisition topologies using serial bus architectures. Detector units can be nodes on a single serial bus (such as FireWire, top), or set up as a tree topology, such is used in most USB implementations (bottom left) or in pass-and-forward ring topologies (bottom right). Ph II, Phase II.

a software system called ORCA (Howe et al. 2004) can be used to control and acquire data from a wide variety of devices, including VME modules, and is written so individuals can extend its functionality. There is also an open-source project for both software and hardware for prototyping PET detectors and imaging systems—OpenPET (Moses et al. 2010). Figure 4.14 depicts one realization of an OpenPET system. Some of the hardware subsystems are being manufactured for sale, but all of the schematics, board layouts, firmware, and software are available to research groups at no charge for their own fabrication. Since it is an open-source project, many different groups are contributing to developing the various options for the system. However, all of these options may not be the best solution for a given set of tasks, and one may have to consider designing and implementing a system of his or her own to meet performance, space, and power requirements.

For many systems, be it a commercial set of components such as VMEbus cards, use of OpenPET, or developing your own electronics, there are standard software tools one can use for development and modification. There have been significant advances in digital signal processors (DSPs), FPGA, and programmable systems on a chip (PoSCs), and most modern systems make heavy use of these powerful and reconfigurable devices. Selection of the tools and design of the software or firmware written with those tools are critical tasks in terms

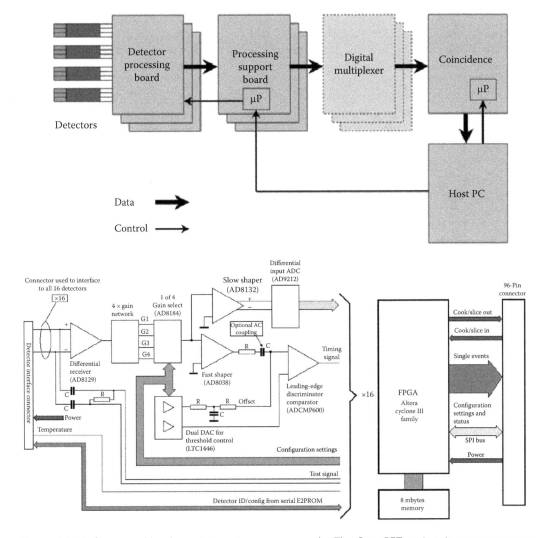

Figure 4.14 Software and hardware integration—one example. The OpenPET project is an open-source approach to both hardware and software for different acquisition topologies. Depicted here is a typical OpenPET implementation for a basic detector block. Note that DAC stands for digital to analog converter and SPI references the standard Small Peripheral Interface bus.

of not only realizing the initial goals for the system, but also supporting that system in the future. On the host computer side, the basic acquisition software can generally be written in a high-level language like C++, given the quality of the mainline compilers. If one is using one of the standard external bus architectures (e.g., USB, FireWire, or PCI Express), it is often possible to use the system APIs to control and get data from your acquisition electronics without having to write any low-level drivers—a major advantage in terms of both development time and ongoing support. For the acquisition nodes, one again has the advantage of using high-level tools provided by the device vendors for the configuration and programming of his or her specific unit. These include the design tools for the logic blocks in devices such as FPGAs and PSoCs, tools for defining soft embedded processors, and editors and compilers for the embedded processor the tools have created. Often, the tools include simulators for all of the logic that has been defined, detailed editing tools for refining where logic blocks are actually placed in the physical device, and pin editors to connect and define the properties of the device pins to the desired logic blocks within them. In all cases, one can usually work in an integrated development environment with a graphics interface for editing, compiling, debugging, and tracking code revisions.

While these tools are powerful and convenient (as well as usually free or a very minimal cost), they can also be a problem. They often have sophisticated optimizers that will rewrite code or, in the case of FPGAs and similar devices, creatively place the various logic blocks in the device based on complex rules that the developer may not be fully aware of. One example is the placement of logic blocks in an FPGA device. For various reasons, the optimizing compiler may put some blocks close to input/output (I/O) pins and others farther away. If the logic is processing time-critical data or having to process many parallel inputs without introducing time skewing, these differences in block placement can lead to subtle errors that may only occur a small percentage of the time. Such problems can be very challenging to isolate and understand and may well require the designer to override the optimizer and force block placements in specific areas of the FPGA device. Of course, there is always the problem of other potential errors in any compiler and optimizer that can be difficult to isolate since the compiler can be changing the order of execution of tasks from what the programmer thought was being defined, or may do some rewriting of code that also produces unexpected results. These sorts of problems lead to longer than expected development times and may even come up after a system is running due to updates in the compilers used and a subsequent code revision for the system that introduces problems due to the changes in the compiler behavior. Thus, any development project—be it totally new or adapting another system—can be faced with unexpected development and support issues, and the project design process has to make allowances for such events.

To illustrate a few of the points we have discussed, let us take a look at one acquisition system that was developed in my laboratory. I choose this system only because it is the one I have the most familiarity with, not because I hold it up as a shining example of what can be done. We were faced with a variety of detector designs (Champley et al. 2009; Lewellen et al. 2007). Most of them utilize some form of statistical estimation process for positioning the event within the detector that we wished to perform as a data reduction step in the acquisition chain. We also wanted to be able to support a wide variety of topologies, including all of those depicted in Figure 4.15. The specification that the acquisition nodes be able to work within different environments, such as strong magnetic and radio frequency (RF) fields, as found in MRI systems, was added. After surveying many options (including standard NIM, CAMAC, VME, and micro telecommunications computing architecture (µTCA) modules; OpenPET; and a variety of commercial and academic general acquisition boards), we decided to undertake development of our own version of a system. In so doing, we knew we were entering into a long development project, but one that would best serve the needs of our laboratory.

The strengths of our laboratory included strong software development skills, excellent collaborations with the FPGA group in our electrical engineering department, and prior experience with adapting a commercial board system to our first preclinical imaging system (Lewellen et al. 2005). The basic design was based on keeping the analog portions of the system to a minimum and moving as much of the pulse processing functions as possible into an FPGA to allow for rapid adaptation to new detector schemes. As a result, the approach is that of continuous digitization of detector pulse information, with all of the pulse integration, timing, and corrections being implemented in the FPGA. The analog subsystem can be very basic, consisting of the detector, a driver to convert the detector pulses into differential line pairs (a signal transmission technique that is good for rejection of noise from the surroundings), and pulse bandwidth limiting as needed for

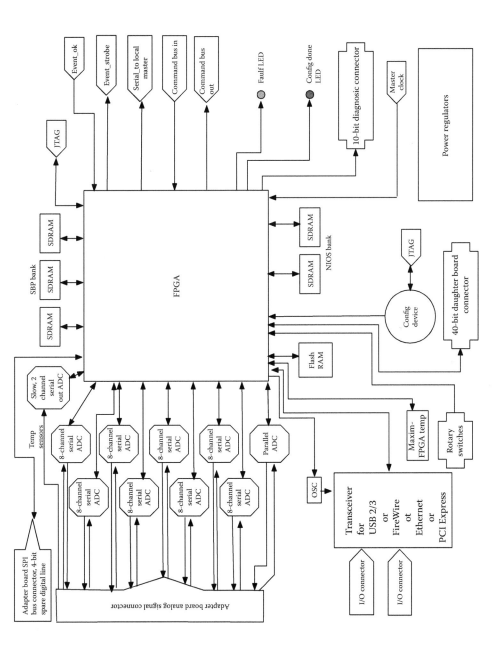

Figure 4.15 An example of an FPGA-based building block for a data acquisition system developed at the University of Washington providing 64 channels of input for basic position decoding and one high-speed input for timing determination, with all of the pulse processing being done within the FPGA. LED, light-emitting diode; SDRAM, synchronous DRAM; temp, temperature; config, configuration.

the ADCs used on the digitizing board. That analog subsystem was kept as separate adapter boards between the basic detector and the digitizing board (what we termed the Phase II board, as listed in Figure 4.13). Since board design and layout is a costly undertaking, particularly if one wishes to minimize the number of layers in the printed circuit board and still be able to make hundreds of connections to the FPGA, we further decided to design one general-purpose board that can be adapted to different tasks based on the components and firmware installed (Lewellen et al. 2011). The final board can support up to 64 channels of 60 MHz ADCs used for basic pulse integration and related tasks and one channel of a much faster ADC (>300 MHz) for processing a common timing signal from the analog subsystem if it is provided. Each Phase II board is then a node in the chain responsible for processing up to 64 channels of data. Those channels could be from a single 64-channel PMT or could be multiple different detectors with fewer signals per detector. For cases where the basic detector provides more than 64 parallel channels of data per event, we can either use an application-specific integrated circuit (ASIC) in the analog subsystem to provide some sort of summing or multiplexing (e.g., row or column summing) or multiple Phase II boards that use a local SPI bus for coordination of tasks. Figure 4.15 depicts the basic block diagram of the board, and as apparent, it is built around a powerful FPGA.

The basic pulse processing blocks that have been developed for the FPGA include those illustrated in Figure 4.16 (Haselman et al. 2009a, 2009b; Johnson-Williams et al. 2011). While many different timing algorithms, such as leading edge and contract fraction, have been implemented in FPGAs, we choose to use a modeled pulse approach. In this approach, a reference pulse shape is used to fit to the measured pulse. Then the reference pulse, which originally generated an effective sampling rate much higher than the standard rate used at run time for pulse processing, is used to find the time when the pulse started. There are tools developed for this arrangement to allow the FPGA to generate this high-quality standard pulse using the "slow" ADCs on the card for each of the ADC inputs. Thus, differences in pulse shape from different sensors on the detector can be included and the optimal reference pulse used at run time. Algorithms are also available for baseline correction by continuously measuring the baseline between pulses and adjusting it as needed. One advantage of continuous pulse digitizing is the ability to also apply different methods for pulse pileup correction. One such method is illustrated in Figure 4.16, where again, a standard pulse shape is used to correct the pulse distortions before final pulse integration and timing determination are done.

Figure 4.17 shows one implementation of a processing chain in the Phase II card FPGA for doing statistical estimation of the X, Y, and Z coordinates of an event in a monolithic crystal coupled to a 64-channel PMT or silicon photomultiplier (SiPM) array. In this case, the detector provides a common pickoff for timing, so that the signal is routed to the high-speed ADC on the card and the FPGA code applies the pileup correction algorithm and then performs the timing determination. The 64 "slow" channels are also pileup corrected and then integrated and used for the position estimation process. Making a high-speed implementation of such an estimation process in an FPGA takes some significant effort to run quickly. In this example, external memories and a decreasing grid search approach were used to get the needed speed. The grid search is done in stages in a pipeline to allow time to load tables from the external memories and still meet the data processing rate goal (of up to 450,000 pulses per second for this application). The data is then packaged into transmission buffers under the control of an embedded soft processor (in this example, an Altera FPGA is used with a NIOS II soft processor). The embedded processor has been designed with direct access to the needed buffers in the FPGA and is interfaced to the bus system to the host processor. The Phase II card was originally intended to be used with FireWire, but with the advent of USB 3, the design was changed to support either USB 2 or 3 bus connections to the host. As noted earlier, the issue of bus selection (type and speed) is not normally a problem of any one mode in the system, but a problem of the combined data rates from all nodes sending data down the same bus system. In some implementations, auxiliary data can be shared between the various nodes to make other decisions on what data is to be sent to the host. For example, each node can impose some degree of energy qualification on the data to reject events that the designer is sure will not be of interest. Other criteria, such as coarse timing windows (e.g., only accept events within 40–60 ns of each other) or geometric restrictions on which detectors are allowed to be paired for an event (e.g., reject events where the line of response is outside the scanner field of view), can be imposed by the nodes sharing data with a central controller that issues event OK or reject commands to the various acquisition nodes. In the example system being used for this discussion, the Phase II card (Figure 4.15) provides specific control lines for such communications, as

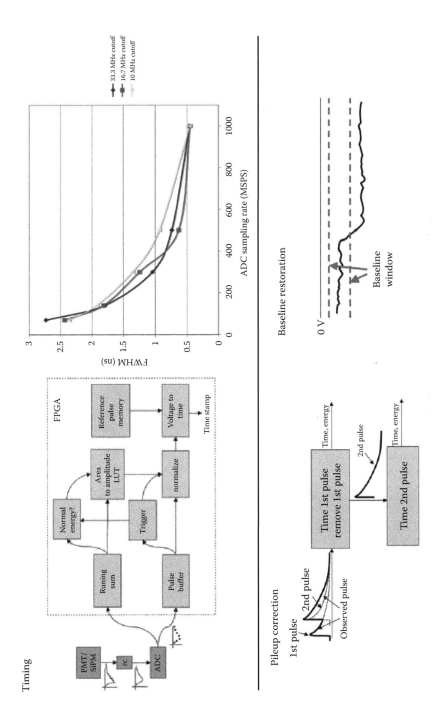

Figure 4.16 Examples of one approach to performing basic pulse processing for timing, pulse pileup, and baseline restoration within an FPGA (and used in the system depicted in Figure 4.15). In this example, the bandwidth limiting of the pulse from the photodetector is accomplished with resistor-capacitor (RC) filter to match the pulse noise to the digitizing speed.

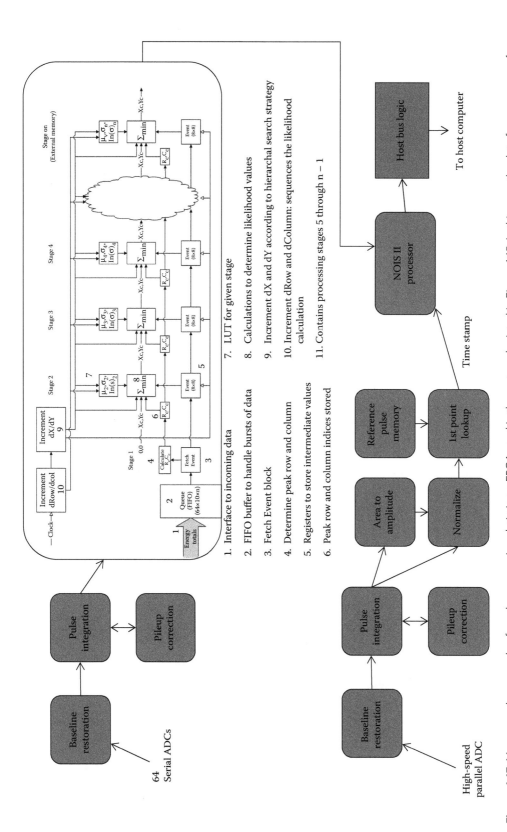

1. Interface to incoming data
2. FIFO buffer to handle bursts of data
3. Fetch Event block
4. Determine peak row and column
5. Registers to store intermediate values
6. Peak row and column indices stored
7. LUT for given stage
8. Calculations to determine likelihood values
9. Increment dX and dY according to hierarchal search strategy
10. Increment dRow and dColumn: sequences the likelihood calculation
11. Contains processing stages 5 through n − 1

Figure 4.17 More complex example of a pulse processing chain in an FPGA used in the system depicted in Figure 4.15. In this case, the data forms an array of sensors on a monolithic scintillator slab and is processed with statistical estimation techniques to determine the position of the event in X, Y, and Z after the digitized pulses from each sensor as corrected for pileup and baseline, and then integrated. A separate processing chain does the timing estimation. FIFO, first in, first out.

Table 4.2 Example of a possible list-mode data packet from a node in an acquisition system

	Raw data	Raw data	Processed data	Processed data
Parameter	Number of bytes	Notes	Number of bytes	Notes
Module ID	2	Bits 12–15: Acquire configuration ID number Bits 8–11: Subnode branch (0..3 for first local master, 0..3 for second-tier local masters) Bits 6..7: Board clock rate flag Bits 0..5: Detector ID	2	Bits 12–15: Acquire configuration ID number Bits 8–11: Subnode branch (0..3 for first local master, 0..3 for second-tier local masters) Bits 0..7: Detector ID
Singles	2	16 bits for the detector pointed to by module ID	2	16 bits for the detector pointed to by module ID
TAC data	1	8 most significant bits	1	8 most significant bits
Time stamp	8	Scalers for board clock rate	8	Scalers for board clock rate
Number of signals	8	Number of digitized detector signals to follow (keyed to acquired configuration ID)	8	Number of digitized detector signals to follow (keyed to acquired configuration ID)
Signal packet 1	2	Up to 16 bits per packet	2	Up to 16 bits per packet
More packets	2	Up to 16 bits per packet	2	Up to 16 bits per packet
Last packet	2	Up to 16 bits per packet	2	Up to 16 bits per packet

Note: This example is one of the formats supported by the Phase II card of Figure 4.15.

well as several SPI bus connectors that can be used for such communications or other control functions, such as commands to logic that might be included in the analog subsystem. One might ask what if the detectors are digital devices sending out bit serial data streams instead of analog pulses. The basic operation of the acquisition system could be the same. In our illustration case with the Phase II card, the 64-channel ADCs are physically integrated circuits with eight ADCs in each chip. The communication between these ADCs and the FPGA is via high-speed-bit serial data streams. Thus, without any modifications other than removing the ADC chips and connecting jumpers so that the digital detector signals can be routed to the serial interface connections to the FPGA that were used for the ADCs, the basic card can support up to eight digital detectors.

This kind of architecture also allows considerable flexibility in the organization of the data to be sent to the host. The simplest format for the acquisition nodes is probably list mode. But even here, the designer can encode a wide variety of data. Table 4.2 shows one scheme that has been implemented for the Phase II card we have been using as an illustration. In this case, the data from each node is sent to the host computer via a serial bus and the data from each node is collected in list mode. The structure in this particular example is designed to support a wide variety of detectors (the detector ID), as well as a wide variety of topologies, such as shown in Figure 4.13, where the detectors may or may not be directly on the bus to the host (the use of the subnode branches listed in the table). With such a structure, the system developers can write general-purpose code for the node and host processors. For example, the standard host acquisition software written in our laboratory checks to see how many nodes are on the bus and then allocates list-mode buffers for each node and collects separate files for each node. During the bus enumeration process, each node informs the host of the type of node it has been configured to be and provides other bookkeeping information. During acquisition, the host runs a thread for each node and each thread checks its node for data, transfers data when the node responds that it is ready, and checks for any error conditions. At the end of acquisition, there are additional steps to ensure each node's data buffer has been transferred, even if it was only partially full at the end of acquisition. Once all the data is on the host, the software sorts the data via the time stamps into a single list-mode file. The software only acquires data from nodes that are directly on the bus to the host, so if there are subnodes, the data for the subnodes is packed into the same list-mode file for the main node and the postacquisition software can sort out the actual detector data using the subnode fields in the module ID bytes in the basic data packet, as defined in Table 4.2.

4.5 SUMMARY

As we have discussed, there are many ways to implement a data acquisition system. One can adapt general laboratory systems using software tools such as LabVIEW and MATLAB and standard commercial modules using a variety of standards (GPIB, µTCA, VME, etc.). This option generally has the advantage of rapid implementation, but usually has the drawbacks of higher cost and compromises in data reduction options or count-rate imitations. The use of a system already developed for another system (university-based or a commercial scanner system) can be advantageous if it conforms to the detector types and gantry geometries to be supported. However, there can be major issues in terms of ease of support (are all the source codes available? how detailed is the documentation?), and this may place major restrictions on future detector designs in terms of how the data is decoded and the ability to preserve the raw detector data for advanced processing. Designing your own system can address issues of flexibility and support of new and innovative detector designs, but has the very significant burden of the development time and cost. Making a final choice of which approach to use for a given system is a major task in itself. This chapter began with a statement of some of the major issues to consider in a basic system. Perhaps the most important first step is to carefully define the goals of the system in terms of both hardware and software tasks and specifications. It cannot be overemphasized that in designing any acquisition system, the total detector or scanner design must be taken into account. What data rates can be expected for the final applications? Where are major data processing steps being done—at the detector level, at an intermittent level in the acquisition system, and by the host computer after the acquisition is completed? Where are corrections for the data done—steps such as timing skew, pileup, detector linearity issues (sensitivity, position estimation, and energy decoding), scatter correction, detector finite-resolution effects, and dead time? Where is it best to allocate limited resources—how much in hardware design and fabrication, firmware design and coding, and postacquisition processing? When adapting or designing such a system, it is often a major advantage to be able to reconfigure the various elements without having to modify the hardware or lay out new boards. The use of many FPGA and similar devices in modern systems reflects the goal to allow major revisions by "simply" changing firmware. But even then, the selection of components such as FPGAs offers challenges since there is a very broad range in price and performance. Does one design for ultimate flexibility with the use of large, expensive FPGAs or design for well-defined cost and performance points with more modest FPGAs, recognizing that additional cards or a card redesign might be necessary at some point in the future? These are questions that each design team must address early in the process. Even when a user is purchasing a fully commercial solution, these same questions must be asked and answered to determine which of the many commercial options solve the immediate goal, as well as issues of long-term flexibility and serviceability. One of the major advantages of modern electronics and components is that one has a wide range of options and the freedom to solve a given problem with a variety of solutions that best fit the budget and capabilities of any single laboratory or commercial vendor.

REFERENCES

Bruyndonckx, P., Wang, Y., Tavernier, S., and Carnochan, P. (2001). Design and performance of a data acquisition system for VUB-PET. *IEEE Trans. Nucl. Sci.*, 150–156.

Champley, K.M., Lewellen, T.K., MacDonald, L.R., Miyaoka, R.S., and Kinahan, P.E. (2009). Statistical LOR estimation for high-resolution dMiCE PET detector. *Phys. Med. Biol.*, 54, 6369–6382.

Frach, T., Prescher, G., Degenhardt, C., De Gruyter, R., Schmitz, A., and Ballizany, R. (2009). The digital silicon photomultiplier—Principle of operation and intrinsic detector performance. In *IEEE Nuclear Science Symposium and Medical Imaging Conference*, Orlando, FL, pp. 1959–1965.

Haselman, M., DeWit, D., McDougald, W., Lewellen, T.K., Miyaoka, R.S., and Hauck, S. (2009a). FPGA-based front-end electronics for positron emission tomography. In *ACM/SIGDA Symposium on Field-Programmable Gate Arrays*, Monterey, CA, pp. 93–102.

Haselman, M., Hauck, S., Lewellen, T.K., and Miyaoka, R.S. (2009b). FPGA-based pulse parameter discovery for positron emission tomography. In *IEEE Nuclear Science Symposium and Medical Imaging Conference*, Orlando, FL, pp. 2956–2961.

Haselman, M.D., Hauck, S., Lewellen, T.K., and Miyaoka, R.S. (2010). FPGA-based pulse pileup correction. In *IEEE Nuclear Science Symposium and Medical Imaging Conference*, pp. 3105–3112.

Howe, M.A., Cox, G.A., Harvey, P.J., McGrit, F., Rielage, K., Wilkerson, J.F., and Wouters, J.M. (2004). Sudbury Neutrino Observatory neutral current detector acquisition software overview. *IEEE Trans. Nucl. Sci.*, 51, 878–883.

Johnson-Williams, N.G., Miyaoka, R.S., Xiaoli, L., Lewellen, T.K., and Hauck, S. (2011). Design of a real time FPGA-based three dimensional positioning algorithm. *IEEE Trans. Nucl. Sci.*, 58, 26–233.

Knoll, G.F. (2010). *Radiation Detection and Measurement*. John Wiley & Sons, New York.

Lewellen, T.K., Janes, M., Miyaoka, R.S., Gillispie, S.G., Park, B., and Herrmannnsfeldt, G. (2005). A firewire based data acquisition system for small volume positron emission tomographs. In *14th IEEE-NPSS Real Time Cofi erence 2005*, Stockholm, pp. 260–264.

Lewellen, T.K., MacDonald, L.R., Miyaoka, R.S., McDougald, W., and Champley, K. (2007). New directions for dMiCE—A depth-of-interaction detector design for PET scanners. In *Nuclear Science Symposium and Medical Imaging Cofi erence*, vol. 5, pp. 3798–3802.

Lewellen, T.K., Miyaoka, R.S., MacDonald, L.R., DeWitt, D., and Hauck, S. (2011). Evolution of the design of a second generation FireWire based data acquisition system. In *IEEE Nuclear Science Symposium and Medical Imaging Cofi erence*, Valencia, Spain, pp. 3994–3998.

Lewellen, T.K., Pollard, K.R., Bice, A.N., and Zhu, J.B. (1990). A new clinical scintillation camera with pulse tail extrapolation electronics. *IEEE Trans. Nucl. Sci.*, 37, 702–706.

Liu, J., Li, H., Wang, Y., Kim, S., Zhang, Y., Liu, S., Baghaei, H., Ramirez, R., and Wong, W.H. (2007). Real time digital implementation of the high-yield-pileup-event-recover (HYPER) method. In *IEEE Nuclear Science Symposium and Medical Imaging Conference*, Honolulu, HI, pp. 4230–4232.

Moses, W.W., Buckley, S., Vu, C., Peng, Q., Pavlov, N., Choong, W.S., Wu, J., and Jackson, C. (2010). OpenPET: A flexible electronics system for radiotracer imaging. *IEEE Trans. Nucl. Sci.*, 57, 2532–2537.

Streun, M., Brandenburg, G., Larue, H., Zimmermann, E., Ziemons, K., and Halling, H. (2002). A PET system based on data processing of free-running sampled pulses. In *IEEE Nuclear Sciences Symposium and Medical Imaging Cofi erence*, Norfolk, VA, pp. 693–694.

SPECT instrumentation

WEI CHANG, MICHAEL ROZLER, AND SCOTT D. METZLER

5.1	Introduction	116
5.2	SPECT instrumentation	117
	5.2.1 Objective	117
	5.2.2 Hardware and software of SPECT systems	117
	5.2.3 Basic issues	117
	5.2.4 System perspective	118
	5.2.4.1 Imaging considerations	118
	5.2.4.2 Geometries of SPECT imaging	119
	5.2.4.3 Major system considerations and performance	119
	5.2.4.4 Secondary system considerations and performance	124
	5.2.4.5 Other instrumentation accessories	125
	5.2.5 Major components	126
	5.2.5.1 Collimator system	126
	5.2.5.2 Detector system	130
	5.2.6 Secondary components	135
	5.2.6.1 Mechanical system	135
	5.2.6.2 Transmission CT	135
5.3	Imaging systems	137
	5.3.1 Clinical SPECT imaging	138
	5.3.1.1 General-purpose and single-purpose SPECT systems	138
	5.3.2 Brain SPECT imaging	138
	5.3.2.1 Consideration for brain SPECT imaging	139
	5.3.2.2 Brain SPECT imaging using general-purpose systems	139
	5.3.2.3 Single-purpose brain SPECT systems	139
	5.3.3 Cardiac SPECT imaging	140
	5.3.3.1 General considerations for cardiac SPECT imaging	140
	5.3.3.2 Using general-purpose dual-head systems for cardiac SPECT imaging	141
	5.3.3.3 Single-purpose cardiac SPECT systems	142
5.4	Future directions	153
	5.4.1 Geometry	153
	5.4.2 Collimation	154
	5.4.3 Detector	154

	5.4.4	Adaptive imaging	154
	5.4.5	Dynamic imaging	154
5.5	Summary		155
Acknowledgments			156
References			156

5.1 INTRODUCTION

Since its introduction in the mid-1970s, SPECT imaging has evolved to be one of the most widely used advanced imaging techniques for clinical diagnosis and management (Kuhl et al. 1976; Budinger and Gullberg 1974; Keyes et al. 1977; Jaszczak et al. 1977). Continuing technological evolution over the years has often kept SPECT advancing in a piecewise and bottom-up manner. To avoid losing sight of the big picture and going astray, the developments of SPECT systems should also be viewed in a top-down perspective occasionally. This chapter describes the instrumentation aspects of SPECT systems from the top-down perspectives and reviews their evolution and trends of development.

SPECT instrumentation has historically been developed along two parallel tracks: general-purpose and single-purpose systems. Currently, general-purpose systems, mostly Anger camera–based dual-head systems, are ubiquitous in clinical nuclear imaging laboratories. Recently, single-purpose systems have been revived in the form of cardiac SPECT systems, after all but disappearing 20 years ago with the decline of brain SPECT imaging. It is the combination of increased clinical demands and new technologies that has led to the development of single-purpose cardiac SPECT systems. While hardware has been mainly driven by detector development, advances in software (facilitated by ever-increasing computing power) have moved iterative processing techniques into mainstream clinical imaging. Once again repeating the bottom-up development cycle, these advances have led to new approaches for special imaging applications. As a result, several new single-purpose SPECT systems have been introduced for cardiac imaging (Patton et al. 2007; Madsen 2007; Slomka et al. 2014).

These new single-purpose SPECT systems employ unconventional approaches and have opened up new directions of instrumentation development. Many recent publications have reported their unprecedented performance in both system sensitivity and spatial resolution, which far exceed the range of traditional concepts (Sharir et al. 2008; Gambhir et al. 2009; Esteves et al. 2009). These performance figures have since been widely promoted commercially and have also led to confusion and controversy in our community. Much of the confusion is caused by the current lack of objective and standardized performance metrics for assessing new SPECT systems. This is because the conventional definition and measurement methodology of spatial resolution are no longer adequate for SPECT systems using iterative reconstruction with resolution recovery techniques.

At this time, SPECT system development is at the juncture facing the question of how to best utilize new technologies to improve imaging performance and increase clinical value. To keep going forward, it is essential to have objective assessments of new imaging systems. For this purpose, it is crucial to have consensus of system performance, particularly in the definitions of system spatial resolution and system sensitivity, so that the methodology of their measurement can be standardized. A potential danger for future development is the current lack of critical assessments of new systems' performance. Obviously, assessing weaknesses critically is the first and necessary step for advances. Only through open, rigorous, and critical discussion based on scientific merits may we find the right direction and set the priorities for development. At this point, it is necessary to understand the situations and clarify the issues. To do these, we have to take a broad view to review our long-term goal and go back to the fundamentals of SPECT instrumentation.

This chapter reviews the basic concepts of SPECT instrumentation and their implications, with a special focus on cardiac SPECT imaging. It serves as a reference for readers who are familiar with the basics of nuclear medical imaging (Chandra 2011; Cherry et al. 2012) and is an update and supplement to the previous review articles (Rogers and Ackermann 1992; Chang 1996; Zeng et al. 2004; Travin 2011). We will not dwell on general and familiar knowledge, but will build upon it to discuss SPECT instrumentation's less explicit meaning and practical implications. This chapter is also intended to fill the gaps between technical developments and clinical applications by explaining the practical implications of the new designs and concepts to clarify current confusion and misconceptions. The topics include objectives, practical considerations, performance parameters, and operations of SPECT systems. We start with the basic requirements, design concepts, detection geometry, major components, and ways of implementation. Toward the end of this chapter, in-depth descriptions and analyses of several clinical cardiac SPECT systems are presented.

5.2 SPECT INSTRUMENTATION

The focus of this chapter is the hardware of SPECT systems. Due to the increased interplay between hardware and software during the image formation process, some aspects of software processing are briefly mentioned as necessary. A thorough discussion of software techniques used in SPECT imaging is presented in Chapter 7.

5.2.1 OBJECTIVE

The ultimate goal of SPECT imaging is to achieve quantitative four-dimensional (4D) mapping of radiotracer distributions in the human body to convey diagnostic information. This goal is realistically within reach (Tsui et al. 1994; Rosenthal et al. 1995; Zeintl et al. 2010). Current SPECT imaging already yields three-dimensional (3D) semiquantitative mapping of radiotracers with limited temporal information. Although the existing capabilities have permitted SPECT imaging to take on important clinical roles, many unfulfilled needs and opportunities for improvements remain. The current development of SPECT instrumentation has pursued two separate objectives. One objective is to improve imaging performance, which should lead to improved diagnostic capability, along with new clinical applications. The other objective is to address other clinical issues or operational concerns, such as to reduce imaging time, patient radiation exposure, complexity of operation, or costs involved, while maintaining the current image quality and diagnostic value (Garcia et al. 2011).

5.2.2 HARDWARE AND SOFTWARE OF SPECT SYSTEMS

Hardware and software are the two major and complementary subsystems in a SPECT system. Hardware acquires projection data; software processes the data to extract, derive, and present diagnostic information in clinically meaningful images. While the connection between the two is fundamental, their roles are different and operations often are conducted serially. Thus, in assessing and optimizing their performance, they should be treated separately, as well as jointly. It is essential to understand the potential and limitations of each subsystem. Although software processing can extract relevant information embedded in the data, it cannot create new information that is not already in the data. Thus, the quantity and quality of the acquired data are determined solely by the hardware. To optimize SPECT imaging, the emphasis should be placed on optimizing the hardware first to yield a large quantity of high-quality data. It is the synergistic effect of hardware and software advances that leads to our optimism that SPECT imaging still has considerable room for improvement to yield new useful diagnostic information.

5.2.3 BASIC ISSUES

The function of SPECT instrumentation is to detect emitted photons with detectors placed around a patient's body to acquire projection data. The ideal data set contains a large quantity of high-quality photon events recorded as a series of projection data from different directions. The quantity determines the statistical precision of the data, while the quality is related to the accuracy of the photon's emission direction. The rate of photon detection per unit activity from a source in the volume of interest is the system sensitivity, while the certainty of the photons' emission directions is related to the system's spatial resolution.

The performance of SPECT systems is mainly characterized by their system sensitivity and system spatial resolution. Collimation plays the most crucial role in SPECT systems since it is the primary determinant of system sensitivity and spatial resolution. These two parameters are inversely related in a given SPECT system; improving one is always at the expense of the other. These two terms are used loosely for now, until they are defined rigorously in Section 5.2.4.3.2.

To achieve a typical spatial resolution of 10 mm at a 10 cm distance, a SPECT system's collimator has to restrict allowed photon paths so that only about 0.01% of emitted photons reach the detector. The detected number of photons available for SPECT is typically two orders of magnitude less than that in PET imaging. Clinical SPECT imaging is always severely photon limited. Under the constraints of patient radiation exposure and imaging time, it takes 5–20 min to acquire sufficient data to produce acceptable images. Long imaging time is a major weakness of SPECT imaging; it makes images vulnerable to patient motion, limits patient throughput, and is too slow to capture fast functional changes of tracer distribution. Because detectability of diagnostic information in typical SPECT imaging is limited more by count density, or signal-to-noise ratio, than by spatial resolution (Budinger 1980; Madsen et al. 1992), it is important that SPECT systems have as high a sensitivity as possible for a given spatial resolution.

Increasing system sensitivity without compromising spatial resolution is thus the key for system designs. In general, an effective and significant sensitivity increase can only come from a fundamental change: improving detection geometry. In fact, detection geometries of existing SPECT systems are not optimized and have left considerable room for improvement. Hence, improving SPECT systems should start with optimizing detection geometry for the imaging applications. For example, one approach is to trade the size of imaging volume for sensitivity or spatial resolution improvement, as in using converging collimation for imaging a small target with relatively large detectors. After the detection geometry is settled for an appropriate imaging volume, the sensitivity or resolution compromises of collimation can be selected based on the requirements of the imaging tasks.

5.2.4 SYSTEM PERSPECTIVE

At the top level of a SPECT system are the clinical imaging applications. The middle level is the hardware concepts and architecture that provide the functionalities to accomplish the imaging; it is reflected in the general design of the components. The bottom level is the detailed designs of the components. The interaction between different components is addressed at all levels. The general considerations of these levels are elaborated in the following sections.

SPECT systems also require additional hardware components for acquiring relevant data to facilitate image acquisition, reconstruction, and corrections. This includes detector movement, patient positioning, gated acquisition, and transmission imaging for corrections of effects of attenuation and scatter. These data and operations are patient specific and have to be acquired, either simultaneously or sequentially, with projection data.

5.2.4.1 IMAGING CONSIDERATIONS

SPECT systems design and evaluation should always start with intended clinical applications. Considerations can be along three fronts:

1. Imaging target: Where is the target in the patient's body? Can an imaging volume be defined for the target? Can the target be identified and placed in the imaging volume reliably? What is the optimal detection geometry for the imaging volume? What system geometry can provide the detection geometry?
2. Clinical considerations: What are the activity distribution, uptake level, and energy range of the relevant tracers? What image features are clinicians looking for? What is the size of the clinical features of interests? How serious are the effects of attenuation given the location of the target? Is the target close to other organs with high tracer concentration? Is projection truncation a serious problem?
3. Patient considerations: Which imaging position would make patients comfortable and less vulnerable to motion? How can patients be made comfortable while remaining still during imaging, given the time frame of the imaging operation?

The answers to these questions help define the requirements and design considerations of clinical SPECT systems.

5.2.4.2 GEOMETRIES OF SPECT IMAGING

SPECT imaging is mainly a matter of geometries. At the top level, it is the detection geometry, which defines the paths of photons to the detector and the upper limit of system performance. At the second level is the system geometry, which is the actual configuration of system components to provide the detection geometry. They are elaborated as follows.

5.2.4.2.1 Detection geometry

Detection geometry is the collective paths, in 3D, through which emitted photons reach the detector system. It defines the quantity and quality of photons detected and determines a system's performance. It is desirable to place as large a detector area as close to the imaging volume as possible to subtend as large a solid angle as possible. Intuitively, a large detector system completely surrounding the patient would be the ultimate detection geometry. Even if such approaches were not cost-prohibitive, variations of patient size and long collimation distance make this geometry impractical and ineffective. As a result, detectors of medium size are used in conjunction with detector and/or collimator motion to provide the detection geometry.

Optimal detection geometry is different for different clinical tasks of SPECT imaging. For example, cylindrical detection geometry has been accepted as optimal for brain imaging. For body SPECT imaging, an adaptive elliptical cylindrical geometry that accommodates a range of body sizes and shapes, such as the body-contouring option of the dual-head geometry, has been widely used. For cardiac SPECT imaging, the optimal detection geometry has been settled over the years to be a large open arc covering the left-front half of the patient's thorax.

5.2.4.2.2 System geometry

System geometry is the actual hardware configuration of a SPECT system, which consists mainly of collimators and detectors, and allows the detection geometry to be realized. As discussed in Section 5.2.4.2.1, detector and collimator motion is often necessary to allow the system geometry to complete the necessary detection geometry for imaging. For example, a dual-head SPECT system with parallel-hole collimators has two system geometries: with the heads opposed or at a right angle (i.e., in an L-shape) to each other. These two system geometries provide the two (360°/180°) detection geometries when their corresponding (180°/90°) rotations are applied.

5.2.4.3 MAJOR SYSTEM CONSIDERATIONS AND PERFORMANCE

In this section, we focus on the four major design considerations and their corresponding performance metrics: imaging volume, sensitivity, geometrical efficiency, and spatial resolution. Because the first three are straightforward parameters, we place special emphasis on clarifying the definitions and distinctions between several different levels of spatial resolution. At the end of the section, we propose ways to combine sensitivity and spatial resolution in unified objective metrics of system performance.

5.2.4.3.1 Imaging volume

The imaging volume of an imaging system is the center of attention and is the first design aspect to be defined. It is often referred to as the field of view (FOV) on the system's transverse plane, but is typically a 3D volume defined by collimation in the system's patient aperture. The imaging volume of general-purpose single- or multihead SPECT systems using a parallel-hole collimator is a large cylindrical volume with the diameter and height of the cylinder equal to the width and axial length of the camera heads, respectively. This large imaging volume is suitable for whole-body SPECT imaging. For imaging a small organ, an effective system design is to trade the size of imaging volume for sensitivity or resolution, so that a larger fraction of the detector area is directed to the target volume; examples are in using a converging collimator for brain imaging, or pinhole collimators for small-animal imaging.

5.2.4.3.2 Sensitivity and spatial resolution

Sensitivity and spatial resolution are the two most important performance metrics of SPECT systems. They are not independent parameters and closely related in a SPECT system. In fact, they always come in pairs in a given system. They are similar concepts to, but more specific than, the quantity and quality of detected photons.

The meaning of spatial resolution has become more complex lately, as a result of iterative reconstruction techniques gaining acceptance in clinical laboratories. Modern iterative reconstruction techniques incorporating *a priori* knowledge of the image formation process are capable of improving and restoring spatial resolution while appropriately suppressing noise. However, there are many variations of iterative algorithms, each with their own set of parameters, which are capable of leading to a different reconstructed image from the same projection data. Until these iterative reconstruction techniques are standardized for system evaluation, spatial resolution depends on the algorithm used and is not a well-defined metric for assessing systems' performance. Confusion, misunderstanding, and controversies have resulted after several performance assessments of new SPECT systems were published. To address and clarify these issues, we need to begin from the conventional definitions of these two terms.

5.2.4.3.2.1 System sensitivity

System sensitivity of SPECT systems is the measured count rate per unit source activity (in cps/MBq or cpm/μCi) for a source model. It is meaningful only when its corresponding spatial resolution performance (defined in Section 5.2.4.3.2.2) and the source model are specified. The source model can be a point source in air, or a clinically relevant extended 3D source model, located at the center of the imaging volume. This definition has been well established for assessing conventional SPECT systems (AAPM 1981; Graham et al. 1995; NEMA 2007). The system sensitivity can be measured experimentally, as well as estimated (either analytically or through simulation), based on hardware design and response of the detector system. Since the system sensitivity is defined per unit acquisition time, idling time during detection should be included as part of the total acquisition time. For example, for systems in which data is acquired for only a fraction of the total imaging time, such as those where acquisition is paused during detector motion, the system sensitivity metric should be corrected for the difference in actual acquisition time and its total imaging time.

5.2.4.3.2.2 System spatial resolution

It is important to recognize that spatial resolution is a broad and general term in SPECT systems; it has several levels of meaning. At the top level is *reconstructed image resolution*, which is the combined result of the hardware's detection and sampling scheme and the software's processing and reconstruction. It is the spatial resolution of the whole system. In the middle level is the *hardware resolution*, which is conventionally defined as the system resolution for a camera–collimator system (Chandra 2011; Cherry et al. 2012). We call it "hardware resolution" here to mark its hardware origin and avoid confusion; it is reflected in the raw projection data before software processing is applied. At the bottom level are the two components, collimator resolution and the detector's intrinsic spatial resolution (ISR), which combine in quadrature to yield the hardware resolution. In the following, we will focus on the two upper levels: reconstructed image resolution and hardware resolution. To characterize SPECT systems, both levels of spatial resolution have specific and significant meaning and thus should be evaluated and presented to characterize the system's spatial resolution performance.

1. *Reconstructed image resolution*: Reconstructed image resolution is the metric that quantifies the level of clarity of the SPECT images. It is the most important one among the many levels of spatial resolution, due to its direct impact on clinical diagnosis. However, it does not present itself explicitly in clinical images and has to be assessed through a special and well-defined measurement and analysis procedure.

   Conventionally, when images of point sources are reconstructed with the standard analytic method, that is, filtered backprojection (FBP) with a ramp filter, the reconstructed image resolution should be the same as its hardware resolution, provided sampling and system alignment are adequate (Graham et al. 1995). With modern iterative processing techniques, reconstructed image resolution can be better than a system's hardware resolution due to the deconvolution effect when resolution modeling is built into the iterative processing. Iterative reconstruction is also the only option available for new systems due to their unconventional detection geometry and sampling scheme. In general, iterative methods' use of accurate modeling of the image formation process allows such algorithms to supplant FBP as the standard reconstruction approach. The consequence is that conventionally defined reconstructed image resolution is no longer adequate to characterize the performance of SPECT systems.

Currently, reconstructed image resolution with the iterative reconstruction technique is not a well-defined term; it depends on the details of the processing algorithm and parameter. Iterative techniques used in commercial systems are mostly proprietary and vary significantly. Thus, the results derived from different processing techniques cannot be compared directly. For example, a reconstructed image of an isolated point source in air can be processed to yield any reconstructed spatial resolution and eventually be processed to be a point represented by a single pixel, if a large enough number of iterations is used (Miller and Wallis 1992). Applying such a large number of iterations in a clinical situation would produce uninterpretable images with excessive noise and artifacts. Iterative reconstruction using basic maximum-likelihood expectation-maximization (MLEM) or ordered-subsets expectation-maximization (OSEM) algorithms is a nonlinear process and has no unique solution for the inverse problem posed by SPECT imaging. The number of iterations is only one of many key parameters that determine the sharpness of the images and the reconstructed image spatial resolution. In addition, the usable number of iterations and reconstructed spatial resolution also depend on surrounding activity distribution, such as source distribution, contrast level, noise content, and background level.

Several papers evaluating new cardiac SPECT systems have reported unprecedented and drastically improved performance in both system sensitivity and reconstructed image resolution (Gambhir et al. 2009; Bocher et al. 2010). These results seem to defy the traditional concept that these two performance parameters cannot be drastically improved at the same time. The explanation of this conflict boils down to the different definitions, measurement methodologies, and processing techniques used in deriving their respective reconstructed image resolution. Since the optimal and objective processing of these techniques has yet to be established, an objective assessment of these systems using the reported results is not possible yet.

It is thus imperative that our community standardizes the definition and measurement methodology of reconstructed image resolution for it to serve as an objective performance metric of SPECT systems. In fact, a candidate to be considered as the standard methodology has already been used in assessing the reconstructed image resolution of a cardiac SPECT system (Erlandsson et al. 2009). It uses an elaborated perturbation technique that involves a clinical realistic cardiac phantom in an experimental measurement.

2. *Hardware resolution*: Hardware resolution can be calculated as the quadrature sum of two components, $R = (R_i^2 + R_c^2)^{1/2}$, where R is the hardware resolution, R_i is the ISR of the detector system, and R_c is the collimator resolution at a standard distance. The collimator resolution, R_c, can be measured or estimated from knowledge of the physical dimensions and design of the collimator, while the detector's intrinsic resolution, R_i, is measurable or well documented by vendors. Thus, the hardware resolution is defined by the hardware of the system and not affected by software techniques used in subsequent processing. It has two components: the two point-spread functions (PSFs) in the transverse and axial planes of the system. In clinical SPECT systems, hardware resolution is typically 5–20 mm full width at half maximum (FWHM) in a distance range of 5–25 cm.

Because hardware resolution is distance dependent, its value in each acquired projection varies with the projection's distance to the imaging volume. To represent a SPECT system's hardware resolution with a single value, one simple approach could be the average of hardware resolutions at the center of the imaging volume from all relevant projections. Because the hardware resolution of a SPECT system is objectively defined and readily measurable, it can serve as a tentative spatial resolution parameter for characterizing SPECT systems until the definition of reconstructed image resolution is standardized. Moreover, a system with better hardware resolution should yield a better reconstructed image resolution under the same conditions, provided sampling and software processing are appropriate.

5.2.4.3.2.3 Relationship between sensitivity and spatial resolution in SPECT systems

In SPECT systems, both system sensitivity and spatial resolution are primarily determined by the collimators used. These two system parameters are directly related to their counterparts—geometric efficiency (GE) and resolution—of the collimator system. Sensitivity is a performance parameter of a detector–collimator combination and is proportional to the GE of the collimator and the stopping power of the detector. For any collimator, its GE and resolution are closely related. Thus, GE and collimator resolution come in pairs; each pair represents a trade-off between these two parameters of a collimator.

The pairing relationship between sensitivity and spatial resolution of a system is best illustrated in a projection image acquired with a point source located at a specific location in the imaging volume. In Figure 5.1, such a projection image is presented as a two-dimensional (2D) histogram of the detected events. The 2D integral of all events in this histogram per unit acquisition time and unit source activity is the system's point source sensitivity at that location for this projection. The combined point source sensitivity of all simultaneous acquired projections in a system is the point source system sensitivity at this source location. Note that the 2D profile of the histogram is the 2D PSF of this projection for this location. Hence, point source sensitivity and spatial resolution are directly related characteristics in the same projection image of a point source. For the system as a whole, system sensitivity and system spatial resolution are similarly related for any extended source distributions, which are aggregates of point sources.

5.2.4.3.3 Objective metrics of system sensitivity

For performance evaluation of SPECT systems, we need objective metrics for their system sensitivity regardless of their software reconstruction technique. Because of the differences in resolution performance between different SPECT systems, direct comparison of system sensitivities without taking into account the resolution differences is not meaningful. The metric for evaluation of performance potential of a system and for intercomparison of systems should be independent of their respective sensitivity–resolution trade-off. We propose two such metrics to put systems on equal footing for evaluation. These metrics are normalized system sensitivity (NSS) and normalized system geometric efficiency (NSGE), as elaborated in the following.

5.2.4.3.3.1 Normalized system sensitivity

The first metric, NSS, is the measured system sensitivity normalized to its 2D hardware resolution for a specific source model. NSS has an absolute numeric value and is a characteristic performance parameter of a SPECT system and also a metric of its specific detection geometry. Hence, all dual-head SPECT systems have basically the same NSS, no matter which set of collimators, high sensitivity or high resolution, it uses.

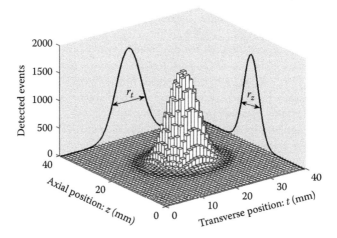

Figure 5.1 2D histogram display of a low-noise projection image of a point source on a detector–collimator system. The two orthogonal profiles projected on the transverse and axial planes are the two characteristic PSFs of the system for this point source location, with their two FWHMs marked. The 2D integral of the histogram, or the sum of all the detected events, divided by its acquisition time and source activity, is the point source sensitivity of the system at this location. This projection image connects the point source sensitivity to the two orthogonal PSFs and their corresponding FWHMs.

The concept of NSS can be easily understood from a single projection image of a SPECT system. A component of NSS, the normalized projection sensitivity (NPS) is defined as $s/(r_t \cdot r_z)$, where s and r_j are sensitivity and hardware resolution in FWHM of a projection image with a particular collimation. The subscripts t and z indicate the two orthogonal directions, transverse (t) and axial (z), of the projection. Referring back to Figure 5.1, the sum of the 2D histogram (i.e., the area integral) of the point source is the sensitivity s_i of this particular projection, while the profile of the histogram is the 2D PSF, from which two orthogonal FWHMs, r_t and r_z, are measured. Because the 2D PSF can be approximated by a 2D Gaussian function, the area integral of the histogram, s, is proportional to the product $r_t \cdot r_z$. This is based on the proportionality between the integral of a one-dimensional (1D) Gaussian function and its standard deviation, which is in turn proportional to its FWHM. In addition, this proportionality is a constant and is independent of the collimator's design and trade-offs. Thus, NPS_i is a characteristic performance parameter of the projection i. The concept of NPS can be expanded to the whole SPECT system that has multiple projections, which are acquired either simultaneously or sequentially. Thus, NSS can be defined as the sum of all the NPS_i, and is the ratio of the total system sensitivity to the product of spatial resolution in the two orthogonal directions of the projections.

$$\mathrm{NSS} \equiv \Sigma_i w_i \mathrm{NPS}_i \tag{5.1}$$

where w_i is the fraction of the total imaging time used in acquiring projection i. NSS is a measurable quantity suitable for representing the absolute system sensitivity of SPECT systems. Its unit is cps/(MBq·mm²). A system's NSS depends mainly on its detection geometry. A SPECT system using any collimators of a given type with different trade-offs would have the same NSS value.

The NSS of SPECT systems should be measured under standardized conditions for each specific imaging application. These conditions, including the source configuration, its activity distribution, and placement in the imaging volume, should be defined to reflect relevant clinical imaging situations and be simple and practical for experimental measurements. For example, the National Electrical Manufacturers Association (NEMA) employs a 20 cm cylindrical phantom of 20 cm in length with uniform activity for system sensitivity measurement, while axially aligned line sources are placed in various transverse locations in the phantom for hardware resolution measurement (NEMA 2007). For cardiac SPECT systems, a spherical or cylindrical phantom of 10 cm size could be used.

5.2.4.3.3.2 Normalized system geometric efficiency

A more mathematical metric directly related to system sensitivity and resolution is NSGE. It is extended from system geometric efficiency (SGE), which was used in assessing detection geometry of a SPECT system (Chang et al. 2009). SGE is defined as the sum of all solid angles of detection for a source model, in units of steradians, of a SPECT system for a given hardware resolution. A source model can be a point source, or an extended source relevant to a target of interest, located at the center of the imaging volume. This definition of SGE is extended from the conventional GE defined for collimators (Cherry et al. 2012), except it is the sum of GEs of all collimators, each from a different projection and weighted for its fraction of acquisition time, of a SPECT system that yields a given average hardware resolution at the center of the imaging volume. Hence,

$$\mathrm{SGE} \equiv \Sigma_i w_i \cdot \mathrm{GE} \quad \text{where } \mathrm{GE} = K\left(d/l\right)^2\left[d/\left(d+t\right)\right]^2 \quad \text{parallel-hole collimator} \tag{5.2}$$

$$= d^2 \cos^3\theta / 16b^2 \quad \text{pinhole collimator} \tag{5.3}$$

where w_i is the same weighting factor as in the previous equation, while d, l, t, and b are standard symbols used for collimator parameters: diameter and length of collimator holes, septal thickness, and distance of the point source from the collimator surface, respectively. Further, the factor K accounts for various hole shapes and is tabulated in Accorsi and Metzler (2006). SGE is a geometrical quantity that can be calculated accurately from detailed knowledge of the system geometry, collimator geometry, and imaging operation of a SPECT system. It is basically the sum of distance-weighted active detector areas in yielding a specific hardware resolution for a source model. Thus, SGE is also an objective metric for estimating a SPECT system's sensitivity, because a system's total solid angle of detection is proportional to its sensitivity.

Similar to NSS, NSGE is the SGE normalized to the general 2D hardware resolution of the system: $NSGE \equiv SGE/(r_t \cdot r_z)$. It is a metric independent of resolution trade-off, and is an absolute and characteristic performance parameter of a SPECT system. It is a useful and effective parameter for guiding a system's design to maximize its sensitivity.

5.2.4.3.3.3 Relationship between NSS and NSGE

Although NSGE and NSS are derived from different approaches, they are proportional to each other for a given SPECT system for the same source model. In fact, NSGE is the major factor in NSS, which also includes other factors, such as a detector's stopping power, photopeak fraction, and energy window. Thus, NSGE complements NSS in assessing system sensitivity of SPECT systems, especially when the SPECT system of interest is not available for experimental measurement. When detailed design parameters are not available, NSGE derived from a generic system design can be an approximate estimate of NSS.

Because the major factor in NSGE is the system's active detector area directed to the imaging volume of interest, the total active detector area per unit imaging volume of a SPECT system usually offers a first clue of its relative NSGE and NSS. This is because SPECT systems for the same application usually employ comparable collimation distances, which lead to similar distance weighting factors.

5.2.4.3.4 Sampling consideration

Sampling theory requires that information of the target should be acquired in sufficient detail to achieve adequate spatial resolution and image quality. These details include projections of sufficient linear and angular sampling; the latter is the number of sampling directions over a sufficiently large angular range. Conventional sampling requirements and their guidelines for SPECT systems are well established (Cherry et al. 2012). Although modern iterative algorithms have been proven to be more robust and forgiving to minor deficiencies in sampling, the basic principles for sampling remain valid and should be observed. Linear sampling and angular sampling requirements are linked and required to meet the Nyquist theorem, which states that the linear sampling interval should be smaller than half of the FWHM of the PSF of the system. When the requirements are not met, reconstructed images would fall short of the intended spatial resolution, image quality, and quantification potential and may lead to imaging artifacts.

The hardware subsystem has to provide a means to achieve adequate angular sampling. When the number of simultaneously acquired projections is not sufficient to meet the angular sampling requirement, the conventional approach is to use detector rotation to add the number of projections as needed. This is why dual-head SPECT systems use elaborate hardware to facilitate the rotation of their heavy detector and collimator systems.

5.2.4.4 SECONDARY SYSTEM CONSIDERATIONS AND PERFORMANCE

Aside from the above-mentioned four major parameters, several secondary parameters, such as energy resolution, count rate capability, and cost are addressed in the following.

5.2.4.4.1 Energy resolution

Energy resolution is a performance parameter of the detector system. It indicates the SPECT system's ability to determine the energy of detected photons and to discriminate scatter events from photopeak events. Only the latter are accepted as detected photons, while the former are rejected because their incoming directions are likely compromised. Energy resolution of SPECT systems is generally specified as the percentage value of the FWHM of the photopeak (i.e., $\Delta E/E$) in the energy spectrum of Tc-99m. The finite energy resolution leads to the inevitable contamination of scattered photons in the acquired data using typical symmetrical energy windows to cover the photopeak. A system with better (numerically lower) energy resolution is desirable since its scatter fraction—the ratio of detected scatter events to total events—should be lower. Scatter fraction in clinical SPECT and PET imaging varies from 20% to 40% depending on imaging situation and patient variations. Scatter events are manifested as elevated background and cause reduced image contrast and quantitative errors or artifacts. In terms of its impact on image quality, scatter contamination is a negative factor that should be corrected or taken into account in image interpretation; however, its importance is secondary to statistical noise and spatial resolution. Thus, energy resolution is secondary to system sensitivity and spatial resolution as a system performance metric. This statement is supported by the excellent quality of PET images, in light of the fact that energy resolution of PET systems has always lagged behind and reached low teens only recently. In practice, system energy resolution is more of an indicator of how efficiently the energy of photons is collected and utilized in an imaging system.

For modern Anger camera–based SPECT systems, the typical energy resolution is 9%–10%. New cadmium-zinc-telluride (CZT) detector–based systems offer an improved average energy resolution of 5%–6%. Although using detectors of better energy resolution can reduce scatter contamination, a system's low-scatter fraction performance requires more than just a low FWHM value; the whole energy spectrum of the detector is relevant. More details are discussed in Section 5.2.5.2.1.

5.2.4.4.2 Count rate capability and dead time

Two other system performance parameters are count rate capability and dead time. All nuclear detectors have a finite dead time associated with detection and position processing of each event. As a result, all detector systems have an upper limit in handling high photon incidence rates properly. Even before a system's count rate is pushed to its limit, an imaging system may misplace or even lose events and create errors in imaging or counting. The count rate performance of the current state-of-the-art Anger cameras has been improved significantly, mainly due to implementation of high-speed digital electronics and real-time digital processing. As a result, the effects of pulse pileup and baseline shift can be effectively corrected or reduced, and legitimate events are recovered to reduce count losses and positioning errors.

The count rate performance of SPECT systems can be tested, similarly to Anger cameras, by comparing the observed versus the incident count rate following the decay of a high-activity source. Modern gamma cameras have been improved to achieve a maximum observed count rate close to 400,000 counts/s, and 20% loss at more than 200,000 counts/s. These systems can operate up to 150,000 counts/s, in low-scatter testing situations, without significant degradation of counting and imaging performance. This capability has far exceeded the count rate requirements of routine clinical SPECT imaging, which ranges from 1,000 to 15,000 counts/s in the photopeak window. For other detector systems used in SPECT, such as CZT or pixelated scintillator coupled to individual photodiode, their count rate performance is at least comparable to, if not higher than, that of Anger cameras, and typically exceeds 1 million counts/s in the whole system (Erlandsson et al. 2009; Bai et al. 2010). Thus, modern SPECT systems have detectors that can handle most high-count-rate situations, even some of those encountered in first-pass dynamic cardiac SPECT imaging or transmission imaging with high-intensity sources.

5.2.4.4.3 Cost

The last, but far from the least, issue for all clinical imaging systems is their cost, which is the denominator of the performance-to-cost ratio and should also be considered an important metric, especially in the current healthcare environment. In fact, in the absence of cost constraints, SPECT systems of much higher performance than that of the state-of-the-art clinical systems can be developed. Striking a balance between cost and performance is the biggest decision that determines the general system design at the planning stage. Needless to say, cost-effectiveness is the design goal of all clinical systems.

5.2.4.5 OTHER INSTRUMENTATION ACCESSORIES

For proper SPECT imaging, additional capabilities and hardware are needed to provide complementary information for imaging and corrections. For example, to provide attenuation correction, it is important to integrate transmission computed tomography (tCT), to be discussed later in Section 5.2.6.2, with SPECT systems. For scatter correction, a multiple-energy-window acquisition should be provided. For cardiac imaging, electrocardiogram (ECG)-gated acquisition is necessary. Furthermore, miscellaneous tools for routine testing and calibrations are needed to ensure reliable data quality, because detector and collimator systems always come with imperfections that cause errors in acquired data. To mitigate these errors so they do not affect image quality, they need to be measured separately and taken into account in image reconstruction. Other practical but crucial considerations include ergonomics, patient safety and comfort, and user-friendly interface. Whether approaching the problem from a designer's or a user's perspective, the performance of the entire system has to be considered, along with those factors that affect patients and technologists.

5.2.5 MAJOR COMPONENTS

The two major components of a SPECT system are the collimator system and detector system. These two key systems interact with and complement each other in many ways. It would be a mistake to consider either of the two without keeping the other also in mind.

5.2.5.1 COLLIMATOR SYSTEM

Since the subject of collimators has been covered in other textbooks, we will provide only an overview from the perspective of SPECT systems. The standard definition of terms and symbols used in Cherry et al. (2012) are followed.

Fundamentally, the collimator system characterizes a SPECT system and largely determines its performance. The basic design concept of collimators has not changed since it was reviewed years ago (Anger 1967). Improvements are limited to variations in geometry, such as in several hybrid collimators, and their collimation quality and manufacturing techniques. Although collimation has long been recognized as the weakest link of general nuclear and SPECT imaging, there is still no alternative to this technology on the horizon.

Collimation is accomplished by restricting photons to narrow allowable paths and absorbing those on other paths. A collimator system defines for each detector element a straight line of sampling into the imaging volume and a narrow conical strip volume of allowable paths for photons coming from the imaging volume along this sampling line. The complete set of these strip volumes constitutes the detection geometry. Each collimator design is the result of a trade-off of GE, collimator resolution, and FOV, which are combined to reflect the trade-off among sensitivity, hardware resolution, and imaging volume of a SPECT system.

5.2.5.1.1 Collimator types

Collimators can be divided into two major groups based on their image formation process or collimation geometry: pinhole collimator and multichannel collimator. A pinhole collimator restricts the sampling lines to those that cross a single point at its front end. It provides a 3D diverging geometry, yielding either projection magnification or minification, depending on target distance. Multichannel collimators pack a large array of narrow mechanical channels in a slab of finite thickness. Depending on the relative orientation of the channels, they can be divided into three subgroups: parallel, converging, and diverging; each is characterized by its focal length, which is ∞, >0, or <0, respectively. Thus, each of the subgroups' magnification factor (M), the ratio of the size of the target in the projection image to its true size, is 1, >1, or <1, respectively. They can provide either 2D or 3D axial sampling. The former restricts photon paths essentially to the system's transverse planes; the latter allows photon paths to cross these planes. Between these two groups is a hybrid of pinhole and multichannel design, called slit-slat collimation.

Combining all these variations, collimators in SPECT systems have five major types: pinhole, parallel-hole, converging, diverging, and slit-slat collimators. Both converging and diverging types have two axial sampling subtypes: 2D as a fan or 3D as a cone. As summarized in Table 5.1, these types have different behaviors with respect to projection magnification, axial sampling geometry, variation of FOV with distance, and variation of point source GE with distance. The mathematical formulas for calculating collimator resolution and GE of these types have been summarized in Cherry et al. (2012). The following descriptive discussion is in the context of collimators' applications in clinical SPECT systems.

5.2.5.1.1.1 Pinhole collimator

A pinhole collimator was the first collimation used on Anger cameras (Anger 1958). It provides a diverging collimation geometry that all incoming photons pass through a circular pinhole of a few millimeters at the

Table 5.1 Projection magnification factor (*M*), axial sampling geometry, and distance dependence of FOV and GE of the five types (including their subtypes) of collimators

Collimator type		Projection magnification (M)		Axial geometry	FOV vs. distance		GE vs. distance
		Transverse	Axial		Transverse	Axial	
Pinhole		<1	<1	3D	+	+	− −
Parallel hole		1	1	2D	=	=	=
Convergent	Fan	>1	1	2D	−	=	+
	Cone	>1	>1	3D	−	−	++
Divergent	Fan	<1	1	2D	+	=	−
	Cone	<1	<1	3D	+	+	− −
Slit-slat		<1	1, >1	2D, 3D	+	=, −	−

Note: The magnification factor, *M*, is always greater than unity for converging collimation but less than unity for diverging collimation. Pinhole and slit-slat can be either magnifying or minifying. When axial magnification is unity or not unity, the sampling geometry is 2D or 3D, respectively. In the third column, the FOV can be constant, increasing, or decreasing at increasing distance from the collimator, as indicated by the symbols =, −, and +, respectively. In the last column, the symbols =, +, ++, −, and − − indicate constant, increasing, large increasing, decreasing, and large decreasing, respectively. In the current context of clinical SPECT imaging, most collimators are used for medium-size imaging volumes located at 5–25 cm distance. Thus, pinhole and slit-slat collimators are only listed with expanded transverse FOV with distance. In the last row, of the slit-slat collimators, the axial slat-stacks are useful for clinical imaging in either parallel or converging design, as indicated.

front end of the collimator. Its focal length, defined as the distance from the pinhole to the detector plane along the central axis of the pinhole, usually varies with detector size and is typically in the range of 5–20 cm.

The most unique and important characteristic of pinhole collimation is its GE's inverse-square response with distance. The imaging volume in front of the pinhole can be divided into two regions along its central axis. In the near region, from the pinhole to its focal point, which is at a distance equal to its focal length, projections are magnified. In the far region beyond the focal point, projections are minified. It is in the first half, or one-third, of the near region that the pinhole is at its best for imaging small targets. It achieves high sensitivity and high hardware resolution at the expense of FOV, because the pinhole provides high GE and its inverse-square decline is limited in this short range. Furthermore, large projection magnification in this range effectively improves ISR, which is coupled with high collimator resolution to yield high hardware resolution. This is why small-animal SPECT systems, even with Anger camera–based detectors of ISR of typically 3.8 cm FWHM, can achieve submillimeter image resolution when a small pinhole is coupled with large magnification.

In the far region of the pinhole collimator, the collimation situation is just the opposite. The GE suffers drastic inverse-square decline. The pinhole collimator's resolution degrades linearly with distance with a rate of the collimator's aspect ratio (i.e., hole size/focal length). When used on Anger cameras, its hardware resolution degrades with distance more than the corresponding decline of collimator resolution, because its effective ISR also deteriorates as projection minification increases with distance. Hence, pinhole collimation is largely limited to imaging small targets in close range and rarely has been used in clinical imaging of medium-size targets in its far region.

5.2.5.1.1.2 Parallel-hole collimator

Due to the limitation of pinhole collimation for clinical imaging, multichannel collimators were developed early on (Anger 1964). Among them, parallel-hole collimators are the most commonly used. All their sampling lines are parallel and typically normal to the collimator's surface. Their broad application and acceptance are due to their intuitive and undistorted projection images, high and distance-independent GE, and an FOV that is constant with distance. They offer favorable all-around performance for SPECT imaging, especially when the imaging volume is large.

The unique and favorable property of parallel-hole collimation is its high GE that is position and distance independent in the imaging volume. While the GE of each individual channel decreases with the inverse square of collimation distance, the number of surrounding channels opening up for photon passage increases with the square of distance to keep the net GE constant. However, this feature holds only when there are sufficient surrounding channels to open up, as in a large parallel-hole collimator. For small parallel-hole collimators, the situation is different; not only is its GE not uniform in its limited FOV, but also it declines beyond a certain distance. If one dimension of the collimator has limited width, the decline of GE with distance is proportional to the distance; if both dimensions are limited in size, the decline is proportional to the square of the distance. In addition, small-size parallel-hole collimators also discriminate against off-axis activities in the dimension of limited width. As for the resolution of parallel-hole collimators, it degrades linearly with distance at a rate equal to the channels' aspect ratio (i.e., hole size/length).

5.2.5.1.1.3 Converging collimator

Converging collimation is a variation of parallel-hole collimation. Its sampling lines converge in the image volume (Moyer 1974). It trades FOV for GE and a slight improvement in collimator resolution. A converging collimator's resolution declines more moderately with distance than that of a comparable parallel-hole collimator. Its hardware resolution's decline with distance is even less due to projection magnification, which makes the effective ISR improve with distance. Examples are converging-fan and converging-cone collimators; the difference between the two is in their focusing—whether to a line or to a point in 3D. However, using converging collimation requires a large detector area, and its application in SPECT systems has been limited by the fact that only a limited number of large detectors can be placed close to an imaging volume.

5.2.5.1.1.4 Diverging collimator

Diverging collimation is the exact opposite of converging collimation in design and function; its sampling lines diverge in the image volume. It has increased FOV with distance at the expense of GE and collimator resolution. This results in projected images that are minified relative to the size of the target. Because the detector area required for each projection is smaller in size than the imaging volume, this collimation geometry is often used when the available detector area is limited. Its shortcomings are the sharp decline of GE and collimator resolution with distance in the imaging volume. It has not had much imaging application. Although they were thought to be historical relics, interest in small and medium-size solid-state and pixelated detectors might bring them back for special applications (Ogawa 2010; Kindem et al. 2010). It should be noted that compromising GE and hardware resolution to suit detector sizes is not a long-term solution; large-size detectors are always preferred. An application of divergent collimation is in system designs that take advantage of projection minification, which is discussed in Section 5.2.5.1.1.6.

5.2.5.1.1.5 Slit-slat collimator

Slit-slat collimation is a hybrid of a pinhole and a multichannel collimation. This collimation was introduced in a research SPECT system (Rogers et al. 1988). It may have potential for new applications in the dedicated imaging systems for breast and heart imaging (Metzler et al. 2006; Chang et al. 2009).

A slit-slat collimator consists of two orthogonally oriented 1D collimators: a slit-plate in the front with a slat-stack sitting behind. The slit-plate contains one or more axially oriented slits (thin air gaps on a plate of lead or tungsten) to provide transaxial collimation. Physically separated and behind the slit-plate, the slat-stack is a stack of flat lead foils or tungsten plates with proper axial spacing to provide axial collimation. Each slit in the plate works with the slat-stack behind it to provide a 2D projection image on the detector system further behind.

The slit performs as a 1D pinhole, which provides, depending on target distance, magnified or minified projections in the transverse planes. The slat-stack can be implemented as parallel, converging, or diverging in the axial plane (Li et al. 2009). When parallel slats are used, a slit-slat collimator provides 2D axial sampling and functions as a converging-fan or a diverging-fan collimator in its near or far regions, similarly defined as that of pinhole collimators. When converging or diverging slats are used in the slat-stack, 3D imaging geometries are formed.

Slit-slat collimators have a hybrid performance of the two independent orthogonal collimators. With parallel slats, its GE declines inversely with distance and is nearly the geometric mean of its pinhole and parallel-hole collimators (Accorsi et al. 2008). Its collimator resolution declines linearly with distance in both directions. This collimator offers a middle-ground performance for imaging medium-size targets at a medium-distance range.

5.2.5.1.1.6 Application of projection minification in SPECT systems

For SPECT systems designed to image a medium-size target, diverging collimation can be used to increase the number of simultaneous projections for a given detector area, as well as SGE. Here, diverging collimation is used in a broad sense for all those using minified projections in the transverse plane; it includes pinhole and slit-slat. This concept for SPECT systems was introduced by a University of Arizona group (Rogulski et al. 1993). Because each minified projection requires less detector area for the same imaging volume, the number of simultaneous projections can be increased on a given size of detector area. This approach may be used to reduce the need for system motion to achieve fast imaging. The net SGE is increased accordingly, as it is proportional to the number of simultaneous projections. Because projection minification would increase effective ISR and degrade hardware resolution, a detector system of higher ISR is needed to accommodate the high spatial frequency content of the projections. Therefore, a net gain of SGE can be achieved in a SPECT system without compromising resolution, provided the detector system has an ISR that is $1/M$ times better than the nonminified situation, or smaller in FWHM by a factor of M, where $M < 1$.

5.2.5.1.2 Other considerations

5.2.5.1.2.1 Septal penetration

The first criterion in choosing a collimator material, as well as in choosing a detector material, is its stopping power. For collimators, the concern is the severity of septal penetration for the energy of photons to be used. For most SPECT imaging, which involves energy no higher than 140 keV, current low-energy collimators made of thin foils are capable of keeping septal penetration to a low level. However, for imaging photons of energy higher than 200 keV, the current commercial medium-energy collimators are not adequate in containing septal penetration, especially for nuclides with multiple higher energies (e.g., I-123, In-111, Ga-67, and I-131). Thus, the septal penetration is an additional source of uncertainty that needs to be accounted for when quantification of activity is important.

5.2.5.1.2.2 Collimator material and x-ray contamination

Collimators are made from high-Z material, such as lead (Pb) or tungsten (W). Tungsten has a higher attenuation coefficient than lead and is more effective as collimation material. The problem in making tungsten collimators is its high cost and difficult machinability. Its use in low-energy collimators is hard to justify. For most SPECT systems, which are designed for 140 keV photons, septa of current lead-based multichannel collimators are already very thin (<0.2 mm for holes of <2 mm). Collimators of thinner septa could at best gain a tiny GE, but at the expense of its septal penetration and structural integrity. As a result, there has been little incentive to develop tungsten multichannel collimators of medium size or larger. A misconception is that using tungsten-based collimators has the advantage of eliminating lead x-rays and is more suitable for Tl-201/Tc-99m dual-isotope imaging. This assertion overlooks the tungsten x-rays, which also get in the wide energy window typically used for Tl-201 imaging. For pinhole collimation, using small knife-edged tungsten pinhole inserts is an effective approach.

5.2.5.1.2.3 Hole pattern

Most multichannel parallel-hole collimators use a hexagonal-hole pattern, due to its structural integrity and low-cost fabrication, which is based on assembling corrugated lead-foil stripes. For pixelated detectors, square-hole collimation is preferred by matching each collimator channel to a detector pixel to realize the intended hardware resolution effectively and prevent photons from hitting the inter-pixel gaps and missing detection. Using a conventional hex-hole collimator on a square pixelated detector would compromise both sensitivity and hardware resolution. Currently, there is a small square-hole tungsten collimator being used on a pixelated detector of a clinical SPECT system (Gambhir et al. 2009). In general, tungsten collimators are expensive and size limited. Until a cost-effective technology for medium-size (~20 cm) square-hole collimators is developed, medium or large-size pixelated detectors still have to use hex-hole collimators. As a result, these detectors cannot perform up to their potential with multichannel collimators.

5.2.5.1.2.4 Quality of manufacturing

How well collimators can be manufactured determines how close the intended performance can be realized. Obviously, nothing can be perfect when it comes to mechanical implementation of engineering specifications. Pinhole collimators are simple to construct with high quality due to the lack of septa. With the presence of septa and channels, multichannel collimators are difficult to construct and cannot be manufactured as perfectly. Although the current technology of manufacturing foil-based parallel-hole collimators can achieve high quality, the technology for converging collimators has not reached the same level. Not surprisingly, 3D (cone) collimators are much more challenging than their 2D (fan) counterparts. Fortunately, minor collimator imperfections and collimation errors can be mitigated by software-based system modeling in image reconstruction provided a detailed and accurate calibration procedure has the deviations mapped out and taken into account in the software.

5.2.5.1.3 Summary and comparisons

The performance of a SPECT system is mainly defined by its collimator system, which is the key to achieving high SGE for a given hardware resolution.

Each type of collimator has its own strengths and weaknesses. They should be used to suit their strength. In clinical SPECT imaging, target distribution could be in the distance range of 5–25 cm. In this range, pinhole collimators suffer low GE. Parallel-hole collimators perform favorably and are suitable for imaging large-size targets. For small or medium-size targets, most of the detector area of a large parallel-hole collimator is not utilized. Converging collimators can be used to improve detector utilization in these situations. Slit-slat collimation provides a compromise for imaging medium-size targets at medium distance.

In terms of rate of change of GE with distance in air, the five collimator types rank in the following order: converging-cone, converging-fan, parallel-hole, slit-slat, and pinhole collimators, as shown in Table 5.1. While converging cone provides increased GE with distance in air, pinhole collimators yield the sharpest decline of the rate among all types. For example, their rate of decline along the pinhole's axis is 20% per centimeter at 10 cm and 10% per centimeter at 20 cm. The different rates of change are reflected in their imposed severity of distance discrimination. As a result, converging collimators are more effective in reaching deep activities, while pinhole collimators favor superficial activities and strongly discriminate deep activities.

A secondary and often overlooked behavior of many collimator types is their discrimination against off-axis activities. In the formulas of the GE of pinhole, converging, diverging, and slit-slat collimators, they all have a $\cos\theta$ term, to either its second or third power, where θ is the off-axis angle of the location of a point source (Cherry et al. 2012). This means that activities are discriminated against if they are located off the central axis of the collimator. For example, when $\theta = 10°$ and $20°$, $\cos^3\theta = 0.95$ and 0.83, respectively. The GE of point sources located off-axis could be discounted by 5%–17%, a small and nonnegligible reduction, relative to that located at the same distance but right on the central axis.

While the GE of collimators can be constant, increasing, or decreasing in air with distance, collimator resolution can only degrade with distance. Their declines are generally linear with distance, with a rate defined mainly by the aspect ratio of the channels or the pinhole.

In clinical imaging, attenuation is the ever-present factor that exacerbates the decline of point source sensitivity with distance. The combined effect of all these factors leads to negative sensitivity gradients in the radial direction of imaging volume. These gradients, if large, mean relatively fewer photons would be detected deep in the imaging volume and are the origin of excessive noise there. They also make the number of detected photons sensitive to the target position in the imaging volume.

5.2.5.2 DETECTOR SYSTEM

The detector system is the second critical component of SPECT systems and is the costliest one, often up to half of the whole imaging system. It captures photons that pass through the collimator and records the 2D coordinates of the photon interaction location to yield projection images. In SPECT systems, stopping power of detector material is not a big issue, due to the relatively low energy of photons in use today. For cost-effectiveness, most types of detector are about three half-value layers thick to stop 85%–90% of 140 keV photons.

The detector system includes three subcomponents: conversion medium, sensors, and data acquisition (DAQ) system. The first two comprise the detector. The conversion medium is made of high-Z and high-density material that stops photons and converts the energy transferred to measurable form, such as carriers of electric charge or scintillation light. The sensors collect these carriers to generate the electric signals that are passed on to the DAQ. The DAQ then processes these signals in real time to derive the spatial coordinates of interaction location along with the energy absorbed from the detected event.

The ISR of conventional Anger camera systems has long been in the 3–4 mm range. Further improving their ISR is generally not cost-effective, because the hardware resolution of a system is mainly limited by the much poorer collimator resolution in the typical imaging distance. However, the design concept of using projection minification in SPECT systems requires new detectors of high ISR to optimize system design and performance. To facilitate special detection geometries, small modular detectors without the dead regions along the detector edges associated with Anger-type cameras are also needed. As a result, several new detectors have been introduced in SPECT systems in the last decade.

Detectors in SPECT systems can be divided into three types: monolithic scintillator based, pixelated scintillator based, and pixelated CZT based, as discussed next. We will cover the latter two types extensively, because they are new. DAQ system will be discussed at the end of the section.

5.2.5.2.1 Detector types

5.2.5.2.1.1 Monolithic scintillator-based detector

The Anger camera–based detector systems have survived 50 years and are still the workhorses in clinical laboratories. Their longevity has many good reasons, which include well-balanced all-around performance, stability, reliability, functionality, and relatively low cost. These reasons make Anger cameras hard to replace and have allowed them to keep their current dominant role for general-purpose imaging, especially for that requiring large-area detectors.

The conversion medium of an Anger camera is a large monolithic scintillator slab. Modern Anger cameras use flat rectangular slabs, up to 60 × 45 cm in size and typically 9.5 mm in thickness. NaI:Tl is the most attractive scintillator to use due to its high light output, low cost, adequate stopping power, and well-matched spectral response with photomultiplier tubes (PMTs). An array of large-size (typically 7.5 cm) PMTs, optically coupled to the slab through a single piece of flat glass as its exit window, converts scintillation light collected by each PMT to an electric pulse. A DAQ system selectively weights and sums these electric pulses to derive in real time the position and energy signals of each event. Commercial Anger cameras today have a typical performance of 90% stopping power, 3.7 mm isotropic ISR, a useful FOV up to nearly 54 × 40 cm, and better than 9.5% FWHM nominal energy resolution for 140 keV photons.

However, several advantageous features of Anger cameras for general-purpose imaging become weaknesses when it comes to special-purpose applications. The large size of the detectors is not really optimal for most clinical imaging, because body contours are mostly curved and convex, which make it difficult, if not impossible, for most of the detector area to maintain close proximity for effective collimation. Curved detector geometries are best facilitated with an assembly of small modular detectors. An example is the curved detectors used in PET systems, which are assembled from a large number of small and identical modular detectors. However, conventional Anger camera technology cannot accommodate small and modular detectors efficiently, because it inherently comes with dead, or non-position-sensitive, regions, which are about half a PMT width all around the edges of each crystal slab.

Another limitation of Anger cameras is that their ISR is limited to be about 3 mm FWHM, regardless of the size of PMTs. This is because scintillation light spreads quite far through multiple internal reflections in the relatively thick NaI:Tl slabs. The range of light spread is proportional to the thickness of the slab and limits its ISR. This limitation prevents Anger cameras from many special imaging applications, where high

ISR is required. To improve ISR, the spreading of scintillation has to be contained. One way to address this issue is to use thin slabs to limit light spread and improve ISR (Milster et al. 1990). However, this approach compromises stopping power and system sensitivity and is therefore not for clinical systems.

5.2.5.2.1.2 Pixelated scintillator-based detector

To contain light spread in thick scintillator slabs to yield high ISR, segmentation and pixelation of detector material was introduced. After proven successful in thick bismuth germanate (BGO) detectors used in PET, this concept was extended to single-photon imaging to develop pixelated NaI:Tl and CsI:Na detectors (Casey and Nutt 1986; Wojcik et al. 1998; Williams et al. 2000). These detectors use a detector slab made up of a large rectangular array of discrete scintillators, physically and optically separated, in square or rectangular pixels of 1–3 mm. As a result, scintillations are confined locally in the narrow and long crystal and can only exit in the far end. Thus, the spread of scintillation photons is better confined to be distributed among an appropriate number of photosensors for identification of the pixel of interaction. The photosensors could be photodiodes, position-sensitive PMTs (PSPMTs), or an array of conventional PMTs. In principle, pixels of very small size can be identified and resolved, if the photosensors are small enough for one-to-one matching.

A variety of scintillators can be used to make these small pixels. NaI:Tl is still the scintillator of choice despite its challenging preparation and requirement for additional canning. Modern NaI:Tl-based pixelated detectors have been improved and can yield better than 10% energy resolution at 140 keV. Currently, NaI:Tl-based detectors are used in a small-animal SPECT system, while CsI:Tl-based pixelated detectors are used in a clinical SPECT system.

Not only can pixelated detectors offer improved ISR, but also, by using small-size pixels, they can be position sensitive in all the surface areas, including the edges and corners. Thus, small or medium-size pixelated detector modules can be used as the building blocks of large or curved detectors. In addition, each module can be designed to function independently to allow multiple modules to operate in parallel to achieve high-count-rate performance in a multimodule system.

In characterizing the spatial resolution of pixelated detectors, the conventional concepts of PSF and FWHM need adjustment, because each event's likely position is not a Gaussian-like function, but a step-function with a pitch equal to the pixel's width. The detected position is equally likely anywhere in the pixel; its uncertainty cannot be more than the size of the pixel. The way for assessing ISR is to quote the pixel's size or its pitch, because they are designed to resolve the majority of the pixels. To quantify how well positions are determined, average peak-to-valley ratios of flood image profiles have been used (Surti et al. 2003).

A downside of using a pixelated detector is its reduced packing fraction, or fill factor, caused by the non-scintillating material packed between the pixels as optical barrier or reflector. The reflector material has no detection capability and causes reduced stopping power and thus detection sensitivity. A typical linear packing fraction of 90% means the width of the reflector material is 10% of the pixel pitch. Such a square pixelated array has a 2D packing fraction of 81%—a potential 19% reduction of detection sensitivity, if all photons hit the detector normally. This kind of reduction is not insignificant and is close to the situation when a parallel-hole collimator with a hex-hole pattern is used on square-pixel detectors, as mentioned in Section 5.2.5.1.2.3.

Another issue is that the cost of pixelated scintillators is significantly higher than that of a conventional monolithic slab, per unit detector area, due to the pixelation process. The cost can increase further if expensive photosensors are needed. For example, pixels of 1–2 mm size may require the use of PSPMTs, which typically cost 10 times more than conventional PMTs for the same area of coverage. Using conventional single-anode PMTs on pixelated NaI:Tl detectors is far more cost-effective. The feasibility of using an array of 5 cm round PMTs to resolve NaI:Tl pixels of $3 \times 3 \times 10$ mm has been demonstrated recently (Rozler et al. 2012).

CsI:Tl-based pixelated detectors have already been marketed in a clinical SPECT system and in a general-purpose gamma camera by Digirad Corp. CsI:Tl has two desirable features as a scintillator. First, it does not have to be canned and can operate in low-humidity housing because it is only slightly hygroscopic. Second, its scintillation matches well with the spectral response of the Si-PIN photodiode—a photosensor. Digirad's current pixelated detectors use square pixels of 6.1 or 3.25 mm pitch with 5 or 6 mm thickness, respectively. Each pixel is directly coupled to a Si-PIN photodiode, which converts scintillations to current that the application-specific integrated chip uses to read out the associated position and energy signals. Their latest detectors achieve a remarkable energy resolution of less than 8% (Kindem et al. 2010). Although these detectors have been promoted as solid-state detectors, only the photosensors are solid state. The fundamental detection mechanism is still through the traditional scintillation conversion in the conversion medium.

The advantages of these Digirad's detectors are their compact size, light weight, and easy maneuverability. The current weakness of these detectors is their low detection sensitivity, which is 15% or 30% less for the two versions of detectors, respectively, than that of standard Anger cameras using collimators of comparable resolution, as reported in their NEMA specifications. This performance can be attributed to the detector's low stopping power, caused mainly by their current packing fraction, and the use of hex-hole collimators.

On the horizon is the prospect of using silicon photomultiplier (SiPM) as a photosensor for pixelated scintillators. SiPM combines the advantages of photodiodes and PMTs. It is compact, robust, and operates at low voltage, while achieving high gain, low noise, and fast response time. Since its incorporation into PET systems is under way, the cost of SiPMs may be reduced in the future to the level justifiable for implementation in detectors of SPECT systems.

5.2.5.2.1.3 Pixelated CZT-based detector

Pixelated solid-state detectors using CZT crystals have been a focus of interest in our community for more than 20 years (Barber and Woolfenden 1996). CZT, a room temperature semiconductor material, can convert a photon's energy directly to charge carriers (as electron–hole pairs) without going through the less efficient scintillation and photoelectron conversions. These charge carriers are collected to read out the position and energy of the signals. Because the energy conversion is very efficient, a huge number of carriers are created in each photon interaction, which results in an electric pulse of excellent energy resolution. Wagenaar (2004) published a classical comprehensive review of CZT detectors for nuclear imaging applications.

The currently popular CZT module, manufactured and marketed by GE Healthcare, is a 5 mm thick monolithic tile of 4×4 cm, with an application-specific integrated circuit (ASIC) board mounted on its back. Although not segmented physically, the tiles are pixelated functionally, through an array of 16×16 electrode pads, each as an anode, into as many square pixels of 2.5 mm pitch. These pixelated detectors are being used in commercial systems for breast imaging and cardiac SPECT imaging.

CZT detectors offer many advantages. First, each CZT tile is position sensitive all the way to its edges. Their compact size and modular nature allow it to be configured flexibly for different system geometries with light weight, reduced shielding and associated cost, and easy maneuverability. The pixel size has potential to be reduced to submillimeters for ultra-high-resolution imaging to provide highly minified projections (Yin et al. 2013). It is its small physical size, small pixel size, and fully functional area that make CZT detectors attractive for imaging systems.

In addition, the energy resolution (4%–6% FWHM) of individual pixels in the current tile is excellent and certainly desirable (Erlandsson et al. 2009). Their energy spectra of commonly used radionuclides are shown in Figure 5.2. However, the excellent FWHM values of the photopeaks do not fully describe CZT's spectral performance. An often overlooked feature is its subpar photofraction, stemming mainly from the slow and incomplete collection of holes. This effect is reflected as an asymmetrical photopeak with a long elevated tail on the low-energy side of its spectrum and its corresponding poor full width at tenth maximum (FWTM) value (Wagenaar 2004; Bocher et al. 2010). As a result, the benefits of CZT's excellent energy resolution and anticipated effective scatter rejection are not fully realized in clinical imaging. This is also why the vendor recommends the use of a relatively wide 20% energy window, rather than a typical window of twice the FWHM, to avoid compromising detection sensitivity. This effect explains the small reduction in scatter fraction, 30% versus 34%, when a CZT detector–based SPECT system is compared with a standard NaI:Tl detector–based system under the same phantom imaging conditions (Erlandsson et al. 2009). The long tail has similar implications for dual-isotope clinical imaging, where Tl-201 or I-123 tracers are used simultaneously with Tc-99m tracers. Although the amount of spillover and scatter (which is not included in the spectra presented in Figure 5.2) from the high-energy tracer into the window of the low-energy tracer can be reduced by using CZT detectors, the reduction is not sufficient to eliminate them and still requires additional corrective processing. To reduce the spectral tail, the manufacturer has recently implemented an electron injection technique, which has achieved limited success, but the photopeaks are still quite asymmetric.

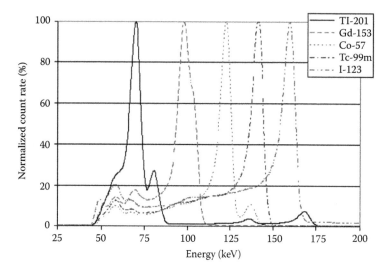

Figure 5.2 Normalized energy spectra of a CZT detector for five different radionuclides: Tl-201 (solid line), Gd-153 (long dashed line), Co-57 (short dashed line), Tc-99m (dot-dashed line), and I-123 (double dot-dashed line). The narrow shape of the photopeaks reflects CZT's excellent energy resolution if defined by its FWHM. All the spectra are asymmetric and have long tails on the low-energy side to reflect non-Gaussian shape and large FWTMs. (From Erlandsson, K., et al., *Phys. Med. Biol.*, 54[9], 2635–49, 2009. Reprinted with permission from IOP Publishing.)

Because each CZT detector tile is monolithic, it does not have physical gaps between pixels. Nonetheless, functional gaps also exist for photons hitting the regions between pixels and cause reduction of detection sensitivity. This is because the charge carriers created by a photon may be shared by multiple anode pads to result in multiple pulse heights in many pixels, which are all short of the photopeak and miss the energy window.

The current CZT detectors still cost far more than most other detectors per unit detector area, mainly due to low yield in manufacturing. Each CZT tile has to go through screening to be selected for meeting performance specifications because their quality is hard to predict. The current high cost is the major concern for implementation in clinical systems, especially for those that require a large detector area. Nonetheless, CZT detectors have the potential to be the future detector of choice, provided their cost can approach that of conventional detectors. This prospect is good due to the intense effort being poured into improving their quality and yield.

5.2.5.2.2 Data acquisition system

The DAQ system is the electronic system that processes raw electric signals provided by the sensors. The DAQ determines the position, energy, and timing information of each event and then presents them as projection images.

There are two types of DAQ systems: direct readout and indirect readout of projection data. In the former, as used in pixelated detectors, the DAQ reads out the three signals, x and y for position and z for energy, of each event directly from each pixel via an ASIC mounted on the back of the detector. The latter is used in Anger camera–based systems, or systems with multiple photosensors involved in each interaction; it processes the simultaneous outputs from the multiple photosensors to algorithmically derive the position and energy of each event and projection image in real time. Modern Anger camera systems use fully digital DAQs, where raw PMT signals are digitized in parallel up front and passed on to firmware in their field-programmable gate arrays (FPGAs) for processing. Advanced approaches use fast (>30 MHz) free-running ADCs to convert all PMT outputs simultaneously to parallel and continuous number streams. The advantage is their flexibility in implementing digital processing techniques, which include de-randomization, baseline correction, adaptive integration, pileup correction, and count recovery. The results are robust operation, high-quality data, and high-count-rate performance. More details of DAQ systems are presented in Chapter 4.

5.2.6 SECONDARY COMPONENTS

Although the collimator and detector systems are the core of SPECT instrumentation, two additional systems warrant discussion to complete the picture. The first is the mechanical system, which supports various operations. The second is a tCT subsystem, which is required to provide attenuation correction for, and fusing of CT images with, SPECT images.

5.2.6.1 MECHANICAL SYSTEM

SPECT systems have a complex set of mechanical components, which form the backbone of the system. The accuracy and precision, as well as reliability and reproducibility, of their operations are essential. The mechanical system consists of two parts: the gantry, which holds all subsystems together and enables their joint operation, and the motion system, which provides motion to complete data sampling and detection geometry.

5.2.6.1.1 Gantry system

Traditionally, clinical SPECT systems use a conventional circular gantry, similar to x-ray CTs, with its central axis horizontally oriented. The gantry is the mounting frame, and often the housing for detector and collimator systems, which are arranged on the transverse plane around a patient lying on a couch along the long axis. The gantry has a mechanical motion system to achieve motion of its detector or collimator systems with multiple degrees of freedom to provide desired detection geometries. The detector system and collimator system can be either integrated in the same unit or separated as two independent components. Although the number of detectors or camera heads varied in early years, only single-head and dual-head systems remain on the current market for general-purpose imaging.

5.2.6.1.2 Motion system

The major function of the motion system is to provide a sufficient number of different projection images of the imaging volume to meet angular sampling requirements. Most SPECT systems have a motion system that varies in complexity. This system includes a series of mechanical components under computer control to rotate its detector or collimator to acquire multiple transaxial projections sequentially over an angular range of the imaging volume. The current general-purpose SPECT systems, such as dual-head systems, use a heavy-duty motion system to rotate the cameras on a vertically oriented transverse plane around a patient lying on the couch. In new single-purpose cardiac SPECT systems, their approaches to motion vary and are presented in Section 5.3.

Additional kinds of motion have been introduced as SPECT systems evolve. Examples are the radial motion of the camera heads for body contouring, translational motion of the gantry or the couch in synchrony with detector motion, sweeping motion of line sources for transmission imaging, and translational motion to move the target into an imaging volume. Providing motion capability in SPECT systems is a complex engineering challenge, due to heavy and bulky hardware, the required precision and reproducibility, and most importantly, patient safety.

Mechanical motion is not desirable in SPECT systems from the point of view of system's design, operation, maintenance, and cost. In fact, motion also prolongs imaging time and limits temporal resolution. Therefore, SPECT systems with little motion are often preferred.

5.2.6.2 TRANSMISSION CT

A fundamental issue in SPECT imaging is the effect caused by tissue attenuation, which renders the images difficult or even impossible to interpret by suppressing the mapped intensity of deep-lying activity. Another issue in interpreting SPECT images is in identifying the precise location of mapped activities due to lack of anatomic landmarks. Both issues can be addressed with a matched set of patient- and slice-specific tCT images. *tCT* is a term that refers to all imaging techniques using external sources and their transmitted radiation to derive attenuation-based tomographic images of body sections. It is used here in the broad sense to include more than conventional diagnostic-quality x-ray CTs.

It has been accepted that SPECT images should be fused with their corresponding tCT images to allow anatomical correlation. At the same time, tCT images can be readily converted to attenuation maps to facilitate attenuation correction of the corresponding SPECT images. Furthermore, tCT images provide *a priori* support information to guide iterative image reconstruction and could also serve as the basis for model-based scatter correction (Welch and Gullberg 1997). For the two sets of images to be matched slice-to-slice for correlation or corrections, tCT and SPECT should be conducted sequentially, if not simultaneously. The key is to keep the patient's pose and the timing of the two imaging procedures as close as possible.

A clinical SPECT system should be complemented by a tCT system. To meet such needs, hybrid SPECT/CT systems, which integrate a SPECT system with a diagnostic-quality x-ray CT to share the same patient couch, have already been marketed by all major manufacturers. For more details, these hybrid SPECT/CTs are discussed in Chapter 14. However, using diagnostic-quality x-ray CTs in hybrid SPECT/CT systems is meant more for clinical image correlation than for attenuation correction. The high cost of hybrid systems is justified mainly in the context of multimodality imaging. Although the current trend is going toward using hybrid systems for whole-body SPECT studies, the reality is that most SPECT systems cannot afford to have a dedicated diagnostic-quality x-ray CT as an underused accessory. The situation is especially different in cardiac SPECT imaging, where tCT imaging is meant more for attenuation correction than for anatomic correlations. Relatively low-cost, low-dose, and low-resolution nondiagnostic tCTs may well have a place in cardiac SPECT systems.

5.2.6.2.1 Attenuation maps for cardiac SPECT imaging

For SPECT images to be interpretable qualitatively, the effect of tissue attenuation needs to be taken into account, either mentally or through quantitatively corrected images, in order to judge the relative activity distribution. A quantitative correction requires that the attenuation maps of the patient's corresponding image slices are available to account for tissue distribution and body size variation (Tsui et al. 1989; LaCroix et al. 1994). This is particularly true for cardiac SPECT imaging, due to varying and nonuniform tissue distribution in the thorax (Bailey et al. 1987; King et al. 1995; Matsunari et al. 1998). On the other hand, cardiac SPECT imaging is also quite different from other SPECT imaging. The overall attenuation effect is less severe, due to the heart's off-center location and the low-density lung tissues surrounding it. Uncorrected cardiac SPECT images still provide important diagnostic value qualitatively. This fact partly explains the lukewarm attitude of many clinical laboratories that do not use tCT routinely, even with the capability. Another reason is that the commercially available tCT techniques have not been optimized and are prone to creating artifacts (Burrell and MacDonald 2006). As a result, these procedures are not reimbursable by insurance due to lack of established positive outcomes. Nevertheless, use of existing attenuation correction techniques for cardiac SPECT imaging has been reported to increase sensitivity, specificity, and normalcy of diagnosis (Garcia and Esteves 2009; Travin 2011). Two joint position statements, issued by the American Society of Nuclear Cardiology (ASNC) and Society of Nuclear Medicine (SNM), have endorsed the use and improvement of tCT techniques for cardiac SPECT imaging (Hendel et al. 2002; Heller et al. 2004).

It is important to recognize that the quality of required attenuation maps is quite modest. The spatial and temporal content of the attenuation maps needs only to match that of the SPECT images (Travin 2011). When a high-end diagnostic-quality CT system is used primarily for derivation of attenuation maps, not only should it be operated in a low-dose mode, but also the high spatial and temporal content need to be smoothed out before their use for attenuation correction. For the purpose of deriving patient-specific attenuation maps, a low-cost nondiagnostic tCT approach makes more sense, as well as being cost-effective. In Section 5.2.6.2.2, we review the instrumentation of nondiagnostic tCTs that are available as accessories of SPECT systems. Although these approaches are fading in popularity lately, their approach is instructive and may pave the way for the development of improved systems in the future.

5.2.6.2.2 Types of tCT

Based on the detector systems, there are two types of tCTs in clinical SPECT systems. One has a special detector system designed exclusively for tCT imaging; the other uses the existing SPECT detector system for tCT imaging. Both types need an external radiation source system (either radionuclide based or x-ray based) to provide the transmission photons. As noted before, the radiation exposure to patients from tCTs is at least an order of magnitude lower than that of diagnostic-quality CTs due to the low-resolution requirement of the attenuation maps.

5.2.6.2.2.1 Approaches with a dedicated detector system

This approach was introduced in the early 1990s (Hasegawa et al. 1990; Lang et al. 1992). An independent low-cost x-ray CT is integrated with a SPECT system on the same patient couch, allowing SPECT and tCT imaging to be conducted sequentially (Blankespoor et al. 1996). Commercial versions fit a low-power x-ray tube between the dual heads of a SPECT system and mount a low-cost x-ray detector system on the opposite side of the patient or couch. Because the tCT imaging can be conducted in either the opposing or L-mode, this approach is suitable for implementation in a dual-head system for general-purpose SPECT imaging. For example, GE Healthcare's Infinia Hawkeye SPECT system offers a four-slice CT that acquires data in sequential axial steps to cover a body section. Philips' BrightView XCT uses a half cone of an x-ray beam directed at an offset flat-panel detector for projection acquisition in a single full-circle rotation. Both approaches deliver nondiagnostic tCT images as attenuation maps. Nonetheless, both approaches require their own dedicated detector systems, which means significant extra cost.

5.2.6.2.2.2 Approaches using the same SPECT detector system

This approach was introduced even earlier and had evolved into using a sweeping line source for simultaneous tCT imaging (Bailey et al. 1987; Tan et al. 1993). It was implemented in commercial dual-head SPECT systems in the mid-1990s and is still in use today. Each camera head has a high-intensity Gd-153 line source mounted on the other side of the patient on a transverse plane, opposite and parallel to the camera's face. As an emission projection is being acquired during each rotational stop of the dual-head system, each of the two line sources of the dual heads sweeps in the axial direction across the plane, transmitting a line of collimated photon beam normal to the opposing camera face, through the patient's body and the parallel-hole collimator. As a result, a transmitted projection builds up during the sweep in the 100 keV energy window of the Gd-153s of each head. As the dual-head system rotates in 30+ steps, a complete set of matched 60+ emission and transmission projections is acquired simultaneously over 180°. This is an adequate tCT approach for dual-head cardiac SPECT imaging, but it did not catch on in the broad market. The appeal of this approach declined as hybrid SPECT/CT became available for whole-body applications. For cardiac imaging, the time-consuming sweeping and rotational motion are against the current trend of fast imaging. The other drawbacks are the required radiation safety monitoring of the line sources and their regular replacement.

A similar tCT approach uses characteristic x-rays emitted from a heavy metal target as transmission photons. Digirad Corp. has developed such a Pb x-ray line source for tCT on its cardiac SPECT system (Bai et al. 2010). The characteristic x-rays are generated inside an expanded x-ray tube housing by irradiating an axially oriented Pb line with conventional x-rays of 140 kVp. The emitted Pb x-rays, nearly monoenergetic with a peak at about 75 keV, are collimated by transversely oriented parallel slats to form a volume of contiguous fan beams for multislice tCT imaging. An advantage of this system is that these x-rays are suitable for detectors of existing SPECT systems in their conventional photon counting mode. It can also provide high and stable photon flux over years of operation without regular replacement and emit radiation only when it is turned on. The cost of this approach is low due to its simple and conventional hardware. It has the advantage of providing high-quality nondiagnostic images and attenuation maps, because the photon flux can be tuned to fit patient size to optimize noise level. To take advantage of the relatively high photon flux, the detector system should have high-count-rate capability. This tCT approach is cost-effective and has potential to be further refined.

5.3 IMAGING SYSTEMS

In this section, the development and evolution of SPECT systems are reviewed to set the stage for the description and discussion of new design concepts and new systems.

SPECT systems were developed right after the introduction of x-ray CT in the early 1970s. Several research groups quickly applied digital computed imaging reconstruction to the "section scanning" technique of Kuhl and Edwards (1963) to develop prototype SPECT systems, as detailed in an anthology (Jaszczak 2006). While Kuhl et al. (1976) overhauled their section scanning approach, several other groups developed Anger camera–based prototype SPECT systems (Budinger and Gullberg 1974; Keyes et al. 1977; Jaszczak et al. 1977). Due to Anger camera's broad range of existing clinical applications and wide acceptance, this latter approach quickly led to the development of general-purpose single-head clinical SPECT systems, which became commercially available in the early 1980s and were applied to clinical myocardial perfusion SPECT imaging (MPI). At the same time, the former approach had taken a parallel track, and maintained a line of development of single-purpose brain SPECT systems, mostly in research institutions, until the demand of clinical brain studies declined in the early 1990s. At this point, the MPI SPECT imaging took center stage after growing through the 1980s. Soon after, L-shaped dual-head systems emerged to meet the clinical demands. In the following 10 years, no new SPECT system was introduced publicly. The situation changed in the last decade as several single-purpose cardiac SPECT systems were developed and introduced commercially. Today, general-purpose clinical SPECT systems, almost exclusively dual-head camera–based systems, are the workhorses in all nuclear medicine imaging clinics, with several different single-purpose cardiac SPECT systems adding up to account for a fraction of the clinical systems in use.

5.3.1 Clinical SPECT Imaging

SPECT imaging accounts for the majority of clinical nuclear imaging routines performed in hospital and clinics these days; the remaining are longitudinal whole-body imaging, other planar or functional imaging for various organs in the body, and PET imaging. Clinical SPECT imaging can also be divided into two categories: cardiac imaging and noncardiac imaging, The former—MPI cardiac SPECT imaging—amounts to the overwhelming majority of all clinical SPECT imaging, while the latter—noncardiac SPECT imaging procedures (e.g., brain, bone, and whole-body tumor imaging)—makes up the minor applications.

5.3.1.1 GENERAL-PURPOSE AND SINGLE-PURPOSE SPECT SYSTEMS

General-purpose SPECT systems are well suited to nuclear medicine clinics where a wide range of procedures are performed. These systems use Anger cameras mounted on a gantry to rotate around the imaging volume to acquire projections. They are matured technology with reliable performance and cost-effectiveness. They are particularly appropriate for imaging large sections of the body (e.g., skeleton, lungs, kidneys, and liver). With the Anger camera's inherent 2D projections, multiple slices are acquired so that a sizable volume is imaged simultaneously. To increase system sensitivity, dual-head and triple-head systems were introduced for brain and whole-body SPECT imaging (Lim et al. 1980, 1986). In the last decade, only single-head and dual-head systems have survived as general-purpose clinical systems, because of their versatility for all kinds of SPECT imaging while still keeping the capability of whole-body longitudinal scanning and simple planar imaging. At the same time, the demands of cardiac SPECT imaging have increased to the point that it has become justifiable to develop optimized single-purpose cardiac systems, even at the expense of versatility.

Customized single-purpose SPECT systems evolved from research brain imaging systems. Thus, we will review brain SPECT systems briefly to provide some general background knowledge of and historical perspectives on SPECT instrumentation.

5.3.2 Brain SPECT Imaging

SPECT imaging started from the brain, not only because the brain has always been the major focus of clinical interests, but also because it is ideally suited for imaging system development from an instrumentation point of view. The brain has many attributes that make it the favorable imaging target, such as its well-defined size and location, its circular symmetry, and its suitability for constraining motion. Although brain SPECT systems are not under active development any more, their design concepts and evolution offer valuable insights for cardiac SPECT systems.

5.3.2.1 CONSIDERATION FOR BRAIN SPECT IMAGING

Due to the near cylindrical symmetry of the head, brain SPECT systems have cylindrical or semispherical detection and system geometry to optimize system sensitivity. To meet the requirement of acquiring a number of different projections, two approaches of rotation are used: either rotate the detector–collimator system around the head, as used in general-purpose systems, or rotate a cylindrical collimator system that is inscribed inside a matched stationary cylindrical detector system. For brain SPECT imaging, high resolution is important; the achievable hardware resolution at the center of the brain is typically about 5–8 mm FWHM. One favorable situation of brain SPECT imaging is that tCT imaging is not critically necessary for deriving its attenuation maps. This is because the required attenuation maps can often be assumed to be uniform inside the head contours, which can be estimated from the raw projections or the corresponding pre-attenuation-corrected images.

5.3.2.2 BRAIN SPECT IMAGING USING GENERAL-PURPOSE SYSTEMS

General-purpose brain SPECT systems use single or multiple camera heads to rotate around the head of a patient to acquire a large number (typically 64 or 128) of projections over 360°. In particular, triple-head whole-body SPECT systems, whose detector heads could move radially to lock in a fixed medium-size triangle, could provide excellent brain imaging. Converging-fan and converging-cone collimators have been adopted on single- or multihead systems to increase system sensitivity. Due to limited demand, the current standard clinical brain SPECT imaging uses a general-purpose dual-head system with converging-fan collimators.

5.3.2.3 SINGLE-PURPOSE BRAIN SPECT SYSTEMS

Single-purpose brain SPECT systems have evolved slowly, despite their early start, and stayed mainly in research institutions. Although several systems had made their way to the marketplace in the 1980s and early 1990s, each had only a handful of installed systems and all turned out to be short-lived. The major design concepts and evolution of single-purpose brain SPECT systems are traced in Section 5.3.2.3.1. For details, several review papers remain good references (Rogers and Ackermann 1992; Chang 1996; Abraham and Feng 2011).

5.3.2.3.1 Evolution of early single-purpose brain SPECT systems

The early single-purpose single-slice systems had used 2π detection geometry from the beginning; all systems had detectors and collimators surrounding the head on the transverse plane. The first SPECT system, Mark IV, used a square-frame system and detection geometry (Kuhl et al. 1976). The square frame had four banks; each bank is a linear array of eight discrete non-position-sensitive detection units, each of which is fitted with a long-focal-length focusing collimator. In imaging, the whole square detector frame and collimator array rotates around the patient's head in small angular steps to acquire four orthogonal projections of a single slice simultaneously. Soon after, two design concepts based on circular stationary rings of discrete detectors with rotating collimators were developed independently at the University of Michigan and Shimadzu, Inc. of Japan (Williams et al. 1979; Kanno et al. 1981). Both collimators were in the form of circular rings concentric to, but physically inside and separated from, their respective detector rings. These ring collimators rotate in small steps so that each detector samples in a slightly different direction sequentially to complete a detector-based fan beam in a large number of steps. The completed Michigan's SPRINT system used a large ring of 78 detectors and a multipinhole ring collimator (Rogers et al. 1982). The Shimadzu system used a medium-size ring of 64 detectors and a unique and innovative turbo fan collimator (Hirose et al. 1982). The Shimadzu system was soon marketed with three independent rings for imaging three axial slices simultaneously (Miura et al. 1984). Another system was introduced, called DCAT, for dynamic imaging of regional cerebral blood flow after the patient inhaled Xe-133 gas (Stokely et al. 1980). This system, similar in geometry to the Mark IV system, used a square frame of four banks of detectors, each having 16 NaI:Tl bars of 14 cm axial length to provide three thick slices simultaneously. Its commercial version—Tomomatic 64—was marketed in the early 1980s.

5.3.2.3.2 Maturing of single-purpose brain SPECT systems

Inspired by the concurrent developments of PET systems, single-purpose brain SPECT systems adopted many of the design features in PET systems to improve performance and contain cost. Cylindrical system and detection geometry were recognized as the preferred choice. This geometry also allows stationary detector systems, which could leave the rotation to a cylindrical collimator with a simplified mechanical and electrical design to achieve better performance while containing cost. In the late 1980s, three brain SPECT systems with stationary cylindrical high-resolution detector systems were introduced. One was a circular cylindrical gamma camera built on a medium-size annular monolithic NaI:Tl crystal; it was later marketed as CeraSPECT in the early 1990s (Genna and Smith 1988). It used a multisegmental cylindrical collimator to fit inside the crystal to acquire multiple projections simultaneously. Another was SPRINT II, the axially expanded version of SPRINT with a large-size polygonal cylindrical detector system formed by 11 2D modular cameras (Rogers et al. 1988). A special feature was the cylindrical slit-slat collimator placed inside the polygonal detector. Soon after, McSPECT was developed using a cylindrical system made of modular bar detectors and a cylindrical collimator of multiple long-focal-length modules (Chang et al. 1992).

Clinical brain SPECT imaging reached its peak in the early 1990s. Two Anger camera–based brain SPECT systems came to the market: Hitachi's four-head square system and GE/CGR's three-head triangular system (Kimura et al. 1990; Kouris et al. 1992). At this point, single-purpose brain SPECT systems have been largely optimized in instrumentation. Good-quality brain SPECT images, of 5–8 mm FWHM resolution at the center of the brain, could be acquired in 15–30 min with a standard dose (25 mCi) of Tc-99m-based radiotracers. However, the emergence of high-resolution MRI quickly rendered brain SPECT imaging uncompetitive for most of its routine applications, even though it is still being used in research institutions. Given the accelerated development of new radiotracers and reconstruction techniques, it is conceivable that a resurgence of functional brain SPECT imaging could take place in the future, because it still offers several unique advantages in special situations of functional imaging, especially when the uptake of a tracer or its clearance in the blood takes more than several hours when PET imaging is not feasible.

5.3.3 CARDIAC SPECT IMAGING

Due to the prevalence of coronary artery disease (CAD) in the United States, planar or projection Tl-201 imaging had been the primary choice for assessing myocardial perfusion since the late 1970s. This was the time when the developers of SPECT technology were looking for clinical applications. Thus, clinical MPI using single-head camera-based SPECT systems was quickly established in the early 1980s. Recently, MPI SPECT has grown in popularity, reaching 10 million procedures annually in the United States at one point, and it accounts for half of all clinical nuclear imaging studies performed (IMV 2008). Therefore, an in-depth analysis of cardiac SPECT imaging and systems is warranted. The instrumentation of cardiac SPECT imaging has also been reviewed recently (Travin 2011; Smith 2013; Slomka et al. 2014).

5.3.3.1 GENERAL CONSIDERATIONS FOR CARDIAC SPECT IMAGING

Cardiac SPECT imaging is very different from SPECT imaging of other organs and body sections. This is because the heart and its SPECT imaging are unique in many ways, which include its size, anatomy, off-centered location, cyclic motion, and imaging resolution requirements. Not all these factors and their variations make SPECT imaging more difficult; in fact, often they are more favorable for imaging. For example, the fact that the heart is not buried deep inside the body to suffer heavy attenuation is a blessing; its high contrast uptake of radioactivity to stand out in a low background area is another. The distribution of the perfusion tracer in the myocardium is also simple and favorable: the distribution is simple in geometry and largely predictable in the form of a hollow half ellipsoid with uniform uptake in the slightly more than 1 cm and relatively uniformly thick left ventricular walls. Perfusion defects of clinical interest are usually larger than 2 cm in size, segmental along the myocardium wall, and generally match well with major coronary artery territories. Due to cardiac and respiratory motion, high-resolution (<10 mm FWHM) cardiac SPECT images are not meaningful in current clinical imaging, unless under dual-gated imaging, which requires high system sensitivity, long acquisition time, and effective motion correction. Thus, the spatial resolution requirement in cardiac SPECT imaging is modest. The typically realized hardware resolution averages about 12–14 mm at the center of the heart, which can be provided by typical low-energy high-resolution (LEHR) parallel-hole collimators at an average imaging distance of 20 cm.

The off-centered location of the heart makes the yield of quantity and quality of photons favorable in the left and anterior directions of patients' thorax. As a result, cardiac SPECT imaging has settled to the detection geometry that covers only the left-anterior half of patients' thorax. In using a single-head SPECT system, projection sampling is accomplished by rotating the head in 30–64 steps to cover the 180° arc from the right anterior oblique (RAO) to the left posterior oblique (LPO) of the left-front thorax.

5.3.3.2 USING GENERAL-PURPOSE DUAL-HEAD SYSTEMS FOR CARDIAC SPECT IMAGING

As cardiac SPECT imaging matured in the mid-1990s, it became clear that the L-shape system geometry formed by two camera heads was the practical approach to provide the required detection geometry with a 180° acquisition arc. This is because the dual-head systems are twice as efficient and effective as a single-head system; they need half the time for imaging, as each head rotates 90° with half the number of steps. The system geometry and operation for cardiac SPECT imaging are shown in Figure 5.3. Most dual-head systems also allow general-purpose imaging by configuring the two heads in opposition for whole-body SPECT imaging and whole-body longitudinal scanning.

In current clinical cardiac SPECT imaging using dual-head systems, the junction of the L-shaped dual-head system is initially placed in front of the patient's thorax. The patient's anterior lower thorax is viewed by the two cameras from the RAO and left anterior oblique (LAO) directions simultaneously through a pair of LEHR parallel-hole collimators. The dual-head system rotates 90° in 14 or 31 additional angular steps on the transverse plane to the left, to acquire a total of 30 or 64 projections over the 180° arc on the left front of the thorax in 15 min. Most vendors provide optional iterative reconstruction software with resolution modeling to cut the acquisition time by half to 7.5 min.

The dual-head imaging approach with parallel-hole collimators has been accepted as the standard for several good reasons. It is simple, intuitive, straightforward, and robust without risking missing the patient's heart. The target distance can be adaptively adjusted to suit each patient thoracic contour by using body contour orbit to improve hardware resolution. The large background area around the heart in the acquired projections is helpful and provides general information of extracardiac activities around the heart.

On the other hand, dual-head systems' L-shaped system geometry is not really optimized for cardiac imaging. Their system sensitivities are compromised due to incomplete detector coverage of the left-front

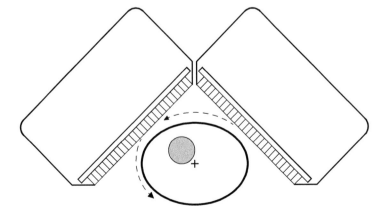

Figure 5.3 Standard system geometry and detection geometry (with rotation indicated by the two arrows) of a dual-head system for imaging a patient. The ellipse (40 × 30 cm) is a phantom representing a large patient's thoracic cross section lying supine on a horizontal couch. The heart is represented by a 10 cm disk located 7 cm to the left front, 45° from the center of the ellipse. Parallel-hole collimators are used on both heads. Also shown in the dashed line is the body contour orbit often used. The imaging operation involves rotating the dual detectors by 90° in small angular steps to cover 180° over the patient's left-front thorax.

thorax. For example, when RAO and LAO projections are covered initially, as shown in Figure 5.3, the LPO direction is left uncovered. In addition, although the total detector area is large, most of the detector area is not directed to the heart region. The large, rigid, and flat heads prevent themselves from being placed close to the heart. This situation cannot be fully mitigated even with the use of body contour orbit, which is determined more by the patient's shoulder, placement of arms, and abdomen size than by the thoracic contour. Furthermore, dual-head systems require rotation to acquire multiple projections; this approach limits framing rate and leads to inconsistent projections acquired at different times. Thus, dual-head systems have limited potential for fast imaging and cannot accommodate dynamic imaging.

5.3.3.3 SINGLE-PURPOSE CARDIAC SPECT SYSTEMS

With the increased clinical demands for cardiac MPI SPECT in the last decade, it became justified to develop single-purpose cardiac SPECT systems to improve performance and reduce imaging time and cost. In addition, clinical imaging has also been facing increasing pressure to address the issues of patient exposure and shortage of radiotracer supply, since cardiac SPECT procedures became a major source of radiation exposure to the general population. Thus, cardiac SPECT systems with high system sensitivity are needed to reduce radiotracer dosage.

Another motivation for high system sensitivity is for the development of the largely untapped area of dynamic myocardium blood flow imaging, which is considered to be the next frontier for cardiac SPECT imaging (Gullberg et al. 2010). To explore this frontier, it is necessary to have SPECT systems capable of imaging with a very fast framing rate of 5–20 s, while providing high enough system sensitivity for a meaningful spatial resolution.

As a result, several single-purpose cardiac SPECT systems have been introduced to the market. These systems are discussed in the following sections along three separate lines: mini-multi-head systems, special collimators on conventional dual-head systems, and unconventional new SPECT systems.

To evaluate the relative merits of these single-purpose systems, the concept of NSGE (Section 5.2.4.3.3.2) with a specific source model can be used to estimate their theoretical performance (Chang et al. 2009). Since dual-head systems are ubiquitous these days, their performance is used as the reference for comparison. Although this NSGE approach could provide objective evaluation of systems, it is difficult to obtain detailed design parameters of commercial systems for accurate estimation. Although generic models can be used, they would be controversial and hard to verify. Thus, we will not quote the NSGE of each system here. We may make general comments of their performance based on other objective observations.

5.3.3.3.1 New concepts for optimized cardiac imaging

Before getting into the details of each individual single-purpose system, we focus on new concepts for optimizing the design of cardiac SPECT systems.

5.3.3.3.1.1 High normalized system sensitivity

Although this is the same simple and most important concept mentioned before, it is new in the sense that it has yet to be taken seriously in new cardiac SPECT systems. The design priority should be to increase NSS to be as high as practically achievable. To do this, we need to have large detection coverage while bringing collimators close to the target to optimize NSGE. A complementary concept is to use minified projections with detectors of high ISR to provide more simultaneous projections and thereby increase system sensitivity.

5.3.3.3.1.2 Cardio-centric geometry

Cardio-centric geometry means to keep the heart at the center of a small imaging volume so that a large number of different projections can be directed to the heart simultaneously. This approach is shared by all new cardiac SPECT systems. It yields multiple projections and increases system sensitivity at the same time for a small or medium-size target. A bonus that comes with the small imaging volume is the reduced number of angular projections required to meet the minimum sampling requirement. Sampling theory requires the number of angular projections to be proportional to the size of the imaging volume and inversely proportional to the image resolution (Cherry et al. 2012). Cardio-centric SPECT systems can thus have a relatively small number of projections, depending on the size of the imaging volume and the resolution intended. For example, conventional dual-head systems typically require about 60 projections for a 40 cm imaging volume. Hence, for a cardio-centric system with a 20 cm imaging volume, 30 projections should be suffice for the typical hardware resolution of 10–12 mm FWHM.

Cardio-centric approach for SPECT imaging also brings its own issues. First, patient positioning is more critical and often difficult due to the small imaging volume and is complicated by the variation of the size and location of the heart, as well as the size and shape of the patient's body. Another issue is the inevitable projection truncation, which causes errors in the reconstructed images due to the resulting inconsistent projections. Fortunately, truncation is usually not a serious issue in cardiac SPECT imaging provided the truncated portions are in the low and uniform background outside the heart (Yu et al. 1997). The currently used iterative reconstruction is fairly effective in handling truncations and keeping errors low. However, there could be situations where introduced errors are significant and could lead to imaging artifacts and quantification errors.

5.3.3.3.1.3 Scout imaging and patient positioning

Before SPECT imaging can be conducted, a patient has to be positioned to have his or her heart properly placed in the imaging volume. This is conventionally done by a technologist with manual adjustments of the patient's position while viewing the real-time monitor—a primitive form of scout imaging. Thus, scout imaging means using a brief preimaging survey to facilitate mechanical adjustment of patient position for imaging. For systems with small imaging volumes, manual positioning by trial and error is difficult, unreliable, and time-consuming. To make the situation more critical, many cardiac SPECT systems have highly nonuniform local GE in the imaging volume. It is thus important to position the heart optimally and reproducibly to benefit from these systems' performance. A scheme of accurate and objective scout imaging is highly desirable, or even necessary, to guide positioning and optimize imaging.

Scout imaging in SPECT should be semiautomated under computer control with operator supervision, similar to those used in CT and MRI. A typical scout imaging is to identify the center of the patient's heart. For example, the center location of the heart can be estimated from briefly acquired projections by real-time computer analysis or operator's judgment. The 3D coordinates of the center of the heart can then be used to set up the subsequent SPECT imaging, by automated mechanical motion to place in the patient's heart in the imaging volume. Thus, proper patient positioning depends on the accuracy of the estimation process, which varies significantly among the current approaches used in different systems.

Scout imaging requires high-sensitivity, low-resolution collimation to keep the presurvey brief. As a result, the same collimators are used for SPECT imaging, unless they can be switched without affecting the patient's position. This is likely the reason that many new cardiac SPECT systems use a high-sensitivity, low-resolution collimator and claim high system sensitivity.

5.3.3.3.1.4 Motion-free imaging operation

Motion of the detector or collimator in SPECT systems during acquisitions of projections is not really a desirable feature. Not only does it cause blurring and prolong imaging, but also it can lead to data inconsistencies among different projections due to timing difference and potential changes of activity and distribution. These kinds of motion are included in a system's imaging operation as a last resort to make up additional projections to meet the sampling requirement.

Eliminating detector or collimator motion during imaging altogether, if possible, allows a system to achieve 4D imaging. SPECT systems for fast imaging should be motion-free, or stationary, during acquisition so that all projections are acquired simultaneously, consistent with each other, and in as short a time frame as needed. Motion-free imaging systems also have many other practical advantages, such as simplicity in system design, accurate and precise operations of electronic and mechanical components, efficient detection without interruptions, and improved patient comfort.

Motion-free SPECT systems are difficult to develop to provide adequate system sensitivity and resolution while also meeting angular sampling requirements. On the other hand, it is not impossible to develop them for special applications with appropriate compromises.

5.3.3.3.2 Mini-multi-head cardiac SPECT systems

Several single-purpose SPECT systems based on dual-head geometry and design concepts were quickly developed and marketed. These systems target clinical applications performed in outpatient clinics and mobile imaging services. Two such approaches are described next.

5.3.3.3.2.1 Mini-dual-head systems

These are scaled-down dual-head systems for dedicated cardiac SPECT imaging. The Siemens c.cam, General Electric Ventri, and Philips CardioMD are examples of these systems. Several small companies have also come up with similar designs. These systems use two medium-size Anger cameras, each with an FOV of about 35×20 cm, with parallel-hole collimators. The two heads are fixed in a rigid L-shape inside its housing or a semicircular cover and generally operate similarly to large dual-head systems. Patient imaging positions could vary from supine to recline or upright. Some of them come with the options of body contouring or tCT imaging using Gd-153 flood sources. These systems perform with a system sensitivity and hardware resolution that are similar to those of their full-size counterparts, except with a slightly smaller imaging volume and reduced size, weight, footprint, and cost.

5.3.3.3.2.2 Cardius series from Digirad

The Cardius platform is a series of mini-multi-head SPECT systems marketed by Digirad Corp. The long axis of their systems is vertically oriented for imaging a patient sitting upright on a chair. The Cardius 2 system was introduced first as a small FOV dual-head system. The Cardius 3 system added an additional head later to increase system sensitivity. The Cardius series has implemented several unique features and is described in more detail here.

The three mini-heads of Cardius 3 are placed on a circular arc on a transverse plane normal to the system's long axis. The system geometry and imaging operation are shown in Figure 5.4. The mini-heads, each having a 20×16 cm FOV, are separated from each other by $67.5°$ on the arc. The nominal cylindrical imaging volume is 20 cm in diameter and 16 cm axially, aligning with the patient chair's rotational axis, which is also the entire imaging system's longitudinal axis. For imaging, the heads are first locked at a selected radial distance, based on estimated thoracic size of the patient. The patient's body is offset on the chair appropriately so that his or her heart is centered on the chair's axis of rotation, which is also the axis of the imaging volume. Then, the chair with the patient begins to rotate $7.5°$ or $3.75°$ in each step, over $67.5°$ in 9 or 19 additional steps, to acquire a total of 30 or 60 projections over $202.5°$, symmetrical to the LAO line of the patient.

The mini-heads use conventional high-resolution parallel-hole collimators or optional long-focal-length converging-fan collimators for projection acquisition. Each head is based on a pixelated-CsI:Ti/Si-PIN array

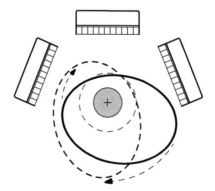

Figure 5.4 System geometry and detection geometry of Digirad's Cardius 3 system, relative to our elliptical phantom. The three small detector heads are separated by $67.5°$, and fixed in positions, on an arc with a radius appropriate for the patient's body size. Either parallel-hole or slightly converging-fan collimators are used. The patient sits upright on a centrally located chair and offset slightly to the right, with his or her heart located on the vertical axis of the chair. The imaging operation is to have the chair rotate over $67.5°$ in small angular steps, as indicated by the arrows, to provide a total of $202°$ projection coverage.

(Section 5.2.5.2.1.2). The array is made up of square pixels with 6.1 mm pitch and 5 mm thickness. These detector heads yield an average energy resolution of 10.5% (Bai et al. 2010).

The Cardius 3 offers an optional tCT approach, using characteristic Pb x-rays (Section 5.2.6.2.2.2), to derive attenuation maps. The x-rays emit from an axial-oriented Pb line housed in a stationary x-ray tube to provide a contiguous volume of transverse fan beam of approximately 30° fan angle. In preparation for tCT imaging, the three mini-heads are manually moved to line up side by side behind the patient on the opposite side of the x-ray unit. The tCT imaging is conducted by rotating the patient on the axis of the chair over about 210°. Because of the high-count-rate performance of the heads, good-quality nondiagnostic tCT images can be derived.

The advantage of the Cardius 3 system is that it provides SPECT imaging at a relatively low cost and even with a tCT option. Although it has three mini-heads with a total of 960 cm^2 detector area, its SGE is only comparable to conventional dual-head systems, because it lacks the body-contouring option and has to use a long target distance as well as the fact its current detector has relatively low sensitivity (Section 5.2.5.2.1.2). A shortcoming of the Cardius 3 system is its difficult manual patient positioning procedure, especially when the optional converging-fan collimators are used. Another weakness is its lack of effective back support and constraints to keep patients sitting upright on the chair. As a result, it is difficult for the patient to remain in the same pose without sagging during the 5–10 min imaging time, let alone to keep the same exact pose for the additional rotation of tCT imaging. Similar to dual-head systems, the relatively long imaging time for patient rotation limits their framing rate and potential for fast imaging, and precludes dynamic imaging.

5.3.3.3.3 Using special cardiac collimators on conventional dual-head systems

A more advanced approach to take advantage of the large detectors of existing dual-head systems is to use special cardiac collimators. These collimators allow more effective use of the detectors by directing more detector area to the heart to achieve high SGE. Another attraction of this approach is its simple implementation and relatively low cost. For users that already have a dual-head SPECT system, this approach requires only two identical collimators and a software package. At the same time, the dual-head systems still retain all the capabilities for other general-purpose imaging. Two such approaches are MP-SPECT and IQ-SPECT.

5.3.3.3.3.1 MP-SPECT

MP-SPECT is a recent one in the series of multipinhole collimator approach that has long been pursued by the Colorado group (Vogel et al. 1978). The idea is to use multiple-pinhole collimators on existing SPECT systems for cardiac imaging. It started out from a seven-pinhole collimator on a single camera years ago, and has evolved by adding detector coverage and pinholes (Funk et al. 2006; Steele et al. 2008). Promoted by Eagle Heart Imaging LLC until a few years ago, the last version uses two identical nine-pinhole collimators to fit on an L-shaped standard dual-head system, as shown in Figure 5.5. MP-SPECT is intended for dynamic imaging; it operates without motion to acquire 18 projections simultaneously in as short a time frame as needed.

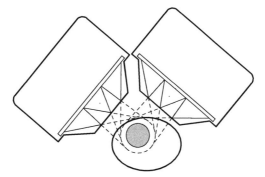

Figure 5.5 System and detection geometry of the MP-SPECT system, relative to our elliptical phantom. A conventional dual-head system, with each head fitted with a nine-pinhole collimator, is placed in the anterior thorax of the patient, with the patient's heart in the 20 cm imaging volume. The imaging operation is motion-free simultaneous projection acquisition through the 18 pinholes.

Each of the collimators has a 3 × 3 array of pinholes on its front end. The central axes of all 18 pinholes converge to the center of an imaging volume of about 20 cm diameter. This center is located at the intersection of the central axes of the two collimators and is approximately 20 cm from the collimators. All 18 pinholes acquire simultaneous and nonoverlapping projections of the imaging volume on the detector plane. Using 8 mm diameter pinholes, the predicted system sensitivity is estimated to be five times that of dual-head cardiac SPECT systems using LEHR collimation (Funk et al. 2006). These large pinholes perform in the high-sensitivity end of the high-sensitivity/low-resolution range.

Although MP-SPECT systems have a total detector area of 4000 cm^2, adapting them for multiple pinhole imaging is constrained by the rigid geometry and performance of the dual-head systems. For example, each of the 16 peripheral projections uses a quite large detector area due to oblique photon incidence. Another limitation is that the design concept of projection minification cannot be used to provide a large number of simultaneous projections, due to the limited ISR of the standard heads in dual-head systems.

Little information on the specific technical design and performance of MP-SPECT has been published and validated by other researchers. Although much improved from its early designs, MP-SPECT has not gone far enough to mitigate its weakness: an inadequately small number of projections in a limited angular coverage. It still falls short of meeting angular sampling requirements in both transverse and axial planes (Budinger 1980). To address this issue, the latest proposed improvement is to increase the number of pinholes to 20, in a 5 × 4 pattern in each collimator, and add a 45° rotation of both heads to provide a total of 80, or 20 × 4, projections over the 180° angular range (Bowen et al. 2013). Although this expansion to 20 projections in four axial rows makes angular sampling more adequate, proper patient positioning would be difficult to achieve.

5.3.3.3.3.2 IQ-SPECT

IQ-SPECT, introduced by Siemens Molecular imaging, is the other approach using existing dual-head systems for high-sensitivity cardiac SPECT imaging. It fits a multifocal collimator (SMARTZOOM®) onto each of the two large FOV heads to acquire a projection of the heart with high GE. It is the extension of the Cardiofocal collimator approach that Siemens proposed previously (Hsieh 1989; Hawman and Haines 1994). This approach has matured recently after implementing iterative reconstruction that incorporates imaging physics on the Siemens Symbia platform (Vija et al. 2010). The design, operation, and performance of the collimator and the IQ-SPECT technology are complex and unconventional. To benefit from their performance and avoid their pitfalls, it is necessary to understand their designs and use them properly. Since it is widely used currently, we provide a more in-depth coverage than what was previously published.

The idea is to achieve high system sensitivity by using converging collimation, but without its major side effect—projection truncation and the resulting artifacts. IQ-SPECT achieves these objectives through the new SMARTZOOM collimators, which also help mitigate other side effects of converging collimation, such as small imaging volume, insufficient axial sampling, and axial distortion.

The design of the SMARTZOOM collimator in the central transverse plane is shown in Figure 5.6a. In a simple and broad glance, it is a multifocal collimator with variable focal length. Although this figure, provided by the vendor, is only approximate in depicting the general design of the SMARTZOOM collimator, it is sufficient to convey the concepts that lead to the enhanced performance. The sampling lines of the collimator's channels on the central transverse plane are marked in Figure 5.6a in the imaging space in front of the collimator up to about 50 cm from the collimator surface. Except for the central channel, the sampling lines of all the other channels on this plane are tilted toward the central axial plane of the collimator. The distance between the intersection point of the sampling line with the central axial plane and the collimator surface is the focal length of the particular channel. The signature design feature is that the focal length increases from 50 cm, at the immediate neighborhood of the center, to 500 cm at both edges of the collimator. In fact, the focal length of a local channel increases as a highly nonlinear (quartic) function of its distance to the central axial plane. These series of multiple intersection points on this transverse plane are also on the central axial plane of the collimator.

In the axial dimension, the collimator has the same general design and the same focal length and function, except the axial length is reduced by about 25% (38 cm instead of the transverse width of 53 cm). Thus, each orthogonal dimension provides an independent multifocal converging-fan collimation. Combined together, it is a 2D multifocal converging-fan collimator, which has rectangular symmetry rather than elliptical symmetry.

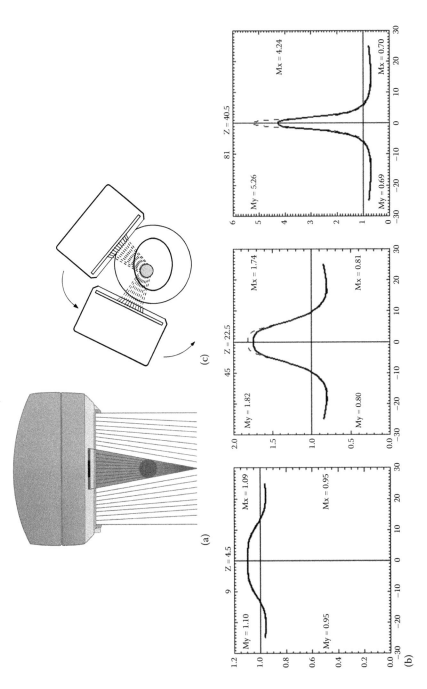

Figure 5.6 IQ-SPECT system of Siemens. (a) SMARTZOOM collimator, mounted on a Siemens camera. It is a variable-focal-length collimator in design, but functionally, it is a hybrid collimator of a converging fan at the central region (shaded area) surrounded by diverging-fan collimation in the peripheral region. In this central transverse plane, the highlighted disk region of 10 cm in diameter, with its center located 28 cm from the collimator and on the central axis, is the sweet spot. Its center is to be placed at the center of the patient's heart in each step of the head rotation. (b) Estimated 1D profiles of LGM for the three planes located at 5, 23, and 41 cm from the collimator, respectively. These profiles are bell shaped, reflecting their GE being shifted toward the center volume in different degrees at the expense of the peripheral volume. The height of the peak, the width of the profile, and the steepness of the slope vary with the distance of each plane. The horizontal reference line of 1.0 in LGM on each plot is the corresponding profile of a parallel-hole collimator that has a constant magnification. (c) System geometry of the IQ-SPECT system relative to our elliptical phantom. The dual heads, each fitted with a SMARTZOOM collimator, rotate around the patient aiming at the patient's heart, which is offset to the left from the rotational axis of the dual-head system, to acquire nontruncated projections of the patient's left-front thorax. To achieve the high gain in detection sensitivity offered by the collimator, the system manages to keep the center of the heart always at the sweet spot during projection acquisition. The large circle in the background is the patient aperture of the gantry. (Courtesy of A. H. Vija, Siemens Healthcare, Molecular Imaging, Erlangen, Germany.)

A close look of the sampling lines of the channels in the peripheral regions of the collimator in Figure 5.6a reveals that these regions should be viewed as a variation of divergent-fan collimator. These channels perform as divergent-fan collimation because their sampling lines actually diverge in the imaging volume, in contrast to the converged sampling lines in the center region of the collimator. Thus, the SMARTZOOM collimator has combined converging and diverging fans in one design. The central region is converging fan, with improved GE and collimator resolution with distance, and is desirable for imaging a small or medium-size target. The peripheral region is diverging fan, which performs oppositely to yield poor GE and collimator resolution, and is only suitable for imaging background around the target. The converging and diverging fans match seamlessly to yield smooth transition in collimation performance between the two regions to provide a full untruncated projection.

To understand the performance of this SMARTZOOM collimator, it is best to examine the variation of local point source geometric efficiency (lpGE) in the imaging volume, which is a large cylindrical volume of 53 cm diameter and 38 cm in axial length. Each collimator effectively creates a central small volume of high GE at the expense of the local GE in the surrounding peripheral volume. The lpGE can be measured by stepping a point source throughout the imaging volume. It can also be estimated from 1D local geometric magnification (LGM) profiles provided by the vendor, because the lpGE is proportional to the product of the two orthogonal LGMs at each location. Three plots of the LGM profiles are shown separately in Figure 5.6b for planes parallel to, and at 5, 23, and 41 cm from, the collimator face. Note that the transverse (solid line) and axial (dashed line) profiles on each plot are nearly identical in shape on the same plane, when the scale of the width and length is normalized. These profiles show that the closer a plane is to the first focal point (at 50 cm), the higher the peak, narrower the width, and steeper the slope of the profile. A horizontal line of 1.0 magnification is a reference representing the LGM profile of a parallel-hole collimator.

In Figure 5.6a, the highlighted spherical volume inscribed in the converging fan can be called the sweet spot, which is about 10 cm in diameter and located at 28 cm from the collimator face on its central axis. We are most interested in the lpGE profile on this 28 cm plane, which is in the middle and representative of other similar planes of the sweet spot. Although this corresponding LGM profile was not provided, it can be estimated and is expected to have a higher peak and narrower width than the middle profile shown for the plane at 23 cm. The lpGE profile derived from the two orthogonal 1D LGMs on this plane would have even narrower relative width and steeper slopes. Hence, the 2D lpGE profile for the plane at 28 cm can be described as follows: It reaches a peak of no more than 5.0 at the center of the sweet spot and remains high within a rectangle of 10 cm (transversely) × 7.5 cm (axially) centered at the peak. The 2D lpGE profile then drops sharply radially outside this rectangle a rate of 8% and 10% per centimeter in the corresponding orthogonal directions in the next 5 and 4 cm, respectively, to the 1.0 reference line on the borders of a larger rectangle of about 18 × 14 cm on this plane. It keeps dropping radially outward with a slower rate below the reference line and remains flat before backing up slightly in the edge regions.

To realize the maximum detection sensitivity, the center of the patient's heart, which could be defined as the center of mass of the activity distribution in the myocardium, should be placed at the center of the sweet spot of each collimator during imaging. The limited size of the sweet spot and the sharp drop of the lpGE outside the sweet spot require patient positioning to be accurate. Because stepped rotation of the dual heads is necessary, IQ-SPECT has to accomplish the complex task of placing the two sweet spots onto the heart for each step of the rotation. The operation of IQ-SPECT is modified from that of dual-head systems to combine stepped rotation with additional fine adjustments of each head. The two heads are separated, as shown in Figure 5.6c, on the transverse plane by 104° on the 28 cm arc centered at the long axis of the system. In imaging, both heads rotate along the arc in synchrony over 98° in 16 steps, each 6.1°, to acquire a total of 34 projections covering 201° of the left-front thorax of the patient.

For imaging, the patient lies either supine or prone on a couch in the circular patient aperture to allow the two heads to conduct complex maneuvering. Because patients' hearts are not on the long axis of the gantry and vary slightly in location in the patients' thorax, each head's radial distance and central axis have to be adjusted at each step. Basically, the two heads have to adjust their central axes by a small lateral or angular movement after each rotational step, to re-aim at the center of the patient's heart. To prepare for this complex rotation and adjustment, the center of the patient's heart is estimated first. This estimation procedure requires the operator to place two on-screen cursers, one for each head, on the real-time display monitor separately to mark the respective centers of the patient's heart on a pair of nearly orthogonal, distortion-corrected real-time projections. A road map for adjustments is then set up and stored in the computer for subsequent execution.

Although the multifocal collimators, with a 1.9 mm hole size and minimum channel length of 40 mm, have medium-sensitivity/high-resolution performance at the standard 10 cm distance, they perform in the sweet spot in the high-sensitivity/low-resolution range. Their relative system sensitivity has been reported from published data. Vija et al. (2010) reported that the peak lpGE at the center of the sweet spot is four times that of a parallel-hole collimator. Zeintl et al. (2011) showed the corresponding planar NEMA-like tests for system specifications. Imbert et al. (2012) reported that the system sensitivity measured with a standard heart phantom placed in the sweet spot is three times that of dual-head systems using LEHR collimators. These results are consistent with our estimated lpGE, as described above, and are the upper limits with the optimal placement of the source models. In clinical imaging, the achievable detection sensitivity depends critically on the accuracy with which the center coordinates of the heart can be marked by the operator.

Another factor that compromises the number of detected photons in imaging operation is the idle time. In the currently recommended 4 min imaging protocol, it has a 9/14 active-duty cycle, which means only 9 s is used for acquisition in each of the 14 s steps (Rajaram et al. 2011). The remaining 5 s is required for rotating and adjusting the position of the heads. The effective sensitivity is thus reduced by one-third to be twice that of a conventional dual-head system for imaging a cardiac phantom. This level of system sensitivity is excellent, provided the sweet spots are placed properly. The effect of this relatively long idle time could be reduced by coupling continuing acquisition during movement of the heads with high framing rate projection acquisition.

On the other hand, IQ-SPECT is relatively forgiving if the patient's heart is placed off the center of the sweet spot because the patient's heart would always be in the large imaging volume. However, this feature does not make positioning less critical because the detected number of photons and spatial resolution could be seriously compromised. The severity of compromise depends on the extent of off positioning. Furthermore, when suboptimal image quality is derived, a question is how the users can rule out off positioning as the cause and repeat imaging with better positioning. IQ-SPECT needs an accurate, objective, and reproducible patient positioning and a verification scheme to ensure its optimal performance in routine imaging.

An inherent limitation of IQ-SPECT is its low framing rate, caused by the necessary large-arc rotational motion of the heads, which limits its potential for fast imaging and precludes it from dynamic imaging.

5.3.3.3.4 Unconventional single-purpose cardiac SPECT systems

Since cardiac SPECT systems cannot be adapted from general-purpose SPECT systems without compromising performance, cardiac SPECT systems should be designed from the ground up to optimize imaging performance and operations. Several novel cardiac SPECT systems have been introduced and discussed in general terms already (Madsen 2007; Patton et al. 2007; Slomka et al. 2009; Garcia et al. 2011; DePuey 2012). In the following, we provide in-depth reviews from the instrumentation perspective. Two current commercial single-purpose cardiac SPECT systems and two additional ones under development are described and analyzed.

5.3.3.3.4.1 D-SPECT

The D-SPECT system has been marketed by Spectrum Dynamics, Inc. for 10 years. It introduced the first major change in design of clinical SPECT systems and implemented several novel features, such as CZT detectors, scout imaging for defining patient-specific imaging volume, and iterative image reconstruction with resolution recovery techniques.

It has nine axially oriented detector columns arranged in an L-shape circumference inside a fixed gantry, whose transverse plane is shown in Figure 5.7. Each detector column has its back pivoted on an axially oriented rod, which serves as its swivel axis and is controlled by a stepper motor. Each column of the detector is made up of an axial array of four standard CZT tiles with 2.5 mm pixels (described in Section 5.2.5.2.1.3), and provides a detection area of 4×16 cm. The front of each detector column has a pixel-matched parallel-square-hole

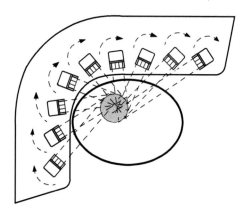

Figure 5.7 System and detection geometry of the D-SPECT system relative to our elliptical phantom. The patient lies on a dental chair half reclined with his or her left-front thorax placed nearly against the L-shape stationary gantry. Nine detector columns are lined up axially inside its gantry along the L. A parallel-hole collimator of 4 cm width is fitted in front of each detector column. Each detector column swivels on its axis to sample projections in a large number of small angular steps across a predetermined imaging volume where the heart is located. Each of the detector columns is a linear array of four standard CZT tiles.

collimator made of tungsten. Each square hole is 2.3 mm in size and 22 mm in channel length. The average energy resolution of the system is 5.5% at 140 keV (Erlandsson et al. 2009).

For imaging, a patient lies on a semireclined dental chair with the L-shaped gantry system placed close to the patient's left-front thorax. A brief scout scan is conducted first, in which each detector column quickly swivels over a default angular range to survey the activity distribution in the general direction of the patient's heart. The result of the survey determines the location and size of a cylindrical imaging volume, from which a custom angular range is defined for the subsequent swivel of each detector column. In clinical imaging, all nine detector columns swivel in synchrony in very small angular (<1°) steps from one side of the imaging volume to the other in 120 steps. A projection of 40 mm transverse width is acquired at each step, which can have weighted dwell time to spend more time on the target than on the background. The system has been reported to have a sensitivity 8–10 times that of a dual-head system using a pair of ultra-high-resolution collimators (Sharir et al. 2008; Gambhir et al. 2009). Based on their physical specifications, these collimators perform in the high-sensitivity/low-resolution range.

The D-SPECT system uses proprietary software for image reconstruction and resolution recovery. Its resolution recovery compensates for the low hardware resolution used in imaging to sharpen the reconstructed images. High-sensitivity collimators are used in this system and lead to the reported high system sensitivity that is much more than the typical values reported by other vendors. Another reason for this high sensitivity is that the performance of the D-SPECT system has been reported under rather vague and not standardized conditions. However, one certainty is that its SGE is limited by the system's relatively small total detector area (576 cm²). This fact is also reflected by the presence of large air gaps between the detector columns. Because the total linear length of air gaps along the transverse circumference of the detector system is much larger than that of the nine detectors (36 cm), considerably more emission photons pass through the air gaps than those crossing paths with the detectors. These air gaps are necessary to provide room for the swivel and shielding of the detector columns. In addition, although the collimators are parallel-hole in structure, they do not really offer the favorable performance of large parallel-hole collimators. As explained in Section 5.2.5.1.1.2, the narrow width of these collimators brings distance and off-axis discrimination to activities in the transverse planes. Moreover, the narrow width of the detector–collimator also means that most of the projections are not acquired at exactly the same time and are bound to have inconsistencies due to changes of tracer distribution with time. Thus, the swivel scanning limits D-SPECT systems' potential for fast, gated, and dynamic imaging.

5.3.3.3.4.2 Discovery 530c

The latest single-purpose clinical cardiac SPECT system is Discovery 530c, introduced by GE Healthcare (Esteves et al. 2009). Its design was inspired by MP-SPECT and can be viewed as its refined implementation with an improved detection geometry and detector system.

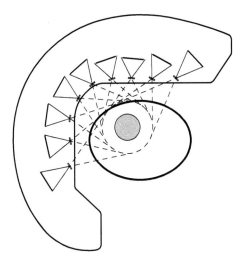

Figure 5.8 System geometry and detection geometry of the Discovery 530c system, relative to our elliptical phantom. Inside the central transverse plane of the L-shaped gantry are nine stationary pinhole–CZT detector units fixed along the L and pointed individually to the center of the 20 cm imaging volume. Each of the units is an 8 × 8 cm CZT detector fitted with a pinhole collimator in the front. There are an additional two rows, and each row has five such units placed axially to and aligned with the odd number of units of the central plane. These 10 units tilt axially toward the center of the imaging volume. The patient lies supine on a horizontal standard CT couch with his or her heart placed in the imaging volume. The imaging operation is motion-free simultaneous projection acquisition by all 19 pinhole–detector units.

The Discovery 530c is made up of 19 stationary units of collimator detector in an L-shaped gantry, as shown in Figure 5.8. Each unit is a pinhole collimator with an 8 × 8 cm square detector plate placed behind and perpendicular to the pinhole's axis. Each detector plate is a 2 × 2 array of the standard CZT tiles. Each of these pinhole–detector units aims its central axis at the center of a fixed imaging volume in the patient aperture. The detector's high ISR is put to good use by a minification factor of 2.5 for the 20 cm diameter imaging volume to be projected onto the 8 cm detectors (Bocher et al. 2010; Kennedy et al. 2014).

The pinhole–detector units are arranged axially inside the gantry in three rows in a 5-9-5 pattern. The central axes of the nine pinholes in the middle row are on the central transverse plane. Each of the two outside row's five units aligns axially with an odd-numbered unit of the middle row. These outside units have their central axes tilted axially toward the center of the imaging volume. Each collimator has a pinhole of 5.1 mm in diameter, and thus performs halfway between a high-sensitivity/low resolution collimator and a medium-sensitivity/medium-resolution collimator.

Discovery 530c has been reported to have a system sensitivity three to five times that of dual-head systems (Bocher et al. 2010). Based on its total size of detector area (1216 cm²), its SGE should be respectable, however, its pinhole collimation imposes a severe (inverse-square) penalty on its system sensitivity in the distance range of 15–25 cm—the target distance from the pinholes to the center of the imaging volume.

During imaging, the patient lies supine or prone on a horizontal couch, with his or her heart placed in the imaging volume for all 19 pinhole–detector units to view and acquire their respective projections simultaneously from the left-front thorax. The system's most important feature is its motion-free imaging operation, which facilitates fast imaging and allows dynamic imaging. A hybrid SPECT/CT—Discovery 570c—had been commercially available for a few years and was simply a Discovery 530c integrated with a diagnostic x-ray CT.

Although this system uses better detectors and detection geometry than MP-SPECT, the current design has not gone far enough to reach its full potential and still leaves plenty of room for improvement. This opinion is also based on the observation of large air gaps between the detectors. For example, the total linear length of the air gaps along the circumference of the detector system in the central transverse plane is about half of that of the all nine detectors in the middle row. In each of the two outer rows, the linear length of air gaps is nearly twice that of the five detectors. Overall, the total area of air gaps in the three rows of detectors is comparable to the total detector area. This means that about half of emission photons escape detection.

In addition, the numbers of angular projections of the system, both transversely and axially, are also on the low side for cardiac imaging. This opinion is supported by several simulation studies (Li et al. 2010; Bowen et al. 2013). Similar to MP-SPECT, Discovery 530c's SGE is limited by pinhole collimation that discriminates against activities at distance and off-axis. This inherent trait favors activities in close range and leads to the reported sharp (>8% per centimeter) local sensitivity gradient in its imaging volume (Kennedy et al. 2014). The implication of this large sensitivity gradient is that the realizable system sensitivity and its reproducibility are sensitive to the placement of the heart. An additional concern is the current high cost of CZT detectors and thus the system. Although the first two issues—the air gaps and the number of angular projections—can be improved by filling more pinhole–detector units in the air gaps, the current high cost of CZT detectors makes this addition unlikely in the short term.

5.3.3.3.4.3 Other emerging cardiac SPECT systems

Two additional cardiac SPECT systems—CardiArc and C-SPECT—have been proposed and warrant discussion due to their unique design concepts in the context of cardiac SPECT instrumentation. Both systems were inspired by the brain SPECT system—SPRINT II—and use a large open-arc detector system and slit-slat collimators. For simplicity in development, the long axes of these systems are vertically oriented for patients to be imaged in a slightly reclined upright position. Although these two systems look similar in outside shape, from the outside their design concepts, implementation, imaging operation, and potential performance are very different.

The design concept of CardiArc is a semicylindrical version of SPRINT II adapted for cardiac imaging (Juni 2003). Its slit-slat collimator system sits in the front of a stationary and nearly horizontally oriented semicylindrical gantry. Behind the collimator system is a semicylindrical gamma camera made up of three 60° arcs of curved monolithic NaI:Tl slabs with their exit window covered by an array of large-size (3 in.) PMTs. The front half of the collimator system is a large 180° slit-arc, which has five axially oriented slits equally spaced 36° apart. During imaging, the slit-arc rotates, while the slat-stack remains stationary, in small angular steps along its semicircular track. Following SPRINT II's original sampling operation, as each of the slits step through a 36° arc, each detector element on the arc is directed by a slit in its front to sample a ray in a slightly different direction sequentially on a transverse plane of the imaging volume. After a large number (about 100) of steps, each detector element completes a set of data that forms a detector-based projection fan. Although technical details have not been disclosed, nor has its performance been confirmed, it is clear that CardiArc has two major limitations. First, its SGE is low because there are only five slits used for acquisition. The second is the time required for the slits to complete the rotation in steps. Not only does this sampling scheme create internal inconsistencies in the acquired projection fan, but also the finite framing rate limits its potential for fast, gated imaging and precludes dynamic imaging.

Currently under development at the prototype stage, the C-SPECT platform (proposed by one of the authors) is optimized for cardiac SPECT imaging with high SGE and expanded functionality (Chang et al. 2009; Rozler et al. 2014). As shown in Figure 5.9, it uses an elliptical open-arc detection and system geometry to achieve cardiac-centric imaging from a large number of directions. It has five different slit-sections connected on a conveyor system and looped around the detector system in the stationary gantry. Each slit-section is a train of multiple discrete lead plates, with some plates containing a slit, forming a transaxial collimator section for an imaging task. Each slit-section has a number (7–18) of slits, each of which casts a projection of a predefined imaging volume (PIV) on the detector system to be acquired simultaneously with other slits of the same slit-section. The curved detector system is essentially continuous and comprised of a transverse array of 14 pixelated NaI:Tl detector modules covered by an array of medium-size (5 cm) PMTs. The active area of the detector system is 2000 cm² (125 × 16 cm) covering a 200° arc with little air gaps (Rozler et al. 2012; Popovic et al. 2014).

In imaging, the patient's heart is moved semiautomatically in a smart chair–computer operation into a specific PIV following a brief scout imaging that identifies the center of the heart. The conveyor system facilitates a collimation exchange operation to set up a collimation of appropriate sensitivity and resolution for imaging (Rozler and Chang 2011; Sankar et al. 2014). There are five choices of collimation, including those for scout imaging, tCT imaging, high-sensitivity SPECT imaging, and high-resolution SPECT imaging for two different PIVs for patients of different body and heart sizes. Each collimation exchange takes 10 s without

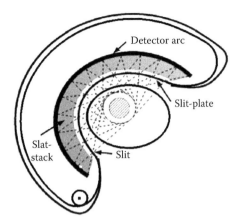

Figure 5.9 System geometry and detection geometry of C-SPECT, relative to the elliptical phantom. It shows a C-shaped continuous detector arc and a matched slit-slat collimator system. The latter conforms to the gantry's patient aperture. The slit-plates and slat-stack are physically separated and function independently. A large number (7–18) of transverse nonoverlapped projections of the heart can be projected and acquired simultaneously through the slits for an imaging volume. Multiple slit-plates connected in a loop on a conveyor belt wrap around the detector system in the gantry. Each slit-plate can be brought up onto the center stage, through rotation of the belt controlled by a stepper motor, for collimation for a specific imaging task.

disturbing the patient, who sits on a slightly reclined chair with firm back support and motion-restraining devices. C-SPECT also has an integrated Digirad's Pb x-ray system for tCT, which works well with the high-count-rate modular detector system in a conventional photon counting operation. The NSGE of the first C-SPECT system, with parallel slats and 16 slits for a 16 cm PIV, is estimated to be 2.2 times that of dual-head systems (Strologas et al. 2012). All SPECT imaging acquisitions are motion-free to facilitate fast, gated, and dynamic imaging.

5.4 FUTURE DIRECTIONS

The direction of future clinical SPECT instrumentation is to keep on improving its quantitative imaging performance to derive objective diagnostic information. Quantification, although difficult, is the strength of ECT that makes it unique. This goal is achievable because all the degradation factors affecting quantification are known and can be dealt with effectively, as well demonstrated in the literature (Tsui et al. 1998). To achieve this goal, more improvements and optimization in both hardware and the reconstruction algorithm are needed. The following sections address the many potential evolution directions of clinical SPECT instrumentation.

5.4.1 GEOMETRY

To achieve high system sensitivity and imaging potential, detection geometry is the key. An optimized system should devote as much active detector area as practically achievable to catch as many quality photons from the imaging volume while keeping collimation distance as short as possible. For brain SPECT imaging, cylindrical or semispherical detection geometry could be optimal. For whole-body SPECT imaging, due to body size variations, multihead systems with adaptive body contour orbiting are practical. For cardiac SPECT imaging, a large (~200°) open-arc body-contour-conforming cylindrical geometry may be optimal. To further increase SGE, axial-converging collimation can be implemented. Two commercial cardiac SPECT systems—IQ-SPECT and Discovery 530c–have already taken this approach. Ultimately, an optimized large detector area design of clinical cardiac SPECT systems with axial-converging detection geometry could potentially push a system beyond an NSGE of 3.0 (Chang et al. 2008).

5.4.2 COLLIMATION

Collimation is the bottleneck in SPECT imaging. It should be noted that different types of collimation behave very differently. Several second-order behaviors of collimation have significant implications on SPECT imaging. For example, more attention should be given to GE's distant and off-axis behavior. Projection minification is a design option that can be used to increase SGE indirectly for a given detector area, provided the detector system has sufficiently high ISR.

Advances in software processing techniques may have shifted the conventional balance between sensitivity and hardware resolution in cardiac SPECT systems toward sensitivity. Which collimation compromise between GE and collimator resolution provides the optimal diagnostic value for a given clinical imaging task needs to be investigated rigorously. The answers are likely to be imaging specific, algorithm specific, and task specific.

Most new cardiac SPECT systems currently use high-sensitivity/low resolution collimators. It is not totally clear whether these collimators are better for diagnostic purposes. An implicit fact is that these existing systems have to use the same collimators for both patient positioning and SPECT imaging, because switching collimators would change the patient's imaging position.

5.4.3 DETECTOR

The detector system captures emission photons to realize its detection geometry. An ideal detector for SPECT systems should have high stopping power for 140 keV photons, high ISR, good energy resolution, and low cost, and be adaptable to different imaging geometries. Detectors that have submillimeter spatial resolution without compromising stopping power and photofraction could allow future designs of SPECT systems to use highly minified projections. Then, hundreds of pinholes could be used with a net increase of SGE and number of simultaneous projections. Among the new detectors, pixelated CZT semiconductor detectors and pixelated-CsI(TI) with photodiodes or SiPMs have the potential to further improve their performance to be detectors of the future. However, their cost is still the major concern, at least for systems that require large-area detectors. One important direction of the development of these detectors is to reduce their cost through improved manufacturing yield and increased production scale.

5.4.4 ADAPTIVE IMAGING

Adaptive imaging has long been used in CT and MRI. This concept was introduced and applied to animal SPECT imaging by the Arizona group and was proposed for clinical cardiac SPECT by Chang (Furenlid et al. 2006; Barrett et al. 2008; Chang et al. 2006). It allows the selection of appropriate imaging parameters based on information derived from an initial scout imaging. Adaptive imaging requires a monitoring system and a collimator exchange mechanism to set up appropriate collimation. Its application to clinical SPECT is still at its beginning. In fact, body contour orbiting used in a multihead system is an early implementation of adaptive imaging. If adaptive imaging can be accomplished practically, clinical imaging can benefit from it to optimize imaging to partly mitigate body size variation and location of the target organ.

5.4.5 DYNAMIC IMAGING

Beyond the 3D quantitative imaging potential, the next breakthrough in clinical SPECT imaging could be in 4D imaging. For functional imaging, temporal changes of a physiological system is often more revealing than its spatial variations. This is especially significant in the current MPI SPECT imaging, which often misses global CADs and causes unreliable prognosis. To address the issues of whether a patient has diffuse atherosclerosis or microvascular dysfunction as opposed to obstructive epicardial stenosis, estimation of myocardial flow reserve (MFR) can provide additional important information (Gullberg et al. 2010; Garcia et al. 2011; Murthy and Di Carli 2012). Here, MFR is the ratio of the absolute myocardial blood flow (MBF) rates between stress and rest imaging, both measured in the first few minutes of tracer injection with high-framing-rate ECT imaging.

Currently, PET imaging is the modality of choice for assessing MBF noninvasively. One of the important research areas in nuclear cardiology lately is to derive these two flow rates using SPECT imaging, so that cost can be reduced and availability can be expanded. However, most current SPECT systems are not fast enough for dynamic SPECT imaging, which requires a 5–20 s framing rate during the first 5 min after a bolus injection of tracers. Although the images derived are necessarily of low resolution, clinically meaningful time–activity curves could be derived to reflect regional MBF. If validated, SPECT dynamic imaging could open a new door for assessing cardiac functions and may offer significant clinical benefits to the cardiac patient population.

Recently, several positive feasibility studies of dynamic cardiac SPECT imaging using new single-purpose systems were reported (Ben-Haim et al. 2013; Wells et al. 2014). Similar preliminary clinical results have demonstrated its promising potential for improving diagnosis and prognosis (Daniele et al. 2011). For dynamic imaging to be developed to yield clinical value, cardiac SPECT systems of much increased NSS and motion-free imaging with more simultaneous projections are needed. Such clinical cardiac SPECT systems are almost within reach, in light of the current trend of continuing improvements in hardware and software.

5.5 SUMMARY

We have reviewed SPECT instrumentation from a system's perspective and have taken a mostly top-down approach in analyzing imaging systems. We have reexamined the fundamentals and focused on the functions and significance of each major component of SPECT systems.

It is important to recognize that the hardware subsystem determines the quality and quantity of acquired data, while software processing can extract information already embedded in the data. Although it becomes clear that new software processing techniques are more powerful than was recognized traditionally, a SPECT system's performance potential is mainly defined and limited by the hardware. Thus, a system with better hardware resolution will yield better reconstructed image resolution, provided the sampling is adequate and the reconstruction is optimized. While awaiting the standardization of the definition and measurement methodology of reconstructed image resolution of SPECT systems, hardware resolution could be used as the tentative reference and the intermediate parameter for systems' spatial resolution performance.

The important performance parameter for the evaluation of SPECT systems is the system sensitivity for a given spatial resolution for a standard source model. We suggest two objective metrics, NSS and NSGE, to quantify the performance of SPECT systems. These two parameters are similar in basic concepts and proportional to each other. The former can be measured experimentally on a SPECT system, while the latter can be calculated based on the design parameters of a SPECT system. Hopefully, they can help clarify the current confusion in our community. These metrics can also help set the standard for system evaluation and potentially guide designs of new systems.

When it comes to the design of SPECT systems, the basic principle is to maximize NSGE through optimizing detection geometry. A general guideline to optimize detection geometry is to have as large a total detector area as practically achievable, and use it efficiently. Projection minification can be used to increase the number of simultaneous projections and thereby system sensitivity, provided the detector has a high enough intrinsic resolution performance. Then the optimized detection geometry can provide different compromises of system sensitivity, hardware resolution, and imaging volume based on the needs of the imaging task. Appropriate data sampling can be worked out through relative motion of the detector, collimator, or target. If fast, gated, or dynamic imaging is the goal, stationary systems offer high performance potential in addition to simplicity, precision, and reliability.

In contrast to PET systems, detector material is not as critical for SPECT systems, because the requirements for stopping power and detection speed are not as demanding. New and novel detectors and their roles in SPECT instrumentation have to be justified not only by their performance but also, by their cost-effectiveness, because cost is particularly important for clinical SPECT applications and the acceptance of SPECT systems in the current healthcare environment.

Using high-sensitivity/low-resolution collimation in SPECT systems for imaging could be advantageous, at least for patient positioning. However, whether this approach improves or compromises diagnostic accuracy needs rigorous investigations. At this point, how much further software processing and high-sensitivity imaging can be pushed to gain diagnostic information is not clear. To take full advantage of software processing power in SPECT imaging, we need to understand its strengths and weaknesses in more depth. Presumably, software processing has its limits, which would likely also depend on the goal of each imaging task.

ACKNOWLEDGMENTS

We thank Dale Stentz, Poopalasingam Sankar, and John Strologas for assistance in the preparation of this chapter. We also thank Drs. Ben Tsui, Mark Madsen, and Hans Vija for helpful discussion and comments.

REFERENCES

Abraham, T., and J. Feng. 2011. Evolution of brain imaging instrumentation. *Seminars in Nuclear Medicine* 41 (3): 202–19.

Accorsi, R., and S. D. Metzler. 2006. Non-diverging analytic expression for the on-axis sensitivity of converging collimators: Analytic derivation. *Physics in Medicine and Biology* 51 (21): 5675–96.

Accorsi, R., J. R. Novak, A. S. Ayan, and S. D. Metzler. 2008. Derivation and validation of a sensitivity formula for slit-slat collimation. *IEEE Transactions on Medical Imaging* 27 (5): 709–22.

AAPM [American Association of Physics in Medicine]. 1981. *Computer-Aided Scintillation Camera Acceptance Testing*, 9. New York: American Institute of Physics.

Anger, H. O. 1958. Scintillation camera. *Review of Scientific Instruments* 29: 27–33.

Anger, H. O. 1964. Scintillation camera with multi-channel collimators. *Journal of Nuclear Medicine* 5: 515–31.

Anger, H. O. 1967. Radioisotope cameras. In *Instrumentation in Nuclear Medicine*, ed. G. Hine, 485–552. London: Academic Press.

Bai, C., R. Conwell, J. Kindem, H. Babla, M. Gurley, R. De Los Santos, R. Old, R. Weatherhead, S. Arram, and J. Maddahi. 2010. Phantom evaluation of a cardiac SPECT/VCT system that uses a common set of solid-state detectors for both emission and transmission scans. *Journal of Nuclear Cardiology* 17 (3): 459–69.

Bailey, D. L., B. F. Hutton, and P. J. Walker. 1987. Improved SPECT using simultaneous emission and transmission tomography. *Journal of Nuclear Medicine* 28 (5): 844–51.

Barber, H. B., and J. M. Woolfenden. 1996. Semiconductor detectors in nuclear medicine: Progress and prospects. In *Nuclear Medicine*, ed. R. E. Henkin, 168–84. Vol. I. St. Louis, MO: Mosby-Year Book.

Barrett, H. H., L. R. Furenlid, M. Freed, J. Y. Hesterman, M. A. Kupinski, E. Clarkson, and M. K. Whitaker. 2008. Adaptive SPECT. *IEEE Transactions on Medical Imaging* 27 (6): 775–88.

Ben-Haim, S., V. L. Murthy, C. Breault, R. Allie, A. Sitek, N. Roth, J. Fantony, et al. 2013. Quantification of myocardial perfusion reserve using dynamic SPECT imaging in humans: A feasibility study. *Journal of Nuclear Medicine* 54 (6): 873–79.

Blankespoor, S. C., X. Xu, and C. K. Kalki. 1996. Attenuation correction of SPECT using x-ray CT on an emission-transmission CT system: Myocardial perfusion assessment. *IEEE Transactions on Nuclear Science* 43: 2263–74.

Bocher, M., I. M. Blevis, L. Tsukerman, Y. Shrem, G. Kovalski, and L. Volokh. 2010. A fast cardiac gamma camera with dynamic SPECT capabilities: Design, system validation and future potential. *European Journal of Nuclear Medicine and Molecular Imaging* 37 (10): 1887–902.

Bowen, J., Q. Huang, J. R. Ellin, T. Lee, U. Shrestha, G. T. Gullberg, and Y. Seo. 2013. Design of 20-aperture multipinhole collimator and performance evaluation for myocardial perfusion imaging application. *Physics in Medicine and Biology* 58: 7209–26.

Budinger, T. F. 1980. Physical attributes of single-photon tomography. *Journal of Nuclear Medicine* 21 (6): 579–92.

Budinger, T. F., and G. T. Gullberg. 1974. Three-dimensional reconstruction in nuclear medicine emission imaging. *IEEE Transactions on Nuclear Science* 21 (3): 2–20.

Burrell, S., and A. MacDonald. 2006. Artifacts and pitfalls in myocardial perfusion imaging. *Journal of Nuclear Medicine Technology* 34 (4): 193–211; quiz 212–14.

Casey, M., and R. Nutt. 1986. A multicrystal two dimensional BGO detector system for positron emission tomography. *IEEE Transactions on Nuclear Science* 33: 460–63.

Chandra, R. 1998. *Nuclear Medicine Physics: The Basics.* 5th ed. Williams & Wilkins.

Chang, W. 1996. Dedicated SPECT systems. In *Nuclear Medicine,* ed. R. E. Henkin, M. A. Boles, G. L. Dillehay, J. R. Halama and S. M. Karesh, 247–53. Vol. I. St. Louis, MO: Mosby.

Chang, W., G. Huang, Z. Tian, Y. Liu, and B. Kari. 1992. Initial characterization of a prototype multi-crystal cylindrical SPECT system. *IEEE Transactions on Nuclear Science* 39 (4): 1084–87.

Chang, W., H. Liang, and J. Liu. 2006. Design concepts and potential performance of MarC-SPECT—A high-performance cardiac SPECT system. Presented at Society of Nuclear Medicine Annual Meeting, San Diego.

Chang, W., C. E. Ordonez, H. Liang, M. Holcomb, Y. Li, and J. Liu. 2008. C-SPECT/CT-II: Design concepts and performance potential. *Journal of Nuclear Medicine* 49 (Suppl. 1): 124P.

Chang, W., C. E. Ordonez, H. Liang, Y. Li, and J. Liu. 2009. C-SPECT—A clinical cardiac SPECT/Tct platform: Design concepts and performance potential. *IEEE Transactions on Nuclear Science* 56 (5): 2659–71.

Cherry, S. R., J. A. Sorenson, and M. E. Phelps. 2003. *Physics in Nuclear Medicine.* 3rd ed. Philadelphia: Saunders.

Daniele, S., C. Nappi, W. Acampa, G. Storto, T. Pellegrino, F. Ricci, E. Xhoxhi, F. Porcaro, M. Petretta, and A. Cuocolo. 2011. Incremental prognostic value of coronary flow reserve assessed with single-photon emission computed tomography. *Journal of Nuclear Cardiology* 18 (4): 612–19.

DePuey, E. G. 2012. Advances in SPECT camera software and hardware: Currently available and new on the horizon. *Journal of Nuclear Cardiology* 19 (3): 551–81.

Erlandsson, K., K. Kacperski, D. van Gramberg, and B. F. Hutton. 2009. Performance evaluation of D-SPECT: A novel SPECT system for nuclear cardiology. *Physics in Medicine and Biology* 54 (9): 2635–49.

Esteves, F. P., P. Raggi, R. D. Folks, Z. Keidar, J. W. Askew, S. Rispler, M. K. O'Connor, L. Verdes, and E. V. Garcia. 2009. Novel solid-state-detector dedicated cardiac camera for fast myocardial perfusion imaging: Multicenter comparison with standard dual detector cameras. *Journal of Nuclear Cardiology* 16 (6): 927–34.

Funk, T., D. L. Kirch, J. E. Koss, E. Botvinick, and B. H. Hasegawa. 2006. A novel approach to multipinhole SPECT for myocardial perfusion imaging. *Journal of Nuclear Medicine* 47 (4): 595–602.

Furenlid, L., M. Freed, J. Hesterman, M. Kupinski, E. Clarkson, and H. Barrett. 2006. Adaptive imaging techniques for nuclear medicine. Presented at Society of Nuclear Medicine Annual Meeting, San Diego.

Gambhir, S. S., D. S. Berman, J. Ziffer, M. Nagler, M. Sandler, J. Patton, B. Hutton, T. Sharir, S. B. Haim, and S. B. Haim. 2009. A novel high-sensitivity rapid-acquisition single-photon cardiac imaging camera. *Journal of Nuclear Medicine* 50 (4): 635–43.

Garcia, E. V., and F. P. Esteves. 2009. Attenuation corrected myocardial perfusion SPECT provides powerful risk stratification in patients with coronary artery disease. *Journal of Nuclear Cardiology* 16 (4): 490–92.

Garcia, E. V., and T. L. Faber. 2009. New trends in camera and software technology in nuclear cardiology. *Cardiology Clinics* 27 (2): 227–36.

Garcia, E. V., T. L. Faber, and F. P. Esteves. 2011. Cardiac dedicated ultrafast SPECT cameras: New designs and clinical implications. *Journal of Nuclear Medicine* 52 (2): 210–17.

Genna, S., and A. P. Smith. 1988. The development of ASPECT: An annular single brain camera for high efficiency SPECT. *IEEE Transactions on Nuclear Science* 35: 654–58.

Graham, L. S., F. H. Fahey, M. T. Madsen, A. Aswegen, and M. V. Yester. 1995. Quantitation of SPECT performance. *Medical Physics* 22 (4): 401–9.

Gullberg, G. T., B. W. Reutter, A. Sitek, J. S. Maltz, and T. F. Budinger. 2010. Dynamic single photon emission computed tomography—Basic principles and cardiac applications. *Physics in Medicine and Biology* 55 (20): R111–91.

Hasegawa, B. H., E. L. Gingold, S. M. Reilly, S.-C. Liew, and C. E. Cann. 1990. Description of a simultaneous emission-transmission CT system. *Proc SPIE* 1231: 50–60.

Hawman, P. C., and E. J. Haines. 1994. The Cardiofocal collimator: A variable-focus collimator for cardiac SPECT. *Physics in Medicine and Biology* 39 (3): 439–50.

Heller, G. V., J. Links, T. M. Bateman, J. A. Ziffer, E. Ficaro, M. C. Cohen, and R. C. Hendel. 2004. American Society of Nuclear Cardiology and Society of Nuclear Medicine joint position statement: Attenuation correction of myocardial perfusion SPECT scintigraphy. *Journal of Nuclear Cardiology* 11 (2): 229–30.

Hendel, R. C., J. R. Corbett, S. J. Cullom, E. G. DePuey, E. V. Garcia, and T. M. Bateman. 2002. The value and practice of attenuation correction for myocardial perfusion SPECT imaging: A joint position statement from the American Society of Nuclear Cardiology and the Society of Nuclear Medicine. *Journal of Nuclear Cardiology* 9 (1): 135–43.

Hirose, Y., Y. Ikeda, and Y. Hegashi. 1982. A hybrid emission CT HEADTOME II. *IEEE Transactions on Nuclear Science* 29: 520–25.

Hsieh, J. 1989. Scintillation camera and three-dimensional multifocal collimator used there within. U.S. Patent 4820924.

Imbert, L., S. Poussier, P. R. Franken, B. Songy, A. Verger, O. Morel, D. Wolf, A. Noel, G. Karcher, and P. Y. Marie. 2012. Compared performance of high-sensitivity cameras dedicated to myocardial perfusion SPECT: A comprehensive analysis of phantom and human images. *Journal of Nuclear Medicine* 53 (12): 1897–903.

IMV Medical Information Division. 2008. Nuclear medicine market summary report. Columbia, MD: IMV.

Jaszczak, R. J. 2006. The early years of single photon emission computed tomography (SPECT): An anthology of selected reminiscences. *Physics in Medicine and Biology* 51 (13): R99–115.

Jaszczak, R. J., P. H. Murphy, D. Huard, and J. A. Burdine. 1977. Radionuclide emission computed tomography of the head with 99mTC and a scintillation camera. *Journal of Nuclear Medicine* 18 (4): 373–80.

Juni, J. E. 2003. Single photon emission computed tomography system. U.S. Patent 6525320. Filed 2003.

Kanno, I., K. Uemura, S. Miura, and Y. Miura. 1981. HEADTOME: A hybrid emission tomograph for single photon and positron emission imaging of the brain. *Journal of Computer Assisted Tomography* 5 (2): 216–26.

Kennedy, J. A., O. Israel, and A. Frenkel. 2014. 3D iterative reconstructed spatial resolution map and sensitivity characterization of a dedicated cardiac SPECT camera. *Journal of Nuclear Cardiology* 21 (3): 443–52.

Keyes, J. W., N. Orlandea, W. J. Heetderks, P. F. Leonard, and W. L. Rogers. 1977. The humogotron: A scintillation-camera transaxial tomograph. *Journal of Nuclear Medicine* 18 (4): 381–87.

Kimura, K., K. Hashikawa, H. Etani, A. Uehara, T. Kozuka, H. Moriwaki, Y. Isaka, M. Matsumoto, T. Kamada, and H. Moriyama. 1990. A new apparatus for brain imaging: Four-head rotating gamma camera single-photon emission computed tomograph. *Journal of Nuclear Medicine* 31 (5): 603–9.

Kindem, J., C. Bai, and R. Conwell. 2010. CsI(Tl)/PIN solid state detectors for combined high resolution SPECT and CT imaging. Presented at Nuclear Science Symposium Conference Record (NSS/MIC), Knoxville, TN.

King, M. A., B. M. Tsui, and T. S. Pan. 1995. Attenuation compensation for cardiac single-photon emission computed tomographic imaging. Part 1. Impact of attenuation and methods of estimating attenuation maps. *Journal of Nuclear Cardiology* 2 (6): 513–24.

Kouris, K., P. H. Jarritt, D. C. Costa, and P. J. Ell. 1992. Physical assessment of the GE/CGR Neurocam and comparison with a single rotating gamma-camera. *European Journal of Nuclear Medicine* 19 (4): 236–42.

Kuhl, D. E., and R. Q. Edwards. 1963. Image separation radioisotope scanning. *Radiology* 80: 653–62.

Kuhl, D. E., R. Q. Edwards, A. R. Ricci, R. J. Yacob, T. J. Mich, and A. Alavi. 1976. The Mark IV system for radionuclide computed tomography of the brain. *Radiology* 121 (2): 405–13.

LaCroix, K. J., B. M. W. Tsui, B. H. Hasegawa, and J. K. Brown. 1994. Investigation of the use of x-ray CT images for attenuation compensation in SPECT. *IEEE Transactions on Nuclear Science* 41 (6): 2793–99.

Lang, T. F., B. H. Hasegawa, S. C. Liew, J. K. Brown, S. C. Blankespoor, S. M. Reilly, E. L. Gingold, and C. E. Cann. 1992. Description of a prototype emission-transmission computed tomography imaging system. *Journal of Nuclear Medicine* 33 (10): 1881–87.

Li, Y., J. Oldendick, C. E. Ordonez, and W. Chang. 2009. The geometric response function for convergent slit-slat collimators. *Physics in Medicine and Biology* 54 (6): 1469–82.

Li, Y., M. Rozler, and W. Chang. 2010. View sampling requirement for cardiac SPECT. Presented at Nuclear Science Symposium Conference Record (NSS/MIC), Knoxville, TN.

Lim, C. B., L. T. Chang, and R. J. Jaszczak. 1980. Performance analysis of three camera configurations for single photon emission computed tomography. *IEEE Transactions on Nuclear Science* 27 (1): 559–68.

Lim, C. B., R. Walker, C. Pinkstaff, and K. I. Kim. 1986. Triangular SPECT system for 3-D total organ volume imaging: Performance results and dynamic imaging capability. *IEEE Transactions on Nuclear Science* 33: 501–504.

Madsen, M. T. 2007. Recent advances in SPECT imaging. *Journal of Nuclear Medicine* 48 (4): 661–73.

Madsen, M. T., W. Chang, and R. D. Hichwa. 1992. Spatial resolution and count density requirements in brain SPECT imaging. *Physics in Medicine and Biology* 37 (8): 1625–36.

Matsunari, I., G. Böning, S. I. Ziegler, I. Kosa, S. G. Nekolla, E. P. Ficaro, and M. Schwaiger. 1998. Attenuation-corrected rest thallium-201/stress technetium 99m sestamibi myocardial SPECT in normals. *Journal of Nuclear Cardiology* 5 (1): 48–55.

Metzler, S. D., R. Accorsi, J. R. Novak, A. S. Ayan, and R. J. Jaszczak. 2006. On-axis sensitivity and resolution of a slit-slat collimator. *Journal of Nuclear Medicine* 47 (11): 1884–90.

Miller, T. R., and J. W. Wallis. 1992. Fast maximum-likelihood reconstruction. *Journal of Nuclear Medicine* 33 (9): 1710–11.

Milster, T. D., J. N. Aarsvold, H. H. Barrett, A. L. Landesman, L. S. Mar, D. D. Patton, T. J. Roney, R. K. Rowe, and R. H. Seacat 3rd. 1990. A full-field modular gamma camera. *Journal of Nuclear Medicine* 31 (5): 632–39.

Miura, S., I. Kanno, Y. Aizawa, M. Murakami, and K. Uemura. 1984. Characteristics of NaI detector in positron imaging device HEADTOME employing circular ring array. *Radioisotopes* 33 (5): 262–68.

Moyer, R. A. 1974. A low-energy multihole converging collimator compared with a pinhole collimator. *Journal of Nuclear Medicine* 15: 59–64.

Murthy, V. L., and M. F. Di Carli. 2012. Non-invasive quantification of coronary vascular dysfunction for diagnosis and management of coronary artery disease. *Journal of Nuclear Cardiology* 19 (5): 1060–72.

NEMA [National Electrical Manufacturers Association]. 2007. *Performance Measurements of Gamma Cameras.* NU 1-2007. Rosslyn, VA: National Electrical Manufacturers Association.

Ogawa, K. 2010. Feasibility study on an ultra-high-resolution SPECT with CdTe detectors. *IEEE Transactions on Nuclear Science* 57 (1): 17–24.

Patton, J. A., P. J. Slomka, G. Germano, and D. S. Berman. 2007. Recent technologic advances in nuclear cardiology. *Journal of Nuclear Cardiology* 14 (4): 501–13.

Popovic, K., M. Rozler, P. Sankar, R. Arseneau, and W. Chang. 2014. A section of a curved pixelated Na(Tl) detector for SPECT/TCT. Presented at Nuclear Science Symposium Conference Record (NSS/MIC), Seattle, WA.

Rajaram, R., M. Bhattacharya, X. Ding, R. Malmin, T. D. Rempel, A. H. Vija, and J. Zeintl. 2011. Tomographic performance characteristics of the IQ-SPECT system. Presented at Nuclear Science Symposium Conference Record (NSS/MIC), Valencia, Spain.

Rogers, W. L., and R. J. Ackermann. 1992. SPECT instrumentation. *American Journal of Physiologic Imaging* 7 (3–4): 105–20.

Rogers, W. L., N. H. Clinthorne, L. Shao, P. Chiao, Y. Ding, J. A. Stamos, and K. F. Koral. 1988. SPRINT II: A second generation single photon ring tomograph. *IEEE Transactions on Medical Imaging* 7 (4): 291–97.

Rogers, W. L., N. H. Clinthorne, J. Stamos, K. F. Koral, R. Mayans, J. W. Keyes, J. J. Williams, W. P. Snapp, and G. F. Knoll. 1982. SPRINT: A stationary detector single photon ring tomograph for brain imaging. *IEEE Transactions on Medical Imaging* 1 (1): 63–68.

Rogulski, M. M., H. B. Barber, H. H. Barrett, R. L. Shoemaker, and J. M. Woolfenden. 1993. Ultra-high-resolution brain SPECT imaging: Simulation results. *IEEE Transactions on Nuclear Science* 40 (4): 1123–29.

Rosenthal, M. S., J. Cullom, W. Hawkins, S. C. Moore, B. M. Tsui, and M. Yester. 1995. Quantitative SPECT imaging: A review and recommendations by the focus committee of the Society of Nuclear Medicine Computer and Instrumentation Council. *Journal of Nuclear Medicine* 36 (8): 1489–513.

Rozler, M., and W. Chang. 2011. Collimator exchange system for adaptive cardiac imaging in C-SPECT. *IEEE Transactions on Nuclear Science* 58 (5): 2226–33.

Rozler, M., H. Liang, and W. Chang. 2012. Development of a cost-effective modular pixelated NaI(Tl) detector for clinical SPECT applications. *IEEE Transactions on Nuclear Science* 59(5): 1831–40.

Rozler, M., P. Sankar, K. Popovic, R. Arseneau, J. Strologas, X. Zheng, S. D. Metzler, and W. Chang. 2014. C-SPECT cardiac SPECT/Tct system: First results from a partial section. Presented at Nuclear Science Symposium Conference Record (NSS/MIC), Seattle, WA.

Sankar, P., M. Rozler, K. Popovic, and W. Chang. 2014. Adjustable resolution/sensitivity slit-slat collimator for task-specific clinical SPECT imaging. Presented at Nuclear Science Symposium Conference Record (NSS/MIC), Seattle, WA.

Sharir, T., S. Ben-Haim, K. Merzon, V. Prochorov, D. Dickman, S. Ben-Haim, and D. S. Berman. 2008. High-speed myocardial perfusion imaging initial clinical comparison with conventional dual detector Anger camera imaging. *JACC Cardiovascular Imaging* 1 (2): 156–63.

Slomka, P. J., D. S. Berman, and G. Germano. 2014. New cardiac cameras: Single-photon emission CT and PET. *Seminars in Nuclear Medicine* 44 (4): 232–51.

Slomka, P. J., J. A. Patton, D. S. Berman, and G. Germano. 2009. Advances in technical aspects of myocardial perfusion SPECT imaging. *Journal of Nuclear Cardiology* 16 (2): 255–76.

Smith, M. F. 2013. Recent advances in cardiac SPECT instrumentation and system design. *Current Cardiology Reports* 15 (8): 387.

Steele, P. P., D. L. Kirch, and J. E. Koss. 2008. Comparison of simultaneous dual-isotope multipinhole SPECT with rotational SPECT in a group of patients with coronary artery disease. *Journal of Nuclear Medicine* 49 (7): 1080–89.

Stokely, E. M., E. Sveinsdottir, N. A. Lassen, and P. Rommer. 1980. A single photon dynamic computer assisted tomograph (DCAT) for imaging brain function in multiple cross sections. *Journal of Computer Assisted Tomography* 4 (2): 230–40.

Strologas, J., and Chang, W. 2012. Assessing the performance of C-SPECT cardiac tomograph using GATE-based Monte Carlo simulations. Presented at Nuclear Science Symposium Conference Record (NSS/MIC), Anaheim, CA.

Surti, S., J. S. Karp, and G. Muehllehner. 2003. Evaluation of pixelated NaI(Tl) detector. *IEEE Transactions on Nuclear Science* 50: 24–31.

Tan, P., D. L. Bailey, S. R. Meikle, S. Eberl, R. R. Fulton, and B. F. Hutton. 1993. A scanning line source for simultaneous emission and transmission measurements in SPECT. *Journal of Nuclear Medicine* 34 (10): 1752–60.

Travin, M. I. 2011. Cardiac cameras. *Seminars in Nuclear Medicine* 41 (3): 182–201.

Tsui, B. M., E. C. Frey, K. J. LaCroix, D. S. Lalush, W. H. McCartney, M. A. King, and G. T. Gullberg. 1998. Quantitative myocardial perfusion SPECT. *Journal of Nuclear Cardiology* 5 (5): 507–22.

Tsui, B. M., E. C. Frey, X. Zhao, D. S. Lalush, R. E. Johnston, and W. H. McCartney. 1994. The importance and implementation of accurate 3D compensation methods for quantitative SPECT. *Physics in Medicine and Biology* 39 (3): 509–30.

Tsui, B. M., G. T. Gullberg, E. R. Edgerton, J. G. Ballard, J. R. Perry, W. H. McCartney, and J. Berg. 1989. Correction of non-uniform attenuation in cardiac SPECT imaging. *Journal of Nuclear Medicine* 30 (4): 497–507.

Vija, A. H., R. Malmin, A. Yahil, and B. Bendriem. 2010. A method for improving the efficiency of myocardial perfusion imaging using conventional SPECT and CT/SPECT imaging systems. Presented at Nuclear Science Symposium Conference Record (NSS/MIC), Knoxville, TN.

Vogel, R. A., D. Kirch, M. LeFree, and P. Steele. 1978. A new method of multi-planar emission tomography using a seven pinhole collimator and an Anger scintillation camera. *Journal of Nuclear Medicine* 19 (6): 648–54.

Wagenaar, D. J. 2004. CdTe and CdZnTe semiconductor detectors for nuclear medicine imaging. In *Emission Tomography: The Fundamentals of PET and SPECT*, ed. M. N. Wernick and J. N. Aarsvold, 269–291. 1st ed. San Diego: Elsevier Academic Press.

Welch, A., and G. T. Gullberg. 1997. Implementation of a model-based nonuniform scatter correction scheme for SPECT. *IEEE Transactions on Medical Imaging* 16 (6): 717–26.

Wells, R. G., R. Timmins, R. Klein, J. Lockwood, B. Marvin, R. A. deKemp, L. Wei, and T. D. Ruddy. 2014. Dynamic SPECT measurement of absolute myocardial blood flow in a porcine model. *Journal of Nuclear Medicine* 55 (10): 1685–91.

Williams, J. J., W. P. Snapp, and G. F. Knoll. 1979. Introducing SPRINT: A single photon ring system for emission tomography. *IEEE Transactions on Nuclear Science* 26: 628–633.

Williams, M. B., M. B. Williams, A. R. Goode, V. Galbis-Reig, S. Majewski, A. G. Weisenberger, and R. Wojcik. 2000. Performance of a PSPMT based detector for scintimammography. *Physics in Medicine and Biology* 45 (3): 781–800.

Wojcik, R., S. Majewski, B. Kross, D. Steinbach, and A. G. Weisenberger. 1998. High spatial resolution gamma imaging detector based on a 5" diameter R3292 Hamamatsu PSPMT. *IEEE Transactions on Nuclear Science* 45 (3): 487–91.

Yin, Y., X. Chen, and H. Wu. 2013. 3-D spatial resolution of 350 m pitch pixelated CdZnTe detectors for imaging applications. *IEEE Transactions on Nuclear Science* 60 (1): 9–15.

Yu, D., W. Chang, T. S. Pan, and S. Loncaric. 1997. A study of reconstruction accuracy for a cardiac SPECT system with multi-segmental collimation. *IEEE Transactions on Nuclear Science* 44: 1403–8.

Zeintl, J., T. D. Rempel, M. Bhattacharya, R. E. Malmin, and A. H. Vija. 2011. Performance characteristics of the SMARTZOOM collimator. Presented at Nuclear Science Symposium Conference Record (NSS/MIC), Valencia, Spain.

Zeintl, J., A. H. Vija, A. Yahil, J. Hornegger, and T. Kuwert. 2010. Quantitative accuracy of clinical 99mTc SPECT/CT using ordered-subset expectation maximization with 3-dimensional resolution recovery, attenuation, and scatter correction. *Journal of Nuclear Medicine* 51 (6): 921–28.

Zeng, G. L. 2004. Single-photon emission computed tomography. In *Emission Tomography: The Fundamentals of PET and SPECT*, ed. M. N. Wernick and J. N. Aarsvold, 127–152. 1st ed. San Diego: Elsevier Academic Press.

PET instrumentation

ANDREW L. GOERTZEN AND JONATHAN D. THIESSEN

6.1	Introduction	163
6.2	General PET instrumentation	164
	6.2.1 Goal of PET instrumentation	164
	6.2.2 Performance considerations	164
	6.2.2.1 Spatial resolution	164
	6.2.2.2 Detection efficiency	170
	6.2.2.3 Timing performance	172
6.3	Detector design for PET imaging	173
	6.3.1 Requirements for PET detector performance	173
	6.3.2 Detector designs	174
	6.3.2.1 Block detector	174
	6.3.2.2 Panel-type detectors	176
	6.3.2.3 Detectors for preclinical and high-resolution PET systems	176
6.4	Data acquisition in PET	180
	6.4.1 Singles event acquisition	181
	6.4.1.1 Location of interaction	181
	6.4.1.2 Energy deposited in interaction	182
	6.4.1.3 Time of event	182
	6.4.2 Coincidence identification methods	182
	6.4.2.1 Delayed coincidence identification	182
6.5	Data sorting and sinograms	183
	6.5.1 Sinogram data organization	183
	6.5.2 2D sinogram organization for a cylindrical PET system	183
	6.5.3 General 2D sinogram organization	184
	6.5.4 3D sinograms	185
6.6	Summary and future directions	188
References		189

6.1 INTRODUCTION

PET imaging is based on the coincidence detection of the two 511 keV photons created following the emission of a positron in the decay of a radioisotope and its subsequent annihilation with an electron. As shown in Figure 6.1, a typical PET system capable of performing this function requires (1) a pair of detectors or detector rings suitable for detecting 511 keV photons, (2) a data acquisition system capable of digitizing the detector signals, (3) a coincidence sorter to identify pairs of 511 keV photon detection events, (4) a method of binning the data into either sinograms or line of response (LOR) bins, and (5) a method of reconstructing the acquired data into images. In addition to these basic requirements, PET systems require several components, such as a patient bed, sometimes referred to as a patient handling system (PHS), in order to position the patient within the PET gantry for imaging and a method to measure the attenuation map of the object being imaged.

6.2 GENERAL PET INSTRUMENTATION

6.2.1 GOAL OF PET INSTRUMENTATION

The goal of a PET imaging system is to detect the 511 keV photons created in the positron annihilation process with a high efficiency and accurate measure of detection position, photon energy, and arrival time in order to allow reliable identification of coincidence photon pairs. The design of systems suitable for this purpose requires a compromise between the various performance parameters outlined in the next section since there is invariably a trade-off between the different parameters. Currently, the most common PET system design is a ring geometry in which multiple rings of scintillation detectors are arranged in a cylindrical geometry about the subject being imaged, as shown schematically in Figure 6.1. This chapter focuses primarily on this common system design.

6.2.2 PERFORMANCE CONSIDERATIONS

6.2.2.1 SPATIAL RESOLUTION

The spatial resolution of a PET system is typically described by the full width at half maximum (FWHM) and full width at tenth maximum (FWTM) values of the point-spread function (PSF) of a point source imaged in the tomograph. In ring geometry systems with scintillator crystal elements aligned along the radial direction,

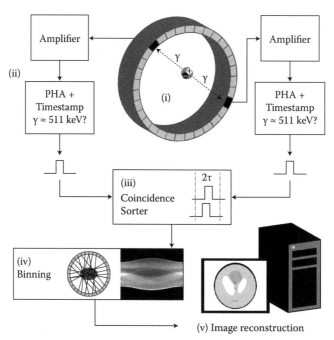

Figure 6.1 A typical PET system consists of (i) a detector ring for detecting 511 keV photons; (ii) a data acquisition system, which can perform pulse height analysis (PHA) to identify likely 511 keV photons and provide a time stamp for each event; (iii) a coincidence sorter to identify pairs of 511 keV photon detection events; (iv) a method of binning the data; and (v) a method of reconstructing the data into images.

there are different sampling properties in different spatial directions (see Figure 6.3). The spatial resolution is thus defined in three directions: (1) radial, or along the radial direction in the transaxial plane; (2) tangential, or along the direction in the transaxial plane perpendicular to the radial direction; and (3) axial, or along the direction perpendicular to the transaxial plane. The spatial resolution of the PET system is determined by a combination of the physical effects of blurring caused by a combination of the physics of the positron emission and annihilation process, the detector response function, and the image reconstruction algorithm.

6.2.2.1.1 Detector response

For detectors with discrete or pixelated detector elements, the coincidence response function (CRF) is determined largely by the solid angle coverage of the pair of detector elements. As shown in Figure 6.2, the response profile at the midway point between the two detectors is a simple triangle function with a FWHM equal to half the detector width d. As the source moves closer to one of the detectors, the response profile changes to become trapezoidal and eventually rectangular.

6.2.2.1.2 Radial elongation or depth of interaction

The detector materials used in PET systems are not perfect absorbers of the 511 keV photons, so that it is possible for the photon to penetrate through several detector elements prior to interacting in a detector. For photons originating from near the center of the field of view (FOV), the photons will be normally incident on the narrow surface of the detector elements, and thus are likely to interact in the detector element that they first pass through. In contrast, as the source of the photons is offset radially, the angle of incidence between the 511 keV photon and the detector surface can be quite large, so that the photon can penetrate through several detector elements before interacting. This process is shown in Figure 6.3, where for radial offsets there is a marked uncertainty in the location of the positron annihilation event due to the radial elongation of the profile. This effect is often termed the depth-of-interaction (DOI) effect since it originates from the uncertainty in the location of the interaction along the length of the detector element. The DOI effect predominantly degrades the spatial resolution in the radial direction while having minimal impact on the tangential and axial resolutions, as shown in Figure 6.3. The FWHM and FWTM radial resolutions increase significantly as the source is moved away from the center of the FOV. This degradation to resolution can be addressed through the use of detectors with DOI capability. The magnitude of the error uncertainty due to DOI, R_{DOI}, has been described as a Gaussian whose FWHM is given by (Moses, 2011)

$$R_{DOI} = \frac{Lr}{\sqrt{r^2 + R^2}} \tag{6.1}$$

where r is the radial offset of the source from the center of the detector ring, R is the radius of the detector ring, and L is the mean depth of penetration of the photon in the detector material and is commonly taken to be 12.5 mm for bismuth germanate (BGO) or lutetium oxyorthosilicate (LSO) scintillators.

6.2.2.1.3 Positron range

The positron emission process results in the positron being emitted from the nucleus with a nonzero kinetic energy, allowing the positron to travel some range prior to annihilating with an electron. The shape of the probability distribution for the location of annihilation relative to the emission location is described by a Lorentzian

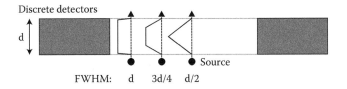

Figure 6.2 Sampling properties of two rectangular detectors for normal incidence photons. As the source moves closer to one of the detectors, the response profile changes from triangular to rectangular.

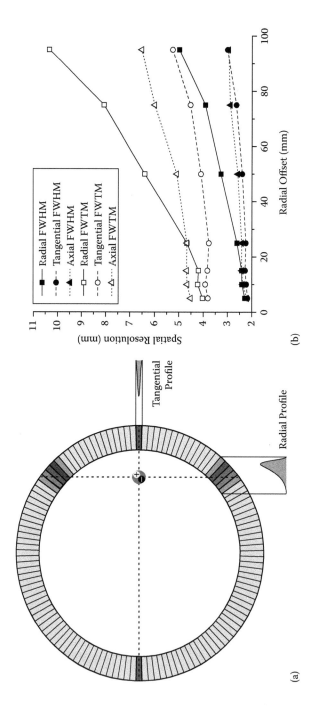

Figure 6.3 (a) Schematic diagram showing the different sampling properties of the PET system in the radial and tangential directions due to the penetration of photons into the detector elements before interacting. This penetration effect results in radial elongation of the response profile, degrading spatial resolution in the radial direction. (b) Dependence of the FWHM and FWTM spatial resolution on radial offset for the radial, tangential, and axial directions of the microPET P4 PET system.

function (Levin and Hoffman, 1999), and contributes an inherent blur to the image formation process. The magnitude of this blur is dependent on the energy of the positron and, as shown in Table 6.1, can vary from 0.102 mm FWHM for ^{18}F to 0.501 mm FWHM for ^{15}O. Due to the Lorentzian shape of the distribution, the FWTM values are typically much greater than the FWHM values, so that the contribution of positron range to spatial resolution is normally better described by considering the root-mean-square (RMS) value of the positron range.

6.2.2.1.4 Photon noncollinearity

At the time when a positron and electron annihilate, the center of mass of the system is not always at rest. As a result, in order to conserve energy and momentum, the two annihilation photons that are created are not traveling exactly 180° apart. This effect is known as photon noncollinearity, and results in a degradation in spatial resolution due to the uncertainty introduced in the location of the true LOR relative to the location of the LOR identified by the two detected photons. The magnitude of the blur introduced by photon noncollinearity scales with the diameter of the PET system according to the equation (Moses, 2011)

$$R_{\text{noncollinearity}} = 0.0044D \tag{6.2}$$

where D is the ring diameter of the PET system. For a typical whole-body PET system diameter of 80 cm, the magnitude of this effect will thus be about 1.8 mm, while for a ring diameter of 15 cm, common in small-animal PET systems, this effect will be 0.3 mm. Figure 6.4 shows the relative contribution of the positron range, photon noncollinearity, and detector size to the spatial resolution of an 80 cm diameter PET system with 4 mm detector size and a 20 cm diameter system with 2 mm detector size. For a low-energy positron emitter, such as ^{18}F, the spatial response of the small-ring-diameter system is dominated by the positron range and detector size, while for the larger ring system, it is dominated by the photon noncollinearity and detector size. For a high-energy positron emitter, such as ^{15}O, the spatial resolution of the small-ring-diameter system is dominated by the positron range, while for the large ring diameter, all components contribute approximately similar amounts.

6.2.2.1.5 Decoding error or block effect

In detectors that employ multiplexing, in which multiple detector elements are read out by a small number of electronic channels, such as in block detector designs, the decoding of which detector element the 511 keV photon interacted in can be imperfect, leading to a blur in the spatial resolution. This effect, commonly called the "block effect," due to the fact that it was characterized for block detector designs that employ light sharing, was reported by St. James and Thompson (2006) to have a magnitude of 1.2 mm for a CTI/Siemens HR+ detector block and 0.7–0.9 mm for a GE Advance detector block, BGO-based scintillator detectors. The magnitude of this effect has not been studied for detector blocks that use newer scintillator materials with greater light output, such as LSO or lutetium-yttrium oxyorthosilicate (LYSO); however, it is likely that the relative magnitude of the effect will be similar due to the similar size and attenuation properties of the crystals still in use.

Table 6.1 Positron range properties of various positron-emitting radioisotopes

Radionuclide	Maximum positron energy (MeV)	FWHM (mm)	FWTM (mm)	Effective range* (mm)
^{11}C	0.96	0.19	1.86	0.92
^{13}N	1.20	0.28	2.53	1.4
^{15}O	1.73	0.50	4.14	2.4
^{18}F	0.64	0.10	1.03	0.54
^{64}Cu	0.65	0.10	1.05	0.55
^{68}Ga	1.90	0.58	4.83	2.8
^{82}Rb	3.36	1.27	10.5	6.1

Source: Adapted from Lecomte, R., *Eur. J. Nucl. Med. Mol. Imaging*, 36, 69–85, 2009.
*Effective range is 2.355 × root-mean-square range.

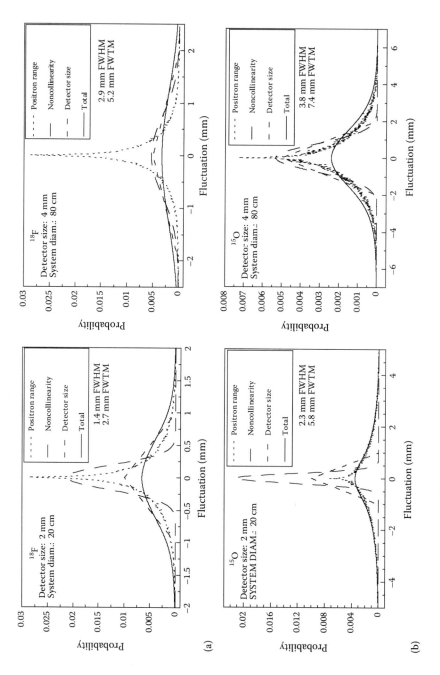

Figure 6.4 Plots of the spatial resolution for (left) 20 cm and (right) 80 cm ring diameter PET systems with 2 and 4 mm detector elements, respectively, for (a) ^{18}F and (b) [15]O radioisotopes showing the relative contributions of the positron range, photon noncollinearity, and detector size. (Adapted from Levin, C.S., and Hoffman, E.J., *Phys. Med. Biol.*, 44, 781–99, 1999. With permission.)

6.2.2.1.6 Sampling

The cylindrical design of a PET system results in nonuniform sampling of the FOV, as demonstrated by the LOR drawings of Figure 6.5. This nonuniform sampling, also called undersampling, is a source of image blurring that degrades the high-frequency components of the signal. The magnitude of this effect was shown by Thompson et al. (2005) to cause the FWHM resolution to fluctuate between 5.45 and 4.55 mm near the center of the FOV of a Siemens/CTI HR+, which uses BGO block detectors with 4.5 mm crystal pitch. Others have commonly used an empirical multiplicative factor of 1.25 (e.g., Moses, 2011) to describe the additional blur. It is likely that as detector technology improves, there will be improvements in sampling uniformity, which will reduce the magnitude of the sampling error.

6.2.2.1.7 Image reconstruction

Current clinical PET systems are typically capable of FWHM spatial resolutions of approximately 5 mm; however, the high noise present in many clinical PET images means that some additional image smoothing is required to create an image that can be reliably interpreted by the nuclear medicine physician. In general, simple Gaussian filtering is used with FWHM kernels of between 3 and 5 mm. It is commonly assumed that the image reconstruction adds a multiplicative blur of 1.25 to the final spatial resolution. In practice, this factor may now be less with the use of reconstruction algorithms that model the PSF of the PET system.

6.2.2.1.8 Total spatial resolution

For simplicity, it is assumed that all contributions to spatial resolution add in quadrature even though not all components are Gaussian in shape. The resulting spatial resolution R_{tot} is given by

$$R_{\text{tot}} = 1.25 \sqrt{\left(\frac{d}{2}\right)^2 + R_{\beta+}^2 + \left(0.0044R\right)^2 + R_b^2 + \frac{\left(Lr\right)^2}{r^2 + R^2}} \tag{6.3}$$

where d is the crystal width, $R_{\beta+}$ is the positron range, R is the detector ring radius, R_b is the block decoding error, L is the mean attenuation length of photons in the detector, r is the offset of the source from the center of the FOV, and the factor of 1.25 describes the additional blur from the reconstruction. As described by Moses (2011), only the positron range and noncollinearity factors are fixed, setting a lower limit on the achievable spatial resolution in PET.

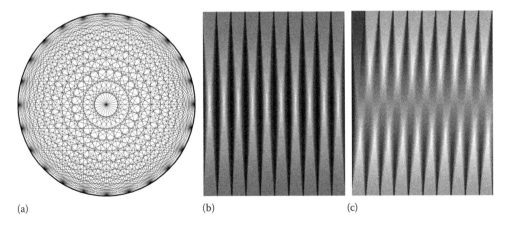

(a) (b) (c)

Figure 6.5 (a) Sampling properties for all LORs in a 24-crystal-ring-geometry PET system. The sampling is clearly nonuniform, leading to errors in the reconstruction process. (b) Geometric CRF from pairs of equally spaced crystals. (c) Geometric response function obtained by adding the interleaved samples of the LOR between a pair of crystals offset by one element. The uniformity is improved; however, the limitations of spatial sampling are still visible. (Left panel adapted from Moses, W.W., *Nucl. Instrum. Methods A*, 648, S236–40, 2011. With permission. Middle and right panels adapted from Thompson, C.J., et al., *Nucl. Instrum. Methods A*, 545, 436–45, 2005. With permission.)

6.2.2.2 DETECTION EFFICIENCY

The detection efficiency of a PET scanner, also commonly referred to as the sensitivity, is one of the most important considerations when building a PET system since the number of detected events has a direct impact on the final image quality due to the Poisson statistical nature of the data. The detection efficiency, or sensitivity, S, for a positron source is given by

$$S = G\varepsilon_D^2 e^{-\mu T} \tag{6.4}$$

where G is the geometric efficiency of the system, ε_D is the intrinsic detector efficiency, μ is the linear attenuation coefficient of the material in which the source is located (e.g., tissue), and T is the thickness of the object. The detection efficiency goes as the square of the intrinsic detector efficiency due to the requirement of detecting two photons to form a coincident pair.

6.2.2.2.1 Geometric efficiency

Geometric efficiency, G, refers to the solid angle coverage of the PET detector system and is the largest single factor affecting the detection efficiency of a PET system. The geometric efficiency will be at a maximum for a point source located at the center of the PET system. For this special case, the geometric efficiency, G_{max}, can be shown to be

$$G_{max} = \frac{l}{2\sqrt{R^2 + \left(\frac{l}{2}\right)^2}} \tag{6.5}$$

where l is the axial length and R is the ring diameter of the PET system. As one might expect, G_{max} approaches 1 as l becomes very large and goes to 0 as l goes to 0 and exhibits an inverse dependence on R. As the point source is moved away from the axial center of the PET system along the center of the transaxial FOV, the geometric efficiency decreases linearly, reaching a value of zero at the edge of the axial FOV. This results in a detection efficiency profile that has a triangular shape when plotted against the axial position, as shown in Figure 6.6a for the Siemens Inveon small-animal PET system (Visser et al., 2009). For a line source positioned parallel to the axial direction of the PET system and positioned at the center of the transaxial FOV, the average efficiency over the complete axial FOV of the PET system, G_{avg}, is then

$$G_{avg} = \frac{G_{max}}{2} \tag{6.6}$$

The detection efficiency of a typical PET system is relatively constant as the source is moved away from the transaxial center of the FOV, as shown in Figure 6.6b and c, reflecting the fact that the geometric efficiency does not change significantly as a function of radial offset due to the cylindrical geometry of the PET detector ring.

The above calculations for G_{max} and G_{avg} assume that all possible detector ring combinations are used in collecting the data. However, in practice the axial acceptance angle can be limited by specifying a maximum ring difference (MRD) between detector rings that can create a coincidence event. Using a MRD that is less than the largest value possible, MRD_{max}, will result in a geometric efficiency that has a trapezoidal shape rather than a triangular shape, as shown in Figure 6.6a. To a first order, the maximum value of the geometric efficiency in this case, G'_{max}, is

$$G'_{max} = G_{max} \frac{MRD}{MRD_{max}} \tag{6.7}$$

and then the average geometric efficiency along the axial length for the trapezoidal efficiency profile, G'_{avg}, is

$$G'_{avg} = G_{max} \left(\frac{MRD}{MRD_{max}}\right)\left(1 - \frac{MRD}{2MRD_{max}}\right) \tag{6.8}$$

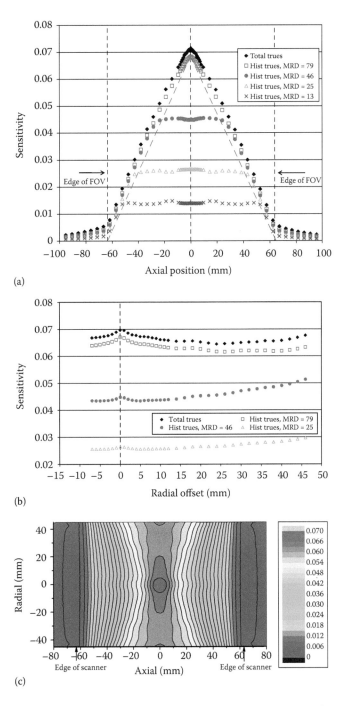

Figure 6.6 Sensitivity images for the Siemens Inveon small-animal PET system. (a) Axial sensitivity at the radial center for various MRDs. The maximum detection efficiency for this 80-ring PET system is for MRD = 79, and as the MRD is limited, there is a corresponding drop in detection efficiency. (b) Radial sensitivity profiles for the middle plane with different MRDs. (c) Sensitivity map for the complete system FOV for an MRD of 79. (From Visser, E.P., et al., *J. Nucl. Med.*, 50, 139–47, 2009.)

6.2.2.2.2 Detector efficiency

The detector efficiency, ε_D, depends primarily on the stopping power of the detector material and its thickness. The detector efficiency is given by

$$\varepsilon_D = \varepsilon_{\text{int}}\varepsilon_{\text{ff}}\varepsilon_E \tag{6.9}$$

where:

1. ε_{int} is the intrinsic efficiency of a detector for stopping the 511 keV photons, given by

$$\varepsilon_{\text{int}} = \left(1 - e^{-\mu_d x}\right) \tag{6.10}$$

 where μ_d is the linear attenuation coefficient of the detector material and x is the detector thickness.

2. ε_{ff} is the fill factor of the detector, which will be 1 for continuous detector materials and less than 1 for pixelated detectors with dead space between detector elements due to reflector materials. For an inter-crystal gap of 0.1 mm, ε_{ff} will be approximately 0.95 for the case of a 4×4 mm^2 detector element size, commonly used in clinical PET systems, but will drop to approximately 0.83 for the case of a 1×1 mm^2 detector element size, as might be used in a dedicated small-animal PET system.

3. ε_E accounts for an energy cutoff or window applied to the detected events. In order to reject scattered events, a common practice in clinical PET is to set an energy window that corresponds to the photopeak region of the energy spectrum. In this case, ε_E is reasonably approximated by the photoelectric fraction of the detector material, PE, given by

$$PE = \frac{\sigma_P}{\sigma_P + \sigma_C} \tag{6.11}$$

 where σ_P is the photoelectric interaction cross section at 511 keV and σ_C is the Compton interaction cross section at 511 keV.

Typical detector efficiency values for commonly used PET detector scintillator materials are given in Table 6.2 for scintillator thicknesses of 10 mm, commonly used in small-animal PET systems, and 20 mm, commonly used in clinical PET systems, and the typical values of ε_{ff} given above. Due to the detector efficiency value being squared in the total system detection efficiency, small differences in the detector efficiency can have significant effects on the overall system detection efficiency.

6.2.2.3 TIMING PERFORMANCE

PET systems rely on the electronic collimation created by the coincidence detection of the two 511 keV photons. In practice, single events are given a time stamp at the detector level and passed to the coincidence processor for identification of coincidence pairs. The uncertainty in the measurement of the time stamp given to the single event is referred to as the timing resolution of the detector and is commonly reported as the FWHM of the timing spread function measured for a pair of detectors. The timing resolution of a detector determines the minimum coincidence window that can be used for determining whether two events form a coincidence pair, with typical coincidence windows being two to three times wider than the timing resolution of the PET detector pair. The most significant impact of the choice of timing window is that it affects the amount of random coincidences in the data as the amount of randoms increases linearly with the timing window used. For this reason, minimizing the timing window directly benefits the overall performance and image quality of a PET system.

In many newer PET systems, the timing resolution is good enough to enable time-of-flight (TOF) data acquisition, in which the detection time difference between the two single events is used to provide additional localization of the event along the LOR (Moses, 2003). For a timing resolution of Δt, the location of the event along the LOR can be localized to a range Δx given by

$$\Delta x = \frac{c}{2}\Delta t \tag{6.12}$$

Table 6.2 Detector efficiencies for several commonly used scintillator materials

Scintillator material	LSO	LYSO	BGO	NaI	GSO	LaBr3
1/µ at 511 keV (mm)	12.3	12.6	11.2	25.9	15.0	22.3
PE at 511 keV	0.34	0.33	0.44	0.18	0.26	0.14
10 mm thickness						
ε_{int}	0.56	0.55	0.59	0.32	0.49	0.36
ε_D ($\varepsilon_{ff} = 1$)	0.19	0.18	0.26	0.058	0.13	0.051
ε_D^2 ($\varepsilon_{ff} = 1$)	0.036	0.033	0.068	0.0033	0.016	0.0026
ε_D ($\varepsilon_{ff} = 0.83$)	0.16	0.15	0.22	0.048	0.11	0.042
ε_D^2 ($\varepsilon_{ff} = 0.83$)	0.025	0.023	0.047	0.0023	0.011	0.0018
20 mm thickness						
ε_{int}	0.80	0.80	0.83	0.54	0.74	0.59
ε_D ($\varepsilon_{ff} = 1$)	0.27	0.26	0.37	0.097	0.19	0.083
ε_D^2 ($\varepsilon_{ff} = 1$)	0.075	0.069	0.13	0.0094	0.037	0.0069
ε_D ($\varepsilon_{ff} = 0.95$)	0.26	0.25	0.35	0.092	0.18	0.079
ε_D^2 ($\varepsilon_{ff} = 0.95$)	0.067	0.062	0.12	0.0085	0.033	0.0062

Source: Data adapted from Lecomte, R., *Eur. J. Nucl. Med. Mol. Imaging*, 36, 69–85, 2009.

where *c* is the speed of light. The best reported timing resolutions at the present time for individual detectors are in the 100–200 ps range (Seifert et al., 2012), which corresponds to positioning uncertainties of 15–30 mm. For the current generation of whole-body PET systems, timing resolutions of 300–600 ps have been reported, which correspond to positioning uncertainties of 4.5–9 cm. While this limited spatial localization will not improve the spatial resolution, it does result in an improvement in the signal-to-noise ratio (SNR) given by (Conti, 2011)

$$SNR_{TOF} = \sqrt{\frac{D}{\Delta x}} \cdot SNR_{non-TOF} \tag{6.13}$$

where SNR_{TOF} is the SNR of the image reconstructed using the TOF information, $SNR_{non-TOF}$ is the SNR of the image reconstructed without the TOF information, D is the diameter of the patient being imaged, and Δx is the positioning uncertainty. For a timing resolution of 500 ps, the ratio between SNR_{TOF} and $SNR_{non-TOF}$ will then be 2.3 for a 40 cm diameter object, resulting in lower noise images. The improvements in SNR from TOF information will most benefit the imaging of large patients, which is a benefit as it is in these patients that there is the greatest amount of scatter and attenuation degrading the SNR. It should be noted that in TOF PET systems, the coincidence timing window may be much larger than the timing resolution of the system in order to allow for the transit time of the 511 keV photons across the FOV of the system.

The timing resolution of a PET detector is largely determined by how quickly and consistently the detector signal rises in response to the creation of photoelectrons and the threshold set for the trigger point. The timing is thus directly impacted by the light output of the scintillator, the photodetection efficiency of the photodetector, and the properties of the preamplifier electronics attached to the photodetector.

6.3 DETECTOR DESIGN FOR PET IMAGING

6.3.1 REQUIREMENTS FOR PET DETECTOR PERFORMANCE

The ideal detector for PET imaging is one that combines the following attributes:

1. High spatial resolution
2. High efficiency for detecting 511 keV photons

3. Good timing resolution to allow use of narrow coincidence timing windows and enable TOF imaging acquisitions
4. Good energy resolution to allow rejection of scattered events

In current practice, the scintillation detector best meets these attributes. This section thus focuses on the application of scintillation detectors to the current practice of PET imaging.

6.3.2 DETECTOR DESIGNS

Early PET systems used an approach of individually coupling a single scintillator crystal to a single photo-multiplier tube (PMT). This one-to-one coupling approach is in many ways ideal since each detector element (i.e., the scintillator crystal) is read out individually. However, this design imposed limitations on the size of scintillator elements that could be used due to limitations on the size of the PMTs used in the detectors. The limitation to how small a PMT could be made led to the investigation of light-sharing detector designs, in which an array of scintillator crystals is read out by an array of photodetectors, with the crystal of interaction determined through analysis of the relative amount of light collected in each photodetector.

6.3.2.1 BLOCK DETECTOR

The first successful demonstration of decoding a large number of scintillator crystals with a PMT array was the block detector design proposed by Casey and Nutt (1986). In the block detector, a two-dimensional (2D) array of scintillator elements is read out by a 2 × 2 array of PMTs. In the original detector described by Casey and Nutt, the 2D BGO scintillator array was coupled to the four PMTs by a light guide that had slots of varying depth that allowed the scintillation light from each crystal in the array to have a unique pattern on the PMT array. In later versions, such as the example shown in Figure 6.7, a block detector from a Siemens/CTI ECAT 953, the scintillator array was cut from a solid block of BGO with varying depths of cuts between adjacent pixels. The cuts were filled with a reflective material, and in this way, the scintillator block itself acted as the light guide to uniquely spread the scintillation light from each crystal. In current versions of the block detector design based on LSO or LYSO scintillators, the design is closer to the original version, with a 2D array of scintillator crystals, separated by a reflector material and coupled to the 2 × 2 PMT array via a light guide. The block detector design is used in the current generation of PET/CT systems manufactured by both Siemens and General Electric. As an example of a current-generation PET block detector, the current Siemens system, the mCT (Jakoby et al., 2011), uses a 13 × 13 array of 4 × 4 × 20 mm³ LSO crystals and is read out by a 2 × 2 PMT array.

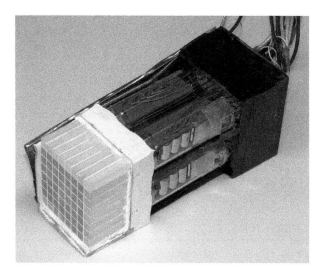

Figure 6.7 Photograph of a block detector from a Siemens/CTI ECAT 953 PET system showing the 8 × 8 BGO scintillator array coupled to a 2 × 2 PMT array.

The principle of operation of a block detector is shown in Figure 6.8. The scintillation light from each crystal creates a unique pattern of signal amplitudes in the four PMTs. This allows the X and Y location of the event to be calculated as

$$X = \frac{(A+B)-(C+D)}{A+B+C+D} \tag{6.14}$$

$$Y = \frac{(A+C)-(B+D)}{A+B+C+D} \tag{6.15}$$

with the total energy of the event, E, given by

$$E = A+B+C+D \tag{6.16}$$

The (X, Y) location of each crystal may not fall on a regular rectangular grid due to nonuniformities in light collection or nonlinearities in the detector gain. For this reason, the response of each detector must be calibrated to map the response of each crystal in the array to a unique set of (X, Y) coordinates. The typical process for performing this calibration is the following:

1. Using a positron emitter as a source, uniformly irradiate the detector to acquire a large number of events in which the amplitude of each PMT is recorded for each event.
2. For each event, calculate the (X, Y) location according to Equations 6.14 and 6.15.

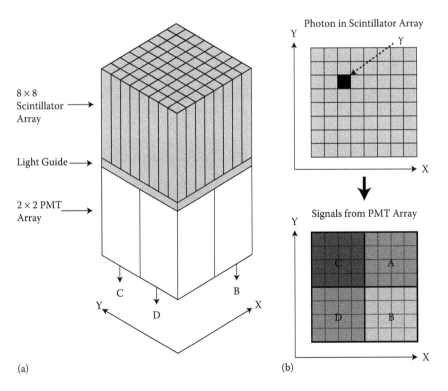

(a) (b)

Figure 6.8 (a) Schematic diagram of a block detector showing an 8 × 8 scintillator element array coupled via a light guide to a 2 × 2 array of PMTs. Note that PMT A is not visible when viewed from this angle. (b) Each crystal in the array creates a unique signal pattern in the four PMTs, allowing the decoding of the crystal of interaction.

3. Discretize the values of (X, Y) into integer values (i, j), where i and j range from 1 to N, where N is the dimension of the lookup table to be used (commonly a power of 2, such as 256).
4. Create a flood histogram image of size $N \times N$ in which the value of each element (x, y) represents the number of events acquired that had a location value of (i, j). An example of a detector flood image is shown in Figure 6.9.
5. Each "blob" in the flood histogram image represents the response of a single scintillator crystal in the array.
6. Segment the detector flood histogram into regions corresponding to the response of each crystal and create a detector lookup table that will be used to assign a crystal number to the (i, j) location of any measured event.
7. Calculate the relative gain or energy response of each crystal by evaluating the location of the 511 keV photopeak in the energy spectrum of each crystal. This allows the energy window used in subsequent acquisitions to be applied on a per-crystal basis.
8. If required, a per-crystal timing calibration can be calculated in a manner similar to the method used to calculate the per-crystal energy response.

While detector designs vary for systems from different vendors and for different applications (e.g., human vs. small-animal imaging), the basic detector calibration steps described above are generally applicable to most PET system designs.

6.3.2.2 PANEL-TYPE DETECTORS

An alternative to the block detector design is to use a panel-type detector in which a large array of scintillator crystals is read out by an array of large PMTs in a manner analogous to large-area gamma cameras that use Anger-type logic. An example of this detector design is the Philips Gemini TF system, which consists of 24 detector panels of the type shown in Figure 6.10. In this case, each panel used 1620 scintillator crystals read out by a hexagonal array of 51 mm diameter PMTs. In general, the calibration procedure for this type of detector system is similar to that described earlier for block detectors, with the exception that the positioning algorithm is modified to account for the difference in both positioning and number of PMTs.

6.3.2.3 DETECTORS FOR PRECLINICAL AND HIGH-RESOLUTION PET SYSTEMS

As discussed in Section 6.2.2.1, a limiting factor to the spatial resolution of a PET system is the scintillator crystal element size used in the detector. Conventional block and panel detector designs use relatively large PMTs (~26 mm square in a block detector or ~51 mm round in a panel detector), which are sufficient for resolving the ~4 mm pitch scintillator crystals used in whole-body PET imaging; however, these are not suitable for resolving the much smaller crystals used in high-resolution imaging systems. For this reason, PET imaging systems designed specifically for high-resolution applications such as small-animal imaging

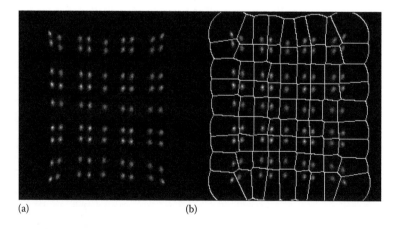

(a)   (b)

Figure 6.9 (a) Example of a detector flood histogram image. (b) Same flood image with region segmentation shown.

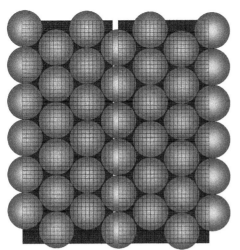 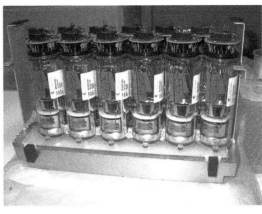

Figure 6.10 Example of a panel-type detector used in the Philips Gemini TF system. In this design, each panel consists of 1620 crystals read out by an array of PMTs. In this system, a total of 24 panels are used. (Adapted from Daube-Witherspoon, M.E., et al., *Phys. Med. Biol.*, 55, 45–64, 2010. With permission.)

or organ-dedicated cameras require modification to the detector design. We describe here some common approaches to create high-resolution PET detectors.

6.3.2.3.1 Block detector designs using position-sensitive or multichannel PMTs

As described above, the large PMTs used in clinical PET systems have a limited ability to resolve the small scintillator crystal elements used in high-resolution PET systems. While a traditional PMT has a single anode output and provides no information about where on the surface of the photocathode the scintillation light was detected, alternative designs, such as position-sensitive PMTs (PS-PMTs) or multichannel PMTs (MC-PMTs), can provide information about where on the surface of the PMT the light was detected. In a MC-PMT, the PMT structure is segmented into multiple independent PMT elements or pixels, each with its own anode output. These elements are typically arranged on a square grid. Examples of this MC-PMT design include the Hamamatsu H7546 family, which is an 8×8 multianode PMT with an active area of 18.1×18.1 mm^2 and anode size of 2×2 mm^2, and the Hamamatsu H8500 series, which is an 8×8 multianode PMT with an active area of 49×49 mm^2 and anode size of 5.8×5.8 mm^2. Coupling a scintillator array to a MC-PMT is then analogous to building a block detector with a large number of small PMTs, enabling the resolving of smaller crystal elements. The outputs of the MC-PMT can be individually sampled or multiplexed so that a smaller number of analog-to-digital converter (ADC) channels are required. A common design is to reduce the number of outputs to a total of four in order to mimic the outputs of conventional block detector designs (Tai et al., 2003; Siegel et al., 1996). MC-PMT-based block detector designs have been used successfully in many small-animal PET systems, including the original microPET system developed at the University of California, Los Angeles (UCLA) by Cherry et al. (1997) and the more recent nanoPET system manufactured by Mediso (Szanda et al., 2011).

In a PS-PMT, the photocathode is typically continuous and the anode structure commonly of multiple wires that form a grid and collect the charge cloud generated. An example of this design is the Hamamatsu R8900-C12 series of PS-PMTs, which have six wires in the X direction and six in the Y direction, giving a total of 12 outputs. Similar to the MC-PMT, the outputs can be individually digitized or multiplexed to reduce the number of signals requiring digitization. An example of the PS-PMT-based detector used in the Siemens Inveon small-animal PET system (Kemp et al., 2009; Bao et al., 2009) is shown in Figure 6.11. In this detector, a 20×20 array of LSO scintillator crystals with a crystal pitch of 1.59 mm is coupled via a multielement light guide (Mintzer and Siegel, 2007) to a Hamamatsu R8900-C12 PS-PMT.

Whether a MC-PMT or a PS-PMT photodetector is used, a common problem is that the active area of the PMT is smaller than the package footprint of the PMT. If the scintillator array is directly coupled to the photocathode and a detector ring assembled, this will result in a situation where there are significant gaps between adjacent detector modules, significantly reducing the geometric detection efficiency of the system and complicating the image reconstruction process. A common solution to this problem has been to use light guides to couple the scintillator array to the PMT, thus allowing the PMTs to fit around the ring of detectors, as shown in Figure 6.12. The light guide can be of a fiber-optic design that simply introduces a distance between the scintillator array and the PMT so that when the detectors are arranged in a ring configuration, the circumference of the ring at the radius of the PMTs is larger than at the radius of the crystals, giving more room for the PMTs. This design was used in the microPET family of animal PET systems manufactured by Concorde Microsystems/Siemens (Tai et al., 2001, 2005) in which an LSO

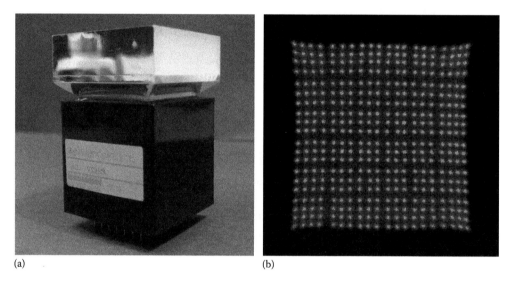

(a)   (b)

Figure 6.11 (a) Photograph of a detector used in the Siemens Inveon animal PET system that uses a PS-PMT coupled to a scintillator array by a multielement light guide. (b) Flood histogram of the 20 × 20 element array. (Adapted from Mintzer, R.A., and Siegel, S.B., in *2007 IEEE Nuclear Science Symposium Conference Record*, IEEE, Piscataway, NJ, 2007, pp. 3418–22. With permission.)

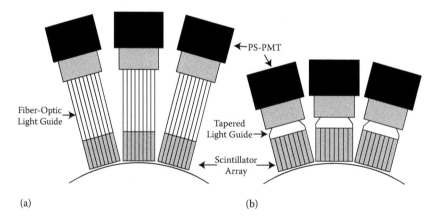

(a)   (b)

Figure 6.12 (a) Example of detector design using fiber-optic light guides. (b) Example of detector design using a tapered light guide. The fiber-optic design requires a larger overall system diameter, while the tapered light guide requires a more complex design.

scintillator array was coupled to a PS-PMT using a 10 cm long fiber-optic bundle built from discrete square cross section plastic fiber. Alternatively, optical fiber bundles made of drawn glass bundles can be used (Chatziioannou et al., 2001; Tai et al., 2003). Another approach to light guide design is to use a tapered light guide, which channels the light from the scintillator array to the PMT and, in doing so, introduces a geometric minimization array pattern. In this way, the active area of the PMT can be smaller than the area of the scintillator array. An example of this is shown in Figure 6.11 for the Siemens Inveon detector. The advantage of the tapered array, as shown in Figure 6.12, is that the overall size of the system detector ring can be kept smaller than when using a nontapered array. Tapered arrays can be assembled from multiple elements like for the Siemens Inveon, or one can use tapered bundles made of drawn glass (Doshi, 2000; Doshi et al., 2001).

While light guides enable the minimization of gaps between detector modules in small-animal PET systems, they also result in some performance degradation due to the loss of efficiency in the collection of scintillation light that they introduce. This loss of light results in a decrease in the energy resolution of the detector and a degradation in the timing performance. More recently, detectors based on silicon photo-multiplier (SiPM) technologies have been introduced (Song et al., 2010; Kolb et al., 2010). These detectors are commonly configured as multipixel arrays that, to a large extent, resemble MC-PMT configurations; however, since they are silicon devices rather than vacuum tube devices, they typically have a much smaller amount of dead space around the detector active area. In future PET systems, it is likely that the SiPM detector will become the detector of choice, thus removing the need for the lengthy fiber bundles required to accommodate the bulky PMT packages. That said, it is likely that many SiPM detector designs will use square or rectangular crystal array shapes and continue to employ some form of analog signal multiplexing to reduce the number of analog outputs. For these reasons, we will likely continue to refer to these detectors as block detectors.

There have been a number of systems built that use a combination of variations on block detector designs and geometry to create a high-resolution PET system. One successful approach is to use a small number of very large-area detectors. For example, the nanoPET system from Mediso (Szanda et al., 2011; Major et al., 2009) is built using only 12 block detectors, each consisting of two Hamamatsu H9500 MC-PMTs and a 39 × 81 array of LYSO:Ce crystals with a pitch of 1.17 mm, giving a block size of approximately 45 × 95 mm². The outputs of the two MC-PMTs in each module are multiplexed together to give only four analog outputs per module. In another approach, the group of Gu et al. (2013) developed a four-detector PET system, named PETbox4, that was subsequently commercialized as the Genisys system by Sofie Biosciences. This system has a detector size similar to that of the nanoPET; however, each detector uses two Hamamatsu H8500 MC-PMTs coupled to a 24 × 50 array of BGO crystals with a pitch of 1.90 mm. Similar to the nanoPET, the outputs of the MC-PMTs are multiplexed down to four analog channels per module. Unlike the nanoPET, the use of only four detectors means that the detector ring opening is much smaller, limiting the system to the imaging of mice only. A key advantage of using large-area block detectors is that the number of analog channels that must be digitized is greatly reduced, thus reducing the cost and complexity of the data acquisition system. A key disadvantage is that the large area of the detector and subsequent large solid coverage will lead to a high event rate, possibly causing event pileup and subsequent loss of performance. In the case of the nanoPET, this effect is mitigated by using fast free-running ADC electronics with minimal pulse shaping to reduce the pulse processing time. In the case of the PETbox4 system, the amount of activity injected into the mouse being imaged is kept purposefully low to avoid pulse pileup effects.

6.3.2.3.2 Panel-type or quadrant-sharing detector for small-animal PET

Several groups have successfully used panel-type detectors to construct high-resolution PET systems for small-animal imaging. For example, the A-PET system developed at the University of Pennsylvania (Surti et al., 2005) used 19 mm diameter PMTs arranged in a hexagonal pattern to resolve 2 mm sized scintillator crystals. The geometry of this system was different from the panel design discussed in Section 6.3.2.2 in that the system used a single continuous annular light guide, with the crystals coupled to the inside surface and the PMTs coupled to the outside surface. In another approach, the MuPET system developed at the University of Texas MD Anderson Cancer Center (Wong et al., 2012; Ramirez et al., 2011) uses a quadrant-sharing design using 19 mm diameter PMTs arranged on a square grid. Unlike the A-PET system, which used a continuous annular light guide, the MuPET system is built using a tapered crystal block design, allowing the outer surface to be a polygon to allow flat coupling of the PMTs. The benefit to panel or quadrant-sharing designs is that there is a relatively small number of PMTs used, allowing each PMT signal to be digitized without the need for analog signal multiplexing, thus reducing system complexity and cost.

6.3.2.3.3 Minimally multiplexed detector designs

An alternative approach to high-resolution PET is to use small photodetector elements that are individually coupled to scintillator elements and read out individually. This approach has been successfully used by the Université de Sherbrooke group to develop the LabPET family of small-animal PET systems (Bergeron et al., 2009). In these systems, a single avalanche photodiode (APD) element is coupled to a phoswich pair of LYSO–lutetium gadolinium oxyorthosilicate (LGSO) scintillator crystals, each 2×2 mm^2 in cross section, as shown in Figure 6.13. In this design, the decay time difference between LYSO and LGSO is used to identify the crystal of interaction, so that effectively there is a 2:1 multiplexing of scintillator crystal to output channel. This high granularity of readout has the potential to allow very high count rates due to the small detector area serviced by each photodetector element and can allow discrimination of intercrystal scattered events. However, this system requires a very large number of ADC channels to individually digitize each output.

6.4 DATA ACQUISITION IN PET

As described in Chapter 4, there are many approaches to converting the analog signals from a PET detector into a digital form. As described earlier in this chapter, there are tremendous variations in the architecture and design of PET systems; however, all share a common set of requirements when it comes to processing data. A central problem in PET data acquisition is that the amount of raw data that the system can generate is very large. This is particularly true for systems that use free-running ADCs to continuously sample the detector outputs at high sample rates of 100 MHz or more. It is therefore essential that the volume of raw data be reduced by preprocessing to extract only relevant information. Another concern is that in whole-body clinical PET systems, the ratio of singles events to coincidence events can be very high. For example, in the Siemens Biograph 16 HiRez PET/CT system (Brambilla et al., 2005) the ratio of singles events to prompt coincidences is approximately 55–60 when there are activity levels of 100–200 MBq in the patient. For example, at an activity of ~170 MBq, the total singles rate in this system

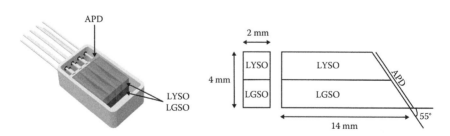

Figure 6.13 Schematic of a LabPET detector module consisting of a LYSO/LGSO crystal pair optically coupled to a single APD. In this module, the decay time difference between LYSO and LGSO is used to determine the crystal of interaction. (Adapted from Bergeron, M., et al., *IEEE Trans. Nucl. Sci.*, 56, 10–16, 2009. With permission.)

is ~10^7 cps. The Biograph 16 has 144 detectors blocks arranged in three rings, so assuming each detector has approximately the same count rate, each detector will have an event rate of ~70 kcps. In contrast, at ~170 MBq the prompts coincidence rate is ~190 kcps. For this system, acquiring singles data and post-processing to identify coincidence events would require 55–60 times the disk storage space of acquiring coincidence events only. The high singles event rate might also require a significantly higher bandwidth data connection between the PET system and the host computer storing the data, increasing the cost and complexity of the system. For example, the 10^7 cps singles rate in the example above would require a bandwidth and storage capability of 40 MB/s if we assume that each singles event is 4 bytes. A typical patient scan on this system requires seven bed positions of 3 min per bed position, giving a total scan time of 21 min or 1260 s. If full singles data are acquired and stored, the data volume will be ~50 GB. In contrast, acquiring only the prompt coincidences would give a data volume of ~0.95 GB, a much more manageable size. While acquiring and storing data in full singles acquisition mode may be feasible, and even desirable, for research PET systems, it does not represent a reasonable solution to data acquisition in a routine clinical scanning environment. For these reasons, it is necessary to implement data selection and reduction strategies within the data acquisition architecture to ensure that irrelevant information is discarded. In general, this process follows these steps:

1. For each interaction in the detector, create a singles event that describes the properties of the detected event.
2. Search the list of singles events for pairs that satisfy the criteria for forming a coincidence event.
3. Store the coincidence events in a usable format.

In this section, we discuss various approaches to implementing the requirements of the data collection process.

6.4.1 SINGLES EVENT ACQUISITION

All modern PET systems employ methods to do real-time identification of singles events from the detector data being collected. Each singles event that is created typically contains the following information: (1) location of interaction, (2) energy deposited in the interaction, and (3) time of event. This information is stored in a singles event "word." It is desirable to keep the amount of information required to a minimum so that the word length can be minimized, as the length of the word directly impacts the number of events that can be transferred in a given amount of time. For this reason, it is not uncommon to have a system that is capable of operating in multiple modes, one for routine imaging where only relevant information is kept, and a diagnostic or calibration mode where the singles event word length is increased in order to allow more information to be transmitted about the event.

6.4.1.1 LOCATION OF INTERACTION

The definition of the location of the event is typically defined according to the type of detector that the event originates from. For systems that use pixelated scintillator elements, the location is defined by identifying the crystal in which the interaction occurred. As described in Section 6.3.2.1, this identification is done through a crystal lookup table that maps the relative signal amplitudes measured in each electronic channel to the originating crystal. For continuous crystals, the location is typically defined by an (X, Y) coordinate mapped to a rectangular grid. For detectors that are DOI capable, there will be an additional location coordinate Z corresponding to the depth of the event within the crystal element. While in principle the coordinates (X, Y, Z) are continuous variables, in practice they are discretized by binning the results into a fixed number of bins. For example, the DOI coordinate Z might use eight DOI bins along a 20 mm length crystal, giving a 2.5 mm DOI bin size. Similarly, the (X, Y) coordinate of a continuous crystal might be binned into a 256×256 array. The reason for this binning is to allow efficient packing of the event into a singles event word.

6.4.1.2 ENERGY DEPOSITED IN INTERACTION

Measuring the energy of a singles event allows thresholding of singles based on the use of an energy window. Different systems take different approaches to applying the energy cut to the singles data. In standard clinical imaging systems, an energy window is specified prior to the scan start (e.g., 425–625 keV for a clinical system or 350–650 keV for an animal PET system), and singles events that fall within this range are kept. Another approach, commonly employed in research systems, is to include the energy information in the singles event word so that energy windowing can be applied later in the data processing and reconstruction stage.

6.4.1.3 TIME OF EVENT

The time stamp of a singles event is required for identifying pairs of singles that form valid coincidence events by applying a timing window to the data. In newer systems that are TOF capable, the time stamp is also used to identify the location along the LOR where the positron annihilation occurred. The requirements for the bit depth of the counter and the granularity of least significant bit of the time stamp depend on the nature of the imaging system performance. In TOF systems, a least significant timing bit of 100 ps or less is required for accurate measurement of the arrival time difference. In non-TOF systems, 500 ps is generally sufficient. In systems that perform real-time coincidence identification, the bit depth of the counter only needs to be sufficient for uniquely identifying the arrival time to within the narrow time frame being considered by the coincidence processor. In contrast, in research systems that acquire and store singles mode data, the time stamps must reference an absolute time.

6.4.2 COINCIDENCE IDENTIFICATION METHODS

Coincidence processors generally consist of two types: hardware and software. In hardware systems, the singles events from the detectors are inspected in real time to identify pairs that form valid coincidence pairs based on defined criteria such as the applied coincidence timing window and physical location of the two detectors that the singles originated from. When a valid coincidence event is identified, the coincidence processor will then package the singles into a coincidence event word and send it to the host PC as a prompt coincidence, which can be either a true, scatter, or random coincidence. Hardware coincidence processors are typically implemented in a field-programmable gate array (FPGA)-based processing system on the PET scanner. An advantage of the hardware-based coincidence processor is that only coincidence data are sent to the host PC, greatly reducing the bandwidth requirements compared with singles mode acquisition. In contrast, a software-based coincidence processor is used on systems that acquire data in singles mode and acts on the host PC by identifying valid coincidence events in the singles data. With the increasing bandwidth capability of system components, future clinical systems using singles mode acquisition and real-time coincidence sorting in software (without saving the singles data) are likely to appear.

6.4.2.1 DELAYED COINCIDENCE IDENTIFICATION

As described in Chapter 8, correction for random coincidences is essential for quantitatively accurate PET imaging. There are two common approaches for estimating the random coincidence rate: measured randoms using a delayed coincidence window and calculated randoms based on the detector singles rate. Measurement methods using a delayed window technique to estimate randoms have the advantage of being relatively simple to implement and are subject to all of the same physical sources of dead time that the randoms in the prompt coincidences are subject to. In this way, the randoms measured with the delayed window can be directly subtracted from the prompts data. The disadvantage of measuring randoms with a delayed window is that the randoms measurement for each LOR represents a Poisson variable, and thus the subtraction of this measurement increases the noise in the data. This noise can be reduced through variance reduction techniques such as Casey smoothing (Casey and Hoffman, 1986), in which the randoms measured in multiple neighboring LORs are averaged to reduce noise. In contrast, estimating random coincidences from the singles data allows essentially noise-free estimates of the random coincidence rates for each LOR, but requires careful correction for system dead time to ensure quantitative accuracy.

6.5 DATA SORTING AND SINOGRAMS

6.5.1 SINOGRAM DATA ORGANIZATION

Coincidence data generated by a PET system contains information about the two locations of interaction of the pair of singles events. For a system with discrete crystal elements, this information is represented by a pair of crystal identification (ID) numbers, while for a system with continuous detectors, the location may be either an (X, Y, Z) coordinate or a detector pixel number. The most commonly used reconstruction algorithms do not directly work on the list-mode data, but rather require the data to be histogrammed into a form where each element of the histogram represents the response of a LOR or the summed response of multiple neighboring LORs. The most common approach used to histogram PET data is the sinogram. The sinogram can be thought of as a Radon transform, or line integral, of the emission data (Radon, 1917, 1986) in which the data along a particular radial offset s and angle φ is mapped into a (row, column) position, as shown in Figure 6.14. For a source distribution that contains a point source, the pattern traced out by the source in the sinogram resembles a sine wave curve.

6.5.2 2D SINOGRAM ORGANIZATION FOR A CYLINDRICAL PET SYSTEM

It is helpful to consider a theoretical single-ring PET system with cylindrical geometry, such as the 32-detector system shown in Figure 6.15, to understand how data are typically mapped into sinogram space and what the sinogram physically represents in PET imaging.

For the example of the 32-detector system shown in Figure 6.15, we can see that the data can be organized into projection angles according to the angle of the LOR for the crystal pair being considered. The LORs for which $\varphi = 0°$ (solid lines) are the LORs for crystal pairs (30, 17), (31, 16), (0, 15), (1, 14), …. The next allowed value of φ is $180°/N$ ($N = 32$ in this case), which corresponds to the crystal pairs (30, 16), (31, 15), (0, 14), (1, 13), (2, 12) …. When organizing the LORs for a cylindrical PET system into a sinogram structure sorted by (s, φ) values, we can see that for a system with N detectors, there will be N possible values of the parameter φ. In practice, it is common to reduce the number of angles in the sinogram by half by interleaving the LORs with angles that are an odd-integer multiple of $180°/N$ (e.g., the dashed lines in Figure 6.15) with the LORs

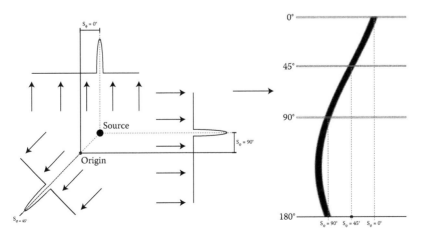

Figure 6.14 (a) Relationship between radial offset s and angle of projection φ for a point source of emission. (b) Sinogram of point source.

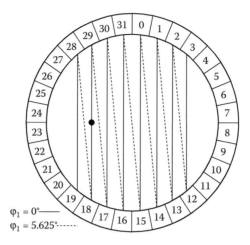

Figure 6.15 A 32-detector cylindrical geometry single-ring PET system.

that correspond to an even-integer multiple of 180°/N (e.g., the solid lines in Figure 6.15). This interleaving, referred to as "mashing," reduces the number of angles in the sinogram to $N/2$ while increasing the number of radial samples for each angle.

The width of the sinogram is determined by the usable FOV of the system. As shown in Figure 6.15, during data acquisition, the coincidence acceptance window is normally limited to only allow coincidences between detectors separated by a minimum angle difference, thus defining an "electronic FOV" for the system. For the 32-detector system considered in Figure 6.15, the minimum detector separation is 8 and the "sinogram FOV" is equal to the electronic FOV. For systems that use block detector designs, the electronic FOV may be larger than the sinogram FOV. For a given detector pair (d_1, d_2), it can be shown that the sinogram angle of the LOR defined by the pair is related to the sum of the detector numbers and the radial offset is related to the difference of the detector numbers, allowing rapid calculation of the sinogram bin. Figure 6.16 shows the sinogram for the 32-detector system of Figure 6.15 mapping each allowed (d_1, d_2) pair to a unique sinogram bin. As can be seen in the sinogram, the response of a single detector (in this case, detector 0) traces a diagonal line across the sinogram, while the response of a point source in the system traces a sine-shaped pattern in the sinogram.

This idealized sinogram representation works well for pure cylindrical geometry systems since it allows the response of each allowed LOR to be uniquely mapped into the sinogram and represents an efficient method of reducing the list-mode data to a form that can be readily handled by analytical reconstruction algorithms. Because each sinogram element represents a unique detector pair, it is relatively simple to apply corrections such as normalization, which depend on the individual detector response. It must be pointed out that a disadvantage of this form is that the columns of the sinogram do not represent equally spaced samples due to the fact that the detectors are arranged around a ring. As can be seen in Figure 6.15, this results in the samples at the edge of the FOV being more closely spaced than at the center of the FOV. This effect, called the "arc effect," must be corrected for either during image reconstruction or through interpolation of the sinogram onto a regularly spaced grid in order to avoid spatial distortions in the reconstructed image.

6.5.3 GENERAL 2D SINOGRAM ORGANIZATION

While the sinogram creation method described in Section 6.5.2 works well for a pure cylindrical geometry system, it poses challenges for polygonal geometries such as those represented by most block detector design systems because the crystals are not each separated by a uniform angular separation. In addition, there are typically gaps between the detector blocks that introduce gaps into both the radial and angular

Angle/Column	0	1	2	3	4	5	6	7	8	9	10	11	12	13	14	15
0	20	20	21	21	22	22	23	23	24	24	25	25	26	26	27	27
	11	10	10	9	9	8	8	7	7	6	6	5	5	4	4	3
1	21	21	22	22	23	23	24	24	25	25	26	26	27	27	28	28
	12	11	11	10	10	9	9	8	8	7	7	6	6	5	5	4
2	22	22	23	23	24	24	25	24	26	26	27	27	28	28	29	29
	13	12	12	11	11	10	10	9	9	8	8	7	7	6	6	5
3	23	23	24	24	25	25	26	26	27	27	28	28	29	29	30	30
	14	13	13	12	12	11	11	10	10	9	9	8	8	7	7	6
4	24	24	25	25	26	26	27	27	28	28	29	29	30	30	31	31
	15	14	14	13	13	12	12	11	11	10	10	9	9	8	8	7
5	25	25	26	26	27	27	28	28	29	29	30	30	31	31	0	0
	16	15	15	14	14	13	13	12	12	11	11	10	10	9	9	8
6	26	26	27	27	28	28	29	29	30	30	31	31	0	0	1	1
	17	16	16	15	15	14	14	13	13	12	12	11	11	10	10	9
7	27	27	28	28	29	29	30	30	31	31	0	0	1	1	2	2
	18	17	17	16	16	15	15	14	14	13	13	12	12	11	11	10
8	28	28	29	29	30	30	31	31	0	0	1	1	2	2	3	3
	19	18	18	17	17	16	16	15	15	14	14	13	13	12	12	11
9	29	29	30	30	31	31	0	0	1	1	2	2	3	3	4	4
	20	19	19	18	18	17	17	16	16	15	15	14	14	13	13	12
10	30	30	31	31	0	0	1	1	2	2	3	3	4	4	5	5
	21	20	20	19	19	18	18	17	17	16	16	15	15	14	14	13
11	31	31	0	0	1	1	2	2	3	3	4	4	5	5	6	6
	22	21	21	20	20	19	19	18	18	17	17	16	16	15	15	14
12	0	0	1	1	2	2	3	3	4	4	5	5	6	6	7	7
	23	22	22	21	21	20	20	19	19	18	18	17	17	16	16	15
13	1	1	2	2	3	3	4	4	5	5	6	6	7	7	8	8
	24	23	23	22	22	21	21	20	20	19	19	18	18	17	17	16
14	2	2	3	3	4	4	5	5	6	6	7	7	8	8	9	9
	25	24	24	23	23	22	22	21	21	20	20	19	19	18	18	17
15	3	3	4	4	5	5	6	6	7	7	8	8	9	9	10	10
	26	25	25	24	24	23	23	22	22	21	21	20	20	19	19	18

Figure 6.16 Mapping of LORs defined by crystal pairs in the 32-detector PET system of Figure 6.15 to a 2D sinogram. The gray shaded boxes represent the LORs that include detector 0, showing how the response of a single detector is a diagonal line in sinogram space. The black shaded boxes represent the point source from Figure 6.15 tracing out a sine-like pattern.

sampling profiles of the sinogram. The general solution to this problem is to interpolate the LORs for each detector pair into the 2D sinogram based on the (s, φ) value represented by the LOR. The main advantage of this approach is that the conventional sinogram structure can be used, facilitating data storage and image reconstruction. However, the key disadvantage of this approach is that creating the sinogram involves an interpolation step, so that the sinogram no longer represents a one-to-one mapping of system LOR to sinogram space. For this reason, if reconstruction algorithms are used that model the PSF or LOR map of the PET system, it may be best not to use the conventional sinogram data structure. In these cases, binning the data according to the unique LOR or reconstructing the data directly from the list mode may be preferred.

6.5.4 3D SINOGRAMS

PET systems are commonly constructed by assembling multiple rings of detectors in order to provide extended axial FOVs. For example, the PET system that is part of the Siemens Biograph mMR (Delso et al., 2011) is made of eight rings of detector blocks, with each detector having an 8×8 array of $4 \times 4 \times 20 \text{ mm}^3$

LSO crystals, for a total of 64 rings of crystals over an axial FOV of 25.8 cm. As described in Section 6.2.2.2, the system sensitivity is highly dependent on accepting the oblique LORs between different crystal rings, so that it is essential to incorporate the data from these oblique LORs. An initial approach one can consider is to simply create a unique 2D sinogram for each possible crystal ring combination, resulting in M^2 2D sinograms for a system with M rings. It should be noted that two 2D sinograms, each covering 180°, are required to uniquely record the data from coincidences originating from crystals in two different crystal rings. This can be understood by considering the 32 crystal rings shown in Figure 6.15 placed in a system with two identical rings. In this case, the LOR defined by a coincidence of crystal 0 in ring 0 with crystal 15 in ring 1 has a different axial angle than the LOR of crystal 15 in ring 0 with crystal 0 in ring 1. Since the number of three-dimensional (3D) sinograms scales as the square of the number of rings, the size of the sinogram data can quickly become very large for large axial FOV systems. As an example, the mMR system with its 64 crystal rings requires 4096 2D sinograms to uniquely define every axial LOR angle. Even a more modest system size of 32 crystal rings would require 1024 2D sinograms. The large number of LORs in 3D PET systems can pose several challenges for sorting data into sinograms and subsequent image reconstruction, including storage space requirements and data sparseness (i.e., few or no counts in many LORs).

A practical method used to reduce the number of sinograms in the 3D data set to manageable amounts is to employ axial binning, commonly referred to as axial mashing. To demonstrate this, we consider a system with 32 crystal rings, as shown in Figure 6.17. As described above, this system design would require $(32)^2 = 1024$ 2D sinograms to uniquely describe each LOR in the system. In practice, the number of sinograms required is determined by setting the span and maximum ring difference (RD) for the acquisition. RD refers to the maximum difference between crystal ring numbers allowed for two singles to form a valid coincidence event. By limiting the RD to a small value, the data collected excludes more oblique angles, thus simplifying the problem of image reconstruction, but at a cost of reduced detection efficiency. Span refers to the number of sinograms that are mashed together to form a single 2D sinogram approximated as having the same axial angle. Choosing a larger span value reduces the number of sinograms in the data set, but at a cost of degraded axial resolution.

The concept of span and RD and how they affect the number of sinograms can best be visualized through the use of a "Michelogram," named for Christian Michel. A Michelogram is a representation of the way in which 2D sinograms are grouped together based on a specified span and RD. For example, for our 32-ring PET system considered in Figure 6.17, binning the data with span 3, RD 31 will result in

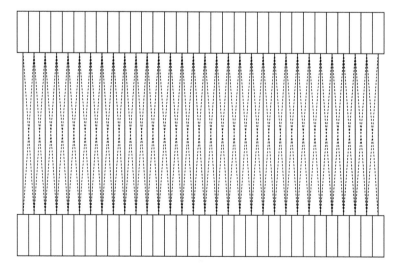

Figure 6.17 Schematic drawing of a 32-ring PET system. The direct (solid lines) and cross (dashed lines) planes, which form the 2D sinograms of a span 3 acquisition, are shown.

703 sinograms, as shown in the Michelogram of Figure 6.18. The Michelogram shows the coincidences between the 32 detector rings, with each allowed coincidence denoted by a •, and 2D sinograms that are mashed together to form a single sinogram denoted by a solid line connecting the dots. The span 3, RD 31 example of Figure 6.18 can be grouped into 21 "segments," where each segment denotes a set of sinograms with similar axial angle. Segment 0, also referred to as the 2D sinograms, is the set of sinograms with RDs of 0 or 1. The positive segments are the sets with axial angle >0, while the negative segments are the sets with axial angle <0.

The concept of sinogram segments is easier to visualize for the case of span 11, RD 27 shown in Figure 6.19. In this case, the higher degree of axial mashing results in only five segments with 223 total sinograms. The segments are easy to see as the diagonal sets in the Michelogram. The 3D axial LORs represented by the different segments are shown in Figure 6.20.

Axial mashing of the 3D data is an efficient way to reduce the overall size of the data set and reduce the noise in the data through averaging the response of multiple axial sinograms together. However, this comes at the price of reduced axial spatial resolution. For a specific system geometry, choosing an optimal span and RD is thus a trade-off between creating a manageable data size and preserving the sampling properties of the system. These choices are influenced by the geometry of the system, which determines the maximum

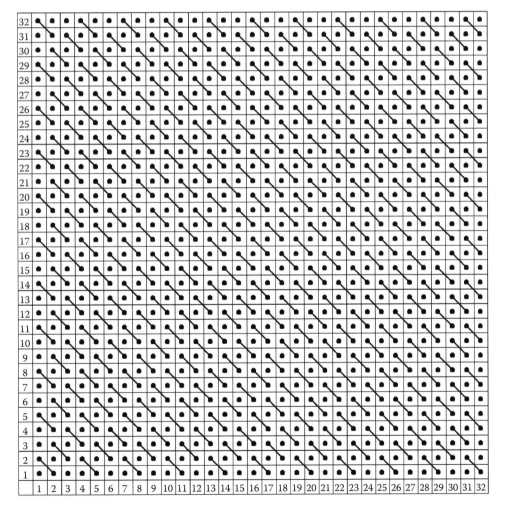

Figure 6.18 Michelogram for 32-ring system with span 3, RD 31 showing 703 sinograms arranged in 21 segments. Segment 0 of this Michelogram, corresponding to the main diagonal from the bottom left to the top right, represents the sinograms for the axial LORs shown in Figure 6.17.

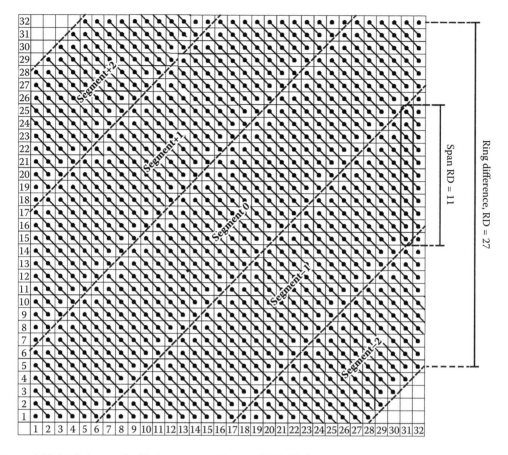

Figure 6.19 Michelogram for 32-ring system with span 11, RD 27 showing 5 segments, 223 sinograms.

axial angle encountered, and the manner in which the system will be used. For example, in general whole-body clinical oncology imaging, one may tolerate a higher degree of mashing than in high-resolution brain imaging.

6.6 SUMMARY AND FUTURE DIRECTIONS

The past four decades has seen continuous improvement in the performance and capabilities of PET system instrumentation, driven by technological advances in scintillators, photodetectors, system electronics, image reconstruction, and computing power. These advances have allowed PET to become established as a reliable, quantitative imaging modality in both clinical and research applications. Looking forward, we can identify several key trends in PET system instrumentation that are likely to have major impact in the field. Among these trends, the most significant at the current time is the move toward silicon-based photodetectors, such as APDs and SiPMs, facilitating the construction of more compact detectors that operate at lower bias voltages and, most importantly, are suitable for use in hybrid PET/MRI systems, potentially making the conventional vacuum tube PMT obsolete as the photodetector of choice. We anticipate that we will see detectors capable of providing DOI information become common, reducing the magnitude of the parallax error, and thus improving spatial resolution across the FOV. This will allow improved system sensitivity through allowing the use of thicker scintillator crystals or smaller ring diameters without resulting in degraded spatial resolution. Finally, we can expect continued improvements in computing power, allowing clinical implementation of more sophisticated real-time reconstruction algorithms that incorporate advanced systems models, improving the final image quality.

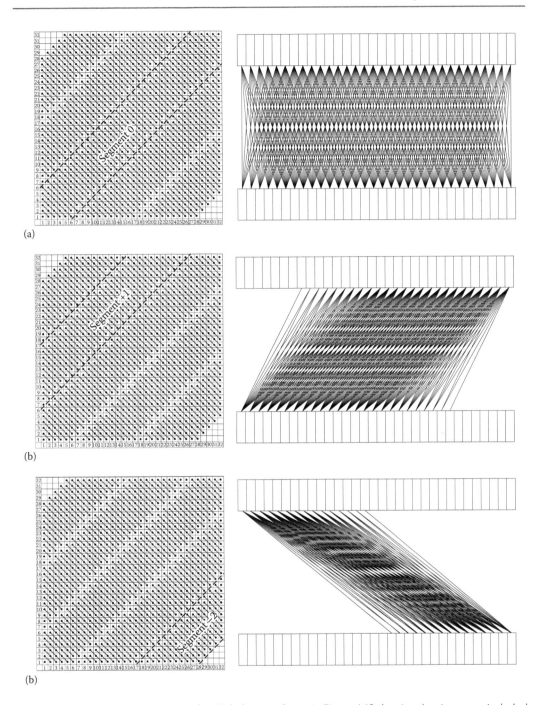

Figure 6.20 3D acquisition based on the Michelogram shown in Figure 6.19 showing the sinograms included in segment 0 (a), segment +1 (b), and segment −2 (c).

REFERENCES

Bao Q, Newport D, Chen M, Stout DB, and Chatziioannou AF. 2009. Performance evaluation of the Inveon dedicated PET preclinical tomograph based on the NEMA NU-4 standards. *J Nucl Med* 50: 401–8.

Bergeron M, Cadorette J, Beaudoin JF, Lepage MD, Robert G, Selivanov V, Tetrault MA, Viscogliosi N, Norenberg JP, Fontaine R, and Lecomte R. 2009. Performance evaluation of the LabPET APD-based digital PET scanner. *IEEE Trans Nucl Sci* 56: 10–16.

Brambilla M, Secco C, Dominietto M, Matheoud R, Sacchetti G, and Inglese E. 2005. Performance characteristics obtained for a new 3-dimensional lutetium oxyorthosilicate-based whole-body PET/CT scanner with the National Electrical Manufacturers Association NU 2-2001 standard. *J Nucl Med* 46: 2083–91.

Casey ME and Hoffman EJ. 1986. Quantitation in positron emission computed tomography. 7. A technique to reduce noise in accidental coincidence measurements and coincidence efficiency calibration. *J Comput Assist Tomogr* 10: 845–50.

Casey ME and Nutt R. 1986. A multicrystal two dimensional BGO detector system for positron emission tomography. *IEEE Trans Nucl Sci* 33: 460–63.

Chatziioannou A, Tai YC, Doshi N, and Cherry SR. 2001. Detector development for microPET II: A 1 ul resolution PET scanner for small animal imaging. *Phys Med Biol* 46: 2899–910.

Cherry SR, Shao Y, Silverman RW, Meadors K, Siegel S, Chatziioannou A, Young JW, et al. 1997. MicroPET: A high resolution PET scanner for imaging small animals. *IEEE Trans Nucl Sci* 44: 1161–66.

Conti M. 2011. Focus on time-of-flight PET: The benefits of improved time resolution. *Eur J Nucl Med Mol Imaging* 38: 1147–57.

Daube-Witherspoon ME, Surti S, Perkins A, Kyba CCM, Wiener R, Werner ME, Kulp R, and Karp JS. 2010. The imaging performance of a LaBr3-based PET scanner. *Phys Med Biol* 55: 45–64.

Delso G, Furst S, Jakoby B, Ladebeck R, Ganter C, Nekolla SG, Schwaiger M. and Ziegler SI. 2011. Performance measurements of the Siemens mMR integrated whole-body PET/MR scanner. *J Nucl Med* 52: 1914–22.

Doshi NK. 2000. Design and development of a dedicated mammary and axillary region positron emission tomography system (maxPET). University of California, Los Angeles.

Doshi NK, Silverman RW, Shao Y, and Cherry SR. 2001. maxPET, a dedicated mammary and axillary region PET imaging system for breast cancer. *IEEE Trans Nucl Sci* 48: 811–15.

Gu Z, Taschereau R, Vu NT, Wang H, Prout DL, Silverman RW, Bai B, Stout DB, Phelps ME, and Chatziioannou AF. 2013. NEMA NU-4 performance evaluation of PETbox4, a high sensitivity dedicated PET preclinical tomograph. *Phys Med Biol* 58: 3791–814.

Jakoby BW, Bercier Y, Conti M, Casey ME, Bendriem B, and Townsend DW. 2011. Physical and clinical performance of the mCT time-of-flight PET/CT scanner. *Phys Med Biol* 56: 2375–89.

Kemp BJ, Hruska CB, McFarland AR, Lenox MW, and Lowe VJ. 2009. NEMA NU 2-2007 performance measurements of the Siemens Inveon (TM) preclinical small animal PET system. *Phys Med Biol* 54: 2359–76.

Kolb A, Lorenz E, Judenhofer MS, Renker D, Lankes K, and Pichler BJ. 2010. Evaluation of Geiger-mode APDs for PET block detector designs. *Phys Med Biol* 55: 1815–32.

Lecomte R. 2009. Novel detector technology for clinical PET. *Eur J Nucl Med Mol Imaging* 36: 69–85.

Levin CS and Hoffman EJ. 1999. Calculation of positron range and its effect on the fundamental limit of positron emission tomography system spatial resolution. *Phys Med Biol* 44: 781–99.

Major P, Hesz G, Szlavecz A, Volgyes D, Benyo B, and Nemeth G. 2009. Local energy scale map for nanoPET/CT system. In *2009 IEEE Nuclear Science Symposium Conference Record (NSS/MIC)*, pp. 3177–80. Piscataway, NJ: IEEE.

Mintzer RA and Siegel SB. 2007. Design and performance of a new pixelated-LSO/PSPMT gamma-ray detector for high resolution PET imaging. In *2007 IEEE Nuclear Science Symposium Conference Record*, pp. 3418–22. Piscataway, NJ: IEEE.

Moses WW. 2003. Time of flight in PET revisited. *IEEE Trans Nucl Sci* 50: 1325–30.

Moses WW. 2011. Fundamental limits of spatial resolution in PET. *Nucl Instrum Methods A* 648: S236–40.

Radon J. 1917. Über die Bestimmung von Funktionen durch ihre Integralwerte längs gewisser Mannigfaltigkeiten. *Berichte Sächsische Akademie der Wissenschaften* 69: 262–77.

Radon J. 1986. On the determination of functions from their integral values along certain manifolds. *IEEE Trans Med Imaging* 5: 170–76.

Ramirez RA, Shaohui A, Shitao L, Yuxuan Z, Hongdi L, Baghaei H, Chao W, and Wai-Hoi W. 2011. Ultra-high resolution LYSO PQS-SSS heptahedron blocks for low-cost MuPET. *IEEE Trans Nucl Sci* 58: 626–33.

Seifert S, van Dam HT, and Schaart DR. 2012. The lower bound on the timing resolution of scintillation detectors. *Phys Med Biol* 57: 1797–814.

Siegel S, Silverman RW, Shao YP, and Cherry SR. 1996. Simple charge division readouts for imaging scintillator arrays using a multi-channel PMT. *IEEE Trans Nucl Sci* 43: 1634–41.

Song TY, Wu H, Komarov S, Siegel SB, and Tai YC. 2010. A sub-millimeter resolution PET detector module using a multi-pixel photon counter array. *Phys Med Biol* 55: 2573–87.

St James S and Thompson CJ. 2006. Image blurring due to light-sharing in PET block detectors. *Med Phys* 33: 405–10.

Surti S, Karp JS, Perkins AE, Cardi CA, Daube-Witherspoon ME, Kuhn A, and Muehllehner G. 2005. Imaging performance of A-PET: A small animal PET camera. *IEEE Trans Med Imaging* 24: 844–52.

Szanda I, Mackewn J, Patay G, Major P, Sunassee K, Mullen GE, Nemeth G, Haemisch Y, Blower PJ, and Marsden PK. 2011. National Electrical Manufacturers Association NU-4 performance evaluation of the PET component of the nanoPET/CT preclinical PET/CT scanner. *J Nucl Med* 52: 1741–47.

Tai YC, Chatziioannou A, Siegel S, Young J, Newport D, Goble RN, Nutt RE, and Cherry SR. 2001. Performance evaluation of the microPET P4: A PET system dedicated to animal imaging. *Phys Med Biol* 46: 1845–62.

Tai Y-C, Chatziioannou AF, Yang Y, Silverman RW, Meadors K, Siegel S, Newport DF, Stickel JR, and Cherry SR. 2003. MicroPET II: Design, development and initial performance of an improved microPET scanner for small-animal imaging. *Phys Med Biol* 48: 1519–37.

Tai YC, Ruangma A, Rowland D, Siegel S, Newport DF, Chow PL, and Laforest R. 2005. Performance evaluation of the microPET focus: A third-generation microPET scanner dedicated to animal imaging. *J Nucl Med* 46: 455–63.

Thompson CJ, James SS, and Tomic N. 2005. Under-sampling in PET scanners as a source of image blurring. *Nucl Instrum Methods A* 545: 436–45.

Visser EP, Disselhorst JA, Brom M, Laverman P, Gotthardt M, Oyen WJ, and Boerman OC. 2009. Spatial resolution and sensitivity of the Inveon small-animal PET scanner. *J Nucl Med* 50: 139–47.

Wong W-H, Li H, Baghaei H, Zhang Y, Ramirez RA, Liu S, Wang C, and An S. 2012. Engineering and performance (NEMA and animal) of a lower-cost higher-resolution animal PET/CT scanner using photomultiplier-quadrant-sharing detectors. *J Nucl Med* 53: 1786–93.

PART 3

QUANTITATIVE IMAGING

7 Methodologies for quantitative SPECT   195
   Irène Buvat
8 Data corrections and quantitative PET   211
   Suleman Surti and Joshua Scheuermann
9 Image reconstruction for PET and SPECT   235
   Richard M. Leahy, Bing Bai, and Evren Asma
10 High-performance computing in emission tomography   259
   Guillem Pratx
11 Methods and applications of dynamic SPECT imaging   285
   Anna M. Celler, Troy H. Farncombe, Alvin Ihsani, Arkadiusz Sitek, and R. Glenn Wells
12 Dynamic PET imaging   321
   Sung-Cheng (Henry) Huang and Koon-Pong Wong

Methodologies for quantitative SPECT

IRÈNE BUVAT

7.1	Introduction	195
7.2	Bias affecting SPECT images	196
7.3	Attenuation	196
7.4	Scatter	199
7.5	Detector response	203
7.6	Partial volume effect	204
7.7	Motion	206
7.8	Measurement	207
7.9	Overall quantitative accuracy achievable in SPECT imaging	208
7.10	Conclusion	209
	References	209

7.1 INTRODUCTION

SPECT has long been considered less accurate than PET as far as quantification is concerned. The main reason is that unlike PET, SPECT has been plagued by the lack of practical attenuation correction for a long time, while attenuation is responsible for the largest bias in quantification when not compensated for. The advent of SPECT–computed tomography (CT) scanners brought a real breakthrough toward accurate SPECT quantification by making attenuation correction both practical and reliable. Many reports now demonstrate that SPECT can accurately estimate tracer uptake, providing that appropriate reconstruction and correction procedures are used. This opens new perspectives regarding the use of SPECT images in applications for which accurate quantification is required. An important example is the use of quantitative SPECT images as an input for dosimetric calculations in radioimmunotherapy protocols, so that the dose–effect relationship can be investigated. Many other clinical investigations could also benefit from reliable quantification in SPECT, including differential diagnosis of neurodegenerative disease, or therapy monitoring in patients with neurodegenerative or cardiovascular diseases.

The purpose of this chapter is to give an overview of the main effects that have to be dealt with to perform accurate SPECT quantification and to present methods that are currently available for achieving reliable measurements from SPECT images. Future developments toward even better accuracy and reduced variability are also discussed.

7.2 BIAS AFFECTING SPECT IMAGES

Accurate quantification in SPECT most often means accurate estimation of tracer uptake, that is, of tracer activity concentration in a given region, from the SPECT images. Although the ultimate goal of image quantitation is to properly estimate a physiological parameter of interest, the step of accurate activity estimation, either at the voxel level or at a regional level, is a requirement to proceed with sophisticated quantitative analysis. This step can even be sufficient to derive informative parameters from images, even without performing advanced data analyses (such as compartmental analysis) that yield physiological parameter estimates. In this chapter, we therefore focus only on the phenomena affecting uptake estimates from SPECT images and on the corrections needed to obtain accurate measurements of local activity concentration.

It is important to understand that in SPECT, the signal intensity in the reconstructed image is *not* proportional to the tracer concentration in the corresponding region unless a number of corrections are performed. In other words, the SPECT image is most often a distorted representation of the actual activity distribution in the body. To make the SPECT image accurately reflect the activity distribution within the body, several effects inherent to the imaging process have to be compensated for. Starting from the patient up to the measurements made on the images, several sources of distortion and quantification errors can be listed:

1. Errors can occur due to the interactions between the gamma photons and matter. SPECT imaging is based on the detection of gamma photons emitted by a radiopharmaceutical in the patient body. These gamma photons may undergo a number of interactions after being emitted, which will either prevent them from being detected, causing activity underestimation, or make it more complicated to establish the relationship between the emission location and the detection spot.
2. The gamma camera used to detect the gamma photons is imperfect, with limited spatial and energy resolutions, making the measured projections different from the signal that actually arrives on the detector.
3. The measurement process may also be a source of quantitative error. Several approaches can be used to make a measurement from an image, and the approach that is used can itself introduce some systematic bias or uncertainty.
4. The patient is not perfectly motionless when performing a SPECT acquisition. Due to a SPECT acquisition duration that is of the order of several minutes, involuntary motions can occur, and even if the patient stays perfectly still, physiological motions, such as respiratory and cardiac motions, cannot be avoided.

In the following, we discuss all these potential sources of bias, give some examples of the resulting errors in SPECT images, explain how the effects can be compensated for, and discuss the performance of the compensation methods.

7.3 ATTENUATION

Attenuation is the largest source of bias in SPECT, given the relatively low energy of the gammas used for SPECT imaging (in the 70–300 keV range) and the high probability that a photon with such energy interacts with matter through the photoelectric effect and Compton scattering. As an example, the number of centimeters of soft tissue needed to stop half of the 140 keV photons emitted by ^{99m}Tc is 4.6 cm. Attenuation therefore considerably reduces the number of emitted photons that escape from the body and have a chance to be detected. The number of photons detected by the gamma camera thus does not reflect the actual number of emitted photons if attenuation is not compensated for. In cardiac imaging, attenuation alone, if not compensated for, would result in an activity underestimation in the cardiac wall of about 90% (El Fakhri et al. 1999). In brain imaging, attenuation is less severe, as the brain represents a smaller attenuating medium than the thorax, but activity underestimation due to attenuation is still greater than 50% (Soret et al. 2003). It is thus essential to compensate for attenuation for accurate quantification.

The physics law describing attenuation is the Beer–Lambert law, given by

$$N(j) = I(i)\exp\left(-\int \mu(i')dr\right)$$ (7.1)

where $N(j)$ is the number of photons detected in projection bin j, $I(i)$ is the number of photons emitted from image voxel i, $\mu(i')$ is the attenuation coefficient value in voxel i', and the integral sums over all image voxel elements located along the projection line between voxel i and projection bin j.

Attenuation depends on the emission energy of the radiotracer. The lower the energy, the greater the attenuation effect. For instance, for ^{201}Tl with emission energies between 69 and 80 keV, the soft tissue thickness needed to stop half of emitted photons is 3.8 cm instead of 4.6 cm for ^{99m}Tc that emits photons of 140 keV. Images acquired with a low-energy radionuclide will thus be more affected by attenuation than images acquired with a higher-energy radionuclide. The linear attenuation coefficient μ in Equation 7.1 at a given energy also depends on the attenuating medium: the denser the tissue, the higher the attenuation effect. Attenuation is higher in soft tissue than in lungs, and is higher in bones than in soft tissues. For instance, for ^{99m}Tc emitting photons of 140 keV, μ is 0.04 cm^{-1} in lung tissue, 0.15 cm^{-1} in soft tissues, and 0.30 cm^{-1} in cortical bone. Last, the attenuation of photons obviously depends on the thickness of attenuation media the photons travel through. In SPECT, photons emitted deep inside the body will be more attenuated than photons emitted at the surface of the body.

The immediately visible consequence of attenuation in SPECT is a distortion in the image, making the observed spatial distribution of activity different from what it actually is. For instance, for a cylindrical phantom filled with uniform activity distribution, the activity reconstructed at the center of the phantom will be less than that reconstructed at the edge of the phantom (Figure 7.1). In clinical studies, the most striking effect of attenuation is observed in cardiac myocardial perfusion imaging and causes what is known as the inferior wall artifact. Because the inferior wall is deeper inside the thorax than the anterior wall, activity emitted from the inferior wall is more severely affected by attenuation than activity emitted from the anterior wall. In myocardial perfusion SPECT images uncorrected for attenuation, one therefore observes a lower activity concentration in the inferior wall that is due to attenuation (Figure 7.2) and that can be misinterpreted as a perfusion defect.

Because attenuation depends on the tissues that the photons go through, accurate attenuation compensation requires a precise mapping of the attenuation coefficients μ of the tissues. In addition, given the attenuation coefficient map, one needs to know exactly how deep within the body a photon was emitted to determine the probability that it has been absorbed. So to accurately correct for attenuation, one has to know where the photons were emitted from, while it is precisely what one wants to estimate in SPECT. This is a catch-22 problem

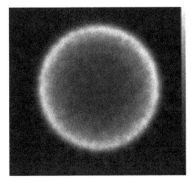 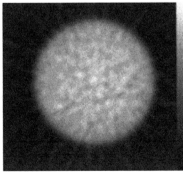

Figure 7.1 Reconstructed transaxial slice across a cylinder filled with uniform activity. Left: Without attenuation correction, the reconstructed activity map appears nonuniform, with a decrease in activity concentration at the center of the phantom, and high activity concentration at the edges. Right: After attenuation compensation, the activity within the phantom is properly recovered as uniformly distributed. (From Zaidi, H., and Hasegawa, B., *J. Nucl. Med.*, 44, 291–315, 2003.)

Tl-201 SPECT

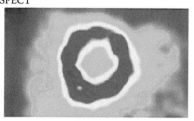

| No attenuation correction | With attenuation correction |

Figure 7.2 Attenuation artifact in the inferior wall of the myocardium on a short-axis SPECT ^{201}Tl reconstructed slice. Without attenuation correction (left), a decrease in activity concentration is seen in the inferior wall and can be wrongly interpreted as a perfusion defect. After attenuation correction, activity is restored in the inferior wall, ruling out the presence of a perfusion defect.

that explains why, in general, no accurate attenuation correction can be applied directly on the projection data to remove the attenuation effect. An iterative process is the most accurate approach to compensate for attenuation, so that the activity map is updated at each iteration until its projections through the attenuation map yield estimated projections close to the measured ones.

To compensate accurately for attenuation, a prerequisite is thus the availability of the attenuation coefficient map, also called the μ map. In most modern gamma cameras, this map is derived using the CT associated with the gamma camera. CT produces images in Hounsfield units (HU). Hounsfield units are attenuation coefficients measured at the energy of the x-ray tube normalized to the attenuation coefficient in water at that same energy:

$$HU(i) = 1000 * \left[\mu(i) - \mu(water)\right] / \mu(water) \qquad (7.2)$$

where $\mu(i)$ is the attenuation coefficient in voxel i at the energy of the CT, and $\mu(water)$ is the attenuation coefficient of water at the energy of the CT. The attenuation map relevant for photon energies used in SPECT can be deduced from the CT by rescaling the HU to account for the dependence of the attenuation coefficient with energy. A linear scaling is sufficient, so that

$$\mu_{E2}(i) = \mu_{E1}(i) \cdot \left[\mu_{E2}(water) / \mu_{E1}(water)\right] \qquad (7.3)$$

where E2 is the energy of interest in SPECT (e.g., 140 keV for ^{99m}Tc scans) and E1 is the average energy of the CT scanner tube.

When a μ map is available, the best approach currently available for attenuation correction consists in modeling attenuation within the system matrix P used in the reconstruction process and using an iterative reconstruction method to invert the resulting system matrix (see Chapter 9). When no attenuation is performed, this system matrix P describing the forward-projection operator calculates the contribution of a given voxel content to a detection bin in a projection based on a geometrical model only. When attenuation is accounted for, the system matrix entries of P, then noted P_{attn}, include the exponential weights shown in Equation 7.1 to estimate the contribution of a voxel $I(i)$ to a projection bin $N(j)$. By modeling attenuation in P_{attn}, the iterative reconstruction algorithm automatically identifies an image that is compatible with the measured projections given that attenuation occurred. The reconstructed images are then intrinsically corrected for attenuation. This is a very elegant solution to the attenuation problem in SPECT, as there is no approximation and the accuracy of the solution is mostly dependent on the convergence of the iterative reconstruction algorithm. The limitations of this approach are mainly associated with practical aspects. For the correction method to be unbiased, the attenuation map has to be perfectly realigned with the emission image. Because CT and SPECT are not simultaneously acquired even in SPECT/CT scanners, slight misalignments can occur and result in significant bias and artifact on the attenuation-corrected images if the misregistration is not

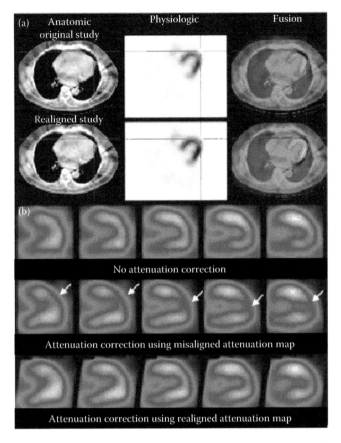

Figure 7.3 Impact of a misalignment between the attenuation coefficient map and the activity map on the resulting attenuation-corrected images. When the attenuation map derived from the CT is misaligned with the SPECT data (top row), attenuation correction introduces some artifacts in the SPECT images, here a misleading perfusion defect at the apex (row 4). After SPECT and CT image registration, the marked apex thinning seen in row 4 is reduced on the attenuation-corrected images (bottom row). (From Fricke, H., et al., *J. Nucl. Med.*, 45, 1619–1625, 2004.)

corrected for (Fricke et al. 2004) (Figure 7.3). Another practical issue is the difference in spatial resolution between the μ map and the SPECT image. Because the CT spatial resolution is better than that of the SPECT image, the μ value derived from the CT in a given voxel might not correspond to the actual attenuation coefficient of the piece of tissue mostly represented in that voxel in the SPECT image. This occurs only at the border between two media with significantly different attenuation, for instance, lung and liver, and can be dealt with by smoothing the μ map derived from the CT so as to make its spatial resolution close to the one of the SPECT image.

Nowadays, attenuation correction as implemented in the vendor scanners is very accurate in SPECT when the gamma camera is associated with a CT, with resulting errors less than 5%. Correcting the SPECT images for attenuation is absolutely essential for accurate quantification, whatever the organ of interest, and is now very reliable. It is also required to avoid artifacts and image distortion such as the inferior wall artifact frequently encountered in cardiac imaging.

7.4 SCATTER

When a photon is emitted by the radiopharmaceutical, it can undergo photoelectric absorption or scatter, either by Compton effect or by Rayleigh effect. Rayleigh scattering, which results in a change of direction of

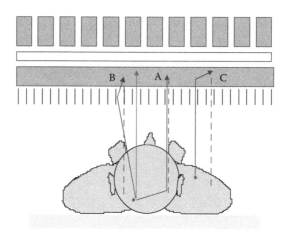

Figure 7.4 Photons that scattered in the patient (a), in the collimator (b), or in the crystal (c) are detected at positions that make it impossible to retrieve the initial emission point (black stars). Indeed, the projection lines (dashed lines) associated with the detection points do not cross the emission points.

the incident photon without any loss of energy, is negligible in SPECT, because of the relatively low probability of Rayleigh interaction in soft tissues at energies relevant for SPECT. Yet, Compton scatter is the dominant interaction in water and soft tissue between 40 keV and 10 MeV, and the scattering cross section increases as the energy decreases. Compton scattering produces a change of direction of the photon, associated with a loss of energy, so that when a photon of energy E is deflected under an angle θ, its resulting energy E' will be given by

$$E' = E \Big/ \Big[1 + E \left(1 - \cos \theta \right) \Big/ \mathrm{m_0} c^2 \Big] \qquad (7.4)$$

Above 100 keV, small deflections are much more likely than large deflections, and the higher the energy of the initial photon, the greater the forward deflection probability. These deflections make the photon change direction and deviate from its initial projection line. After a scattering event, the photon travels in another direction, and thus conveys poor information regarding its initial trajectory. If it goes through the collimator and is detected, it will increment a detection bin corresponding to a projection line crossing the position of the latest scatter interaction the photon underwent, instead of a projection line that would cross the photon emission location (Figure 7.4). Therefore, the photon will be assigned a position corresponding to its latest scatter interaction and not to its emission location. The detection of scattered photons will thus lead to images including photons located at a wrong location. The presence of these photons decreases the contrast of the image. For instance, because of scatter, activity can be detected in a dense medium that favors scatter but which is void of any activity. Scatter photons cause quantitative errors since they yield reconstructed signal that is not located at the right position.

Most scattering occurs in the patient, but there is also scatter in the collimator and in the crystal of the camera. The respective importance of these three contributions of scatter depends on the emission energy of the radionuclide, the patient size (more or less scattering medium), and the collimator features (more or less scattering medium). For instance, for a low-energy general-purpose (LEGP) collimator, scatter in the collimator contributes to only 2% of the ^{99m}Tc point-spread function (PSF) describing the response of the detector, but this proportion can be higher for higher-energy isotopes (Dewaraja et al. 2000).

Given that the scattered photons lose part of their energy, a gamma camera with a perfect energy resolution could distinguish scattered from unscattered photons based on the detected photon energy. Yet, current gamma cameras still have limited energy resolution, around 9% in NaI:Tl-based cameras and of the order of 5% for cadmium-zinc-telluride (CZT)–based gamma cameras. Scatter photons cannot be eliminated using energy discrimination only. Still, the better the energy resolution of the camera, the better the rejection of scattered photons using a spectral window centered on the emission energy.

Using conventional NaI:Tl-based gamma cameras and a 15% or 20% wide energy window (126–154 keV for ^{99m}Tc), the proportion of recorded scattered photons is still high (about 20%–30% of all photons detected in the energy window). This means that one-fifth to one-third of photons will be located at a wrong position in the SPECT image if no scatter correction is used. Using Monte Carlo simulations, it is possible to identify scattered photons and demonstrate that the scatter photons detected in the energy window used for acquisition (also called photopeak window) have mostly scattered once, but that some of them have scattered twice.

There is no exact solution to the scatter correction problem, and this is why many approaches have been proposed in the last 30 years (see Buvat et al. 1994; Hutton et al. 2011 for reviews).

One of the most popular, most effective, and easiest approaches to implement was proposed in 1984 by Ronald Jaszczak et al. (1984) and is known as the double energy window method. It consists in performing the acquisition in two energy windows simultaneously: the usual photopeak energy window centered on the emission energy of the radionuclide of interest, and a lower energy window, chosen so that only scattered photons are recorded in that window, but still as close as possible to the photopeak energy window. For instance, for ^{99m}Tc, the lower energy window is usually set to 92–125 keV, just next to the main energy window often set to 126–154 keV. The method then assumes that the image L acquired in the lower energy window is identical to the image of scattered photons within the photopeak window except for a scaling factor. The correction thus consists in subtracting the lower energy window image L weighted by a scaling factor k from the photopeak image N:

$$N_{sc}(j) = N(j) - k \cdot L(j) \tag{7.5}$$

where j denotes the projection pixel, and N_{sc} is the projection corrected for scatter.

This scaling factor k can be determined using Monte Carlo simulations or phantom experiments involving a scattering medium and a region with any radioactivity. Without scatter correction, some activity is detected in that theoretically devoid of activity region, and the scaling factor needed to get a mean activity of zero in that radioactivity-free region is adjusted. This method is very simple to implement. Yet, the underlying assumption makes it theoretically wrong. Indeed, Equation 7.4 clearly shows that the scattered photons have an energy that depends on their scattering angle. The most deflected photons have a lower energy than photons that have scattered under a very low angle. As a result, scattered photons detected in the lower energy window image L will be, on average, farther from their emission location than scattered photons detected in the photopeak window image N, because the former have lost more energy than the latter. The correction therefore tends to remove too many photons far from the real source of photons, and not enough where the photons are actually emitted. The net result is that the image contrast is artificially enhanced, which is satisfactory for an observer point of view, but which is not quantitatively accurate. Still, this method has proven to be quite robust and accurate for ^{99m}Tc, when using 92–125 keV and a scaling factor of 0.5. A drawback of this method is that the energy window setting and the scaling factor have to be tuned for every radionuclide.

A similar method, called the triple energy window method, is also based on the use of multiple energy windows and has been proposed to overcome the limitation of the double energy window method. This method assumes that in each pixel, the energy spectrum of the scattered photons detected within the photopeak energy window has an area under the curve identical to that of a trapezoid, with a base equal to the energy window width and sides equal to the values of the total energy spectrum on both sides of the photopeak window (Figure 7.5). To estimate the area under this trapezoid, two additional images acquired in two narrow energy windows are recorded and the number of scattered photons in voxel j is estimated using

$$D(j) = W\left[N_1(j) + N_2(j)\right]/2w \tag{7.6}$$

where W is the width (in keV) of the photopeak energy window, w is the width of each narrow energy window located on both sides of the photopeak window, $N_1(j)$ is the content of voxel j in the lowest narrow energy

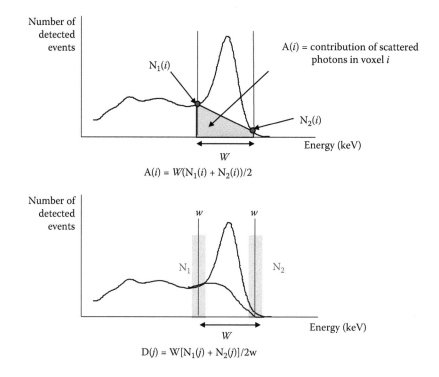

Figure 7.5 The triple energy window scatter correction assumes that in each projection pixel j, the number of scattered photons can be estimated as the area $A(j)$ under a trapezoid with a base equal to the width W of the photopeak energy window and the heights equal to the energy spectrum values $N_1(j)$ and $N_2(j)$ on each size of the photopeak energy window (top). From a practical point of view, this area $A(j)$ can be estimated by calculating $D(j)$ involving the number of events $I_1(j)$ and $I_2(j)$ recorded in two narrow energy windows, in addition to the photopeak energy window (bottom).

window, and $N_2(j)$ is the content of voxel j in the highest narrow energy window. This $D(j)$ contribution is then subtracted from voxel j to get an estimate of the scatter-free projection:

$$N_{sc}(j) = N(j) - D(j) \qquad (7.7)$$

An advantage of this approach compared with the dual energy window method is that there is no need for calibrating a scaling factor. The scaling factor is automatically determined by the width of the photopeak and narrow energy windows. The method is then easily applicable for different radionuclides without specific calibration. A significant drawback with respect to the dual energy window method is that the corrected images N_{sc} are noisy because the scatter estimate D is based on two narrow energy windows that record low numbers of counts. Noise can yet be reduced by filtering the N_1 and N_2 images (Ichihara et al. 1993; Hashimoto et al. 1997).

The dual and triple energy window approaches operate on the projections, before reconstruction: scatter is subtracted from the projections and the estimated scatter-free projections N_{sc} are then reconstructed. A different approach consists in modeling the scatter component within the reconstruction algorithm. This avoids the amplification of the noise observed when reconstructing projections from which scatter has initially been subtracted. Instead of removing scatter events from the data before reconstructing the images, the ambition is actually to estimate the original position of the photons that scattered before being detected. Many models have been proposed to estimate scatter and account for it within the reconstruction (Hutton et al. 2011). They are based on either Monte Carlo simulations or experiments that make it possible to determine the scatter response functions (also called scatter kernels) at various thicknesses in a homogeneous or heterogeneous attenuation medium (Beekman et al. 1999). Using these models and an activity map estimated at each iteration of an iterative reconstruction, the spatial distribution of the scattered photons that would be generated by the estimated activity map can be calculated, and added to the denominator of the update equation of the maximum-likelihood expectation maximization (MLEM) or ordered subset expectation maximization (OSEM) algorithm (see Equation 9.20 in Chapter 9) to be accounted for in the comparison with the actual projection measurements. In addition to the better noise handling associated with this approach, another advantage is that the Poisson nature of the original projections is retained as the original projections are used. On the contrary, projections resulting from a scatter subtraction (using the double or triple energy window method) have their statistical properties modified, which makes the use of some reconstruction algorithms inappropriate, as these algorithms (e.g., MLEM; see Chapter 9) include assumptions regarding the statistical properties of the projections. The main disadvantage of these modeling approaches is that, unlike the energy-based methods (dual and triple energy window approaches), they do not account for scatter photons coming from activity emitted outside the field of view of the gamma camera. Indeed, the estimated scatter contribution is based on an estimated activity distribution within the field of view of the camera.

For most common SPECT tracers, these scatter corrections yield reasonable accuracy. Scatter correction remains more challenging for radionuclides with multiple primary emissions at different energies (e.g., ^{123}I, ^{131}I, ^{111}In, and ^{67}Ga) where scatter originating from higher-energy photopeak emissions contaminates measurements in lower photopeak energy windows (Dewaraja et al. 2000; Dobbeleir et al. 1999). In these particular cases, energy-based methods, as well as reconstruction-based correction approaches, can also be used, but the issue is complicated by the fact that it is often necessary to account for scatter in both the collimator and the patient.

7.5 DETECTOR RESPONSE

Attenuation and scatter are mostly associated with photon interactions within the patient. The imperfect energy resolution of the gamma camera complicates the scatter correction problem, as described above. In addition, the imperfect spatial resolution of the gamma camera introduces a blur in the images that yields quantitative inaccuracy. Because of the limited spatial resolution of a gamma camera (typically of the order of 6 mm for a high-resolution collimator distance of 10 cm from the point source to the collimator), the image of a point source is an enlarged spot, resulting in blurred projections. In SPECT, the detector response is mostly dependent on the collimator features. The hole diameter and length of the collimator define a solid angle that makes the spatial resolution depend on the distance between the source and the detector. For parallel-hole collimators, there is a linear relationship between the spatial resolution characterized by the full width at half maximum (FWHM) of the PSF and the distance between the source and the detector. This implies that a source that is off-centered in a phantom or in the body will be seen as spots of different sizes in different projections. Therefore, if this change in spatial resolution as a function of the source-to-detector distance is not modeled during the image reconstruction, the reconstruction algorithm will not be able to properly reconstruct the source. This effect yields distortions in the reconstructed images, in which spherical structures will appear ellipsoidal (Kappadath 2011). This also leads to nonstationary spatial resolution in the reconstructed images: the spatial resolution is not the same in different regions of the images (e.g., in the center and at the periphery), which complicates other corrections, such as partial volume correction.

Given that the spatial resolution of a gamma camera can be precisely measured, the detector response can be easily modeled within the SPECT reconstruction process. Point source measurements have to be performed to fully characterize the PSF as a function of the position in the field of view. For a parallel-hole collimator, as the FWHM of the PSF varies linearly as a function of the distance between the point source and the detector, a few measurements are sufficient to get a good estimate of the PSF variations with the source–detector distance. For fan-beam and cone-beam collimators, the spatial resolution is a more complicated function of the three-dimensional (3D) source position location in the field of view, but it can still be experimentally determined. A compensation for the PSF of the detector can then be achieved by modeling the PSF effect within the forward projector P used for reconstruction (see Chapter 9). Instead of accounting for the projection geometry only in the P calculation, the spread caused by the PSF as a function of the position of the source in the field of view can be analytically modeled in the projection space. The inversion of P by iterative reconstruction then results in an image compatible with the measured projections given that the gamma camera has an imperfect spatial resolution. It is important to note that the modeling of the PSF within P modifies the convergence speed of the algorithm. Therefore, the number of iterations should not be the same, depending on whether the PSF is modeled within the reconstruction or not. This correction approach is now implemented on all recent gamma cameras, and its use has two major benefits. First, the spatial resolution in the reconstructed images is enhanced, and smaller structures are better visualized. Second, the spatial resolution in the reconstructed images is far more stationary; that is, there are fewer variations of the PSF FWHM across the field of view than when not compensating for the PSF. This latter feature is desirable because it facilitates subsequent partial volume correction.

A current remaining issue associated with the correction for the detector response is the possible observation of Gibbs artifacts (Zeng et al. 2011). These artifacts may be mitigated by tuning the PSF model toward an undercorrection, that is, assuming that the PSF is not as broad as actually measured. Another approach to reduce the Gibbs artifacts consists in using the appropriate PSF model but then smoothing the reconstructed images, as described in PET imaging (Stute and Comtat 2013).

7.6 PARTIAL VOLUME EFFECT

The so-called partial volume effect results from two phenomena: the limited spatial resolution in the reconstructed images as presented above and the sampling of the reconstructed images using a voxel grid (Figure 7.6). The limited spatial resolution blurs the images. This blur causes cross-contamination between adjacent structures. A high-activity structure will spill out into the nearby lower-activity region, and part of the activity of that low-activity region will actually spill into the high-activity structure. This results in a mixture of counts coming from different regions in a given voxel. The sampling effect, also called tissue fraction effect, has the same consequence. Because the voxel edges do not exactly correspond to edges of physiological structures, many voxels in a SPECT image actually contain activity from several tissue types. The net result is that a voxel signal does not purely reflect the activity in a tissue type but rather is composed of a mixture

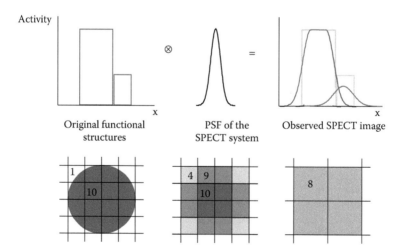

Figure 7.6 Illustration of partial volume effect. Top: Effect of the blur introduced by the PSF of a SPECT imaging system. The blue structure spills in the red one, and conversely. Because the red structure is small in size with respect to the width of the PSF of the SPECT imaging system, the activity level in that red structure is underestimated (height of the solid red curve less than the height of the light red rectangular object). Bottom: Effect of voxel sampling, also known as tissue fraction effect. When a voxel includes two tissue types (left: dark blue with an activity concentration of 10 and white with an activity concentration of 1), the voxel value is a weighted average of the activity in each tissue (central picture). If a given tissue (dark blue) is always present with other tissues in a voxel, then the activity in that tissue cannot be easily recovered (bottom right).

of activity coming from different adjacent structures. Assuming a high-activity compartment A (dark blue in Figure 7.6) in a low-activity surrounding compartment B (white in Figure 7.6), part of the activity of A will be detected outside A, due to both the limited spatial resolution and the tissue fraction effect; hence, the activity of A will be underestimated. The combination of limited spatial resolution and the tissue fraction effect introduces quantitative bias and a loss of contrast in the images.

The severity of the partial volume effect in SPECT highly depends on the size of the structure of interest, the contrast between compartments, the spatial resolution in the SPECT image, and the voxel size. All actions that enhance spatial resolution reduce the severity of the partial volume effect. As a rule of thumb, it can be remembered that the partial volume effect introduces biases in activity measurements of a compartment of interest when the smallest dimension of that compartment is less than three times the FWHM of the PSF in the reconstructed images. The partial volume effect can thus often be neglected in large organs with relatively uniform activity distribution, such as the healthy liver, as soon as measurements are performed in regions that do not encompass the edges of the organs. The partial volume effect is prominent in small compartments, such as the striata in brain imaging, the myocardial wall in cardiac imaging, and small lesions (tumors, nodes, and small metastases) in oncology.

A first approach that can be used to reduce partial volume is to enhance the spatial resolution of the reconstructed images using deconvolution. Iterative deconvolution can be performed, for instance, using the Van Cittert algorithm (Van Cittert 1931) or the Lucy–Richardson algorithm (Zeng et al. 2011). In these approaches, the reconstructed SPECT image X is modeled as the convolution of the unblurred image I with the 3D PSF F of the imaging system, where $\otimes$ denotes the 3D convolution operator:

$$X = I \otimes F \tag{7.8}$$

The Van Cittert deconvolution procedure consists in estimating I iteratively using

$$I^{(n)} = I^{(n-1)} + \alpha\left(X - I^{(n-1)} \otimes F\right) \tag{7.9}$$

where $I^{(n)}$ is the nth estimate of I, $I^{(0)}$ is estimated by X, and a is a parameter of order 1 that impacts the convergence rate.

Deconvolution is not a partial volume correction per se because the noise present in image X is amplified and prevents from achieving a complete recovery of the unblurred image I. Still, by enhancing the spatial resolution in the reconstructed images, deconvolution helps in reducing the bias introduced by the partial volume effect.

There is no simple solution to partial volume, and many compensation methods have been proposed (see Erlandsson et al. 2012 for a review). A simple approach consists in using recovery coefficients (RCs), that is, multiplying the measured value by the inverse of a scalar RC to restore the value that would have been measured if there were no partial volume effect. The RC is defined as the ratio of the measured activity to the true activity. The RC depends on the size and shape of the structure of interest, the contrast between the structure of interest and the surrounding structure(s), the local spatial resolution in the images, and the voxel size. They can be tabulated or calculated specifically given the size and shape of the structure of interest and the contrast. In situations in which the activity map can be described as piecewise constant, RC accounting for the shape of the structure of interest and contrast significantly improves the quantification accuracy (e.g., Soret et al. 2006). In intricate activity distribution patterns, though, the RC approach is usually not sufficient.

A more sophisticated partial volume correction approach consists in describing the image by a limited number C of compartments in which the activity is supposed to be constant. Assuming the PSF is known, the spill-in and spill-out between each compartment and the others can be calculated and stored in a $C \times C$ matrix called a geometric transfer matrix (GTM) (Rousset et al. 1998). Then, the measured values in the different compartments can be expressed as a vector equal to the product of the GTM matrix, with a vector composed of the unknown true uptake values in each compartment. An inversion of this matrix system gives the unknown true uptake value in each compartment. This approach is easy to implement and has been quite popular for brain imaging, where it is reasonable to describe the brain activity distribution as a piecewise constant 3D function. Its applicability to more complex activity distributions requires the extension of the method so that each voxel is seen as a compartment by itself. The corresponding method is known as the Müller-Gärtner method (Müller-Gärtner et al. 1992). In this method, one compartment is seen as a target compartment in which activity is estimated on a voxel-by-voxel basis, while the other neighboring compartments are used to determine the spill-in and spill-out activities affecting the target compartment.

Many other approaches for partial volume correction have been described (Erlandsson et al. 2012). However, while PSF modeling within the reconstruction is now available on all modern gamma cameras, thus reducing the severity of partial volume effects, subsequent partial volume correction is not offered yet and has not been broadly evaluated in clinical routine. Still, in small regions, any partial volume correction improves the quantitative accuracy with which activity is measured, as the initial biases caused by partial volume are often large. Making partial volume correction widely available is now necessary to encourage a more systematic quantitative interpretation of SPECT images.

7.7 MOTION

SPECT acquisitions usually lasts more than 10 min. The data can therefore be affected by both involuntary and physiological periodic motions, which can bias subsequent quantitative measurements. In particular, if motions occur during the SPECT acquisition, they will create inconsistent projection data; that is, all the projections will not represent a view of the same scene, making the reconstructed image a mixture of various activity distributions seen during the acquisition. Motion usually causes blur in the SPECT images. If a region with high tracer uptake is affected by motion, its spatial extent will be overestimated, while its activity concentration will be underestimated, as the real activity will be distributed over a larger region.

Involuntary motions can be limited in brain imaging by using a fixation device to maintain the brain in a fixed position, and this is still the most frequent method used to reduce motion in brain SPECT studies, although brain motion detection and correction methods have been developed (Kyme et al. 2003). In other body parts, involuntary motion is limited by appropriate fixation and is not explicitly taken care of.

Physiological periodic motions mostly include breathing and cardiac motions. Both can be monitored so as to "freeze" motion using gating. Gating sorts the acquired events in different "frames" as a function of their arrival time upon the detector with respect to a periodic physiological signal describing motion. This signal is the electrocardiogram of the subject for cardiac motion, and can be provided by various external devices, such as a pneumatic belt for respiratory motion. A period of the physiological signal is split into G gates. During the first period, each of the G images corresponding to the G gates is created and populated, and during the following periods, these G images are updated by new events (Figure 7.7). As a result, the frame corresponding to a single gate is less affected by motion than the image recorded during the whole cycle.

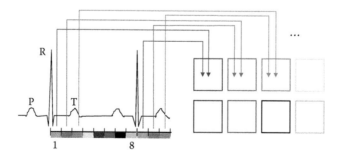

Figure 7.7 Illustration of electrocardiogram (ECG) gating. The ECG is recorded during the SPECT acquisition and divided into a number of frames, called gates. Here, $G = 8$ gates are used. For each cycle, the events detected during the first gate populate the first image of the gated image series, the events detected during the second gate populate the second image, and so on. At the end of the acquisition, each image g of the gated image series is the sum of all events detected during the gth portion of the cycles. The same principle applies to respiratory gating where the ECG signal is replaced by a respiratory signal.

Cardiac gating is routinely used in myocardial SPECT scans and in blood pool SPECT, not only for motion compensation purposes but also mostly because it allows for the characterization of the myocardial mechanical function. No motion correction is thus performed, but the analysis of separated gates allows the observer to actually analyze myocardial motion and wall thickening in myocardial SPECT or to calculate the ejection fraction in blood pool SPECT, which are all of first importance for patient management. The separate analysis of the different cardiac gated images makes it possible to study the tracer myocardial uptake without the confounding effect of motion. Respiratory gating is not yet used in SPECT. However, some methods of respiratory motion correction based on respiratory gating that have been developed for PET (Pépin et al. 2014) are also effective in SPECT (Bitarafan-Rajabi et al. 2015; Smyczynski et al. 2016). Note that even double cardiac and respiratory gating is feasible in PET (Slomka et al. 2015), and could ultimately be used in SPECT if applications would benefit from it. Unlike cardiac gating, a limitation of respiratory gating is caused by irregular breathing, even in healthy subjects, that complicates effective and robust gating over all respiratory cycles. Also, gated SPECT acquisitions should ideally benefit from a gated attenuation map, so that each volume corresponding to a specific gate is corrected with a perfectly aligned attenuation map acquired at the same respiratory or cardiac position. Given that gated CT increases the dose delivered to the patient, the application of respiratory gating has not found its way to the clinics.

7.8 MEASUREMENT

Quantitative SPECT images are expressed in kBq cm^{-3} and the conversion of the reconstructed signal (often seen as a number of counts in SPECT) into activity concentration requires a calibration procedure that determines the sensitivity of the imaging system and, ideally, a reconstruction-dependent constant (IAEA 2014). This procedure consists in performing a planar acquisition of a point source with known activity and measuring the total number of counts in the image of that source to determine the sensitivity of the camera. An additional acquisition involving a phantom mimicking the patient features of interest (e.g., a cardiac phantom or a liver phantom) should also be performed using the exact same acquisition and quantification protocol as the one used for patients so that a factor accounting for the reconstruction and correction algorithms can be determined by comparing the activity concentration set in the regions of interest of the phantom and the signal measured in the reconstructed images. A calibration factor Q expressed in cps kBq^{-1} is derived. To facilitate quantitative interpretation of the SPECT images, a convenient approach is to convert images expressed in kBq cm^{-3} into standardized uptake value (SUV) images, by dividing the measured activity concentration $I(i)$ in each voxel i of the image by the injected activity (Act) normalized by the patient weight expressed in grams:

$$SUV(i) = I(i)\left(\text{kBq cm}^{-3}\right) * m(g)\Big/Act(\text{kBq}) \tag{7.10}$$

Assuming the patient density is that of water (1 g cm^{-3}), SUVs are then dimensionless and offer a practical way to compare tracer uptake between patients even when the injected activity and the body size strongly differ. Another advantage of SUV is that if the tracer is distributed uniformly throughout the patient, then the SUV would be equal to 1 in each and every voxel.

Even with an adequate calibration procedure, the reliability of a measurement made from a SPECT image actually depends on how this measurement is performed. As an example, if one is interested in estimating the liver activity, several approaches can be used. The most intuitive method is to draw a volume of interest in the liver and calculate the average uptake in that region. The accuracy and variability of the measurement will actually depend on the way the region is drawn and on which index is calculated within that region. Regarding the region drawing, a critical aspect is whether the edges of the organ of interest are included in the region. Indeed, SPECT images are blurred, and an accurate delineation of organ borders is impossible. The CT overlaid over the SPECT image as available when using SPECT/CT scanners facilitates organ delineation, but this approach implicitly assumes that the contours of the anatomical region as reflected by the CT image correspond to the contours of the tracer uptake in the SPECT image, which is not necessarily true. In addition, organ edges in the SPECT images are affected by spill-in and spill-out because of the partial volume effect; hence, the edge region is prone to biased activity estimates. For large organs with relatively homogeneous uptake, it is thus preferable to exclude the borders from the region to get a more robust estimate of the average uptake in the region. For small organs, such as metastases, nodes, and spleen, that are usually strongly affected by the partial volume effect, contours might be difficult to delineate, even using the overlaid CT. Measures other than the average uptake might thus be preferred, such as the maximum uptake over the region of interest, which has the advantage not to depend highly on the contours that have been drawn. In practice, the reproducibility of a SPECT measurement is often more important than its accuracy. The reproducibility of a quantification protocol intended to guide patient management should ideally be characterized using what is known as a test–retest procedure, involving repeating the same measurement from two different scans performed within a short period of time so that the patient can be assumed to be in the exact same pathophysiological state (Tavares et al. 2013). The comparison of the quantitative results from the two measurements then gives a good indication regarding the reproducibility of the quantification procedure, and hence its reliability.

7.9 OVERALL QUANTITATIVE ACCURACY ACHIEVABLE IN SPECT IMAGING

As described before, many phenomena impact the reliability of a measurement made from SPECT images. One can thus wonder which corrections are crucial, and what to expect as far as quantitative accuracy is concerned in a given setting. Whatever the setting, a first short answer is that attenuation correction should always be performed. Accurate attenuation correction is now widely available thanks to the large availability of SPECT/CT scanners and is a prerequisite for accurate quantification. A more complete answer depends on the size of the structure of interest in which uptake is to be estimated from the SPECT images. One can distinguish two cases: For functional structures whose smallest dimensions exceed 3 cm and that have a relatively uniform tracer uptake, the second most important correction to be applied is scatter correction. The combination of attenuation and scatter corrections ensures sound activity concentration estimates in large regions. For smaller structures, such as the striata in brain studies, the myocardial wall in cardiac scans, or bone lesions, the second most important correction after attenuation correction is partial volume correction. The images should first be reconstructed using a compensation for the detector response function so as to enhance the spatial resolution and reduce the biases due to the partial volume effect, and ideally a partial volume correction should be subsequently applied. In small structures, the importance of scatter correction is often less than that of partial volume correction, but activity recovery within 10% requires both on top of attenuation correction. Motion correction is still sort of a luxury in SPECT and would become useful if all the other phenomena were first properly handled.

In the clinics, compensations for attenuation, scatter, and detector response are now available in most modern cameras. The advent of SPECT/CT has been a decisive step toward quantitative SPECT, by considerably facilitating the implementation of attenuation correction. The principle of accurate attenuation correction in SPECT does not require the availability of a SPECT/CT scanner, but the CT provides a fast and convenient means to measure the attenuation coefficient maps required for accurate attenuation correction. Vendors are also now supplying software implementing scatter and detector response corrections on top of attenuation correction, offering the user all needed tools to interpret SPECT images quantitatively. Still, the reliability of an imaging protocol intended to produce quantitative values used for scan interpretation should always be assessed using phantoms first, and possibly using test–retest protocols. The use of phantoms is especially recommended to understand the accuracy of the measurements and their sensitivity to various parameters involved in the corrections or image reconstruction.

Using highly realistic simulations and phantom experiments, many studies have shown that SPECT can yield highly accurate uptake quantification, with errors less than 10%, at least using ^{99m}Tc-labeled tracers, but also using radionuclides with more complicated decay schemes (Bailey and Willowson 2013; van Gils et al. 2016). All these studies involved optimized imaging and quantification protocols, using well-tuned corrections and reconstructions, demonstrating that accurate SPECT quantification is achievable but needs sophisticated procedures. Vendors have made tremendous efforts over the past years to make accurate quantification available for clinical routine applications. It is likely that these efforts will continue in the coming years and, as a result, that the quantitative interpretation of SPECT images will become more and more widespread.

7.10 CONCLUSION

The availability of SPECT/CT scanners has immensely contributed to making SPECT a quantitative imaging modality with accuracy now similar to that achieved in PET. Because SPECT still suffers from poorer spatial resolution and sensitivity compared with PET, sophisticated approaches have to be used to get quantitatively accurate SPECT images. Such approaches have been described in the literature, and most of them can now be implemented on patient data using vendor software. These recent advances in SPECT quantification should greatly serve applications for which quantification is a prerequisite, such as imaging-based dosimetry and patient monitoring. Brain, cardiac, and cancer imaging can all benefit from a more accurate quantitative accuracy in the images, especially using advanced image analyses such as performed in cardiac SPECT or brain SPECT that use the SPECT activity map estimate as input.

REFERENCES

Bailey DL, Willowson KP. An evidence-based review of quantitative SPECT imaging and potential clinical applications. *J Nucl Med* 54:83–89, 2013.

Beekman FJ, de Jong HW, Slijpen ET. Efficient SPECT scatter calculation in non-uniform media using correlated Monte Carlo simulation. *Phys Med Biol* 44:N183–N192, 1999.

Bitarafan-Rajabi A, Rajabi H, Rastgou F, Firoozabady H, Yaghoobi N, Malek H, Langesteger W, Beheshti M. Influence of respiratory motion correction on quantification of myocardial perfusion SPECT. *J Nucl Cardiol* 22:1019–1030, 2015.

Buvat I, Benali H, Todd-Pokropek A, Di Paola R. Scatter correction in scintigraphy: The state of the art. *Eur J Nucl Med* 21:675–694, 1994.

Dewaraja YK, Ljungberg M, Koral KF. Accuracy of 131I tumor quantification in radioimmunotherapy using SPECT imaging with an ultra-high-energy collimator: Monte Carlo study. *J Nucl Med* 41:1760–1767, 2000.

Dobbeleir AA, Hambÿe AS, Franken PR. Influence of high-energy photons on the spectrum of iodine-123 with low- and medium-energy collimators: Consequences for imaging with 123I-labelled compounds in clinical practice. *Eur J Nucl Med* 26:655–658, 1999.

El Fakhri G, Buvat I, Pélégrini M, Benali H, Almeida P, Bendriem B, Todd-Pokropek A, Di Paola R. Respective roles of scatter, attenuation, depth-dependent collimator response and finite spatial resolution in cardiac SPECT quantitation: A Monte Carlo study. *Eur J Nucl Med* 26:437–446, 1999.

Erlandsson K, Buvat I, Pretoruis PH, Thomas BA, Hutton BF. A review of partial volume correction techniques for emission tomography and their applications in neurology, cardiology and oncology. *Phys Med Biol* 57:R119–R159, 2012.

Fricke H, Fricke E, Weise R, Kammeier A, Lindner O, Burchert W. A method to remove artifacts in attenuation-corrected myocardial perfusion SPECT introduced by misalignment between emission scan and CT-derived attenuation maps. *J Nucl Med* 45:1619–1625, 2004.

Hashimoto J, Kubo A, Ogawa K, Amano T, Fukuuchi Y, Motomura N, Ichihara T. Scatter and attenuation correction in technetium-99m brain SPECT. *J Nucl Med* 38:157–162, 1997.

Hutton B, Buvat I, Beekman F. Review and current status of SPECT scatter correction. *Phys Med Biol* 56: R85–R112, 2011.

IAEA [International Atomic Energy Agency]. *Quantitative Nuclear Medicine Imaging: Concepts, Requirements, and Methods.* IAEA Human Health Reports No. 9. Vienna: IAEA, 2014.

Ichihara T, Ogawa K, Motomura N, Kubo A, Hashimoto S. Compton scatter compensation using the triple-energy window method for single- and dual-isotope SPECT. *J Nucl Med* 34:2216–2221, 1993.

Jaszczak RJ, Greer KL, Floyd CE Jr, Harris CC, Coleman RE. Improved SPECT quantification using compensation for scattered photons. *J Nucl Med* 25:893–900, 1984.

Kappadath SC. Effects of voxel size and iterative reconstruction parameters on the spatial resolution of 99mTc SPECT/CT. *J Appl Clin Med Phys* 12:3459, 2011.

Kyme AZ, Hutton BF, Hatton RL, Skerrett DW, Barnden LR. Practical aspects of a data-driven motion correction approach for brain SPECT. *IEEE Trans Med Imaging* 22:722–729, 2003.

Müller-Gärtner HW, Links JM, Prince JL, Bryan RN, McVeigh E, Leal JP, Davatzikos C, Frost JJ. Measurement of radiotracer concentration in brain gray matter using positron emission tomography: MRI-based correction for partial volume effects. *J Cereb Blood Flow Metab* 12:571–583, 1992.

Pépin A, Daouk J, Bailly P, Hapdey S, Meyer ME. Management of respiratory motion in PET/computed tomography: The state of the art. *Nucl Med Commun* 35:113–122, 2014.

Rousset OG, Ma Y, Evans AC. Correction for partial volume effects in PET: Principle and validation. *J Nucl Med* 39:904–911, 1998.

Slomka PJ, Rubeaux M, Le Meunier L, Dey D, Lazewatsky JL, Pan T, Dweck MR, Newby DE, Germano G, Berman DS. Dual-gated motion-frozen cardiac PET with flurpiridaz F 18. *J Nucl Med* 56:1876–1881, 2015.

Smyczynski MS, Gifford HC, Dey J, Lehovich A, McNamara JE, Segars WP, King MA. LROC investigation of three strategies for reducing the impact of respiratory motion on the detection of solitary pulmonary nodules in SPECT. *IEEE Trans Nucl Sci* 63:130–139, 2016.

Soret M, Koulibaly PM, Darcourt J, Buvat I. Partial volume effect correction in SPECT for striatal uptake measurements in patients with neurodegenerative diseases: Impact upon patient classification. *Eur J Nucl Med Mol Imaging* 33:1062–1072, 2006.

Soret M, Koulibaly PM, Darcourt J, Hapdey S, Buvat I. Quantitative accuracy of dopaminergic neurotransmission imaging using 123I SPECT. *J Nucl Med* 44:1184–1193, 2003.

Stute S, Comtat C. Practical considerations for image-based PSF and blobs reconstruction in PET. *Phys Med Biol* 58:3849–3870, 2013.

Tavares AA, Batis JC, Papin C, Jennings D, Alagille D, Russell DS, Vala C, et al. Kinetic modeling, test-retest, and dosimetry of 123I-MNI-420 in humans. *J Nucl Med* 54:1760–1767, 2013.

Van Cittert PH. The effect of slit width on the intensity distribution of spectral lines II [in German]. *Z Phys A* 69:298–308, 1931.

van Gils CA, Beijst C, van Rooij R, de Jong HW. Impact of reconstruction parameters on quantitative I-131 SPECT. *Phys Med Biol* 61:5166–5182, 2016.

Zaidi H, Hasegawa B. Determination of the attenuation map in emission tomography. *J Nucl Med* 44:291–315, 2003.

Zeng GL. Gibbs artifact reduction by nonnegativity constraint. *J Nucl Med Technol* 39:213–219, 2011.

Data corrections and quantitative PET

SULEMAN SURTI AND JOSHUA SCHEUERMANN

8.1	Calibrations for improved quality of collected data	211
	8.1.1 Energy calibration	211
	8.1.2 Timing calibration	212
8.2	Corrections for accurate image reconstruction	214
	8.2.1 Attenuation correction	214
	8.2.2 Scatter correction	219
	8.2.3 Randoms correction	224
	8.2.4 Dead-time correction	226
	8.2.5 Normalization	228
8.3	Calibration of reconstructed image to emission activity level	231
8.4	Summary	231
References		232

PET imaging is regarded as a quantitative imaging modality that provides an accurate measure of physiological function within a patient. However, several physical effects, as well as data collection procedures, can lead to bias and artifacts in the reconstructed image. Corrections to PET data are therefore needed for an accurate clinical interpretation of the patient image, as well as to obtain physiological information from the static (e.g., standardized uptake value [SUV]) or dynamic (kinetic modeling) image. Corrections to PET data can be broadly split into three categories depending on where in the data acquisition and image generation chain the correction is applied. The three categories are (1) calibrations at the detector level, which affect the quality of collected events; (2) corrections as part of image reconstruction, which remove or reduce bias or nonuniformities in the image; and (3) calibrations after image reconstruction, which allow for measuring activity levels in the patient.

8.1 CALIBRATIONS FOR IMPROVED QUALITY OF COLLECTED DATA

Data calibrations for collected events can require hardware solutions, as well as software lookup tables, that help improve the intrinsic quality of the coincident events that are used for reconstructing the PET image.

8.1.1 ENERGY CALIBRATION

To obtain good and uniform system energy resolution in a PET scanner, corrections need to be made for variations in the measured signal for a fixed amount of deposited energy. For a fixed amount of energy deposition in a crystal by an annihilation photon, there are three primary sources of variation in the signal measured from a single photomultiplier tube (PMT) or a group of PMTs comprising a detector in a PET scanner: differences in the gains of individual PMTs, differences in the light output of individual crystals, and finally, differences in the number of scintillation photons detected in a PET detector due to the relative position of individual crystals in the detector. As shown by Cherry et al. (1995), the variation in the total number of collected photons can be as high as a factor of three between center and edge crystals in a block detector. All three of these factors lead to a significant degradation in measured system energy resolution, requiring the use of a wide energy gate for collected events and, consequently, leading to an increase in the relative number of scattered coincidences in the collected data. Differences in PMT gain factors can also lead to distortions in the measured interaction position, and hence a degradation in the system spatial resolution.

The PMT gains are typically measured before their incorporation in the PET detector and can be adjusted either by adjusting preamplifier outputs or by saving the gain values in a calibration table for use during energy and position calculations. To correct for the systematic variation in collected light due to crystal light output or crystal position within a detector, calibration data are typically acquired with either a point source (^{68}Ge or ^{22}Na) or a uniform cylinder placed at the center of the scanner. Position gates are applied for events within individual crystals to measure the energy spectra for interactions within each crystal. Scale factors (or energy calibration factors) that align energy photopeak for all crystals at a fixed, predefined value can then be determined and stored in a lookup table. For each detected event during patient imaging, the measured energy for an interaction in a given crystal is then corrected using this energy calibration factor. In Figure 8.1a and b, we show energy centroid flood maps over a portion of a full scanner before and after energy calibrations, respectively. The variation in measured energy is <20% between a crystal near a PMT center and a crystal near the PMT edge. The system energy resolution improves from 28% to 18% after energy calibrations, as shown in Figure 8.1c.

8.1.2 Timing calibration

Just as in the case of energy resolution, good and uniform system timing resolution is obtained after correction for several effects that can affect the measurement of signal arrival times: variations in PMT transit times, differences in crystal scintillation behavior, electronics effects such as pulse amplification and signal delay, and variations in the path length of scintillation photons before they reach a PMT photocathode, which is a function of the interaction crystal position within the detector. All these factors lead to degradation in the system coincidence timing resolution by adding a bias in the measured signal arrival time, which adversely affects the time-of-flight (TOF) imaging capability of a PET scanner. Even in a non-TOF PET scanner, the degraded timing resolution will require the use of a wider coincidence timing window to collect all true coincidences, which in turn increases the relative number of random coincidences collected during data acquisition. Hence, timing calibration is needed to maintain good and uniform system timing resolution in a PET scanner.

Individual PMT transit times can be adjusted in hardware by making changes in the supplied high voltage for the different dynode stages of a PMT. However, quite often PMT dynode high-voltage adjustments will also impact the PMT gain, and therefore significant care is needed when making these corrections (Liu et al., 2004; Davidson et al., 2011). Several techniques can be used to perform timing calibrations that correct for variations or bias in signal arrival times from each crystal. The simplest technique is to place a point source at the center of the scanner and measure the TOF histogram for all possible lines of response (LORs). An alignment of the centers of each TOF histogram to a common value (zero for a centered point source) produces a timing calibration table for all possible LORs. Due to a very high number of LORs in a clinical scanner and the need to acquire data in coincidence, this procedure requires a very long data acquisition time. Hence, iterative algorithms have been developed to reduce the amount of data needed. In these methods, an assumption is made that the absolute time biases for all crystals are independent, and hence, the measured TOF bias for an LOR formed by any two crystals is simply the difference in the absolute time biases of the two crystals. With this assumption, there is no longer a requirement that each crystal be measured in coincidence with every other crystal, and instead, each crystal can be measured in coincidence with a larger group of crystals in the opposing detector. This reduces the need for a very long data acquisition time. For each crystal, A, in

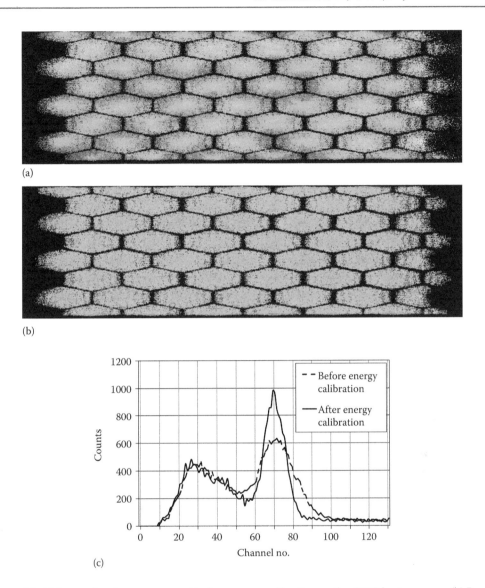

(a)

(b)

(c)

Figure 8.1 (a) Energy flood map measured before energy calibration on the GPET brain scanner. (b) Energy flood map measured after energy calibration on the GPET brain scanner. (c) System energy spectrum measured on the GPET scanner before and after energy calibration. After energy calibration, the system energy resolution is 18%. (These figures were originally published in Karp, et al., *J. Nucl. Med.*, 44, 1340–1349, 2003. Copyright by the Society of Nuclear Medicine and Molecular Imaging, Inc. All rights reserved.)

coincidence with a group of crystals on the opposing detector side, a TOF offset histogram is generated using these coincident LORs and calculating the measured versus true TOF difference for each LOR. The TOF bias for crystal A is then estimated as the mean or peak location of this offset histogram. This process can be repeated iteratively where the bias for each crystal A is estimated iteratively using $bias_{i+1} = bias_i - \lambda^*$peak location, where λ is a relaxation parameter and the initial estimate of bias is zero for all crystals. The process is iterated until the TOF offset histograms for all crystals are centered around zero, and the crystal bias (crystal timing offset) values are saved as a timing offset calibration table that can be used in real time or offline during patient imaging. In Figure 8.2a, we show timing offset flood maps over a portion of a full scanner before timing offset calibrations. The major source of bias in the timing offsets shown here is the difference in timing at the PMT level, as can be seen from the structure in the timing offset map. Figure 8.2b shows timing resolution flood maps over a portion of a full scanner after timing calibrations, which is fairly uniform and has a

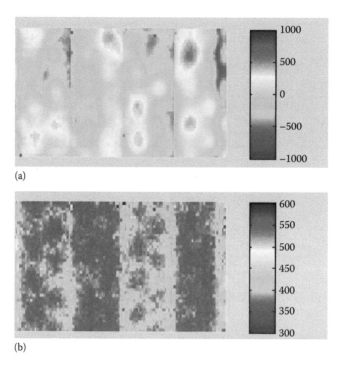

(a)

(b)

Figure 8.2 (a) Timing offset map for a portion of the LaPET scanner showing an offset range of ±1 ns. The major source of the timing variation is due to the difference in the transit times of individual PMTs that have not been adjusted in hardware. (b) Timing resolution map for a portion of the LaPET scanner shown after a software-based crystal-by-crystal timing calibration has been performed. Very small variations are observed in the timing resolution with a system timing resolution of 375 ps. (These figures were originally published in Daube-Witherspoon, M. E., et al., *Phys. Med. Biol.*, 55, 45–64, 2010. Copyright Institute of Physics and Engineering in Medicine, published on behalf of IPEM by IOP Publishing Ltd. All rights reserved.)

system timing resolution of 375 ps. Data for timing calibration are typically acquired with a simple source, such as a uniform phantom, rotating point, or line source, or by placing a small ^{22}Na source in a small brass block at the center of the scanner, where the real TOF difference is easily known. However, as shown recently (Werner and Karp, 2013), any data, including patient data, can be used with this technique since a non-TOF reconstructed image can be used to obtain a good estimate of the true TOF difference along a given LOR. In this case, the TOF offset or bias of crystal A is estimated as the value that maximizes the cross-correlation between the true and measured TOF differences for all LORs formed between crystal A and a small group of crystals in the opposing detector. Once again, this process can be performed iteratively to achieve a stable estimate for all crystal timing offsets.

8.2 CORRECTIONS FOR ACCURATE IMAGE RECONSTRUCTION

The events collected during a PET scan are affected by several physical factors that add some form of bias or nonuniformity to the reconstructed image. Corrections for these effects can be patient specific, scanner specific, or just imaging protocol specific.

8.2.1 ATTENUATION CORRECTION

In PET imaging, where the signal (positron annihilation followed by emission of coincident annihilation photons) is generated within the patient, animal, or object being imaged, there is a high probability for one or both of the annihilation photons to be absorbed or scattered away from the true coincident path that passes

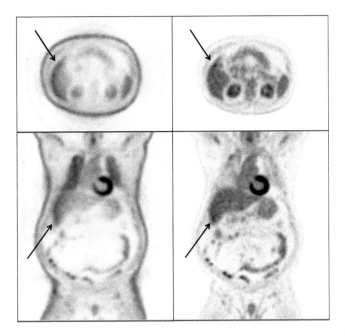

Figure 8.3 Transverse (top row) and coronal (bottom row) slices of an ^{18}F-F-FDG image of a patient without (left column) and with (right column) attenuation correction. The arrows point to a small lesion in the liver that is difficult to see in the image without attenuation correction, but is more apparent in the attenuation-corrected image. (Images acquired courtesy of the Hospital of the University of Pennsylvania PET Center.)

through the positron annihilation point. Physically, the probability of interaction for photons is a function of the photon energy (511 keV in PET), object size, and object composition (or atomic number) along the photon path. In brain imaging, where the head size is in the range of 25 cm, as many as half the coincident events will be lost or attenuated, while in whole-body imaging the attenuation factor can increase to as high 90% depending on the patient size. Since photon interaction probability is also a function of the material composition through which the photon travels, the attenuation effects will be nonuniform over all LORs, and if left uncorrected, will lead to nonuniformities in the reconstructed image. Figure 8.3 shows an ^{18}F-FDG patient study reconstructed without and with attenuation correction. Without attenuation correction, the liver uptake looks very nonuniform, with the lateral portion having much higher uptake than the central portion, while the lungs appear to have high uptake. Attenuation correction removes the liver nonuniformities and reduces the amount of uptake seen in the lungs, making the measured uptake more accurate in the different regions. In addition, a small lesion near the bottom of the liver is more easily visible in the attenuation-corrected image. Figure 8.4 is another ^{18}F-FDG patient study reconstructed without and with attenuation correction. After attenuation correction, a lesion in a vertebral body is observed that is not visible in the image without attenuation correction.

For attenuation correction, we make use of the fact that an event in PET represents the detection of two coincident events emitted back to back. In Figure 8.5, we show a schematic of a PET scanner where the two annihilation photons travel distances d_1 and d_2 through the patient before reaching the PET detector. The probability for detecting both of these photons will be a product of their individual transmission probabilities:

$$P = e^{-\mu d_1} e^{-\mu d_2} = e^{-\mu(d_1+d_2)} = e^{-\mu D}$$

where μ is the linear attenuation coefficient of the object being imaged and D is the total path length $(d_1 + d_2)$ through the object for the two photons. The total transmission probability is therefore independent of the emission point along the LOR, and depends only on the total path length D for the LOR. Hence, the transmission probability or, alternately, the attenuation correction factor (ACF) can be measured for every LOR by

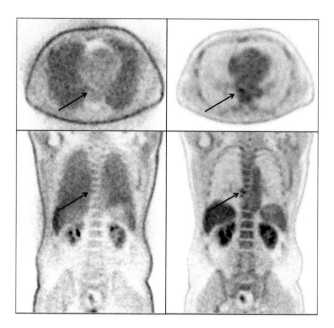

Figure 8.4 Transverse (top row) and coronal (bottom row) slices of an ^{18}F-F-FDG image of a patient without (left column) and with (right column) attenuation correction. The arrows point to a lesion in a vertebral body that is difficult to see in the non-attenuation corrected (NAC) image. (Images acquired courtesy of the Hospital of the University of Pennsylvania PET Center.)

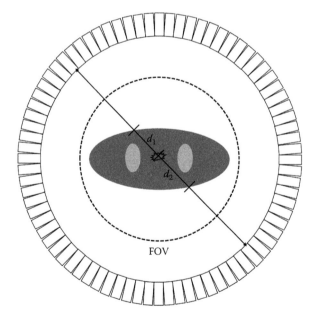

Figure 8.5 Path length for two 511 keV photons emitted from the same annihilation event. The two photons travel distances d_1 and d_2 within the patient.

using a source placed externally to the patient or object and collecting transmission data. Transmission scans should acquire data fast compared with emission scans, be accurate, and acquire a high number of counts in order to reduce noise propagation in image reconstruction.

Before the advent of PET–computed tomography (CT), dedicated PET scanners used an external radioactive source to acquire transmission data. The most common transmission imaging technique used in dedicated

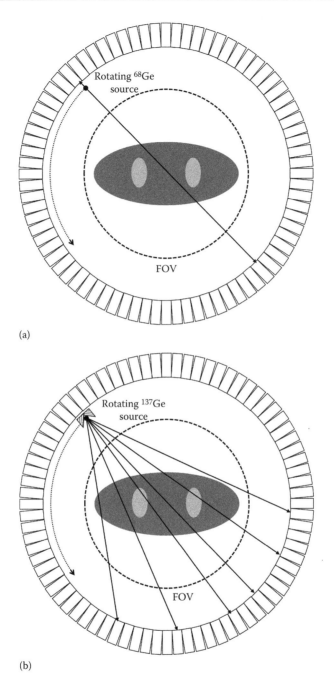

Figure 8.6 (a) Rotating ^{68}Ge point or rod source collecting coincidence transmission data. (b) Rotating, collimated ^{137}Cs point source collecting transmission data in singles mode.

PET scanners used a rotating, β^+-emitting, ^{68}Ge point or rod source (Carroll et al., 1983) (Figure 8.6a). In this technique, data are acquired in coincidence between a detector close to the transmission source and another on the opposite side of the ring. Knowledge of the source location together with the end points of the LOR formed between the two coincident detectors provides a constraint where all three of these points need to lie on a straight line. One benefit of this constraint is that it allows one to perform a transmission scan in the presence of emission activity (postinjection scan) in the patient without data corruption, greatly reducing the amount of time a patient spends on the scanner bed (Daube-Witherspoon et al., 1988; Carson et al.,

1989). In addition, the constraint that the source position and end points of the LOR lie on a straight line also provides the ability to reject scattered events in the transmission data, and hence improves the accuracy of the transmission scan. To acquire a high number of counts in a short duration, a high-activity source is needed, which, however, can lead to significant dead time in the detector nearest to the source. A solution to this problem has been the use of two or three lower-activity rotating sources simultaneously to acquire the transmission data. Another solution is the use of a rotating, collimated ^{68}Ge source attached to a small, dedicated detector (Watson et al., 2001). Coincidences are measured between the dedicated detector and a PET detector on the opposite side of the scanner ring. With this approach, it has also been shown that transmission data can be collected simultaneously with the emission scan. A recent variation on this concept of simultaneous emission and transmission imaging has been the use of a β^+-emitting ring source placed within the scanner detector ring, but beyond the transverse imaging field of view (FOV) (Mollet et al., 2012). Knowledge of the transmission ring location, together with the good TOF information obtained from the current generation of PET scanners, makes it possible to separate the collected coincident events into emission and transmission data. The accuracy of this separation will, however, depend on the coincidence timing resolution achieved in the TOF scanners.

An alternative technique for performing fast postinjection transmission scans is to acquire data in singles acquisition mode with a rotating, shielded point source (Figure 8.6b) (deKemp and Nahmias, 1994). The interaction point of the single photon on the opposing side of PET detectors, together with knowledge of the source position, defines individual LORs. In order to perform postinjection transmission scans, a single-photon emission source such as ^{137}Cs (662 keV photons) (Karp et al., 1995; Smith et al., 1997) can also be used, with the scanner energy resolution allowing a discrimination between the 662 keV transmission photons and the 511 keV annihilation photons from emission activity within the patient. An advantage of this technique over the coincidence transmission imaging is that a much higher-activity source can be used, and with proper shielding any concerns for dead time in a detector very close to the source are reduced. ACFs in both coincidence and singles-based transmission imaging are directly measured by taking the natural logarithm of the ratio between data obtained using the transmission source, with and without the patient in the scanner. With the ^{137}Cs technique, the directly measured ACFs are for 662 keV photons and scaling is necessary to obtain the correct ACFs for the 511 keV photons detected in emission data. Alternately, image segmentation can first be used to partition the transmission image into a few well-defined regions. After image segmentation, the correct 511 keV ACFs for each region can then be uniformly assigned (Smith et al., 1997). Coincident ^{68}Ge transmission scans with rotating sources are typically acquired for 15–30 min per bed position, and due to dead-time issues, the collected data are noisy. However, the emission and transmission scans are acquired at the same energy, and so there is a very low bias in the estimated ACFs. With the singles-based ^{137}Cs source, transmission scans are 5–10 min long and less noisy, but there is some bias in the measured ACF due to the difference in energies of the emission and transmission photons.

With the advent of PET/CT scanners, there has been a shift away from dedicated transmission imaging to using the CT image for estimating the PET ACFs (Alessio et al., 2004). CT scans are acquired with x-ray photons in the energy range of 30–130 keV, and so any ACFs obtained from a CT image need to be scaled for the 511 keV emission photons. However, while Compton scatter dominates as the primary interaction of 511 keV photons within a patient, for the x-ray photons used in CT imaging, photoelectric interactions dominate. The linear attenuation coefficient for Compton scattering is a function only of the material density, while the linear attenuation coefficient for photoelectric interactions is a function of the material density as well as its composition. Hence, a single scaling factor for the ACFs obtained from the CT image cannot be used to measure 511 keV emission photon ACFs. Instead, the CT image is first segmented into different regions based on the Hounsfield unit values. Several conversion methods have been developed, which are then used to perform appropriate scaling for the different segmented regions (lung, adipose tissue, cortical bone, etc.) within the patient (LaCroix et al., 1994; Blankespoor et al., 1996; Burger and Buck, 1996; Bai et al., 2003; Kinahan et al., 1998). CT scans are very fast (1 min or less) and have very little noise compared with the transmission scans with an external radioactive source. However, due to the need for a careful scaling of the ACFs to 511 keV photon energy, there is a potential for bias. For example, the use of a contrast agent during the CT scan can also lead to an incorrect estimate of the PET ACFs if appropriate scaling procedures are not used. The very fast CT scans can also lead to artifacts in the PET image due to differences in the respiratory pattern during the separate CT and PET data acquisitions. Finally, beam-hardening effects of the x-ray photons used for CT can also lead to bias in the PET image when using CT for estimating the ACFs. Despite some of these issues with CT-based attenuation correction, use of dedicated PET/CT where the CT image is used to estimate the PET ACFs has become a standard for clinical imaging. A more detailed discussion of this topic can be found in Chapter 13.

8.2.2 SCATTER CORRECTION

The primary interaction of 511 keV photons inside a patient is elastic scattering off an electron through Compton scatter. While undergoing this process, the 511 keV photon loses some energy and also changes its direction, as described by the equation

$$E_{scat} = \frac{E_{incident}}{1 + \frac{E_{incident}}{m_e c^2}\left(1 - \cos(\theta_{scat})\right)}$$

where $E_{incident}$ and E_{scat} are the energies of the incident and scattered photons, respectively, θ_c is the scattering angle, and $m_e c^2$ is the rest mass energy of the electron. In PET, either one or both of the coincident photons can undergo one or several Compton scatters before reaching the detectors. As shown in Figure 8.7, due to the change in direction of the photon after Compton scatter, the assigned LOR does not pass through the annihilation or emission point, thereby leading to a bias in the collected data, and consequently in the image if it is not corrected. This bias leads to a reduced contrast in the image and an incorrect estimate of activity.

In Figure 8.8, we plot simulated energy spectra showing separately the unscattered (or true events), single scattered events (where only one of the two photons undergoes a single scattering event), and multiple scatter events (which include all non-single-scatter events). From Figure 8.8a, for a 20 cm diameter cylinder and a scanner with 12% energy resolution, we see that applying a lower energy gate (LLD) at around 440 keV allows

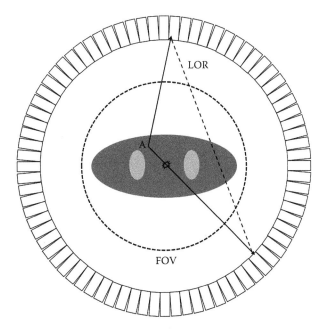

Figure 8.7 Schematic showing the emission of two coincident photons where one photon undergoes scatter at point A within the patient. The assigned LOR does not pass through the annihilation point, hence leading to a bias in the collected data.

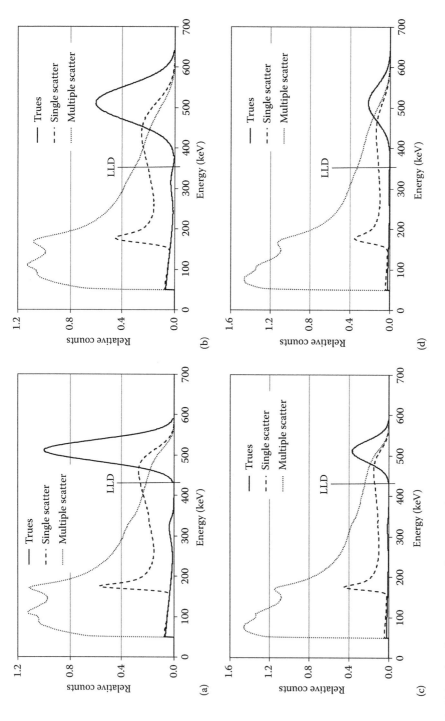

Figure 8.8 (a) Simulated energy spectra for true, single scatter, and multiple scatter 511 keV photons detected in a 20 cm diameter by 40 cm long cylinder. The LLD value sets the lower energy gate for collected events in the scanner. (b) Simulated energy spectra for true, single scatter, and multiple scatter 511 keV photons detected in a whole-body scanner with 12% energy resolution for a 20 cm diameter by 40 cm long cylinder. (c) Simulated energy spectra for true, single scatter, and multiple scatter 511 keV photons detected in a whole-body scanner with 20% energy resolution for a 20 cm diameter by 40 cm long cylinder. (d) Simulated energy spectra for true, single scatter, and multiple scatter 511 keV photons detected in a whole-body scanner with 12% energy resolution for a 35 cm diameter by 40 cm long cylinder. (d) Simulated energy spectra for true, single scatter, and multiple scatter 511 keV photons detected in a whole-body scanner with 20% energy resolution for a 35 cm diameter by 40 cm long cylinder.

for the collection of all true photopeak coincidences, together with some scattered events that are primarily single scatter events. The scatter fraction (SF), which is the ratio of all scattered coincidences to all coincidences, is 35% with a 1.5:1 split between single and multiple scatter events. Figure 8.8b shows the results for the same 20 cm diameter cylinder but in a scanner with 20% energy resolution. In order to collect all true photopeak coincidences, the energy gate now needs to be lowered to 350 keV, which increases the SF to 54% and decreases the ratio of single to multiple scatter events to 1:1. These results shows that the SF in a scanner is a strong function of the energy resolution, and most of the scattered events are of the single scatter type for a high LLD. Figure 8.8c and d shows the energy spectra, but now with a larger 35 cm diameter phantom. The SF increases to 54% and 73% for scanners with 12% and 20% energy resolution, respectively. The ratio of singles to multiple scatter events decreases to 0.7:1 and 0.6:1 for scanners with 12% and 20% energy resolution, respectively. These results show that for a larger phantom or patient size, SF increases in the scanner, leading to an even bigger need for an accurate scatter correction.

Several techniques have been developed over the years for an accurate subtraction of the scattered coincidences   from the measured data. An early technique known as the tail-fitting technique was based on the observation that for most objects the background of scattered events contributes (approximately) a broad, inverse parabolic shape to the projection data. Tail-fitting techniques (Karp et al., 1990; Cherry and Huang, 1995) use this information, together with the knowledge that any events in the sinogram that lie beyond the object boundary are scattered events, to perform a simple parabolic or Gaussian fit to events in the tails of the sinogram that lie beyond the object boundary. The advantage of tail-fitting methods lies in the simplicity of their application. However, the need to smooth noisy data in the sinogram tails before fitting, and the fact that it represents a smooth, low-frequency estimate for the scatter, makes the tail-fitting technique not sensitive to local variations in the scatter distribution and can lead to errors when imaging heterogeneous regions with varying density. In addition, in TOF PET the scatter distribution also varies in the TOF dimension and the tail-fitting technique cannot be extended beyond some simple situations to estimate this distribution.

Convolution subtraction or integral transformation techniques for scatter correction (Bailey and Meikle, 1994; Bergstrom et al., 1983; Hoverath et al., 1993; Lercher and Wienhard, 1994; Shao and Karp, 1991) estimate the scatter distribution (s) in a measurement as a convolution of the true data (t) with an *a priori* defined distribution of scatter within the scanner (h), $s = t \otimes h$. An estimate of the SF is then used to scale this scatter distribution for the measured data. Since the true coincidence data, t, is unknown, this process can be repeated iteratively using the measured data p (includes all events) as the initial guess, to obtain a stable estimate of the true coincidence data using the formula

$$t^{(n)} = p - SF \times \left(t^{(n-1)} \otimes h \right)$$

The scatter distribution, s, can be estimated as a two-dimensional (2D) function where the second dimension is the TOF domain, thereby allowing the extension of the convolution subtraction technique to TOF PET (Bendriem et al., 1986). Since the convolution subtraction technique depends on an estimate of the scatter distribution (h) acquired through measurements typically performed with point or line sources at several positions within the scanner, its accuracy can be limited in clinical situations, especially in the case of fully three-dimensional (3D) scanners with activity present outside the FOV.

A different class of techniques exists that utilizes the energy spectrum of the collected events to estimate the scatter coincidences. These techniques make use of the fact that events with deposited energy below the photopeak have a higher probability of being scattered events, while those with deposited energy above the photopeak are primarily true coincidence events. The dual energy window (DEW) technique (Adam et al., 2000) uses data from the default photopeak energy window (PEW) over which the data are collected, together with another nonoverlapping lower energy window (LEW) that lies below the default energy window (see Figure 8.9). The true events in PEW, t_{PEW}, are then estimated using

$$t_{PEW} = \frac{r_{scat} \times p_{PEW} - p_{LEW}}{r_{scat} - r_{true}}$$

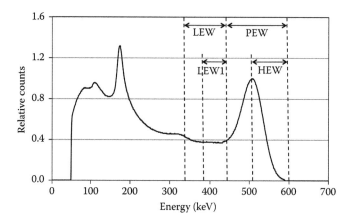

Figure 8.9 Simulated energy spectrum for all 511 keV photons detected in a whole-body scanner with 12% energy resolution for a 20 cm diameter by 40 cm long cylinder. The PEW, HEW, and lower energy windows (LEW and LEW1) are shown to illustrate the different energy windows used in the various energy-based scatter estimation algorithms.

where p_{PEW} and p_{LEW} are the total counts in the PEW and LEW, respectively, r_{scat} is the ratio of scattered events in the LEW to PEW, and r_{true} is the ratio of true events in the LEW to PEW. The r_{scat} and r_{trues} values are determined separately using point and line sources in air and water. Under the condition where $r_{scat} \gg r_{true}$, t_{PEW} is calculated as

$$t_{PEW} = p_{PEW} - \frac{p_{LEW}}{r_{scat}}$$

While the DEW was demonstrated to perform well for uniform distributions (Grootoonk et al., 1996), other work has suggested that the technique can be error-prone for more complex phantom distributions (Adam et al., 2000; Harrison et al., 1991). In addition, while the scale factors have been shown to be independent of the object size and fairly constant transaxially, the effect of phantoms representing average to large-size patients, as well as the presence of activity outside the FOV, has not been investigated. The triple energy window (TEW) technique (Shao et al., 1994) is a direct extension of the DEW where in addition to the PEW and LEW, a third energy window that is a subset of the LEW at the higher energies is also used (labeled as LEW1 in Figure 8.9). Under the condition where $r_{scat} \gg r_{true}$, t_{PEW} is now calculated as

$$t_{PEW} = p_{PEW} - M \times \left(\frac{p_{LEW}}{r_{scat}} \right)$$

where M is the modification factor that accounts for variations due to object size and distribution and is defined as

$$M = \left(\frac{r_{object}}{r_{calib}} \right)^b$$

Here, r_{object} and r_{calib} are the ratio of total counts in LEW and LEW1 in the object and a calibration phantom (uniform cylinder), respectively. The relaxation factor, b, controls the amount of feedback and needs to be optimized for different classes of studies. Compared with the DEW technique, the TEW technique provides a better estimate for changes in object size and source distribution.

A different energy window–based method labeled the estimation of trues method (ETM) uses data collected in the photopeak window and a high energy window (HEW), which is a subset of PEW with the lower value of the energy gate lying above the photopeak (Figure 8.9). The idea behind this technique is that the events in the HEW are primarily true coincidence events, and by properly scaling the data in this window and subtracting it from the counts collected in the PEW, one can obtain an estimate of the scattered events. However, this estimate will be noisy and some smoothing of the scatter estimate is needed. Previous studies have shown that the ETM works very well for a range of activity distributions in scanners with good energy resolution (Adam et al., 2000). However, a primary limitation of this technique is the noisy estimate of the true coincidence events in the HEW, which can be especially relevant for dynamic imaging with very short data acquisition times.

The energy-based scatter estimation techniques described up to this point use primarily the energy information in a few limited energy windows without utilizing the full energy and spatial distribution information for scattered events. Recently, new methods have been proposed that make use of this information to ascribe a weight to every event in an LOR that defines the probability of it being a scatter event. One method uses average Monte Carlo simulations over various activity and source distributions to produce a trues fraction lookup table (Chen et al., 2003). Another technique (Popescu et al., 2006) uses the 2D energy information available for all coincidence events in a list-mode data acquisition to calculate the relative weights for three classes of scatter events (both photons scatter, first photon scatters, or second photon scatters) and true events. In this technique, a group of events collected in a region close to a point of interest in the projection space is used to determine the relative weight components of the event being scatter or a true event using a statistical estimator. This technique requires an accurate characterization of the scattered and true coincidence events' energy spectra in the scanner and, while promising as shown in simulations, has not been implemented on a scanner.

The most accurate estimation of scattered coincidences in a data set can only be obtained if a full Monte Carlo simulation (Levin et al., 1995; Holdsworth et al., 2001, 2002) of the imaging environment is performed. This will include an accurate modeling of the scanner geometry and shielding, as well as the detector parameters, which will have an impact on the collected events; an *a priori* knowledge of the patient activity distribution inside and outside the FOV; and the attenuation map. All these patient and scanner-specific requirements make the full Monte Carlo techniques computationally exorbitant and slow, and are currently difficult to implement in a clinical environment.

Finally, in recent years, the most popular and successful technique for scatter correction in PET has been the model-based single scatter simulation (SSS) (Ollinger, 1996; Watson et al., 1997; Accorsi et al., 2004), which is based upon the observation that in PET scanners with good energy resolution (and hence a higher energy threshold), the dominant form of scattered events is single scatter events (see Figure 8.8). The SSS technique starts with an initial estimate of the emission image without any scatter correction, while the attenuation image is used to distribute scatter points within the patient. The Klein–Nishina equation is then used to obtain an estimate of the number of counts contributed to each LOR by every scatter point within the patient based on the emission activity distribution. In this manner, an estimate of the total scatter distribution is obtained for all possible LORs. While the SSS method provides an estimate of the scatter distribution, it does not provide an absolute measure of the number of scattered events in every LOR. In order to scale the scatter distribution obtained from SSS to an absolute measure, the tails of the scatter estimate are scaled to the number of counts present beyond the object boundary in the sinogram for an absolute estimate of the scattered events. Since this scatter calculation (first iteration) is based on an initial emission image without any scatter correction, the SSS algorithm needs to be repeated for a few (typically three or four) iterations using the scatter estimate from the previous iteration for a more accurate initial emission image. Figure 8.10 is a flowchart describing the SSS technique for estimating the scattered events in PET data. With the advent of TOF PET, the SSS technique was easily extended in the TOF dimension, since, for each scatter event, there is a precise measure of the distance traveled by each photon, and hence the TOF for each scattered event (after convolving it with the scanner timing resolution) is naturally available (Watson, 2007; Werner et al., 2006). A primary limitation of the SSS technique is the assumption that all scattered events are single scatter, which breaks down for scanners with poor energy resolution, especially those operating in a fully 3D mode. Current and previous generations of PET scanners with an energy resolution of 15% or less and operating in the fully 3D

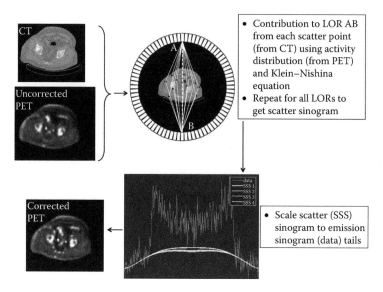

Figure 8.10 General flowchart showing the steps in calculating a scatter estimate using the SSS algorithm. Points A and B are the two end-points for the detected LOR, AB. Several iterations are needed before a stable solution is reached.

mode have generally performed well when using the SSS technique for scatter estimation. Another limitation of SSS is the collection of scattered events originating from outside the imaging FOV. This can be a problem for single-bed-position imaging studies; however, for multibed studies that are typical of clinical whole-body scans, emission images from adjacent bed positions can be used to accurately estimate scattered events originating from outside the FOV for each bed position. Finally, a limitation, which can arise when imaging large patients who fill most of the transverse imaging FOV, is the very short tails of the emission sinogram (beyond the patient boundary), which prevents an accurate scaling of the scatter estimate to the emission data. Despite some of these limitations, model-based SSS techniques have become standard for scatter correction in PET, and are utilized in all fully 3D PET scanners due to their accuracy and fast calculation.

8.2.3 RANDOMS CORRECTION

In order to detect coincident events in a PET scanner, whenever a photon is detected in one of the PET detectors, i, coincidence electronics search for another photon detected in one of the other detectors, j, within a time τ (coincidence timing window) of the first photon. Practically, the coincidence determination is performed in a field-programmable gate array (FPGA) where τ is defined by the number of system clock cycles within which a second photon is detected to form a coincident event. For a typical scanner transverse FOV of 60 cm diameter, the TOF difference between two coincident photons emitted at the edge of the FOV will be 2 ns. Hence, the coincidence timing window τ has to be at least 2 ns in order to collect all true coincidence events generated within the imaging FOV. In practice, the nonzero timing resolution of a PET detector leads to a convolution of the 2 ns TOF difference with a Gaussian with full width at half maximum (FWHM) equal to the scanner timing resolution. Hence, the coincidence timing window is larger than 2 ns, typically 2.5–3 ns in the current generation of TOF scanners with a timing resolution of around 500–600 ps. Due to the finite size of the coincidence timing window, uncorrelated single photons from two different annihilation events will have a nonzero probability of being detected within this coincidence timing window as well, with the probability increasing as the singles rate in the scanner increases. Because the two photons are not generated from a single annihilation event, such events are called random coincidences. Figure 8.11 shows a schematic describing the detection of a true coincident event as well as a random coincident event. The random coincidence rate, R_{ij}, between two detectors i and j is given by

$$R_{ij} = 2\tau S_i S_j$$

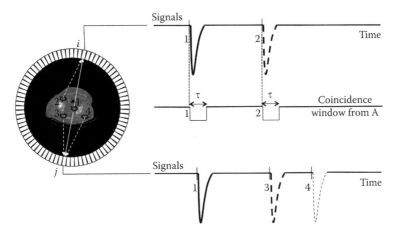

Figure 8.11 Schematic showing collection of coincident events in detectors *i* and *j* in a PET scanner. Solid lines are signals from true coincident events, dashed lines are from single events, and thick lines in the two detector signal chains show a detected coincident event. Event 1 represents a positron annihilation where the two coincident 511 keV photons are detected in detectors *i* and *j* (true coincidence). Events 2–4 are positron annihilations that occur close to event 1 temporally, but where only one of the two photons is detected in either detector *i* or *j* (single events). The coincidence logic determines photons from event 1 as a valid coincident event. In addition, event 2 in detector *i* and event 3 in detector *j* are also in coincidence, and hence an incorrect, or random, coincident event is detected.

where S_i and S_j are the single-photon count rates in the two detectors, and τ is the coincidence timing window, and the factor of two accounts for the probability that any of the two photons can be detected first in the PET scanner. Since the photons that form a random coincidence are generated from two unrelated annihilation events, they add a very slowly changing bias in the image that will affect image contrast, as well as the measured activity uptake. Hence, correction techniques are need to produce accurate PET images.

The simplest technique that has been used in the past is tail fitting, which was also used for scatter correction. For random coincidences, the tails of the emission sinogram beyond the object boundary are fit to a constant value or a very slowly changing parabola, which is then subtracted from the full sinogram. In practice, this technique could also be combined for a joint randoms and scatter estimation (Karp et al., 1990). However, limits of the tail-fitting algorithm, as described earlier when the patient fills most of the imaging FOV, are still detrimental, and hence this technique is rarely used in commercial scanners nowadays.

Random coincidence rate R_{ij} between the two detectors *i* and *j* can also be estimated if a direct measure of the singles rate in each detector is available and using the relationship between the randoms and singles rate defined earlier. Since single-photon count rates in a PET scanner are much higher than the coincidence photon count rates, the random coincidence estimate obtained this way is not very noisy due to high statistics. However, in order to obtain an accurate estimate, a proper modeling of detector dead time in the individual detectors, as well as variability in timing between detector pairs, needs to be performed.

The most common technique for randoms estimation is the delayed window technique that is routinely used in most commercial PET scanners. This technique makes use of the fact that the two photons forming a random coincident event are not related to each other spatially or temporally. Hence, by using an additional coincidence timing window that is delayed by a time τ_d relative to the detection of the first photon, one can get an accurate estimate of the random coincidences without any true coincidences being collected in this data acquisition channel. In Figure 8.12, we show schematically how a delayed coincidence timing window can be used to estimate the random coincidences in the two detectors *i* and *j*, where coincidences in the delayed window are formed by events falling within a coincidence timing window of τ ns that is delayed by τ_d ns relative to the arrival of the first photon. The data collected in the delayed window sinogram can be subtracted from the emission sinogram to obtain an accurate measure of true and scattered coincidences. Relative to the singles-based randoms estimation technique, the delayed coincidence window technique is very accurate since it acquires data at the same rate as the true coincidence data, and hence suffers from the same

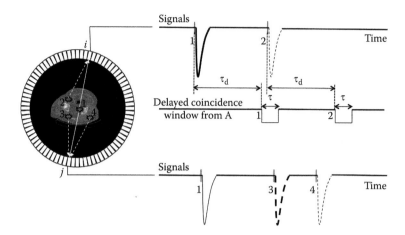

Figure 8.12 Schematic showing the electronics chain where the coincidence window for events from detector *i* is delayed by a fixed amount (t_d) relative to the true arrival time of the photon. Solid lines are signals from true coincident events, dashed lines are from single events, and thick lines in the two detector signal chains show a detected coincident event. Here, the true coincident photon in detector *j* from annihilation event 1 is lost, but a random coincident event formed by a photon from event 1 in detector *i* and event 3 in detector *j* is measured. Coincidences measured in the delayed window are all random and are labeled as delayed coincidences.

dead-time effects. However, the collected counts in each LOR can be very small, so the noise propagated into the randoms-corrected emission sinogram may be high. Noise propagation due to randoms correction can be reduced if the delayed window data are collected separately and variance reduction techniques utilized before their subtraction from the prompt events. Straightforward smoothing of the delayed data can be employed in scanners that have infinite symmetry such that the efficiency for all detectors (crystals) is the same in the full scanner. Most, if not all, PET scanners employ a modular detector design where several flat detector modules (such as block detectors) are used to form a polygonal scanner geometry. In these scanners, there will be a variation in detection efficiency for different LORs based on the crystal position. Hence, straightforward smoothing over all LORs is not appropriate in these systems. An alternative is the Casey averaging technique (Casey and Hoffman, 1986), where the number of random coincidences in an LOR formed between two detectors *i* and *j* (R_{ij}) is calculated by

$$R_{ij} = \frac{R_{iB} \times R_{jA}}{R_{AB}}$$

where R_{iB} is a sum of all coincidences between detector *i* and a group of similar detectors *B* that include detector *j*, R_{jA} is a sum of all coincidences between detector *j* and a group of similar detectors *A* that include detector *i*, and R_{AB} is a sum of all coincidences between detectors in groups *A* and *B*. The equivalency of this relationship was shown by Casey and Hoffman (1986), where they also show that the ratio of the variance in this noise-reduced estimate, as opposed to the direct estimate, is $(2N + 1)/N^2$, where *N* is the number of detectors in each group, such as *A* or *B*. Hence, by using a variance reduction technique, one can obtain an accurate, as well as less noisy, estimate of the random coincidences from the data collected in the delayed window technique, which can then be subtracted from the prompt data before or during image reconstruction.

8.2.4 DEAD-TIME CORRECTION

Like all radiation detectors, PET scanners suffer from dead-time effects at high data count rates, which manifest themselves in two ways: pulse pileup effects that degrade data quality and can lead to a loss in image quality, and dead-time effects that lead to a loss in collected events. Pulse pileup effects arise when two or more single events occur close to each other both spatially and temporally so that the scintillation pulses

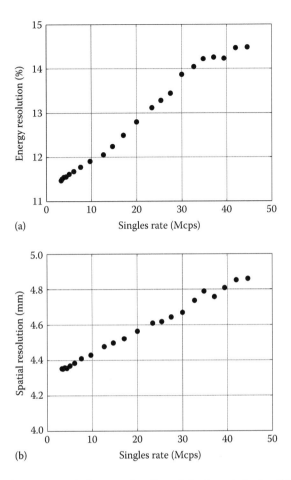

Figure 8.13 (a) Measured energy resolution as a function of singles rate in the Philips Gemini TF PET/CT. (b) Measured spatial resolution as a function of singles rate in the Philips Gemini TF PET/CT. (These figures were originally published in Surti, S., et al., *J. Nucl. Med.*, 48, 471–480, 2007. Copyright by the Society of Nuclear Medicine and Molecular Imaging, Inc.)

overlap, leading to a miscalculation of the energy as well as interaction position. In some situations, the total measured energy will be above the energy window, leading to a rejection (loss) of the event, while in other situations, the image quality will be compromised due to a degraded energy, spatial, or timing resolution. Figure 8.13 shows measured energy and spatial resolution as a function of singles rate acquired on a clinical PET/CT scanner. Both energy and spatial resolution degrade as the singles rate increases.

In addition to the loss of events due to energy rejection of pulse pileup events, there are two other sources for loss of coincident events in a PET scanner. At high count rates, there is an increasing probability for more than two scintillation photons to be detected within a single coincidence timing window. Since the system electronics cannot discriminate between these photons to determine a valid coincident event, these events are typically rejected, leading to a loss in collected coincidences. In addition, the scanner data acquisition system typically has a processing time for every event detected. At high count rates, the electronics processing time is not negligible, leading to a loss in coincident events at high count rates. Figure 8.14 shows measured true coincidence rate in a clinical PET/CT as a function of singles rate. The extrapolated true coincidence rate shows the rate that we expect based on scanner sensitivity. The difference between the measured and extrapolated true coincidence rates represents the system dead time.

Since a PET image provides a quantitative measure of the activity uptake within the patient, an accurate correction for dead-time effects needs to be performed. Pulse pileup effects can be reduced in PET scanners by using a fast scintillator and designing a PET detector with reduced light spread. In addition, dedicated

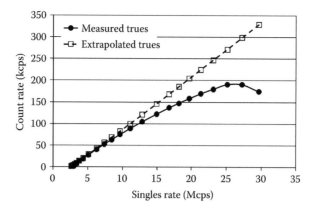

Figure 8.14 Measured true coincidence rate as a function of singles rate in the Philips Gemini TF PET/CT measured for a 27 cm diameter by 70 cm long line source cylinder. The extrapolated curve shows the rate expected from the sensitivity of the scanner. The measured trues coincidence rate at a high singles rate is lower than the extrapolated rate due to dead-time effects.

electronics have been developed that make use of the signal shape to reduce the impact of pileup from events that occur close (temporally and spatially) to the event of interest (Wong and Li, 1998). A fast scintillator and data acquisition architecture with reduced processing times will also help reduce dead-time effects. Despite the hardware solution to reduce loss of counts at high rates, scanner dead-time calibration needs to be performed in order to have a linear scanner performance at all activity levels. A standard technique used for dead-time calibration involves imaging a uniform activity–filled cylinder at a very high activity level (or count rate) and acquiring data as the activity decays. In this way, a lookup table can be derived based on the measured and expected coincidence rate as a function of singles rate in the scanner (similar to the plot shown in Figure 8.14). For a more accurate measure, the dead-time calibration table could also be generated for individual detector modules in the scanner instead of a single value for the whole system.

8.2.5 NORMALIZATION

Data normalization in PET refers to corrections for various nonuniformities in the data collection process that lead to a varying LOR sensitivity. If uncorrected, these nonuniformities will lead to artifacts and bias in the reconstructed images. The sources of these LOR nonuniformities can be separated into two distinct categories: (1) variations in crystal efficiency and (2) geometric effects. Variation in crystal efficiency can arise due to random variations in the intrinsic efficiency of individual crystals, as well as systematic variations in collected light and timing for each crystal, which can be reduced with accurate energy and timing calibrations, as described earlier (also called "block" profile effect). The geometric factors affecting LOR uniformity arise from effects related to the change in detector solid angle and change in the angle of incidence of annihilation photons at the detector surface for increasing LOR radial position. As shown schematically in Figure 8.15, the radial profile systematically increases in counts with increasing LOR radial position. This is primarily due to the fact that at increasing radial positions, the LORs reach the detector surface at increasing oblique angles, and therefore have to pass through an increasing detector thickness. However, in scanners employing block or other forms of modular detectors to form a polygonal scanner, if a photon enters near a detector edge, it will have less crystal material to travel through, and hence the efficiency will be reduced relative to photons entering near the center of that block (also called the crystal interference effect).

The simplest approach to estimating the normalization component for each LOR is the direct inversion technique, where data are collected for every LOR with the same source and the measured counts in each LOR are normalized to the same average value. The measurement can be performed with a rotating point or line source of ^{68}Ge, a planar sheet source, or a uniform cylinder (typically 20 cm in diameter). The disadvantage of this technique is the need for a very high number of counts to achieve reasonable count statistics per LOR for direct inversion, leading to long scan times with a low-activity source. In addition, scatter in the uniform

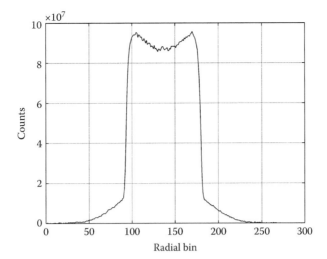

Figure 8.15 Measured radial profile summed over all direct sinogram slices and projection angles for data acquired with a 20 cm diameter uniform cylinder. Data were acquired on a Philips Gemini TF PET/CT scanner at the Hospital of the University of Pennsylvania. (This figure was originally published in Surti, S., et al., *J. Nucl. Med.*, 48, 471–480, 2007. Copyright by the Society of Nuclear Medicine and Molecular Imaging, Inc.)

cylinder can be confounding, since accurate scatter correction is needed for an estimate of the normalization factors. In order to overcome these disadvantages, component-based normalization methods (Hoffman et al., 1989; Ollinger, 1995; Casey et al., 1995; Badawi and Marsden, 1999; Badawi et al., 2000) that make use of variance reduction techniques (such as the Casey averaging described earlier) (Casey and Hoffman, 1986; Hoffman et al., 1989) to reduce scan time and improve statistical accuracy of the data are more routinely used nowadays. The normalization coefficient n_{ij}^{uv} for an LOR formed between crystals i and j in detector rings u and v, respectively, can be separated into

$$n_{ij}^{uv} = \left(\varepsilon_i^u b_i^u c_i^u\right) \times \left(\varepsilon_j^v b_j^v c_j^v\right) \times \left(g_{ij}^{uv} h_{ij}^{uv}\right)$$

where ε_i^u, b_i^u, and c_i^u are the factors for crystal efficiency, transverse block profile effect, and axial block profile effect for crystal i in detector ring u, respectively. Also, g_{ij}^{uv} and h_{ij}^{uv} are the transverse and axial geometric factors for an LOR formed between crystal i in detector ring u and crystal j in detector ring v, respectively. Data collection is performed using a planar or cylindrical source.

Crystal efficiency and transverse block effect components are estimated jointly by summing all counts between detector i in scanner ring u and a fan group of similar detectors opposite of it (C_i^u). For a sufficiently large number of detectors in the opposing fan group, and by repeating this calculation for each detector i in scanner ring u, it can be shown that

$$\varepsilon_i^u \times b_i^u \approx \left(\frac{C_i^u}{\overline{C_i^u}}\right)$$

where $\overline{C_i^u}$ is the mean over all detectors i in scanner ring u.

The transverse geometric factor, g_{ij}^{uv}, is estimated from the data after correcting for crystal efficiency and the transverse block effect, and by using counts from all LORs formed between scanner rings u and v, which defines a single 2D sinogram. Within this sonogram, an average C_{ij}^{uv} is calculated for counts in LORs that have the same radial position and the same crystal positions within the detector as crystals i and j. The g_{ij}^{uv} factor is then defined to be

$$g_{ij}^{uv} = \left(\frac{\overline{C_{ij}^{uv}}}{C_{ij}^{uv}} \right)$$

where $\overline{C_{ij}^{uv}}$ is an average of counts over all radial positions for LORs that have the same crystal positions within the detector as crystals i and j.

The correction factor for the axial block profile effect, c_i^u, which is just the relative efficiency of each scanner detector ring, u, and is independent of crystal, i, within the rings, is calculated by

$$c_i^u = c^u = \sqrt{\frac{\overline{C^u}}{C^u}}$$

where C^u is the total counts for all LORs within scanner ring u (direct plane), and $\overline{C^u}$ is the mean of C^u over all scanner rings u (direct planes). The axial geometric factor, h_{ij}^{uv}, is independent of the crystal positions within the ring (i and j) and can be estimated from the data, after correcting for the block axial effect, by

$$h_{ij}^{uv} = h^{uv} = \sqrt{\frac{\overline{C^{uv}}}{C^{uv}}}$$

where C^{uv} is the total counts for all LORs formed between crystals in scanner rings u and v, and $\overline{C^{uv}}$ is the mean of C^{uv} over all combinations of scanner rings u and v.

Figure 8.16 shows an example of reconstructed image without and with normalization correction for a uniform cylinder. The image without normalization correction shows ring artifacts that are removed after a component-based normalization correction.

Recently, it has been observed that TOF reconstructed images are less susceptible to errors or even absence of normalization correction in the image reconstruction process. Based on this observation, one can use a TOF image without normalization correction to forward project and produce an estimate of the true sinogram (Werner and Karp, 2014). Comparison of this sinogram to the measured sinogram can be used to produce an initial estimate of the normalization factors in a manner analogous to the direct inversion techniques. By repeating this procedure iteratively (using the estimated normalization coefficients in the new TOF reconstruction), an accurate measure of the normalization factors can be achieved. Since this technique uses a TOF reconstructed image of any object to obtain the initial estimate, no prior calibration data

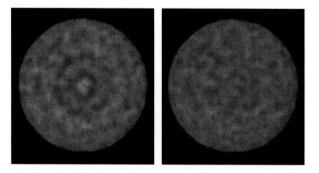

Figure 8.16 Reconstructed transverse view of 20 cm diameter uniform cylinder data without (left) and with (right) normalization correction. Data were acquired on a Philips Gemini TF PET/CT scanner at the Hospital of the University of Pennsylvania. (This figure was originally published in Surti, S., et al., *J. Nucl. Med.*, 48, 471–480, 2007. Copyright by the Society of Nuclear Medicine and Molecular Imaging, Inc.)

acquisition is necessary, and clinically one could use the patient data to obtain the normalization sonogram, as well as the corrected, reconstructed image.

8.3 CALIBRATION OF RECONSTRUCTED IMAGE TO EMISSION ACTIVITY LEVEL

The reconstructed PET image with all the above corrections provides an accurate measure of relative uptake within different tissue regions in the reconstructed image. For routine imaging where the relative uptake in tissue defines the image contrast, this image provides enough information for a qualitative interpretation.

In situations such as dynamic studies where the image values are compared to activity concentration measured from blood samples for kinetic modeling, an accurate measure of the activity in image voxels is needed. For this purpose, a calibration step is performed where a cylinder with uniform activity distribution is imaged in the PET scanner. The acquired data are reconstructed with full corrections, and the mean activity uptake per voxel measured. In parallel, an aliquot from the cylinder is measured in the well counter that is used for measuring the blood samples. A calibration factor is then derived as the ratio between the aliquot activity concentration measured in the well counter and the counts per second per voxel in the calibration phantom image. This technique is known as cross-calibration, where the uptake in the reconstructed image is calibrated against a well counter. However, for an absolute calibration, this technique is susceptible to the accuracy of the well counter measurement, as well as the accuracy of all corrections performed on the PET data.

For an absolute calibration, an accurate measurement of scanner sensitivity needs to be performed, which provides a measure of counts per second in collected PET data relative to activity (in kBq or mCi) in the FOV. In particular, for this measurement a source that does not require any data corrections is needed. The technique prescribed by Bailey et al. (1991) using a line source with multiple metal sleeves, and currently used for sensitivity measurements according to the National Electrical Manufacturers Association NU2-2007 protocols (NEMA, 2008), can be useful in this scenario. With this sensitivity calibration factor, the counts per second per voxel in a fully corrected, reconstructed image can then be converted into kilobequerel (or millicurie) per voxel.

The SUV is a metric most commonly specified when referring to the amount of tracer uptake in a clinical image. The SUV is the ratio of the average activity concentration in a specific region of an image (voxel, region of interest [ROI] or volume of interest [VOI], or organ system) to the average activity concentration in the entire patient or phantom being imaged. Most frequently, the patient weight is used as a surrogate for volume in the activity concentration calculation, with the assumption that the density of a person is approximately 1.0 g/ml. This gives the SUV calculation as

$$SUV = \frac{\text{Measured Activity Concentration}}{\text{Injected Activity}/\text{Weight}}$$

In addition to the accuracy and validity of the data corrections applied, there are many factors that will influence the SUV calculation, including accurate measurement of the patient's weight, the activity injected, and the time of the activity measurement.

8.4 SUMMARY

Over several decades of development, the techniques used for correcting PET data have been well established, leading to quantitative images. While the calibration methods for energy and timing at the detector level can vary slightly in implementation, the techniques used for data corrections (attenuation, scatter, randoms, dead time, and normalization) have converged to a fairly standard set of methods for all commercial PET scanners. For example, attenuation correction is routinely performed using the CT image from the PET/CT systems, the SSS technique is used for scatter estimation, the delayed window technique with some smoothing is utilized for randoms estimation, and component-based methods are used for normalization. The adoption of these techniques is driven by an evolution in the underlying PET technology, as well as the practicality and ease of using them in a clinical environment where fast image reconstruction and image accuracy are highly desired. For instance, widespread adoption of PET/CT since its introduction has led to a demise of stand-alone PET scanners, and hence use of the CT image for attenuation correction has become routine. Similarly, current developments in PET/MR scanners have reopened active areas for research in using the MR image for attenuation correction, underlining the role of new technology development in guiding the data correction techniques used for quantitative PET.

REFERENCES

Accorsi, R., Adam, L. E., Werner, M. E., and Karp, J. S. 2004. Optimization of a fully 3D single scatter simulation algorithm for 3D PET. *Phys. Med. Biol.*, 49, 2577–2598.

Adam, L. E., Karp, J. S., and Freifelder, R. 2000. Energy-based scatter correction for 3-D PET scanners using NaI(Tl) detectors. *IEEE Trans. Med. Imaging*, 19, 513–521.

Alessio, A. M., Kinahan, P. E., Cheng, P. M., Vesselle, H., and Karp, J. S. 2004. PET/CT scanner instrumentation, challenges, and solutions. *Radiol. Clin. North Am.*, 42, 1017–1032.

Badawi, R. D., Ferreira, N. C., Kohlmyer, S. G., Dahlbom, M., Marsden, P. K., and Lewellen, T. K. 2000. A comparison of normalization effects on three whole-body cylindrical 3D PET systems. *Phys. Med. Biol.*, 45, 3253–3266.

Badawi, R. D., and Marsden, P. K. 1999. Developments in component-based normalization for 3D PET. *Phys. Med. Biol.*, 44, 571–594.

Bai, C., Shao, L., Da Silva, A. J., and Zhao, Z. 2003. A generalized model for the conversion from CT numbers to linear attenuation coefficients. *IEEE Trans. Nucl. Sci.*, 50, 1510–1515.

Bailey, D. L., Jones, T., and Spinks, T. S. 1991. A method for measuring the absolute sensitivity of positron emission tomographic scanners. *Eur. J. Nucl. Med.*, 18, 374–379.

Bailey, D. L., and Meikle, S. R. 1994. A convolution-subtraction scatter correction method for 3D PET. *Phys. Med. Biol.*, 39, 411–424.

Bendriem, B., Soussaline, F., Campagnolo, R., Verrey, B., Wajnberg, P., and Syrota, A. 1986. A technique for the correction of scattered radiation in a PET system using time-of-flight information. *J. Comput. Assist. Tomogr.*, 10, 287.

Bergstrom, M., Eriksson, L., Bohm, C., Blomqvist, G., and Litton, J. 1983. Correction for scattered radiation in a ring detector positron camera by integral transformation of the projections. *J. Comput. Assist. Tomogr.*, 7, 42–50.

Blankespoor, S. C., Xu, X., Kaiki, K., Brown, J. K., Tang, H. R., Cann, C. E., and Hasegawa, B. H. 1996. Attenuation correction of SPECT using x-ray CT on an emission-transmission CT system: Myocardial perfusion assessment. *IEEE Trans. Nucl. Sci.*, 43, 2263–2274.

Burger, C., and Buck, A. 1996. Tracer kinetic modeling of receptor data with mathematical metabolite correction. *Eur. J. Nucl. Med.*, 23, 539–545.

Carroll, L. R., Kertz, P., and Orcut, G. 1983. The orbiting rod source: Improving performance in PET transmission correction scans. In *Emission Computed Tomography—Current Trends*, ed. P. D. Esser, pp. 235–247. New York: Society of Nuclear Medicine.

Carson, R. E., Daube-Witherspoon, M. E., Jacobs, G. I., and Herscovitch, P. 1989. Validation of postinjection transmission measurments for PET. *J. Nucl. Med.*, 30, 825.

Casey, M. E., Gadagkar, H., and Newport, D. 1995. A component based method for normalization in volume PET. In *Proceedings of the 3rd International Meeting on Fully Three-Dimensional Image Reconstruction in Radiology and Nuclear Medicine*, Aix-les-Bains, France, pp. 67–71.

Casey, M. E., and Hoffman, E. J. 1986. Quantitation in positron emission computed-tomography. 7. A technique to reduce noise in accidental coincidence measurements and coincidence efficiency calibration. *J. Comput. Assist. Tomogr.*, 10, 845–850.

Chen, H. T., Kao, C. M., and Chen, C. T. 2003. A fast, energy-dependent scatter reduction method for 3D PET imaging. In *2003 IEEE Nuclear Science Symposium and Medical Imaging Conference*, Portland, OR, pp. 2630–2634.

Cherry, S. R., and Huang, S. C. 1995. Effects of scatter on model parameter estimates in 3D PET studies of the human brain. *IEEE Trans. Nucl. Sci.*, 42, 1174–1179.

Cherry, S. R., Tornai, M. P., Levin, C. S., Siegel, S., and Hoffman, E. J. 1995. A comparison of PET detector modules employing rectangular and round photomultiplier tubes. *IEEE Trans. Nucl. Sci.*, 42, 1064–1068.

Daube-Witherspoon, M., Carson, R. E., and Green, M. V. 1988. Postinjection transmission attenuation measurments for PET. *IEEE Trans. Nucl. Sci.*, 35, 757–761.

Daube-Witherspoon, M. E., Surti, S., Perkins, A. E., Kyba, C. C. M., Wiener, R. I., and Karp, J. S. 2010. Imaging performance of a LaBr$_3$-based time-of-flight PET scanner. *Phys. Med. Biol.*, 55, 45–64.

Davidson, Z. S., Wiener, R. I., Newcomer, F. M., Vanberg, R., and Karp, J. S. 2011. High voltage photodetector calibration for improved timing resolution with scintillation detectors for TOF-PET imaging. Presented at 2011 IEEE Nuclear Science Symposium and Medical Imaging Conference, Valencia, Spain.

deKemp, R. A., and Nahmias, C. 1994. Attenuation correction in PET using single photon transmission measurement. *Med. Phys.*, 21, 771–778.

Grootoonk, S., Spinks, T. J., Sashin, D., Spyrou, N. M., and Jones, T. 1996. Correction for scatter in 3D brain PET using a dual energy window method. *Phys. Med. Biol.*, 41, 2757–2774.

Harrison, R., Haynor, D., and Lewellen, T. 1991. Dual energy window scatter corrections for positron emission tomography. In *1991 IEEE Nuclear Science Symposium and Medical Imaging Conference*, Santa Fe, NM, pp. 1700–1704.

Hoffman, E. J., Guerrero, T. M., Germano, G., Digby, W. M., and Dahlbom, M. 1989. PET system calibrations and corrections for quantitative and spatially accurate images. *IEEE Trans. Nucl. Sci.*, 36, 1108–1112.

Holdsworth, C. H., Levin, C. S., Farquhar, T. H., Dahlbom, M., and Hoffman, E. J. 2001. Investigation of accelerated Monte Carlo techniques for PET simulation and 3D PET scatter correction. *IEEE Trans. Nucl. Sci.*, 48, 74–81.

Holdsworth, C. H., Levin, C. S., Janecek, M., Dahlbom, M., and Hoffman, E. J. 2002. Performance analysis of an improved 3-D PET Monte Carlo simulation and scatter correction. *IEEE Trans. Nucl. Sci.*, 49, 83–89.

Hoverath, H., Kuebler, W. K., Ostertag, H. J., Doll, J., Ziegler, S. I., Knopp, M. V., and Lorenz, W. J. 1993. Scatter correction in the transaxial slices of a whole-body positron emission tomograph. *Phys. Med. Biol.*, 38, 717–728.

Karp, J. S., Muehllehner, G., Mankoff, D. A., Ordonez, C. E., Ollinger, J. M., Daube-Witherspoon, M. E., Haigh, A. T., and Beerbohm, D. J. 1990. Continuous-slice PENN-PET: A positron tomograph with volume imaging capability. *J. Nucl. Med.*, 31, 617–627.

Karp, J. S., Muehllehner, G., Qu, H., and Yan, X.-H. 1995. Singles transmission in volume imaging PET with a Cs-137 source. *Phys. Med. Biol.*, 40, 929–944.

Karp, J. S., Surti, S., Daube-Witherspoon, M. E., Freifelder, R., Cardi, C. A., Adam, L. E., Bilger, K., and Muehllehner, G. 2003. Performance of a brain PET camera based on Anger-logic gadolinium oxyrorthosilicate detectors. *J. Nucl. Med.*, 44, 1340–1349.

Kinahan, P. E., Townsend, D. W., Beyer, T., and Sashin, D. 1998. Attenuation correction for a combined 3D PET/CT scanner. *Med. Phys.*, 25, 2046–2053.

LaCroix, K. J., Tsui, B. M. W., Hasegawa, B. H., and Brown, J. K. 1994. Investigation of the use of x-ray CT images for attenuation compensation in SPECT. *IEEE Trans. Nucl. Sci.*, 41, 2793–2799.

Lercher, M. J., and Wienhard, K. 1994. Scatter correction in 3-D PET. *IEEE Trans. Med. Imaging*, 13, 649–657.

Levin, C. S., Dahlbom, M., and Hoffman, E. J. 1995. A Monte-Carlo correction for the effect of Compton-scattering in 3-D PET brain imaging. *IEEE Trans. Nucl. Sci.*, 42, 1181–1185.

Liu, Y., Li, H., Wang, Y., Xing, T., Xie, S., Uribe, J., Baghaei, H., Ramirez, R., Kim, S., and Wong, W. H. 2004. A gain-programmable transit-time-stable and temperature-stable PMT voltage divider. *IEEE Trans. Nucl. Sci.*, 51, 2558–2562.

Mollet, P., Keereeman, V., Clementel, E., and Vandenberghe, S. 2012. Simultaneous MR-compatible emission and transmission imaging for PET using time-of-flight information. *IEEE Trans. Med. Imaging*, 31, 1734–1742.

NEMA [National Electrical Manufacturers Association]. 2008. *Performance Measurements of Positron Emission Tomographs*. NEMA Standards Publication NU 2-2008. Rosslyn, VA: NEMA.

Ollinger, J. M. 1995. Detector efficiency and Compton scatter in fully 3D PET. *IEEE Trans. Nucl. Sci.*, 42, 1168–1173.

Ollinger, J. M. 1996. Model-based scatter correction for fully 3-D PET. *Phys. Med. Biol.*, 41, 153–176.

Popescu, L. M., Lewitt, R. M., Matej, S., and Karp, J. S. 2006. PET energy-based scatter estimation and image reconstruction with energy-dependent corrections. *Phys. Med. Biol.*, 51, 2919–2937.

Shao, L. X., Freifelder, R., and Karp, J. S. 1994. Triple energy window scatter correction technique in PET. *IEEE Trans. Med. Imaging*, 13, 641–648.

Shao, L. X., and Karp, J. S. 1991. Cross-plane scattering correction—Point-source deconvolution in PET. *IEEE Trans. Med. Imaging*, 10, 234–239.

Smith, R. J., Karp, J. S., Muehllehner, G., Gualtieri, E., and Benard, F. 1997. Singles transmission scans performed post-injection for quantitative whole-body PET imaging. *IEEE Trans. Nucl. Sci.*, 44, 1329–1335.

Surti, S., Kuhn, A., Werner, M. E., Perkins, A. E., Kolthammer, J., and Karp, J. S. 2007. Performance of Philips Gemini TF PET/CT scanner with special consideration for its time-of-flight imaging capabilities. *J. Nucl. Med.*, 48, 471–480.

Watson, C. C. 2007. Extension of single scatter simulation to scatter correction of time-of-flight PET. *IEEE Trans. Nucl. Sci.*, 54, 1679–1686.

Watson, C. C., Eriksson, L., Casey, M. E., Jones, W. F., Moyers, J. C., Miller, S., Hamill, J., Van Lingen, A., Bendriem, B., and Nutt, R. 2001. Design and performance of collimated coincidence point sources for simultaneous transmission measurements in 3-D PET. *IEEE Trans. Nucl. Sci.*, 48, 673–679.

Watson, C. C., Newport, D., Casey, M. E., Dekemp, R. A., Beanlands, R. S., and Schmand, M. 1997. Evaluation of simulation-based scatter correction for 3-D PET cardiac imaging. *IEEE Trans. Nucl. Sci.*, 44, 90–97.

Werner, M. E., and Karp, J. S. 2013. TOF PET offset calibration from clinical data. *Phys. Med. Biol.*, 58, 4031–4036.

Werner, M. E., and Karp, J. S. 2014. Detector efficiency calibration from clinical listmode TOF PET data. Presented at 2014 IEEE Nuclear Science Symposium and Medical Imaging Conference, Seattle, WA.

Werner, M. E., Surti, S., and Karp, J. S. 2006. Implementation and evaluation of a 3D PET single scatter simulation with TOF modeling. In *2006 IEEE Nuclear Science Symposium and Medical Imaging Conference*, San Diego, pp. 1768–1773.

Wong, W. H., and Li, H. 1998. A scintillation detector signal processing technique with active pileup prevention for extending scintillation count rates. *IEEE Trans. Nucl. Sci.*, 45, 838–842.

Image reconstruction for PET and SPECT

RICHARD M. LEAHY, BING BAI, AND EVREN ASMA

9.1	Introduction	235
9.2	Radon transforms, sinograms, and projections	236
	9.2.1 Radon and x-ray transforms	236
	9.2.2 PET data formation	237
	9.2.3 SPECT data formation	238
9.3	Analytic 2D reconstruction methods	239
9.4	Analytic 3D reconstruction methods	241
	9.4.1 3D parallel-beam reconstruction methods for PET	241
	9.4.2 3D SPECT reconstruction	243
9.5	Model-based image reconstruction	243
	9.5.1 Introduction	243
	9.5.2 Statistical image reconstruction components	244
	9.5.2.1 Basis function selection	244
	9.5.2.2 System modeling	245
	9.5.2.3 Noise modeling	246
	9.5.2.4 Objective functions	247
	9.5.2.5 Numerical optimization	251
9.6	Conclusions	253
	References	253

9.1 INTRODUCTION

Image reconstruction algorithms are used to form images of radiotracer biodistributions from PET and SPECT emission data. These algorithms can be classified into two main groups: analytical and statistical or model-based reconstruction. Analytical approaches are based on inverting the mathematical relationships between a function and its line integrals or projections. Statistical or model-based approaches use computational models of the physical and statistical aspects of the data acquisition process, possibly also incorporating prior information about the radiotracer biodistribution, to arrive at an image that best explains the data.

Image reconstruction can be performed either as a series of two-dimensional (2D) reconstructions or in a "fully three-dimensional" (3D) manner. In 2D image reconstruction, data are first separated into a stack of 2D datasets, each of which corresponds to a single image slice. These 2D datasets are then reconstructed slice by slice to form a set of 2D images that are stacked to form the final 3D image. In fully 3D image reconstruction, all data are used together to directly form a 3D image.

The use of septa between detector rings in earlier PET systems separated data into a stack of independent 2D slices. Similarly, parallel collimators in SPECT systems allow reconstruction to be posed as a set of 2D problems. The later development of fully 3D septa-less PET systems and SPECT systems with converging and diverging collimators made the reconstruction problem fully 3D in the sense that it cannot be directly decoupled into a set of 2D problems.

Under some simplifying assumptions, 2D image reconstruction is equivalent to the mathematical problem of recovering a 2D function from its line integrals or projections, which are often referred to collectively as the sinogram. This problem was first solved by Radon (1917). With the development of x-ray computed tomography (CT) in the early 1970s (Hounsfield, 1973), Radon's results were rediscovered in the form of the filtered backprojection (FBP) algorithm (Shepp and Logan, 1974). Analytic extensions of the theory of line integrals to 3D resulted in the development of fully 3D FBP methods for both parallel projections (for PET) and cone-beam projections (for SPECT) (Feldkamp et al., 1984; Kinahan and Rogers, 1989; Defrise and Clack, 1994). Methods based on FBP and its 3D extensions remain the basis for reconstruction of most x-ray CT images today and are still in widespread use in PET and SPECT.

Data acquisition in emission tomography involves the counting of coincident 511 keV photon pairs for PET or single gamma rays for SPECT. The limited number of these events detected in a single scan results in photon-limited noise in the data. The Poisson distribution of this noise is not explicitly modeled in the analytical reconstruction methods. In addition, the physics of PET and SPECT event detection limits the accuracy of the line integral model implicit in analytical methods. These two factors motivated the development of model-based statistical reconstruction methods that can specifically include models for photon-limited noise and an accurate system response model (Shepp and Vardi, 1982). The original maximum-likelihood (ML) method of Shepp and Vardi is based on the application of the expectation maximization (EM) methodology to emission imaging (Dempster et al., 1977). The images formed using EM showed significant improvements in noise handling compared with FBP, but slow convergence made the algorithm impractical. The problem of slow convergence of EM was later addressed by the introduction of ordered subsets EM (OSEM), which iteratively updates the reconstructed image using only a subset of the data at each iteration (Hudson and Larkin, 1994). As with FBP, many extensions and variations on EM and OSEM have been developed over the past few decades.

In this chapter, we give an introduction to both analytical and statistical image reconstruction techniques, with references to the literature for interested readers to explore this interesting and still active area of research and development in more depth.

9.2 RADON TRANSFORMS, SINOGRAMS, AND PROJECTIONS

9.2.1 RADON AND X-RAY TRANSFORMS

The basic assumption in analytical reconstruction methods is that each measurement is proportional to the integral of the activity distribution along a line (the line of response [LOR]) in 2D or 3D space. The set of one-dimensional (1D) integrals along parallel lines intercepting a 2D or 3D image is called the x-ray transform (Defrise, 1995). By comparison, the Radon transform of an N-dimensional (n-D) function is defined as the set of all integrals over $(N - 1)$-D hyperplanes through the image. Therefore, for 2D images, the x-ray and Radon transforms are equivalent, while in 3D, the x-ray transform consists of 1D line integrals, but the Radon transform is made up of planar integrals.

The Radon transform of a 2D function $f(x, y)$ is given by

$$p(s,\phi) = \int_{-\infty}^{\infty} f(s\cos\phi - l\sin\phi, s\sin\phi + l\cos\phi)dl \tag{9.1}$$

and is illustrated in Figure 9.1. The variables (s, ϕ) represent, respectively, the displacement of the LOR from the origin and its rotation relative to the y axis of the fixed coordinate system (x, y). In the next section, we

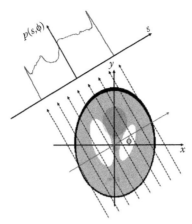

Figure 9.1 Illustration of the relationship between image $f(x, y)$ and its 2D Radon transform $p(s,\phi)$.

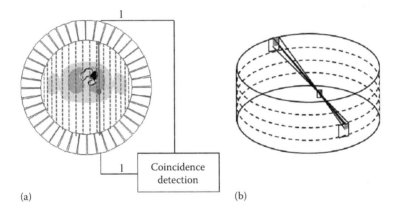

Figure 9.2 Coincidence detection for a single-ring PET scanner (a) and illustration of the LOR indicating the sensitivity between a pair of detectors within a fully 3D PET scanner (b).

describe how we recover $f(x, y)$ from its Radon transform, but first we describe how PET and SPECT data are mapped into this line integral model.

9.2.2 PET DATA FORMATION

A PET scanner is usually composed of multiple detector rings. Figure 9.2 illustrates a single ring in which coincidence events correspond to the detection of collinear pairs of 511 keV gamma rays resulting from positron–electron annihilation. Raw data can be saved in a "list-mode" format in which each event is recorded separately. More typically, PET scanners record the total number of events between each detector pair, which corresponds approximately to the line integral along an LOR joining the two detectors. These data are stored in a 2D array or "sinogram," with each element corresponding to a single LOR indexed by radial displacement, s, and rotational angle, ϕ, the two coordinates of the Radon transform in Equation 9.1. As illustrated in Figure 9.2, the decreasing angle between the detector surface and the LOR as we approach the edge of the field of view (FOV) results in a nonuniform sampling in radial displacement, s, which must be accounted for during reconstruction.

In time-of-flight (TOF) PET, the difference between the arrival times of the two photons in the coincidence event is also measured, and this additional information can be used to limit the possible locations along the LOR where the event originated. This information can be either saved in the list-mode file, or used to divide sinograms into multiple TOF-bin sinograms, each corresponding to a separate difference in arrival times. In this case, the Radon transform equation is modified as follows:

$$p(s,\phi,t) \approx \int_{-\infty}^{\infty} f(-s\sin\phi + l\cos\phi, s\cos\phi + l\sin\phi)h(t-l)dl \tag{9.2}$$

where t is the TOF variable recording the difference between photon arrival times and $h(t)$ is a kernel that represents uncertainty in the TOF measurement t along the LOR. This kernel is usually assumed to be a Gaussian function with full width at half maximum (FWHM) determined by the scanner's timing resolution. For example, a 400 ps timing resolution is equivalent to an FWHM of approximately 6 cm ($\Delta x = C^*\Delta t/2$).

Modern PET scanners are typically constructed by stacking several rings of block detectors, where each block consists of a 2D array of scintillators. The resulting system contains an approximately cylindrical arrangement of detectors, as shown in Figure 9.2. Coincident 511 keV photon pairs can be detected between any pair of detectors whose LOR passes through the patient port. This arrangement allows efficient collection of multiple sinograms that include both the transaxial 2D sinograms for each ring of detectors and the set of oblique sinograms, each corresponding to LORs between two different rings of detectors. Jointly, these sinograms are a fully 3D dataset that requires more complex reconstruction algorithms than those for reconstruction from a single 2D transaxial sinogram.

9.2.3 SPECT DATA FORMATION

In SPECT, high-energy gamma rays are emitted from a radioactive tracer and detected using a 2D planar gamma camera. A collimator is needed to restrict the direction from which incoming photons can enter the gamma camera. The collimator is composed of a sheet of dense material such as lead or tungsten, with holes through which the gamma rays pass. Figure 9.3 illustrates a SPECT detector panel with a parallel-hole collimator. In a typical SPECT system, a gamma camera and parallel-hole collimator are rotated around the patient to acquire projection data from multiple different angles. The 2D Radon transform for each transaxial 2D plane will be measured along a single line of camera pixels in the plane of rotation, with different angles ϕ collected as the camera is rotated around the patient. The combined planar projection images from the SPECT camera therefore provide a stacked set of 2D Radon transforms or sinograms from which the 3D emission image can be reconstructed slice by slice. Alternative collimators use fan-beam or cone-beam geometries to modify the FOV or improve sensitivity or resolution, as illustrated in Figure 9.3 (Moore et al., 1992). Converging fan-beam and cone-beam collimators are used to image organs such as the heart or brain, while diverging collimators are used when imaging objects that are large relative to the gamma camera. Multiple-pinhole collimators, which also acquire data in a cone-beam geometry, have been developed for use in cardiac, brain, and small-animal SPECT imaging (Jaszczak et al., 1994). Alternative geometries that

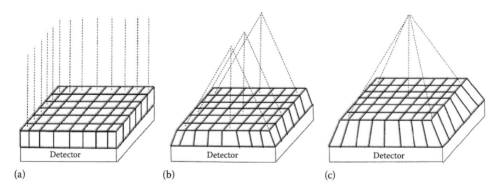

(a)   (b)   (c)

Figure 9.3 SPECT data acquisition using a detector panel with (a) a parallel-hole collimator, (b) a fan-beam collimator, or (c) a cone-beam collimator.

combine rotating collimators with cylindrical gamma-ray detectors have also been explored, but to date have not been widely adopted.

Fan-beam SPECT data can be re-sorted into equivalent parallel projections and reconstructed using the same methods as for parallel-beam collimation. However, as we describe below, extensions of parallel-beam FBP to 2D fan beam and 3D cone beam have been developed that avoid the need for re-sorting.

9.3 ANALYTIC 2D RECONSTRUCTION METHODS

The most important result in 2D image reconstruction is the central slice theorem, which equates the 2D Fourier transform $F(\omega_x, \omega_y)$ of $f(x, y)$ to the 1D Fourier transform, with respect to the s coordinate, of the Radon transform $p(s, \phi)$, as illustrated in Figure 9.4:

$$F(\omega_s \cos\phi, \omega_s \sin\phi) = P(\omega_s; \phi) \tag{9.3}$$

This result shows that the 1D Fourier transform of the Radon transform at angle ϕ gives a slice of the 2D Fourier transform of the image at the same angle ϕ. This result is directly used in the Fourier method of image reconstruction by first computing the 1D Fourier transform at each projection angle to find samples of the 2D image Fourier transform along radial lines through the origin. Interpolation of these samples onto a regular rectangular grid and applying an inverse 2D Fourier transform will reconstruct the image.

A more elegant solution to the reconstruction problem avoids the use of Fourier transforms by using the central slice theorem to manipulate Equation 9.2 to obtain the FBP equations in which the data are first filtered in 1D along the radial sampling direction s:

$$\tilde{p}(s, \phi) = \int p(s - s', \phi) g(s') ds \tag{9.4}$$

where $g(s)$ is the impulse response of the filter with frequency response $G(\omega) = |\omega|$, frequently referred to as the "ramp filter." This frequency response arises from the Jacobian of the transformation from polar coordinates

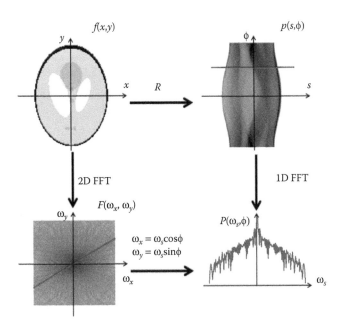

Figure 9.4 2D central slice theorem. (FFT, Fast Fourier Transform).

in which the 2D image Fourier transform is sampled in the Fourier method, to a rectangular coordinate system. The filtered projections are then "backprojected" to recover the image:

$$f(x,y) = \int_0^\pi \tilde{p}(x\cos\phi + y\sin\phi, \phi)d\phi \tag{9.5}$$

This step is referred to as backprojection because the mapping between the image coordinates (x, y) and those of the filtered projections $(x\cos\phi + y\sin\phi, \phi)$ can be viewed geometrically as backprojecting each filtered projection along the parallel lines over which the line integrals were originally formed.

Practical implementations of FBP discretize the integrals in Equations 9.4 and 9.5 by summing over radial and angular samples and windowing the ramp filter frequency response for noise control in the reconstructed image (Shepp and Logan, 1974). Frequently used window functions in FBP include Shepp–Logan, Butterworth, and Hann windows (Farquhar et al., 1997; Tsui and Frey, 2006). This algorithm is still used for reconstruction of 2D images in both PET and parallel-collimated SPECT. Figure 9.5 illustrates the performance of FBP for a simulated SPECT NURBS-based cardiac-torso (NCAT) phantom using different window functions.

TOF information introduces some degree of redundancy in the PET data, as revealed in the TOF version of the central slice theorem:

$$F(-\omega_t \sin\phi + \omega_s \cos\phi, \omega_t \cos\phi + \omega_s \sin\phi)H(\omega_t) = P(\omega_s, \phi, \omega_t) \tag{9.6}$$

where $H(\omega_t)$ is the 1D Fourier transform of the TOF resolution kernel $h(t)$. Equation 9.6 shows that in principle, the entire Fourier transform, and therefore the entire image, can be recovered from TOF data for a single projection angle. In practice, this is not possible because timing resolution in the current generation of PET scanners, on the order of 400 ps, limits the spatial resolution with which events can be resolved along each LOR. Equivalently, poor TOF resolution results in a fast drop in $H(\omega_t)$ as ω_t increases, making it difficult to recover accurate estimates of the image Fourier transform for large ω_t. The central slice theorem for TOF data can be used as the basis for developing FBP algorithms. Since there is redundancy in TOF data, there are multiple possible FBP algorithms in this case, each of which would produce identical solutions in the case

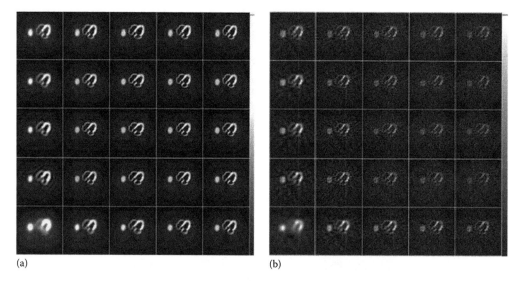

(a)   (b)

Figure 9.5 Images reconstructed from simulated NCAT phantom (a) noiseless and (b) noisy data. The top four rows were reconstructed using the Butterworth window with orders 2, 4, 8, and 32, respectively. The bottom row used the Hann window. Left to right: Cutoff frequencies of 0.1, 0.2, 0.3, 0.4, and 0.5 cycle/pixel, respectively. (From Tsui, B., and Frey, E., in *Quantitative Analysis in Nuclear Medicine Imaging*, Springer, Berlin, 2006, pp. 82–106.)

of perfectly accurate and noiseless data. In practice, the TOF FBP algorithm can be optimized using data weighting schemes to shape the noise characteristics in the reconstructed image (Watson, 2007).

For 2D SPECT data acquired using parallel-beam collimators, the 2D FBP approach described above can be applied directly to reconstruct each transaxial plane. Interestingly, FBP algorithms can also be derived for fan-beam collimators. So, rather than re-sorting fan beam into equivalent parallel projections, we can instead apply a change of variables from parallel- to fan-beam coordinates in the FBP equations (Equations 9.4 and 9.5). This results in an equivalent pair of equations that allow filtering and backprojection in the native coordinates of the fan-beam data (Besson, 1996).

9.4 ANALYTIC 3D RECONSTRUCTION METHODS

9.4.1 3D PARALLEL-BEAM RECONSTRUCTION METHODS FOR PET

For 3D PET, coincidence data are recorded between detectors in different rings, as well as within the same ring. This greatly improves sensitivity, but also increases the dimensionality of the data and the complexity of the reconstruction problem. The sinogram representation can be extended to fully 3D data using a four-dimensional (4D) function, $p(s, \phi, z, \theta)$, by introducing additional parameters for the oblique angle θ between two detector rings, and the axial displacement z of the midpoint between the two rings from the center of the scanner, as illustrated in Figure 9.6. An alternative but equivalent representation for fully 3D data is the x-ray transform $p'(x_r, y_r, \phi, \theta)$, in which the data are grouped into 2D planar parallel projections of $f(x, y, z)$, each with coordinates (x_r, y_r). The orientation of the set of parallel LORs for each planar projection is defined by two rotation parameters: ϕ, the rotation in the transaxial plane (orthogonal to the central axis of the cylinder containing the detectors), and θ, the oblique angle of the LORs relative to the transaxial plane, as illustrated in Figure 9.6.

The central slice theorem extends directly to 3D PET when using the x-ray projection format $p'(x_r, y_r, \phi, \theta)$: the 2D Fourier transform of each planar projection provides one 2D slice through the 3D image Fourier transform. This result can be used to derive a 3D version of FBP (Colsher, 1980), which requires 2D filtering of planar projections prior to backprojection. The finite number of detector rings results in limited axial coverage of the PET scanner, so that oblique projections ($\theta \neq 0$) will be truncated, preventing direct application of these 2D filters. To overcome this problem, we can make use of the fact that, as with TOF PET data, fully 3D PET data are redundant. In principle, it is sufficient to know $p'(x_r, y_r, \phi, \theta)$ for $\theta = 0$ only (this is equivalent to having a stack of 2D sinograms, one per transaxial slice). The additional data ($\theta \neq 0$) increase the sensitivity of the PET scanner and therefore lead to improved signal-to-noise ratio (SNR) in the final image. The missing data for $\theta \neq 0$ can be estimated by reprojection of an initial estimate of the image computed from the complete nonoblique ($\theta = 0$) data only. Gaps in the truncated data are filled in with the results of this reprojection to yield a full set of untruncated data. These are then used for 3D FBP. This approach is the basis for the 3D reprojection (3DRP) method, which was for several years the standard reconstruction algorithm for 3D PET (Kinahan and Rogers, 1989).

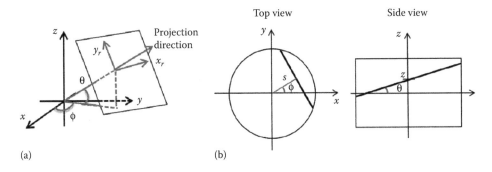

Figure 9.6 3D PET can be stored in two different but equivalent formats: (a) x-ray projection or (b) sinogram.

An alternative approach to fully 3D reconstruction is to exploit redundancy in the data through a class of methods referred to as "rebinning." As we noted above, it is possible to form a 3D volume as a stack of 2D slices or images, each reconstructed from the 2D PET sinogram for that slice. In other words, 3D images can be reconstructed from sinogram data $p(s, \phi, z, \theta)$ known for $\theta = 0$ only. However, sinogram data measured at oblique angles, $\theta \neq 0$, should also be used in order to maximize the SNR in the reconstructed images. Rebinning methods exploit redundancy in 3D PET data by calculating an equivalent set of 2D sinograms based on the analytic relationship between the redundant (3D) and nonredundant (2D) sinograms. Importantly, this rebinning must be done in such a way as to retain the SNR advantages of the 3D data in the rebinned 2D data.

Single-slice rebinning (SSRB), the simplest form of rebinning, generates a set of 2D sinograms by simply adding together sinograms over a small range of oblique angles at each transaxial plane. Despite being a very simple approximation, it is surprisingly effective (Daube-Witherspoon and Muehllehner 1987). More accurate rebinning methods can be derived from the relationship between the Fourier transforms of the 2D and 3D sinogram data (Defrise et al., 1997). Once 3D data are rebinned into 2D, the PET image can then be constructed slice by slice using a 2D reconstruction algorithm such as FBP or the EM algorithm described below. Figure 9.7 shows examples of patient data reconstructed using Fourier rebinning (FORE) in combination with three different 2D reconstruction algorithms.

Rebinning techniques can also be used to map TOF data to their non-TOF counterpart in a way that preserves the additional SNR benefits of TOF (Tomitani, 1981; Watson, 2007; Ahn et al., 2011). Cho et al. (2008, 2009) developed a generalized projection slice theorem and proposed a unified framework for exact and approximate mappings between different representations of the data, allowing us to explore and optimize the use of both TOF and 3D PET information. For example, in the TOF FORE algorithms developed by Cho et al. (2009), 2D non-TOF data can be computed from a weighted average of the TOF 3D data after taking appropriate Fourier transforms, with the weights chosen to optimize SNR. This huge reduction in dimensionality of

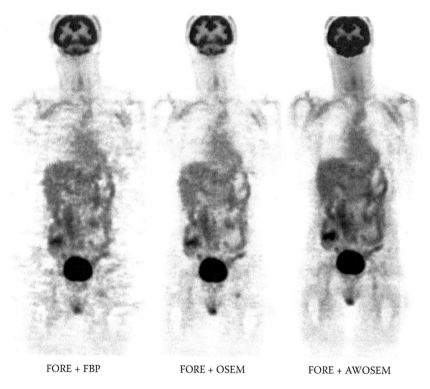

FORE + FBP   FORE + OSEM   FORE + AWOSEM

Figure 9.7 Fluorodeoxyglucose patient images reconstructed using 2D algorithm after FORE: (a) FBP, (b) OSEM, or (c) attenuation weighted OSEM (AWOSEM). (From Lartizien, C., et al., *J. Nucl. Med.*, 44, 276–290, 2003.)

the data translates to significant reductions in the computational cost associated with subsequent reconstruction of the PET image. Figure 9.8 shows a patient dataset reconstructed from fully 3D TOF data and from non-TOF 2D and 3D rebinnings of these data. The similarity of the three images reflects the ability of rebinning to reduce data dimensionality without significant loss of SNR.

9.4.2 3D SPECT RECONSTRUCTION

SPECT data using parallel and fan-beam collimators can be organized as a stack of 2D data, and the algorithms described in Section 9.3 can be used to reconstruct each 2D slice separately. When converging or diverging cone-beam collimators are used, however, reconstruction must be performed directly in 3D space to account for the presence of oblique line integrals through the object. A direct extension of FBP to cone-beam data, the Feldkamp algorithm (FDK) (Feldkamp et al., 1984) uses a set of cone-beam projections collected by rotating the detector around the patient so that the cone vertices trace out a circular orbit. FDK combines 1D filtering of the cone-beam projections with a 3D backprojection step. While this method can perform reasonably in practice if the angle of the cone is small, Feldkamp reconstruction will always be approximate, producing increasingly large artifacts away from the plane containing the cone vertices. In fact, it can be shown that when the cone vertices are restricted to a circular orbit, the data are incomplete and the image cannot be reconstructed exactly. Development of alternative geometries for cone-beam data collection have been driven by "Tuy's complete data condition": all 2D planes passing through the object must intersect the cone vertex trajectory at least once (Tuy, 1983). This is violated by the circular orbit, but satisfied, for example, with helical trajectories. In this and other complete data cases, exact FBP-like algorithms can be derived (Defrise and Clack, 1994), although these geometries are more commonly encountered in cone-beam x-ray CT rather than SPECT imaging systems.

9.5 MODEL-BASED IMAGE RECONSTRUCTION

9.5.1 INTRODUCTION

While analytic reconstruction algorithms have been widely used in nuclear medicine, they lack an explicit model to account for the photon-limited noise in the data that arise from counting individual radioactive emission events. In addition, the line integral models that they assume do not accurately account

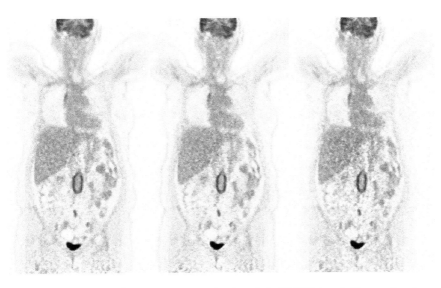

Figure 9.8 FDG patient images showing reconstruction from fully 3D PET data (left), as well as from rebinned non-TOF 3D (center) and non-TOF 2D (right) data. (From Bai, B., et al., *Phys. Med. Biol.*, 59, 925–949, 2014.)

for the physical properties and limited detector resolution of PET and SPECT systems. Statistical image reconstruction algorithms, on the other hand, are capable of accurately modeling data noise, as well as the physics of data acquisition in arbitrary geometries. For this reason, many statistical image reconstruction algorithms have been proposed over the last two decades, and they are now routinely used in clinical PET and SPECT studies.

Model-based statistical image reconstruction methods consist of the following five elements:

1. *Basis function selection*: The continuous image is represented as a linear combination of basis functions; in most cases the voxel, which represents tracer uptake over a small cubic volume of tissue. This allows for a discrete representation of the image as a vector of basis function coefficients. For example, in the case of voxels, these coefficients are the amount of uptake in each voxel. Since data are also acquired discretely, the image reconstruction problem then deals with discrete representations in both data and image domains.

2. *System model*: The system model includes the effects of the scanner geometry on data acquisition, as well as physical effects, such as attenuation, normalization for varying detector efficiencies, system dead time, scattered events, and for PET, random coincidence events.

3. *Noise model*: The noise model describes how measured data deviate from their expected value through the data probability distribution. Counting of individual events in PET and SPECT leads to a Poisson distribution model in most cases. The use of an accurate noise model can lead to an improved trade-off between resolution and SNR, as well as more accurate quantitation in reconstructed images.

4. *Objective function*: System and noise models are combined to determine the likelihood of observing measured data for a given image. The objective function to be optimized is then a combination (i.e., weighted sum) of the data likelihood and penalty terms that are designed to penalize structure in the reconstructed images that deviates from our prior knowledge about the tracer distribution, for example, images that have negative intensity, are not piecewise smooth, or differ greatly from corresponding anatomical images. Regularization through introduction of these penalty terms tends to make the reconstruction problem better conditioned; in other words, the reconstructed images are less sensitive to noise in the data and avoid noise amplification problems that can occur in methods based only on maximization of the data likelihood.

5. *Numerical optimizer*: The numerical optimizer is a mathematical optimization algorithm that computes the reconstructed image that maximizes the objective function.

Once considered slow and only used for research studies, these methods are now applied in nuclear medicine clinics every day for tumor detection and staging, assessment of therapy response, and other applications. By combining an appropriate noise model with an accurate system model, one can improve image resolution and noise properties, which in turn can increase the sensitivity and specificity of clinical studies. In recent years, there has also been a great deal of research into regularized reconstruction algorithms in which we can effectively control the image properties and optimize them for different tasks through the choice and weighting of the penalty function. In the following sections, we investigate these statistical image reconstruction components in greater detail.

9.5.2 STATISTICAL IMAGE RECONSTRUCTION COMPONENTS

9.5.2.1 BASIS FUNCTION SELECTION

In PET and SPECT image reconstruction, the data are recorded in discrete form and the image is typically discretized using a collection of basis functions:

$$f(\vec{r}) = \sum_{j=1}^{N} x_j b_j(\vec{r}) \tag{9.7}$$

where N is the total number of image voxels and $\vec{r}$ denotes the Cartesian coordinate in continuous image space. The most commonly used basis functions, $b_j(\vec{r})$, are cubic voxels. Cubic voxels assume that activity values are constant within each voxel and have the advantage of easily understood basis function parameters: voxel dimensions across all three dimensions. Other basis functions have also been successfully used in PET and SPECT reconstruction, such as Kaiser–Bessel windows (Matej and Lewitt, 1996; Yendiki and Fessler, 2004), polar grids (Cabello and Rafecas, 2012), and detector response functions or "natural pixels" (Buonocore et al., 1981).

9.5.2.2 SYSTEM MODELING

In the absence of noise, the mean data in PET and SPECT can be expressed as a linear function of the image, as represented by the coefficients x_j of the selected basis function:

$$\bar{y}_i = \sum_{j=1}^{N} p_{ij} x_j + \bar{r}_i \tag{9.8}$$

where p_{ij} are the elements of the system matrix P containing the probabilities that events originating in voxel j are detected in detector i, and $\bar{r}_i$ denotes the sum of the expected number of random and scattered events for PET and the mean of scattered and background events for SPECT. This relationship can be expressed in matrix–vector format as $\bar{y} = Px + \bar{r}$. System modeling involves computation of the matrix P that accurately represents data acquisition by the scanner. One approach to system modeling in PET is the factored system matrix model (Qi et al., 1998):

$$P = P_{\text{norm}} P_{\text{blur}} P_{\text{attn}} P_{\text{geom}} P_{\text{range}} \tag{9.9}$$

where P_{range} models blurring due to positron range in image space (Bai et al., 2003; Fu and Qi, 2010); P_{geom} is the geometric probability matrix that depends on the solid angles subtended by each voxel at the detector pairs involved in each LOR; P_{attn} is a diagonal matrix containing the attenuation factors; P_{blur} models the blurring in sinogram space due to photon pair noncollinearity, intercrystal penetration, and scattering; and P_{norm} is a diagonal matrix containing calibration and detector sensitivity normalization factors. These matrices are computed through some combination of geometric calculation, Monte Carlo modeling, and experimental detector response measurement.

A similar factored system matrix can be written for SPECT. The calculation of attenuation factors is more involved in SPECT because attenuation depends on the position of the source along the ray, and therefore the attenuation component of the system matrix is not diagonal. In addition, resolution loss at the detectors depends on a combination of the detector response and the collimator design (Metzler et al., 2002).

Matrix–vector multiplications involving the system matrix and its transpose are the most time-consuming components of statistical image reconstruction. To make model-based reconstruction practical, methods have been developed to reduce the time of forward projection (multiplication by P) and backprojection (multiplication by P^T). These algorithms exploit the sparseness of P; further reductions in storage requirements resulting from the many symmetries in the scanner and sinogram geometry; and use of fast processors, such as graphics processing units (GPUs), to achieve high performance at low cost. Chapter 10 describes some of these methods for fast forward and backprojection.

Detector response or sinogram blurring models can be included in the system matrix for improved resolution recovery (Qi et al., 1998). The point-spread function (PSF) that models sinogram blurring can be calculated analytically (Huesman et al., 2000) or from Monte Carlo simulations (Qi et al., 1998), or can be estimated from measured point source data (Panin et al., 2006; Tohme and Qi, 2009). When measured point source data are used, either the PSFs can be estimated using a physical model for the measurements (Tohme and Qi, 2009), or the measurements can be fit to a parametric model, such as a set of asymmetric Gaussian functions (Panin et al., 2006). It has also been shown that for FORE data, the PSF can be estimated from point source data (Tohme and Qi, 2009; Bai et al., 2014).

Another more recent approach to resolution recovery is to use an image space PSF model to account for the resolution-degrading effects in data acquisition and image reconstruction:

$$P = P_{\text{norm}} P_{\text{attn}} P_{\text{geom}} P_{\text{psf}} \tag{9.10}$$

The image space PSF matrix P_{psf} can be estimated from an initial reconstruction without resolution recovery and is straightforward to implement as a blurring operation in image space. Recently, shift-variant PSFs have been designed to model the increased degradation of image resolution toward the edge of the FOV (Rahmim et al., 2013).

Finally, we note that when rebinning methods are used to reduce data size and speed up image reconstruction, the system model needs to be modified to reflect the effects of rebinning (Alessio et al., 2006; Bai et al., 2014; Tohme and Qi, 2009).

9.5.2.3 NOISE MODELING

The events detected in PET and SPECT result from the decay of unstable radioactive nuclei, which emit either a positron (in PET) or one or more gamma rays (in SPECT). In PET, the positron annihilates with an electron shortly after it is emitted and the annihilation creates two back-to-back 511 keV photons. In SPECT, high-energy photons are directly emitted as gamma rays during radioactive decay. Some of these emitted photons are scattered and lose energy or are completely attenuated as they travel through the human body. Radiation detectors assembled outside the body detect the photons that survive and leave the patient. The timing and energy deposited in the detector by the photons are recorded as an "event" provided that photon energies (and the timing between the two photons in PET) fall within predefined windows. Other chapters explain the physics (Chapter 1), radiation detection (Chapters 2–4), and scanner systems (Chapters 5 and 6) in much greater detail.

Radioactive decay of the tracer inside the patient is a random process, and the number of nuclei that decay within a given time follows a Poisson distribution. Each decay event either is independently detected or goes undetected, a process that can be modeled as a Bernoulli random variable. The combination of the Poisson emission distribution and a Bernoulli detection process produces sinogram measurements (i.e., the total number of events detected over a given time window) that also follow a Poisson distribution provided the injected activity levels are sufficiently low that dead-time and pileup effects are small. As a result, the joint probability distribution of a sinogram dataset vector y given as a function of the image x, or equivalently, the mean data vector $\bar{y} = Px + \bar{r}$, is

$$P(y \mid \bar{y}) = \prod_{i=1}^{M} \frac{e^{-\bar{y}_i} \bar{y}_i^{y_i}}{y_i!} \tag{9.11}$$

where M denotes the total number of LORs. In nuclear medicine applications, the data are photon limited with a relatively poor SNR, and therefore the use of appropriate statistical noise models is very important. Most statistical reconstruction methods use this Poisson noise model. For data precorrected for physical effects such as dead time, attenuation, scatter, and randoms (in PET), the Poisson nature of the data is lost and a Gaussian noise model may be appropriate (Fessler, 1994):

$$P(y \mid \bar{y}) = \prod_{i=1}^{M} \frac{1}{\sigma_i \sqrt{2\pi}} \exp\left[\frac{-(y_i - \bar{y}_i)^2}{2\sigma_i^2} \right] \tag{9.12}$$

where σ_i^2 denotes the estimated variance of the measurement at the ith LOR. This Gaussian model can also be used in cases of high-count, low-noise data as an accurate approximation of the Poisson model.

A common practice in PET is to subtract an estimate of the random events before storing the sinogram to reduce the bandwidth needed for data transfer and storage (Hoffman et al., 1981). The randoms-subtracted data can be written as $y_i = p_i - r_i$, where p_i and r_i are independent Poisson random variables denoting the number of prompt (true and random coincidences) and delayed (random coincidences only) events at the ith LOR, respectively. This difference between two independent Poisson random variables is no longer Poisson and has a numerically intractable distribution. While one could use the aforementioned Gaussian distribution as an approximate distribution, Yavuz and Fessler (1998) noticed that a simple but good approximation is to add $2\bar{r}_i$ to the data and to model the result as a Poisson random variable with mean and variance equal to $\bar{y}_i + 2\bar{r}_i$. Here, $\bar{r}_i$ denotes the mean of the delayed (random) events that can be estimated from the data. Other more accurate models for randoms precorrected data are described by Yavuz (2000) and Li and Leahy (2006).

As discussed previously, FORE is commonly used to reduce the size of the dataset and reconstruction time. Unlike Poisson data, the mean and variance of FORE data are not equal and the Poisson model no longer applies. Liu et al. (2001) used a simple scaling to match the mean and variance of the rebinned data. A similar approach was proposed for rebinned TOF data (Bai et al., 2014). After applying these scaling factors, the Poisson noise model can then be used in the reconstruction of rebinned data. However, the rebinning operator does introduce correlation between samples. In principle, noise models should account for such noise correlations, but development of a tractable formulation in this case is difficult (Alessio et al., 2007).

9.5.2.4 OBJECTIVE FUNCTIONS

Once we have the system and noise models, an ML estimate of the image can be computed by finding the maximizer of the logarithm of the likelihood function:

$$\check{x} = \arg\max_{x \geq 0} L(x) = \ln P(y \mid \bar{y}), \; \bar{y} = Px + \bar{r} \tag{9.13}$$

Maximizing the logarithm of the likelihood is equivalent to maximizing the likelihood because the logarithm is a monotonically increasing, one-to-one function, and the nonnegativity constraint is necessary because radioactivity concentrations cannot be negative. The log-likelihood functions (ignoring image-independent constants) under the Poisson and Gaussian noise models are given by

Poisson log-likelihood:
$$L(x) = \sum_{i=1}^{M} y_i \ln \bar{y}_i(x) - \bar{y}_i(x) \tag{9.14}$$

Gaussian log-likelihood:
$$L(x) = -\sum_{i=1}^{M} \left(y_i - \bar{y}_i(x) \right)^2 \Big/ 2\sigma_i^2 \tag{9.15}$$

ML estimators have attractive properties, such as consistency (they are asymptotically unbiased) and efficiency (they asymptotically achieve the minimum variance among all unbiased estimators); however, for the typical levels of noise seen in clinical studies, the ML estimator is unstable and produces noisy images of poor diagnostic quality. The reason for this is that ML estimators will find the image that best explains the data without any constraint (other than positivity) on the quality of the image. Because of the inherent ill-posedness of the PET and SPECT image reconstruction problems, large changes in the estimated image can be required to make small improvements in the fit to the data. As a result, small modeling errors or small changes in the noise level can result in large changes (or noise) in the reconstructed image.

Noise in ML images can be controlled in practice by stopping the numerical optimizer before convergence (Veklerov and Llacer, 1987) or by postsmoothing of the image after many iterations (Llacer et al., 1993). An alternative approach is to deal directly with the instability of the ML estimates by modifying the formulation of the optimization problem using regularization. Regularization adds a penalty term to the log-likelihood, which penalizes images with undesirable attributes such as high noise levels. Maximizing the sum of the log-likelihood and a regularizing function is often referred to as penalized maximum likelihood (PML). These regularization-based modifications of ML can also be viewed in a Bayesian framework where the regularizing function is the log of a prior distribution on the unknown PET or SPECT image. This prior represents our prior expectations about the image, such as smoothness, piecewise smoothness, or similarity in edge structure to a coregistered anatomical image. The PML and Bayesian formulations are equivalent when the reconstructed image is computed using either PML or maximum *a posteriori* (MAP) estimation from the objective function:

$$\check{x}_{MAP} = \arg\max_{x \geq 0} \Phi(x) = L(y \mid x) - p(x) \tag{9.16}$$

where $L(y|x)$ is the log-likelihood function and $p(x)$ is the log-prior (or penalty) function.

The prior function allows us to use other information about the image, such as smoothness, or anatomical information to improve image quality. The effect of the prior is to choose among those images that have likelihood values similar to the one that is most preferred with respect to the prior.

9.5.2.4.1 Prior functions

There are many ways of designing the prior or penalty function for PET and SPECT image reconstruction. One simple method is to ignore the statistical spatial dependence between voxels and treat each voxel separately. Independent Gaussian (Huesman et al., 2000) and Gamma models (Lange et al., 1987) have been proposed. For these models, the mean image needs to be estimated, which can be difficult and introduce significant bias. Several methods have been developed to estimate the mean image (Alenius and Ruotsalainen, 1997; Hsiao et al., 2003).

The independent voxel models are of limited value since the information we typically seek to capture in the prior is some degree of piecewise smoothness in the image. In order to model the local smoothness of the image, we can use a Markov random field (MRF) model or Gibbs distribution (Besag, 1974), whose general form is given by the probability density function (PDF)

$$p(x|\beta) = \frac{1}{Z} e^{-\beta U(x)} \tag{9.17}$$

where Z is a normalization factor, $U(x)$ is the Gibbs energy function that increases with image roughness, and β is a hyperparameter that determines how quickly the PDF decreases with increasing $U(x)$.

The Gibbs distribution has the Markov property that the conditional probability of any voxel value in the image depends only on the values of the voxels in a local neighborhood of that voxel. In other words, given its neighbors, each voxel is conditionally independent of all other voxels. This important property allows us to model desired image properties by specifying an image prior in terms of local voxelwise interactions and also leads to tractable MAP reconstruction algorithms.

In image reconstruction, the Gibbs energy function $U(x)$ is usually expressed as the sum of potential functions defined on pairwise voxels:

$$U(x) = \sum_{j=1}^{N} \sum_{k \in N_j, k > j} \varphi_{jk}(x_j - x_k) \tag{9.18}$$

where N_j denotes the neighborhood of voxel j and the potential function ϕ_{jk} is nonnegative and monotonically nondecreasing in $|x_j - x_k|$. Note that $U(x)$ has its minimum value of 0 for constant images and increases with image roughness so that the associated probability density decreases, indicating that, *a priori*, noisy or unsmooth images are less likely than smoother images.

The potential function $\phi_{jk}(x_j - x_k)$ determines the properties of the prior by deciding how the size of the difference between neighboring voxels affects the PDF. Among the most widely used choices is the quadratic prior $\phi_{jk}(x_j - x_k) = \omega_{jk}(x_j - x_k)^2$, where ω_{jk} allows for different voxel pairs to be weighted differently. The advantage of the quadratic prior is that it tends to produce the most natural-looking images; however, it is limited in its abilities to identify sharp changes in image intensity. Figure 9.9 compares analytical FBP reconstruction with MAP reconstruction using the quadratic prior of monkey brain phantom data. The superior image quality of MAP is clear.

A large number of alternative, nonquadratic prior functions have been explored that all share the goal of encouraging the reconstruction of generally smooth images, but without heavily penalizing the presence of true edges that represent sharp changes in tracer density across tissue boundaries. These include the generalized p-Gaussian model (Bouman and Sauer, 1996) and the Huber prior (Qi et al., 1998).

Recently, total variation (TV) regularization, which has become popular for CT image reconstruction (Sidky and Pan, 2008), has also been applied to PET and SPECT image reconstruction (Panin et al., 1999; Bai, 2012; Wang and Qi, 2013), as well as more broadly to the context of sparse imaging (Candes et al., 2006). The TV regularizer is equivalent to a Gibbs distribution with $\phi_{jk}(x_j - x_k) = |x_j - x_k|$.

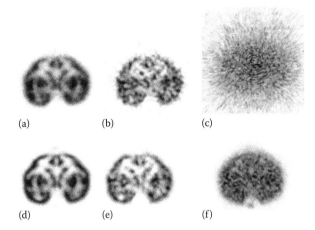

(a) (b) (c)

(d) (e) (f)

Figure 9.9 FDG monkey brain phantom image from the University of California, Los Angeles (UCLA) microPET scanner: (a–c) FBP and (d–f) MAP. Panels a and d are reconstructed from a 60 min scan, panels b and e from a 1 min scan, and panels c and f from variance images computed from 60 separate 1 min scans. (From Chatziioannou, A., et al., *IEEE Trans. Med. Imaging*, 19, 507–512, 2000.)

Another prior that has recently been adapted for use in clinical PET image reconstruction (Asma et al., 2012) is the relative difference prior (RDP), originally proposed for activity-dependent smoothing (Nuyts et al., 2002). The log-prior RDP is given by

$$\log p\left(x\right)=\beta\sum_{j}\sum_{k\in N_j}\omega_{jk}\frac{\left(x_j-x_k\right)^2}{x_j+x_k+\gamma\left|x_j-x_k\right|} \tag{9.19}$$

The idea behind RDP is that a fixed voxelwise difference is more critical when it corresponds to a significant fraction of the voxel values and less critical when it represents only a small fraction. Therefore, for small values of γ, this prior behaves similar to a quadratic prior, except that regions with high activity are penalized less and vice versa. At large values of γ, the penalty becomes a very good approximation to the edge-preserving TV prior. As a result, by choosing intermediate values of γ, one can control the trade-off between the natural-looking images produced by the quadratic-like behavior and the improved quantitation associated with the TV-like, edge-preserving behavior of the prior. The ability to control this trade-off is particularly useful in clinical imaging where one aims to improve quantitation without producing nonnatural, cartoonish images. Representative images reconstructed with RDP are shown in Figure 9.10.

The above prior functions are all convex. In order to further encourage the formation of sharp edges in the image, nonconvex functions have also been proposed and investigated (Geman and McClure, 1985). These nonconvex priors present challenges because reconstruction algorithms will converge only to a local rather than globally optimal solution, meaning that the final image depends on the initial estimate used in the iterative algorithm that computes the MAP estimate.

Finally, we note that when prior functions include data-dependent terms to control image properties (Fessler and Rogers, 1996), they are no longer truly priors and the estimator is no longer a true MAP estimator, and the approach can be more accurately viewed as PML estimation with a data-dependent penalty. The most common manner in which data-dependent penalties are used is in the selection of the weighting ω_{jk} in the Gibbs potential functions $\phi_{jk}(x_j-x_k)=\omega_{jk}(x_j-x_k)^2$. Interestingly, it can be shown that a constant value of ω_{jk} will lead to a spatially variant resolution in the reconstructed image. However, it is possible to compute spatially variant and data-dependent ω_{jk} values that will guarantee approximately spatially invariant resolution throughout the image (Fessler and Rogers, 1996; Qi and Leahy, 2000).

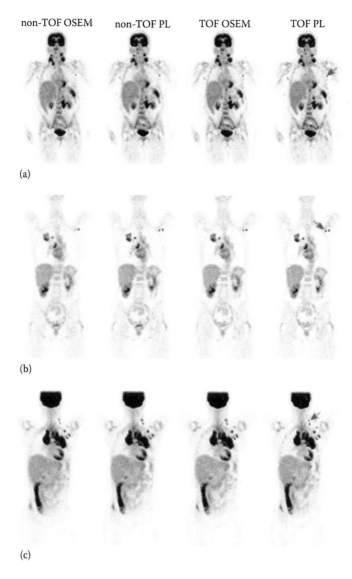

Figure 9.10 Representative non-TOF and TOF images from three different patients reconstructed using the RDP and OSEM. Red arrows indicate some of the FDG-avid features. (From Ahn, S., et al., *Phys. Med. Biol.*, 60, 5733–5751, 2015.)

9.5.2.4.2 Anatomical priors

In many clinical imaging scenarios, high-resolution anatomical information is available from coregistered MR or CT images. Recently, simultaneous PET/MR scanners that provide anatomical MR information with near-perfect registration and excellent soft-tissue contrast have become commercially available. Prior functions that incorporate such anatomical information can be designed to guide the reconstruction of functional images (Vunckx et al., 2012; Bai et al., 2013). There are two main approaches to incorporating anatomical information:

1. Use of edge or region information to reduce or eliminate penalties on voxelwise differences across organ or tissue boundaries (Gindi et al., 1993)
2. Maximization of an information-based similarity measure between the anatomical and reconstructed functional images, such as the Kullback–Leiber (KL) distance, joint entropy, or mutual information (Somayajula et al., 2011; Bai et al., 2013)

Both of these approaches have been shown to improve quantitation in regions for which the boundary information was present in the anatomical image.

We note that while anatomical and functional images clearly give very different views on the human body, it is also true that functional images, whether they represent metabolism, blood volume, or receptor binding, will exhibit a spatial morphology that reflects the underlying anatomy. It is therefore reasonable to assume that most tracers exhibit distinct changes in activity across tissue boundaries, while inside each region the distribution is smooth, unless there is evidence to the contrary in the functional data themselves. The idea behind anatomical prior use is not to force changes in activity across anatomical boundaries, but rather to view such changes as more likely.

9.5.2.5 NUMERICAL OPTIMIZATION

There are many algorithms that can be used to find the ML estimate of the image, including coordinate ascent or gradient-based methods. One of the earliest algorithms used for ML PET and SPECT image reconstruction is the EM algorithm (Dempster et al., 1977). EM is a general framework for computing the ML solution through the specification of a "complete" but unobservable dataset. EM alternates between two steps. The first step, called the E-step, calculates the conditional expectation of the complete data given the observed data and the current image estimate. The second step, called the M-step, maximizes the conditional expectation of this function with respect to the image.

EM was first applied to PET by Shepp and Vardi (1982) and Lange and Carson (1984) by choosing the complete data as the number of events detected by the ith detector pair that were emitted from the jth voxel. Following the general approach of Dempster et al. (1977), the EM algorithm reduces in this case to the single and simple recursive update equation:

$$x_j^{k+1} = \frac{x_j^k}{\sum\limits_{i=1}^{M} p_{ij}} \sum_{i=1}^{M} \frac{p_{ij} y_i}{\sum\limits_{j=1}^{N} p_{ij} x_j^k + \bar{r_i}} \tag{9.20}$$

This algorithm is straightforward to implement given the system matrix, P, with each iteration consisting of a single forward and backprojection calculation.

It can also be shown that EM is a special case of the majorize–minimize (MM) or functional substitution method. At each iteration, MM methods maximize a surrogate function $\Psi(x, x^n)$ instead of the original objective function $\Phi(x)$. The surrogate function is chosen such that it is easier to maximize than $\Phi(x)$. Provided the surrogate function satisfies a simple pair of constraints in relation to the original objective, the MM method converges to the maximum of the original function (Lange and Fessler, 1995; Hunter and Lange, 2004; Jacobson and Fessler, 2007).

The EM algorithm converges monotonically to the global maximum of the log-likelihood function, and the image is guaranteed to be nonnegative if initialized with a nonnegative image (Vardi et al., 1985). While these properties and ease of implementation made EM a popular algorithm, it converges very slowly, possibly requiring hundreds of iterations for effective convergence.

Hudson and Larkin (1994) observed that the convergence of the EM algorithm could be significantly sped up by dividing the projection data into nonoverlapping blocks, or subsets, and using only a single data subset at each EM update. They called this method OSEM. In early iterations, OSEM can speed up the reconstruction by approximately a factor equal to the number of subsets. As a result, OSEM reconstruction times became practical for clinical applications, leading to its rapid adoption for use in clinical PET and SPECT.

The speedup of OSEM is due to the fact that far away from the solution, the approximate gradient of the likelihood computed from a subset of the data provides a reasonable search direction for increasing the log-likelihood (the EM algorithm can be recast in terms of the gradient of the log-likelihood with respect to the image). However, as we get closer to the maximum, the error in the gradient due to use of only subsets of the data can cause the image to enter a limit cycle. This is illustrated in Figure 9.11.

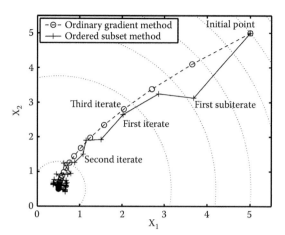

Figure 9.11 Simple 2D example of the ordered subset method showing the trajectory from initialization toward the maximizer of the objective function. Note the fast initial convergence of the ordered subset method, but eventual limit cycle behavior. (From Ahn, S., and Fessler, J.A., *IEEE Trans. Med. Imaging*, 22, 613–626, 2003.)

Hudson and Larkin (1994) recommended "subset balance"; that is, the subsets should be chosen such that the detection probability of each voxel is equal for each subset. In practice, subset balance is difficult to achieve due to differences in sensitivity and attenuation. Typically, the projections in each subset are chosen with maximum angular separation to avoid directional artifacts. With consistent data and under the condition of subset balance, OSEM can be shown to converge to the ML solution (Hudson and Larkin, 1994). However, in general data are not consistent due to noise and OSEM is not convergent, as illustrated in Figure 9.11.

The practical utility of OSEM, coupled with the limitation that the method does not usually converge to an ML solution, has motivated a great deal of research into the development of OSEM-like algorithms that do converge. One way to ensure OSEM converges is to gradually reduce the number of subsets to one as iterations proceed. Alternatively, one can use OSEM in the early iterations and switch to an alternative convergent algorithm to ensure convergence (Li et al., 2005).

Another approach is to use a subset-independent step size that is slowly reduced to zero to ensure convergence. One such example is the row-action maximum-likelihood algorithm (RAMLA) (Browne and De Pierro, 1996). Unlike OSEM, RAMLA converges to an ML solution if the log-likelihood function is strictly concave (Browne and De Pierro, 1996); however, the convergence rate can be very slow. Yet another approach to achieve convergence is through the use of an augmented cost function (Ahn and Fessler, 2003). Despite convergence issues, the original OSEM algorithm remains the most widely used algorithm for ML reconstruction in clinical PET and SPECT.

For MAP estimation, most of the optimization algorithms used for ML can be extended to maximize the MAP objective function. When EM is applied to MAP, the M-step has a closed-form solution only when the prior function is spatially independent. For spatially coupled priors, an iterative method such as gradient or coordinate ascent can be applied in the M-step (Hebert and Leahy, 1989). Green proposed a "one-step-late" (OSL) approach where the partial derivatives of the prior function are evaluated using the current estimate (Green, 1990). However, the OSL method does not in general converge to the MAP solution and the estimated image is not guaranteed to be nonnegative. Another approach to MAP optimization is to apply the MM methodology and design separable surrogate functions for the prior function (De Pierro, 1995), which lead to closed-form updates.

Standard gradient-based methods have also been applied to the MAP estimation problem. For example, the preconditioned conjugate gradient algorithm has been used for PET image reconstruction (Mumcuoglu et al., 1996) where the preconditioner is critical to the convergence speed of the algorithm. A simple diagonal preconditioner derived from the EM algorithm has been shown to be effective (Mumcuoglu et al., 1994). The ideal preconditioner is the inverse of the Hessian matrix (Luenberger, 1984), and several methods have been proposed to approximate it, such as using the inverse of the diagonal of the Hessian matrix (Johnson et al., 2000), Fourier-based preconditioners (Fessler and Booth, 1999), and matrix factorization (Chinn and Huang, 1997).

Unlike in the EM algorithm, the nonnegativity constraint needs to be handled explicitly in gradient-based methods. This can be achieved by several strategies, including restricting the step size (Kaufman, 1987), performing bent line searches that involve a secondary line search (Kaufman, 1993), or using an active set approach (Mumcuoglu et al., 1996). Penalty functions (Mumcuoglu et al., 1994) and interior-point methods (Johnson et al., 2000) have also been used.

The convergence rates of MAP algorithms are typically much faster than those of pure ML methods due to the improved conditioning of the inverse problem, and good-quality images can be reconstructed using tens of iterations (Qi et al., 1998).

9.6 CONCLUSIONS

In this chapter, we have described the basic algorithms for 2D and 3D reconstruction of PET and SPECT data. Analytic FBP reconstruction methods were the standard approach for clinical applications for many years, but recently have largely been replaced by iterative model-based techniques. Currently, OSEM remains the most popular statistical method, mainly due to low computational cost, although MAP or PML methods have more recently been made available for commercial preclinical (Chatziioannou et al., 2000) and clinical (Asma et al., 2012) systems.

In this chapter, we have focused on the reconstruction of a single image from 2D and 3D sinogram data. An alternative approach is to reconstruct images from list-mode data in which each detected event is recorded separately (Parra and Barrett, 1998; Huesman et al., 2000; Nichols et al., 2002; Reader et al., 2002; Li et al., 2007). List-mode reconstruction is especially attractive when the number of counts per LOR is low or when a large number of attributes of the data can be stored and used for reconstruction (e.g., arrival time, photon energy, and TOF information). If histogrammed into sinograms, they would have many zero entries, leading to inefficient data storage and access. The list-mode approach may therefore be more efficient, although some reordering of the list-mode data, in terms of the spatial arrangement of the LORs relative to the image, is preferable when computing forward and backprojections. Alternatively, histogrammed sinogram data could be stored in sparse format to reduce storage size and costs of forward and backprojection.

Another class of image reconstruction methods are designed to reconstruct parametric images directly from measurements (Kamasak et al., 2005; Karakatsanis et al., 2013; Zhu et al., 2014), instead of the traditional two-step approach, where the kinetic parameters are estimated from time–activity curves computed from a sequence of multiple temporal frames of reconstructed PET images. The model-based framework based on ML or MAP estimation described above for static PET imaging extends naturally to this dynamic formulation (e.g., see Zhu et al., 2014.)

In summary, image reconstruction methods for PET and SPECT are now relatively mature. Both analytic and model-based statistical methods are available to compute accurate quantitative images of tracer uptake for a wide range of tracers and system geometries for both PET and SPECT. Analytic methods have the advantage of linearity, which makes interpretation and quantitative analysis more straightforward, while model-based methods can usually achieve superior resolution or SNR, but at the expense of using nonlinear methods that make analysis of image properties more difficult (but still tractable). However, tomographic reconstruction remains a rich area for research, with continuing developments ranging from fundamental results related to the ability to reconstruct images from limited data (Clackdoyle and Defrise, 2010) to model-based reconstruction of parametric images from dynamically acquired list-mode data (Zhu et al., 2014).

REFERENCES

Ahn, S., Cho, S., Li, Q., Lin, Y., Leahy, R.M. 2011. Optimal rebinning of time-of-flight PET data. *IEEE Trans. Med. Imaging* 30, 1808–1818.

Ahn, S., Fessler, J.A. 2003. Globally convergent image reconstruction for emission tomography using relaxed ordered subsets algorithms. *IEEE Trans. Med. Imaging* 22, 613–626.

Ahn, S., Ross, S.G., Asma, E., Miao, J., Jin, X., Cheng, L., Wollenweber, S.D., Manjeshwar, R.M. 2015. Quantitative comparison of OSEM and penalized likelihood image reconstruction using relative differences for clinical PET. *Phys. Med. Biol.* 60, 5733–5751.

Alenius, S., Ruotsalainen, U. 1997. Bayesian image reconstruction for emission tomography based on median root prior. *Eur. J. Nucl. Med.* 24, 258–265.

Alessio, A., Sauer, K., Kinahan, P. 2007. Statistical image reconstruction from correlated data with applications to PET. *Phys. Med. Biol.* 52, 6133–6150.

Alessio, A.M., Kinahan, P.E., Lewellen, T.K. 2006. Modeling and incorporation of system response functions in 3-D whole body PET. *IEEE Trans. Med. Imaging* 25, 828–837.

Asma, E., Ahn, S., Qian, H., Gopalakrishnan, G., Thielemans, K., Ross, S.G., Manjeshwar, R.M., Ganin, A., GE Healthcare. 2012. Quantitatively accurate image reconstruction for clinical whole-body PET imaging. In *Annual Summit and Conference of the Asia-Pacific Signal and Information Processing Association*, Hollywood, CA, pp. 1–9.

Bai, B. 2012. An interior-point method for total variation regularized positron emission tomography image reconstruction. *Proc. SPIE* 8313, 83136B1–83136B6.

Bai, B., Li, Q., Leahy, R.M. 2013. Magnetic resonance-guided positron emission tomography image reconstruction. *Semin. Nucl. Med.* 43, 30–44.

Bai, B., Lin, Y., Zhu, W., Ren, R., Li, Q., Dahlbom, M., DiFilippo, F., Leahy, R.M. 2014. MAP reconstruction for Fourier rebinned TOF-PET data. *Phys. Med. Biol.* 59, 925–949.

Bai, B., Ruangma, A., Laforest, R., Tai, Y.C., Leahy, R.M. 2003. Positron range modeling for statistical PET image reconstruction. In *IEEE Nuclear Science Symposium and Medical Imaging Conference Record*, pp. 2501–2505. Piscataway, NJ: IEEE.

Besag, J. 1974. Spatial interaction and the statistical analysis of lattice systems. *J. R. Stat. Soc. Ser. B Methodol.* 36, 192–236.

Besson, G. 1996. CT fan-beam parametrizations leading to shift-invariant filtering. *Inverse Probl.* 12, 815–833.

Bouman, C.A., Sauer, K. 1996. A unified approach to statistical tomography using coordinate descent optimization. *IEEE Trans. Image Process.* 5, 480–492.

Browne, J., De Pierro, A.B. 1996. A row-action alternative to the EM algorithm for maximizing likelihood in emission tomography. *IEEE Trans. Med. Imaging* 15, 687–699.

Buonocore, M.H., Brody, W.R., Macovski, A. 1981. A natural pixel decomposition for two-dimensional image reconstruction. *IEEE Trans. Biomed. Eng.* 69–78.

Cabello, J., Rafecas, M. 2012. Comparison of basis functions for 3D PET reconstruction using a Monte Carlo system matrix. *Phys. Med. Biol.* 57, 1759–1777.

Candes, E.J., Romberg, J., Tao, T. 2006. Robust uncertainty principles: Exact signal reconstruction from highly incomplete frequency information. *IEEE Trans. Inf. Theory* 52, 489–509.

Chatziioannou, A., Qi, J., Moore, A., Annala, A., Nguyen, K., Leahy, R., Cherry, S.R. 2000. Comparison of 3-D maximum a posteriori and filtered backprojection algorithms for high-resolution animal imaging with microPET. *IEEE Trans. Med. Imaging* 19, 507–512.

Chinn, G., Huang, S.-C. 1997. A general class of preconditioners for statistical iterative reconstruction of emission computed tomography. *IEEE Trans. Med. Imaging* 16, 1–10.

Cho, S., Ahn, S., Li, Q., Leahy, R.M. 2008. Analytical properties of time-of-flight PET data. *Phys. Med. Biol.* 53, 2809–2821.

Cho, S., Ahn, S., Li, Q., Leahy, R.M. 2009. Exact and approximate Fourier rebinning of PET data from time-of-flight to non time-of-flight. *Phys. Med. Biol.* 54, 467–484.

Colsher, J.G. 1980. Fully three-dimensional positron emission tomography. *Phys. Med. Biol.* 25, 103–115.

Clackdoyle, R., Defrise, M. 2010. Tomographic reconstruction in the 21st century. *IEEE Signal Process. Mag.* 27(4), 60–80.

Daube-Witherspoon, M.E., Muehllehner, G. 1987. Treatment of axial data in three-dimensional PET. *J Nucl. Med.* 28, 1717–1724.

De Pierro, A.R. 1995. A modified expectation maximization algorithm for penalized likelihood estimation in emission tomography. *IEEE Trans. Med. Imaging* 14, 132–137.

Defrise, M. 1995. A factorization method for the 3D X-ray transform. *Inverse Probl.* 11, 983–994.

Defrise, M., Clack, R. 1994. A cone-beam reconstruction algorithm using shift-variant filtering and cone-beam backprojection. *IEEE Trans. Med. Imaging* 13, 186–195.

Defrise, M., Kinahan, P.E., Townsend, D.W., Michel, C., Sibomana, M., Newport, D.F. 1997. Exact and approximate rebinning algorithms for 3-D PET data. *IEEE Trans. Med. Imaging* 16, 145–158.

Dempster, A.P., Laird, N.M., Rubin, D.B. 1977. Maximum likelihood from incomplete data via the EM algorithm. *J. R. Stat. Soc. Ser. B Methodol.* 39, 1–38.

Farquhar, T.H., Chatziioannou, A., Chinn, G., Dahlbom, M., Hoffman, E.J. 1997. An investigation of filter choice for filtered back-projection reconstruction in PET. In *Nuclear Science Symposium and Medical Imaging Conference*, Albuquerque, NM, pp. 1042–1046.

Feldkamp, L.A., Davis, L.C., Kress, J.W. 1984. Practical cone-beam algorithm. *J Opt. Soc. Am. A* 1, 612–619.

Fessler, J.A. 1994. Penalized weighted least-squares image reconstruction for positron emission tomography. *IEEE Trans. Med. Imaging* 13, 290–300.

Fessler, J.A., Booth, S.D. 1999. Conjugate-gradient preconditioning methods for shift-variant PET image reconstruction. *IEEE Trans. Image Process.* 8, 688–699.

Fessler, J.A., Rogers, W.L. 1996. Spatial resolution properties of penalized-likelihood image reconstruction: Space-invariant tomographs. *IEEE Trans. Image Process.* 5, 1346–1358.

Fu, L., Qi, J. 2010. A residual correction method for high-resolution PET reconstruction with application to on-the-fly Monte Carlo based model of positron range. *Med. Phys.* 37, 704–713.

Geman, S., McClure, D. 1985. Bayesian image analysis: An application to single photon emission tomography. In *Proceedings of the American Statistical Association, Statistical Computing Section*, pp. 12–18. Washington, DC: American Statistical Association.

Green, P.J. 1990. Bayesian reconstructions from emission tomography data using a modified EM algorithm. *IEEE Trans. Med. Imaging* 9, 84–93.

Hebert, T., Leahy, R. 1989. A generalized EM algorithm for 3-D Bayesian reconstruction from Poisson data using Gibbs priors. *IEEE Trans. Med. Imaging* 8, 194–202.

Hoffman, E.J., Huang, S.-C., Phelps, M.E., Kuhl, D.E. 1981. Quantitation in positron emission computed tomography. 4. Effect of accidental coincidences. *J. Comput. Assist. Tomogr.* 5, 391–400.

Hounsfield, G.N. 1973. Computerized transverse axial scanning (tomography). Part 1. Description of system. *Br. J. Radiol.* 46, 1016–1022.

Hsiao, T., Rangarajan, A., Gindi, G. 2003. A new convex edge-preserving median prior with applications to tomography. *IEEE Trans. Med. Imaging* 22, 580–585.

Hudson, H.M., Larkin, R.S. 1994. Accelerated image reconstruction using ordered subsets of projection data. *IEEE Trans. Med. Imaging* 13, 601–609.

Huesman, R.H., Klein, G.J., Moses, W.W., Qi, J., Reutter, B.W., Virador, P.R. 2000. List-mode maximum-likelihood reconstruction applied to positron emission mammography (PEM) with irregular sampling. *IEEE Trans. Med. Imaging* 19, 532–537.

Hunter, D.R., Lange, K. 2004. A tutorial on MM algorithms. *Am. Stat.* 58, 30–37.

Jacobson, M.W., Fessler, J.A. 2007. An expanded theoretical treatment of iteration-dependent majorize-minimize algorithms. *IEEE Trans. Image Process.* 16, 2411–2422.

Jaszczak, R., Li, J., Wang, H., Zalutsky, M., Coleman, R. 1994. Pinhole collimation for ultra-high-resolution, small-field-of-view SPECT. *Phys. Med. Biol.* 39, 425–437.

Johnson, C.A., Seidel, J., Sofer, A. 2000. Interior-point methodology for 3-D PET reconstruction. *IEEE Trans. Med. Imaging* 19, 271–285.

Kamasak, M.E., Bouman, C.A., Morris, E.D., Sauer, K. 2005. Direct reconstruction of kinetic parameter images from dynamic PET data. *IEEE Trans. Med. Imaging* 24, 636–650.

Karakatsanis, N.A., Lodge, M.A., Tahari, A.K., Zhou, Y., Wahl, R.L., Rahmim, A. 2013. Dynamic whole-body PET parametric imaging. I. Concept, acquisition protocol optimization and clinical application. *Phys. Med. Biol.* 58, 7391–7418.

Kaufman, L. 1987. Implementing and accelerating the EM algorithm for positron emission tomography. *IEEE Trans. Med. Imaging* 6, 37–51.

Kaufman, L. 1993. Maximum likelihood, least squares, and penalized least squares for PET. *IEEE Trans. Med. Imaging* 12, 200–214.

Kinahan, P.E., Rogers, J.G. 1989. Analytic 3D image reconstruction using all detected events. *IEEE Trans. Nucl. Sci.* 36, 964–968.

Lange, K., Bahn, M., Little, R. 1987. A theoretical study of some maximum likelihood algorithms for emission and transmission tomography. *IEEE Trans. Med. Imaging* 6, 106–114.

Lange, K., Carson, R. 1984. EM reconstruction algorithms for emission and transmission tomography. *J. Comput. Assist. Tomogr.* 8, 306–316.

Lange, K., Fessler, J.A. 1995. Globally convergent algorithms for maximum a posteriori transmission tomography. *IEEE Trans. Image Process.* 4, 1430–1438.

Lartizien, C., Kinahan, P.E., Swensson, R., Comtat, C., Lin, M., Villemagne, V., Trébossen, R. 2003. Evaluating image reconstruction methods for tumor detection in 3-dimensional whole-body PET oncology imaging. *J. Nucl. Med.* 44, 276–290.

Li, Q., Ahn, S., Leahy, R. 2005. Fast hybrid algorithms for PET image reconstruction. In *Nuclear Science Symposium and Medical Imaging Conference Record*, pp. 1851–1855. Piscataway, NJ: IEEE.

Li, Q., Asma, E., Ahn, S., Leahy, R.M. 2007. A fast fully 4-D incremental gradient reconstruction algorithm for list mode PET data. *IEEE Trans. Med. Imaging* 26, 58–67.

Li, Q., Leahy, R.M. 2006. Statistical modeling and reconstruction of randoms precorrected PET data. *IEEE Trans. Med. Imaging* 25, 1565–1572.

Liu, X., Comtat, C., Michel, C., Kinahan, P., Defrise, M., Townsend, D. 2001. Comparison of 3-D reconstruction with 3D-OSEM and with FORE+OSEM for PET. *IEEE Trans. Med. Imaging* 20, 804–814.

Llacer, J., Veklerov, E., Coakley, K.J., Hoffman, E.J., Nunez, J. 1993. Statistical analysis of maximum likelihood estimator images of human brain FDG PET studies. *IEEE Trans. Med. Imaging* 12, 215–231.

Luenberger, D.G. 1984. *Linear and Non-Linear Programming*. Reading, MA: Addison-Wesley.

Matej, S., Lewitt, R.M. 1996. Practical considerations for 3-D image reconstruction using spherically symmetric volume elements. *IEEE Trans. Med. Imaging* 15, 68–78.

Metzler, S.D., Bowsher, J.E., Greer, K.L., Jaszczak, R.J. 2002. Analytic determination of the pinhole collimator's point-spread function and RMS resolution with penetration. *IEEE Trans. Med. Imaging* 21, 878–887.

Moore, S.C., Kouris, K., Cullum, I. 1992. Collimator design for single photon emission tomography. *Eur. J. Nucl. Med.* 19, 138–150.

Mumcuoglu, E.U., Leahy, R.M., Cherry, S.R. 1996. Bayesian reconstruction of PET images: Methodology and performance analysis. *Phys. Med. Biol.* 41, 1777–1807.

Mumcuoglu, E.U., Leahy, R., Cherry, S.R., Zhou, Z. 1994. Fast gradient-based methods for Bayesian reconstruction of transmission and emission PET images. *IEEE Trans. Med. Imaging* 13, 687–701.

Nichols, T.E., Qi, J., Asma, E., Leahy, R.M. 2002. Spatiotemporal reconstruction of list-mode PET data. *IEEE Trans. Med. Imaging* 21, 396–404.

Nuyts, J., Bequé, D., Dupont, P., Mortelmans, L. 2002. A concave prior penalizing relative differences for maximum-a-posteriori reconstruction in emission tomography. *IEEE Trans. Nucl. Sci.* 49, 56–60.

Panin, V.Y., Kehren, F., Michel, C., Casey, M. 2006. Fully 3-D PET reconstruction with system matrix derived from point source measurements. *IEEE Trans. Med. Imaging* 25, 907–921.

Panin, V.Y., Zeng, G.L., Gullberg, G.T. 1999. Total variation regulated EM algorithm [SPECT reconstruction]. *IEEE Trans. Nucl. Sci.* 46, 2202–2210.

Parra, L., Barrett, H.H. 1998. List-mode likelihood: EM algorithm and image quality estimation demonstrated on 2-D PET. *IEEE Trans. Med. Imaging* 17, 228–235.

Qi, J., Leahy, R.M. 2000. Resolution and noise properties of MAP reconstruction for fully 3-D PET. *IEEE Trans. Med. Imaging* 19, 493–506.

Qi, J., Leahy, R.M., Cherry, S.R., Chatziioannou, A., Farquhar, T.H. 1998. High-resolution 3D Bayesian image reconstruction using the microPET small-animal scanner. *Phys. Med. Biol.* 43, 1001–1013.

Radon, J. 1917. On determination of functions by their integral values along certain multiplicities. *Ber. Sachsische Akad. Wiss. Leipzig Germany* 69, 262–277.

Rahmim, A., Qi, J., Sossi, V. 2013. Resolution modeling in PET imaging: Theory, practice, benefits, and pitfalls. *Med. Phys.* 40, 064301.

Reader, A.J., Ally, S., Bakatselos, F., Manavaki, R., Walledge, R.J., Jeavons, A.P., Julyan, P.J., Zhao, S., Hastings, D.L., Zweit, J. 2002. One-pass list-mode EM algorithm for high-resolution 3-D PET image reconstruction into large arrays. *IEEE Trans. Nucl. Sci.* 49, 693–699.

Shepp, L.A., Logan, B. 1974. The Fourier reconstruction of a head section. *IEEE Trans. Nucl. Sci.* 21, 21–33.

Shepp, L.A., Vardi, Y. 1982. Maximum likelihood reconstruction for emission tomography. *IEEE Trans. Med. Imaging* 1, 113–122.

Sidky, E.Y., Pan, X. 2008. Image reconstruction in circular cone-beam computed tomography by constrained, total-variation minimization. *Phys. Med. Biol.* 53, 4777–4807.

Tohme, M.S., Qi, J. 2009. Iterative image reconstruction for positron emission tomography based on a detector response function estimated from point source measurements. *Phys. Med. Biol.* 54, 3709–3725.

Tomitani, T. 1981. Image reconstruction and noise evaluation in photon time-of-flight assisted positron emission tomography. *IEEE Trans. Nucl. Sci.* 28, 4581–4589.

Tsui, B., Frey, E. 2006. Analytic image reconstruction methods in emission computed tomography. In *Quantitative Analysis in Nuclear Medicine Imaging*. Berlin: Springer, pp. 82–106.

Tuy, H.K. 1983. An inversion formula for cone-beam reconstruction. *SIAM J. Appl. Math.* 43, 546–552.

Vardi, Y., Shepp, L.A., Kaufman, L. 1985. A statistical model for positron emission tomography. *J. Am. Stat. Assoc.* 80, 8–20.

Veklerov, E., Llacer, J. 1987. Stopping rule for the MLE algorithm based on statistical hypothesis testing. *IEEE Trans. Med. Imaging* 6, 313–319.

Vunckx, K., Atre A., Baete, K., Reilhac A., Deroose C.M., Van Laere K., Nuyts, J. 2012. Evaluation of three MRI-based anatomical priors for quantitative PET brain imaging. *IEEE Trans. Med. Imaging* 31, 599–612.

Wang, G., Qi, J. 2013. Edge-preserving PET image reconstruction using trust optimization transfer. In *12th International Meeting on Fully Three-Dimensional Image Reconstruction in Radiology and Nuclear Medicine*, Lake Tahoe, CA, pp. 70–73.

Watson, C.C. 2007. An evaluation of image noise variance for time-of-flight PET. *IEEE Trans. Nucl. Sci.* 54, 1639–1647.

Yavuz, M. 2000. Statistical tomographic image reconstruction methods for randoms precorrected PET measurements. PhD thesis, University of Michigan, Ann Arbor.

Yavuz, M., Fessler, J.A. 1998. Statistical image reconstruction methods for randoms-precorrected PET scans. *Med. Image Anal.* 2, 369–378.

Yendiki, A., Fessler, J.A. 2004. A comparison of rotation-and blob-based system models for 3D SPECT with depth-dependent detector response. *Phys. Med. Biol.* 49, 2157–2168.

Zhu, W., Li, Q., Bai, B., Conti, P., Leahy, R. 2014. Patlak image estimation from dual time-point list-mode PET data. *IEEE Trans. Med. Imaging* 33, 913–924.

10

High-performance computing in emission tomography

GUILLEM PRATX

10.1	Introduction	260
10.2	Parallelism in PET and SPECT	261
	10.2.1 Building blocks for data-parallel algorithms	261
	10.2.2 Sinogram correction	262
	10.2.3 Image reconstruction	262
	10.2.3.1 Fast Fourier transform	262
	10.2.3.2 Backprojection	263
	10.2.3.3 Iterative reconstruction	264
	10.2.3.4 List-mode reconstruction	265
	10.2.4 Monte Carlo simulation	265
10.3	GPU platform	266
	10.3.1 Short history of the GPU	266
	10.3.2 Graphics pipeline	267
	10.3.3 GPU as a coprocessor	270
	10.3.4 Cooperation between threads	272
	10.3.5 Allocating resources	274
	10.3.6 Efficient memory operations	275
	10.3.7 Advanced concepts	277
10.4	Applications of GPU computing	277
	10.4.1 Backprojection using texture mapping	277
	10.4.2 Back- and forward projection using CUDA	278
	10.4.3 Multi-GPU reconstruction	279
	10.4.4 List-mode projection operations	279
	10.4.5 Monte Carlo simulation	280
10.5	Other considerations	281
	References	282

10.1 INTRODUCTION

The ECAT II, one of the very first commercial PET systems, has a simple design: its 66 detectors were arranged in a single partial ring to measure coincidence events along 363 lines of response (Phelps et al. 1978). For image reconstruction, it came equipped with a DEC PDP-11/45, a computer capable of executing 189,000 instructions per second with only 32 KB of memory. Thirty-five years later, at the time of this writing, PET systems have changed tremendously. They have tens of thousands of detectors, spanning multiple rings. Their image reconstruction uses iterative algorithms that accurately model the coincidence detection process, including scatter, attenuation, resolution blurring, and time of flight. With these advances, computing requirements for processing and reconstruction have exploded. A state-of-the-art PET system, such as the Philips Gemini TF, comprises 28,336 detector elements and performs the reconstruction entirely in list mode to preserve the full spatial and temporal resolution of the measurements (Surti et al. 2007). For practical reconstruction times, the system comes equipped with a cluster of four computers, each with two six-core CPUs—a total peak performance of 640.8 billion floating-point operations per second (FLOPS) (Table 10.1). Stunningly, this amounts to a 3 million–fold increase in the utilization of computing for PET over a span of 30 years, a 60% yearly increase.

Demand for fast computation is exploding, whether it is for scientific or consumer applications. Computation-intensive applications are now starting to appear on consumer devices, such as voice and gesture recognition, computer vision, and artificial intelligence. This need for faster computation is driving the microprocessor industry to find new ways of increasing the performance of their devices. The performance of a computer task depends on how fast the processor is executing instructions. Until the early 2000s, the paradigm that dominated computing was that processors issued their instructions one at a time, and therefore, faster computation meant a faster internal clock. However, clock speeds have reached the physical limit imposed by energy dissipation. In response, the microprocessor industry has shifted its focus to a new paradigm: general-purpose processors should handle higher workloads by executing multiple instructions at the same time. Instead of faster clock frequency, modern processors embed multiple parallel processing units, each performing computation in parallel. Recently released processors are predominantly based on such multi- and many-core architectures. These new parallel architectures can provide faster performance provided that software is designed to run their workload in parallel.

Scientific computing is also adapting to the shift from sequential to parallel computing. Many scientific computing packages now exploit the availability of multiple computing cores for improved performance. These scientific packages complement the rich ecosystem of parallel computing tools that have been developed for clusters of commodity computers (e.g., MPI and OpenMP). Parallel computing tools have found use in many medical imaging applications, including emission tomography reconstruction (Martino et al. 1994).

One of the most exciting developments in high-performance computing has been the invention and evolution of the *graphics processing unit* (GPU). While the original goal of the GPU was to accelerate graphics computation for three-dimensional (3D) video games, over the years, it has matured into a general-purpose coprocessor for massively parallel computation (Owens et al. 2008). It is an inexpensive platform with a rich ecosystem of developer toolkits and packages. Its hardware capabilities, although designed for computer graphics, can be very useful for accelerating medical imaging applications.

Table 10.1 Characteristics of two PET systems and their image reconstruction hardware

PET system	Year	Detectors	Features	Reconstruction platform	Peak performance
ECAT	1977	66	Single ring	PDP-11/45	0.189 MIPS
Philips Gemini TF	2007	28,336	3D acquisition	Intel Xeon E5645 (8X)	640.8 GLOPS
			List mode		
			Time of flight		

Note: MIPS, million instructions per second; GFLOPS, billion floating-point operations per second.

Increasingly, research and commercial software for PET and SPECT imaging is based, at least in part, on GPU hardware acceleration. As such, knowing the basics of GPU computing should be a priority for anyone wanting to develop efficient code for image processing and reconstruction. Fortunately, programming the GPU is easy to learn. An abundance of tools has been developed to help the programmer write high-level code that is easy to maintain, yet uses the computational power of thousands of parallel computing units.

This chapter is organized as follows. Section 10.2 describes how to parallelize emission tomography computation on a generic hardware platform using standard building blocks. The rest of this chapter focuses more specifically on the GPU platform. Section 10.3 explains the architecture of the GPU and presents various strategies for optimizing performance. Section 10.4 reviews several important applications of emission tomography on GPU hardware. Section 10.5 concludes the chapter with a few practical considerations.

10.2 PARALLELISM IN PET AND SPECT

10.2.1 BUILDING BLOCKS FOR DATA-PARALLEL ALGORITHMS

Most data-parallel algorithms can be decomposed into a set of generic building blocks (Asanovic et al. 2006). The advantage of doing so is that there are methods available to implement these blocks on a distributed computing architecture with high efficiency. The simplest building block in the parallel computing toolbox is the *map* operation. This operation simply applies a function to an array of input data, producing an array of output data of the same size (Figure 10.1). It is usually the most straightforward building block to implement because its does not require communication between multiple parallel units.

Another common building block is the *reduce* operation, also known as a reduction (Figure 10.1). This operation combines many input elements into fewer elements, with each input element contributing to no more than one output element. Reductions are an important type of computation and are used for applications such as computing high-level statistics from a dataset.

Two other operations frequently used for image reconstruction are *gather* and *scatter* operations. These two operations are mathematically equivalent but lead to different distributed implementations. A gather operation partitions the computation according to the output. For each output element, it reads, processes, and combines corresponding inputs (Figure 10.1). Therefore, the focus of a gather operation is backward. In opposition, a scatter operation is forward looking. It partitions the data according to the input and, for each input element, computes contributions to multiple output elements, which are accumulated since an output may receive contributions from more than one input. In a serial execution model, a gather operation is implemented using a nested loop: an outer loop over the output elements and an inner loop over the input elements. A scatter operation is the reverse: the outer loop is over the input and the inner loop over the output. On a parallel architecture, the outer loop is typically distributed over multiple processing elements.

The last two common building blocks are *scan* and *search* operations. Scan operations are used for sorting arrays and producing histograms. Search operations are used for finding a particular value among an array of

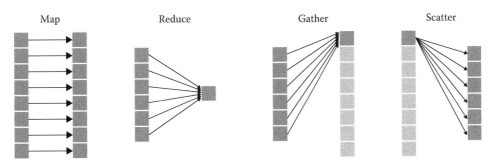

Figure 10.1 Depiction of four of the computing building blocks used to represent data-parallel algorithms.

data. Both operations can be parallelized for efficient processing of very large datasets, but are not frequently used in medical imaging applications.

In the rest of this section, we identify those building blocks used in emission tomography algorithms. This analysis is independent of the specific hardware used to run the parallel computation. To keep our description general, we call *processing element* a generic piece of hardware capable of executing a sequence of arithmetic and memory operations. A processing element may be a CPU or GPU core.

10.2.2 SINOGRAM CORRECTION

Data acquired from PET and SPECT systems are inherently parallel. They are composed of many similar elements, such as individual prompt events (for a list-mode acquisition) or sinogram elements (for a sinogram acquisition). As such, applying corrections to these data is inherently a parallel task.

Prior to performing filtered backprojection, a PET sinogram must be corrected for randoms, scatter, attenuation, and normalization. These corrections are applied component-wise, with each component processed independently. The corrections can be modeled as multiplicative and additive components, noted a and b, respectively. Sinogram correction is a typical example of a map operation; therefore, it is easily parallelizable.

Figure 10.2 shows the difference between a sequential and a parallel program. The sequential program processes elements sequentially, using an index to enumerate all the elements. In contrast, the equivalent parallel program defines a unique index for each processing element, which is updated so that each sinogram element is processed exactly once. Note that in this example, we assume that the sinogram and correction factors are stored in a memory location accessible to all processing elements. Later in this chapter, we demonstrate an implementation of this example on a GPU using hundreds of parallel cores.

10.2.3 IMAGE RECONSTRUCTION

10.2.3.1 FAST FOURIER TRANSFORM

The fast Fourier transform (FFT) is used extensively in medical imaging applications such as computed tomography (CT) and magnetic resonance imaging. It can be applied to one-dimensional (1D) vectors or k-dimensional (k-D) arrays. A k-D FFT is equivalent to multiple 1D FFTs that are performed along each dimension and for each row of elements. Hence, transforming a N^k matrix requires kN^{k-1} independent 1D FFTs. Since these computations are independent, they are considered map operations, where the inputs are different rows of the matrix. The parallelization of these 1D FFTs is straightforward. Each processing element is responsible for transforming one or more rows. In a shared memory architecture, the processing elements can access the entire matrix. We note that for some hardware architectures, memory access may be slower along certain dimensions because of interleaved memory access. In addition, in a distributed memory

Serial execution

Parallel execution

```
i=0;
while (i<N) {
  s2[i] = s[i]/a[i]-b[i];
  i=i+1;
}
```

Core 1
```
i=0;
while (i<N) {
  s2[i] = s[i]/a[i]-b[i];
  i=i+4;
}
```

Core 2
```
i=1;
while (i<N) {
  s2[i] = s[i]/a[i]-b[i];
  i=i+4;
}
```

Core 3
```
i=2;
while (i<N) {
  s2[i] = s[i]/a[i]-b[i];
  i=i+4;
}
```

Core 4
```
i=□;
while (i<N) {
  s2[i] = s[i]/a[i]-b[i];
  i=i+4;
}
```

Figure 10.2 Comparison between serial and parallel execution, shown for a computer algorithm that applies multiplicative and additive corrections to a sinogram.

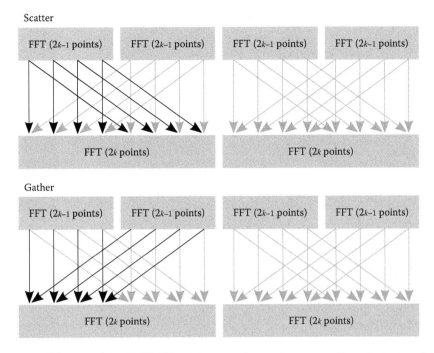

Figure 10.3 Parallelization of the 1D FFT. The dark arrows show tasks executed by a single thread, while the gray arrows are tasks executed by other parallel threads.

architecture, each processing element can only see a fraction of the full matrix. Therefore, data must be exchanged each time the matrix is transposed (i.e., $k - 1$ times).

A 1D FFT can also be performed in a distributed fashion. The 1D FFT procedure is recursive: a transform of size 2^N can be computed by performing two transforms of size 2^{N-1}. This procedure suggests a simple way of distributing computation, by distributing it according to either the input (scatter) or the output (gather). Figure 10.3 shows how intermediary computation can be distributed in either a scatter or gather manner. This mapping is repeated $N - 1$ times.

10.2.3.2 BACKPROJECTION

In simple terms, backprojection is an image reconstruction operation that consists in smearing sinogram elements uniformly along lines of response to produce an image. Mathematically, backprojection can be expressed as a matrix-vector multiplication:

$$x = A^T y \tag{10.1}$$

where y are the sinogram measurements, x is the output image, and A is the system matrix describing the measurement process. Equation 10.1 can be further expanded as

$$x_j = \sum_{i=1}^{N} a_{ij} y_i \tag{10.2}$$

where a_{ij} are the coefficients of the system matrix. In a serial execution program, this matrix–vector multiplication can be performed using a nested loop over the image elements (index i) and sinogram elements (index j). A simple parallel implementation of backprojection distributes the outer loop to parallel processing elements, while the inner loop is performed serially. Because the outer loop can be over either image voxels or sinogram elements, backprojection can be performed in either a gather or scatter manner.

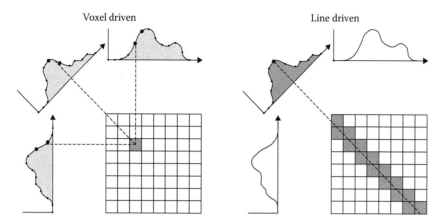

Figure 10.4 Comparison between voxel- and line-driven backprojection of sinogram data. Shading represents voxels updated by a single thread.

Computation is called *voxel driven* when it is parallelized in the image domain, with the outer loop over image voxels (Figure 10.4, left). Each processing element is assigned a voxel and *gathers* sinogram elements that correspond to lines of response intersecting that voxel. For each voxel written to memory, the processing element reads multiple sinogram elements. The dual formulation is the *line-driven* backprojection, which partitions computation in the sinogram domain (Figure 10.4, right). Each processing element is responsible for smearing a sinogram element along the corresponding line of response through the image, in a *scatter* fashion. For each sinogram element read from memory, the processing element writes multiple image voxels back to memory.

As seen in the previous example, a gather formulation requires a large number of read operations but only one write operation per processing element. In contrast, a scatter formulation requires one read operation but multiple write operations. Gather operations are preferable for parallel processing, because they avoid data write conflicts. These conflicts arise when multiple processing elements attempt to update the same memory address at the same time. Most memory systems require special hardware to handle simultaneous write requests. Furthermore, memory reads are cached and, for this reason, generally more efficient than writes. As we will see in more detail in Section 10.3, a cache is a short-term memory that helps accelerate memory transactions by guessing which memory elements will be needed in the future.

10.2.3.3 ITERATIVE RECONSTRUCTION

Iterative reconstruction methods such as expectation maximization, ordered subsets expectation maximization, and maximum a posteriori reconstruction present a better trade-off between noise and spatial resolution than filtered backprojection. Forward- and backprojection operations, which are common to all iterative reconstruction algorithms, represent the principal target for parallelization due to their high computational burden.

The expectation maximization algorithm, taken here as an example, can be expressed as

$$x_j^{(n+1)} = \frac{x_j^{(n)}}{\sum_{i=1}^{N} a_{ij}} \sum_{i=1}^{N} \frac{y_i}{\sum_{j=1}^{P} a_{ij} x_j^{(n)}}$$

(10.3)

Briefly, this algorithm first computes the forward projection of a previous image estimate $x^{(n)}$. The component-wise ratio of the measured data y to the forward projection is then propagated back into the image domain by backprojection and used as a multiplicative correction factor for $x^{(n)}$. Finally, a normalization factor is applied component-wise in the image domain. All component-wise computations used in this algorithm are map operations, straightforward to implement on a parallel architecture.

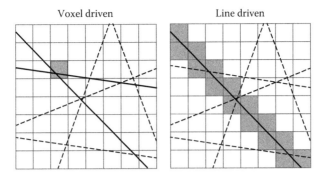

Figure 10.5 Comparison between voxel- and line-driven projections for list-mode data. Shading represents voxels updated by a single thread.

Recall that backprojection is mathematically represented by multiplication by A^T. Forward projection is simply multiplication by the system matrix A. Similar to backprojection, forward projection can be line driven or voxel driven, but with opposite partitioning of the input and output. A *voxel-driven* forward projection *scatters* voxel values into the sinogram elements it intersects. It partitions computation in the image domain, that is, the input. Conversely, a *line-driven* forward projection *gathers* voxel values along lines of response, and writes the result to the corresponding sinogram bins. Forward projections are computed more efficiently in a line-driven manner, and thus are different from backprojection in this regard.

10.2.3.4 LIST-MODE RECONSTRUCTION

Image reconstruction in PET and SPECT is most commonly performed using sinograms. Sinograms provide compact data storage and are compatible with a wide range of existing reconstruction algorithms. However, the only way to store temporal or time-of-flight information using a sinogram is to create a different sinogram for each time gate or each time-of-flight bin. This leads to sparse data storage, especially when the number of events is less than the total number of sinogram elements.

List-mode processing is a method of storing PET and SPECT data on an event-by-event basis, using a long list. List mode preserves the full spatial and temporal resolution of the measurements. Furthermore, the expectation maximization algorithm can be modified to reconstruct images directly from list-mode measurements, without the intermediate step of binning the events into a sinogram. List-mode processing is most useful for time-of-flight and dynamic PET. For the latter application, it also allows for retrospective gating of the data into different breathing and cardiac phases.

The difference between list-mode and sinogram processing is in the implementation of the projection operations. While sinogram processing can be implemented using either voxel-driven or line-driven operations, voxel-driven operations are not efficient in list mode (Figure 10.5). List-mode events are not arranged in any particular order, but are rather stored in the order they were acquired. Finding which lines intersect a given voxel is computationally challenging, as it requires searching through the entire list of events. Given this, list-mode backprojection must be performed in a line-driven fashion using scatter operations. Implementation of such methods must be carefully designed to avoid errors due to data write hazards. Furthermore, because list-mode events are unorganized, the reconstruction algorithm must access memory randomly, which is inefficient. In Section 10.4, we will see various strategies to mitigate these issues on a GPU.

10.2.4 MONTE CARLO SIMULATION

Monte Carlo methods are extensively used in nuclear medicine to simulate imaging systems involving large numbers of independent physical particles. These methods compute the histories of billions of individual particles, resulting in high accuracy but also high computational requirements. The most straightforward way of accelerating Monte Carlo simulation is to partition computation over groups of particle histories, since these histories can be computed independently of one another. In a standard parallel implementation, individual processing elements are tasked with computing the history of a group of particles, including secondary particles, if any (e.g., fluorescent x-rays, recoil electrons, and photoelectrons).

Monte Carlo simulation relies heavily on pseudo-random numbers. To avoid correlation between parallel simulations, the initialization is a crucial step. A list of distinct seeds should be distributed to each of the parallel processing units prior to starting computation. For each random seed and time interval, a simulation is executed in parallel and produces an output; thus, Monte Carlo simulation is considered a map operation. The outputs produced by parallel Monte Carlo tasks can be aggregated by parallel reduce operations. A word of caution is warranted, however: although Monte Carlo simulation is easily broken down into parallel tasks, it is sometimes challenging to run these parallel tasks efficiently on the certain computing devices. Later in this chapter, we will see practical implementations of Monte Carlo simulation on a GPU.

Having now concluded this overview of the various types of parallel computing operations, we focus in the rest of this chapter on PET and SPECT reconstruction using the GPU.

10.3 GPU PLATFORM

10.3.1 SHORT HISTORY OF THE GPU

Early computers could run applications either in text mode or using a graphical interface. Text-mode applications have nearly disappeared today, but their use was once very common due to their very low computational requirements. Graphical applications quickly became more popular because they could provide a more sophisticated user interface, even though they used the CPU more heavily. As graphical applications became more widespread, the portion of CPU time dedicated to graphics kept growing. Hardware manufacturers thus saw an opportunity for dedicated two-dimensional (2D) graphics cards that could free up valuable CPU time. With the rising popularity of immersive 3D video games, graphics cards that could also accelerate 3D graphics were introduced. The development of these technologies was driven by companies such as Silicon Graphics (SGI), 3D-FX, NVIDIA, and ATI. An important milestone was achieved when SGI developed an open language (OpenGL) to express graphical operations within computer programs, as it allows for standardization of computer code among various hardware manufacturers.

Eventually, highly specialized GPUs became faster than general-purpose CPUs, at least in terms of raw compute power, and researchers started to wonder whether GPUs could be used to run computing tasks other than graphics rendering. Noting that backprojection is similar to texture mapping, researchers at SGI were able to perform backprojection on a graphics workstation by disguising computation as graphics operations (Cabral et al. 1994). (This is explained in more detail in Section 10.4). The GPU backprojection technique they developed was 100 times faster than the equivalent CPU version. To put it into perspective, it took CPUs 10 years of Moore's law exponential growth to beat this first GPU implementation.

However, early GPU computing remained limited because GPUs could only perform integer operations and only few problems could be disguised as graphics computation. This changed with the introduction of the first programmable GPU in 2003. Unlike previous GPUs, which could only execute predefined functions in a predefined order, these new GPUs were able to run custom programs called *shaders* that were written and compiled by the developer using a new GPU-specific language (Owens et al. 2007).

With the later introduction of floating-point precision arithmetic, programmable GPUs became able to perform most types of data-parallel computation, including iterative reconstruction and image segmentation (Rumpf and Strzodka 2001; Xu and Mueller 2005). GPU programming remained complicated because computation still had to be programmed using a graphics interface. A few research groups developed toolkits (e.g., Brooks) that could translate general-purpose computation into rendering tasks, but those toolkits were limited in their performance and capabilities. GPU computing really became mainstream when hardware manufacturers allowed software developers to directly tap into the computational resources of the GPU, without having to reformulate computation as graphics tasks. The ability to program the GPU in a standard language (e.g., C++), via a compute-specific interface, marked the beginning of a new era for parallel computing. GPUs have since been used for a variety of compute-intensive applications, including

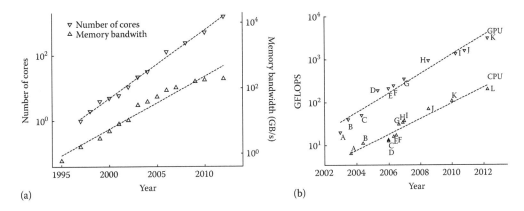

Figure 10.6 Trends in GPU computing. (a) Evolution in the number of cores and memory bandwidth from 1995 to 2012. (b) Evolution in overall performance, measured in billion floating-point operations per second (GFLOPS), for GPUs and CPUs. GPUs: (A) NVIDIA GeForce FX 5800, (B) FX 5950 Ultra, (C) 6800 Ultra, (D) 7800 GTX, (E) Quadro FX 4500, (F) GeForce 7900 GTX, (G) 8800 GTX, (H) GTX 280, (I) GTX 480, (J) GTX 580, and (K) GTX 680. CPUs: (A) Athlon 64 3200+, (B) Pentium IV 560, (C) Pentium D 960, (D) 950, (E) Athlon 64 X2 5000+, (F) Core 2 Duo E6700, (G) Core 2 Quad Q6600, (H) Athlon 64 FX-74, (I) Core 2 Quad QX6700, (J) Core i7 965 XE, (K) Core i7-980X Extreme, and (L) Xeon E5-2687W. (Reproduced from Pratx, G., Xing, L. *Med Phys* 38:2685–2697, 2011. With permission.)

financial modeling, fluid mechanics, protein folding, and image processing (Owens et al. 2008; Pratx and Xing 2011).

A remarkable fact about GPUs is that their performance has kept increasing rapidly over the years, outpacing computing platforms. Overall, performance growth has been driven by the spectacular increase in the number of cores and memory bandwidth (Figure 10.6). The number of FLOPS achievable with a GPU has doubled every 1.3 years, compared with 1.6 years for CPUs, and recently, GPUs have even broken the symbolic barrier of 1 trillion FLOPS (single precision) on a single chip.

10.3.2 GRAPHICS PIPELINE

While modern GPU computing applications are now all built using compute-specific application programming interfaces (APIs), it is useful to understand how graphics rendering works because a medical imaging application may need to display graphics. Furthermore, general-purpose GPU computing uses concepts directly derived from computer graphics.

The graphics pipeline is a concept that describes how the various components of the GPU are linked together to provide fast graphics. The term *pipeline* indicates that data flows through multiple processing stages, with geometrical vertices entering the GPU on one end, and output images being progressively painted on the other end. Typically, a 3D scene (e.g., in a video game) is represented by a collection of 3D triangular meshes, which are filled with color or texture. Textures are bitmap images that are drawn onto a 3D surface to increase the perceived complexity of a 3D scene. For instance, a foliage texture may be drawn onto the 3D model of a tree.

Typically, a single GPU can draw 1 billion triangles in less than 1 s. Designed to meet the requirements of video games, the GPU has evolved toward an architecture that favors throughput over latency. With the wide availability of high-definition screens, throughput is a higher priority for GPUs because it determines the level of detail of a 3D scene, whereas latency determines the frame rate, which is of lesser importance because the human visual system is not sensitive to frame rates above 50 Hz.

The GPU uses both *task parallelism* and *data parallelism* to achieve high processing throughput. The graphics pipeline decomposes graphics computation into a sequence of stages that expose task parallelism. Task parallelism is achieved when data at different stages of the pipeline is processed simultaneously. Taking laundry as a simple analogy, a task-parallel system can perform different tasks (e.g., washing, drying, and ironing) on different loads simultaneously (Figure 10.7). Task parallelism requires dedicated hardware

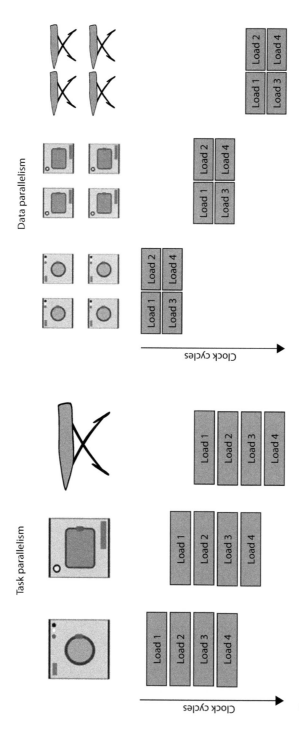

Figure 10.7 Illustration of task and data parallelism. Task parallelism is achieved when the same task is performed on multiple data at the same time. Data parallelism is achieved when multiple tasks are performed at the same time.

for each stage of the pipeline. However, a process can only be broken down into a finite number of stages. Therefore, the GPU also uses data parallelism to achieve high throughput. Data parallelism is achieved when the same task is performed simultaneously on multiple data elements. In the laundry analogy, it is analogous to washing multiple loads using multiple machines (Figure 10.7). Here, the entire processing hardware is simply replicated as many times as needed.

This organization of the GPU has been very successful for computer graphics applications. The hardware implementation of the GPU is highly efficient because each stage of the graphics pipeline is implemented with special-purpose hardware. While a given triangle might take hundreds to thousands of clock cycles to make its way through the pipeline and be rendered, at any time tens of thousands of vertices and fragments are in flight in the pipeline. At any stage, the hardware of the GPU exploits data parallelism by processing multiple elements at the same time.

The graphics pipeline consists of five main stages, two of which are fully programmable (Figure 10.8). A stream of triangular vertices, representing objects in a 3D scene, enters the GPU from the computer's main memory. At the output end of the pipeline, a 2D raster image is slowly synthesized. As an illustration, we will follow a triangle—that is, three vertices—as it makes its way through the pipeline. We will assume that each vertex in the triangle is of a different shade of gray (Figure 10.8).

Upon entering the GPU, these three vertices are transformed by vertex shaders, which are programmable parallel processing units (Figure 10.8). The role of the vertex shaders is to simulate how a virtual camera would project the triangle coordinates into its focal plane. Typically, the projection is a perspective transformation, but other user-defined projections are possible as well. Next, the triangle must be discretized into a set of discrete fragments. In computer graphics, a fragment is defined as a small data structure that contains all the information needed to update a pixel in the framebuffer, such as pixel and texture coordinates, depth, and color. The conversion of a triangle into a set of fragments is called rasterization. During this process, newly created fragments inherit properties (e.g., color) from their three parent vertices, using bilinear interpolation to blend the contribution of each. In the case of the example triangle, the inside of the triangle is filled by a linear gradient of gray shading.

The stream of fragments produced during rasterization is then processed by parallel *fragment shaders* (Figure 10.8). Fragment shaders can fetch data from textures, calculate lighting effects, determine occlusions,

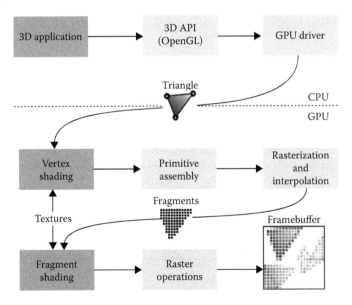

Figure 10.8 GPU pipeline. The GPU can render a 3D scene (represented by a triangular mesh) by drawing each triangle individually. These triangles can be modified in parallel by programmable vertex shaders. After rasterization, each triangle is converted to a set of fragments. These fragments can be modified by fragment shaders and are eventually written to the framebuffer to form a 2D image. (Reproduced from Pratx, G., Xing, L. *Med Phys* 38:2685–2697, 2011. With permission.)

and combine various layers to simulate transparency. They are responsible for putting the finishing touches on the triangle before it is written to the framebuffer. Due to the large number of fragments, this stage concentrates most of the GPU's compute resources. The processed fragments are used to update the framebuffer according to user-defined rules that specify how multiple overlapping triangles should be combined with respect to occlusions and transparency.

The graphics pipeline is programmed using a graphics library such as OpenGL or DirectX. These libraries allow the user to define their 3D models as combinations of triangular meshes and textures. To customize the rendering of a scene, the user can also write shader programs in a high-level language such as Cg or HLSL. Those languages provide a rich set of features, which include control flow, vector arithmetic operations (up to 4D), and memory operations. While technically feasible, general-purpose computation using those rendering interfaces has been supplanted by more practical compute-specific interfaces, which will be presented in the next section.

10.3.3 GPU AS A COPROCESSOR

Modern computers are heterogeneous computing systems, with the CPU (the *host*) the main processor and the GPU (the *device*) a massively parallel coprocessor. Both host and device have their own dedicated memory. The basic idea behind GPU computing is to move data-parallel tasks from the CPU to the GPU for faster processing. Because the host and device cannot directly access each other's memory, input data must be transferred to the device memory before computation can start; any GPU output must also be transferred back to the host memory afterwards. These data transfers, which are initiated by the CPU, transit via the PCI Express bus at a speed much lower than typical memory transactions.

A wide range of software tools are available for programming the GPU. At the lowest level, the programmer can use an API such as CUDA or OpenCL to finely control the device resources and capabilities. For historical reasons, CUDA has the largest user base in the researcher community. CUDA gives fine control over NVIDIA GPUs but is incompatible with AMD and Intel GPUs. The other API, OpenCL, is an open language for which vendors provide packages that work over a variety of platforms, including GPUs and multicore CPUs. Potentially, OpenCL can function in a heterogeneous computing system that embeds multiple technologies. It is generally thought that OpenCL is not as fast as CUDA and has coarser control over the GPU hardware. The rest of this chapter focuses on the CUDA interface, but the concepts can be easily adapted to OpenCL.

CUDA and OpenCL both extend the C and C++ languages by defining a GPU-specific syntax. At compilation, a preprocessor separates GPU instructions, which are compiled by a special GPU compiler, from standard C or C++ instructions, which are compiled by the general-purpose C/C++ compiler available on the host. The C/C++ binary is then linked with GPU runtime libraries that coordinate GPU and CPU computation.

Programming the GPU can also be done without writing GPU-specific code. Several general-purpose C/C++ libraries exist that provide GPU-accelerated functions for common tasks (Figure 10.9). On the CUDA platform, those libraries include cuFFT, for performing the FFT; cuBLAS, for linear algebra; cuSPARSE, for sparse matrix computations; cuRAND, for pseudo-random number generation; NPP, for image and video processing; and Thrust, an extension of the C++ Standard Template Library (STL). These libraries allow the developer to implement massively parallel applications with minimum programming effort and little knowledge of GPU programming. Moreover, these libraries can be included in a larger project that uses the CUDA API.

To illustrate how the GPU can be used as a coprocessor for parallel processing, Figure 10.10 shows how sinogram correction can be implemented in CUDA.

A program that runs in parallel on the device is called a *kernel*. Kernels are defined inline, as standard C functions. A—global—identifier precedes the function declaration to signal the compiler that this function runs on the GPU. The function can take arguments: here, four pointers to memory arrays on the device. It should be understood that device pointers only make sense in the context of a device kernel. They cannot be used on the host to directly access the device memory.

Upon the launch of a kernel, multiple processes are created that execute multiple instances of the kernel (called *threads*) in parallel. CUDA defines device-specific variables that are available for the programmer

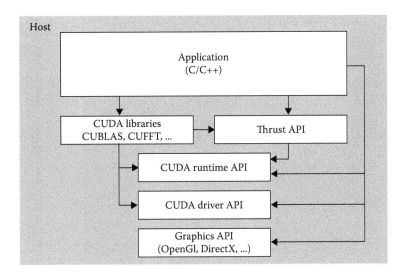

Figure 10.9 Depiction of the various interfaces available for programming the GPU. A C++ application may call a high-level API such as CUBLAS, CUFFT, or Thrust; a low-level runtime or driver API; or a graphics API such as OpenGL.

to query the properties of these threads. In this example, we use threadIdx.x to obtain the index of the thread being executed and distribute data between multiple instances of the same kernel. If four threads are launched, threadIdx.x will take a value between 0 and 3. Hence, thread 0 will process elements 0, 4, 8, 12, and so forth. The thread index can be multidimensional, which is useful when working with 2D images.

Memory storage on the GPU is more complex than on the CPU, with multiple types of memory available. In the example above, we stored arrays using a type of memory called *global memory*. Global memory is allocated in the GPU's external memory and is accessible for read and write operations by all the threads. Although convenient, global memory has high latency because it is located off the GPU chip. Other types of memory that are on-chip have much lower latencies.

Code executed on the host is contained in main() and given in Figure 10.10. First, the program allocates memory on the GPU using cudaMalloc, a GPU-specific function. This function is similar to the standard malloc function, but it returns a pointer to device memory. Only pointers to device memory can be dereferenced inside a device kernel, using the standard C syntax, for example, a[i]. Next, data is copied from the host to the device's memory using the function cudaMemcpy. The arguments of this function are two pointers, one to a device memory location and another to a host memory location, and an integer defining the size of the array. Once the data transfer has completed, four instances of the kernel (threads) are launched on the GPU by calling the kernel function. The only difference with standard C is that the number of desired threads is indicated between <<< and >>>. The exact role of these two numbers is explained in more detail later in this section. Each thread is executed on a dedicated processor on the device and performs one-fourth of the total workload. Once the device has completed, control returns to the host and the output data is transferred back to the host. The program terminates by freeing the device memory, which is no longer needed.

This simple example illustrates some of the capabilities of GPU kernel programs. CUDA kernels are very similar to C programs. They can access memory, execute loops, and branch according to conditional statements. In the following sections, we will see capabilities that are specific to GPUs. We will also use the following nomenclature: we call *warp* a small group of threads (usually 32 threads), *block* a group of warps, and *grid* a group of blocks.

The previous example showed how to execute computation in parallel with no data exchange between threads. However, it is sometimes desirable for threads to communicate with one another. For example, the execution of a thread may be conditional upon computations performed by other threads. The GPU provides various mechanisms for enabling efficient cooperation between threads.

```
#define N    65536    // number of bins in sinogram
#define P    4        // number of parallel threads

// GPU kernel
__global__ void sinocorrect( int *s, int *b, int *c ) {
    int i = threadIdx.x;
    while (i< N) {
        s2[i] = s[i]/a[i] - b[i];
        i = i + P;
    }
}

int main( void ) {
    // host memory
    int s[N], s2[N], a[N], a[N];

    // pointers to device memory
    int *dev_s, *dev_s2, *dev_a, *dev_b;

    // [...] Load sinogram in s and corrections in a and b

    // allocate GPU memory
    cudaMalloc( (void**)&dev_s, N * sizeof(int) );
    cudaMalloc( (void**)&dev_s2, N * sizeof(int) );
    cudaMalloc( (void**)&dev_a, N * sizeof(int) );
    cudaMalloc( (void**)&dev_b, N * sizeof(int) );

    // copy the arrays 's', 'a' and 'b' to GPU memory
    cudaMemcpy( dev_s, s2, N * sizeof(int), cudaMemcpyHostToDevice );
    cudaMemcpy( dev_a, a, N * sizeof(int), cudaMemcpyHostToDevice );
    cudaMemcpy( dev_b, b, N * sizeof(int), cudaMemcpyHostToDevice );

    // call the GPU kernel
    sinocorrect<<<1,P>>>( dev_s, dev_a, dev_b, dev_s2 );

    // copy the array 's2' back from the GPU to the CPU
    cudaMemcpy( s2, dev_s2, N * sizeof(int), cudaMemcpyDeviceToHost );

    // free the memory allocated on the GPU
    cudaFree( dev_s );  cudaFree( dev_s2 );
    cudaFree( dev_b );  cudaFree( dev_c );

    return 0;
}
```

Figure 10.10 Example of CUDA programming. This sample includes a GPU kernel (sinocorrect) that applies a correction to a sinogram s. The CPU portion of the code allocates memory on the GPU, transfers data, starts computation, and then reads the results back.

10.3.4 COOPERATION BETWEEN THREADS

The basic unit of processing in a GPU is called a *streaming multiprocessor* (SM). Each SM is a multicore processor with dedicated on-chip memory storage (Figure 10.11). For higher parallelism, GPUs can embed several of these SMs. A high-performance GPU such as the GeForce 680 GTX has eight SMs, each containing 192 cores. Less expensive GPUs are also available that have only one or two SMs. The division of computing hardware into SM units allows manufacturers to market devices that have different levels of performance yet operate within the same software framework.

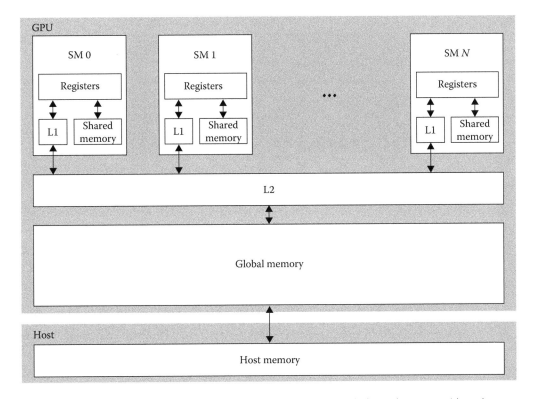

Figure 10.11 Memory architecture of the GPU. Each SM has access to dedicated resources (shared memory and registers), as well as global resources (global memory). Two levels of cache (L1 and L2) are provided by the GPU to accelerate memory transactions.

Each SM contains three types of on-chip memory storage: *registers*, *shared memory*, and *L1 cache* (Figure 10.11). Registers are private variables allocated by the compiler to each thread. For instance, a register may be used to store a counter within a loop. Shared memory is a block of on-chip memory that is associated with a thread block; only the threads within this block can access it. Shared memory facilitates cooperation between threads in the same block by allowing data to be quickly exchanged. The L1 cache, managed by the device, enables faster access to global memory by exploiting spatial and temporal locality at the SM level. A L2 global cache also handles memory transactions from all SMs.

The programming abstraction of the GPU differentiates between two levels of parallelism, within an SM and between SMs. Given a parallel task, the developer must identify threads that cooperate with one another and group them together in a *thread block*. Thread blocks execute instructions independently of one another. The GPU queues and schedules these blocks on different SMs, in arbitrary order (Figure 10.12). The advantage of this design is that a parallel kernel can scale seamlessly to devices with an arbitrary number of SMs, since thread blocks are executed independently of one another. However, threads can only cooperate if they belong to the same block. Physically, the members of a thread block reside on the same SM for their entire lifetime. They can cooperate by accessing block-specific shared memory. While multiple blocks may reside on the same SM, threads belonging to different blocks cannot access each other's shared memory. Hence, interblock communication is only possible using slower global memory. Threads within a block can also synchronize their execution using the—synchthreads function, which acts as a barrier at which all threads in the block must wait before any are allowed to proceed. This function can be used, for instance, to ensure that all threads have finished writing to shared memory before reading back.

Thread-block dimensions are defined at kernel launch using the syntax kernel_name<<<a,b>>>, where a is the number of blocks and b the number of threads per block. In the example above, the kernel was launched using one block of four threads. In the next section, we discuss how these numbers should be adjusted for optimal performance.

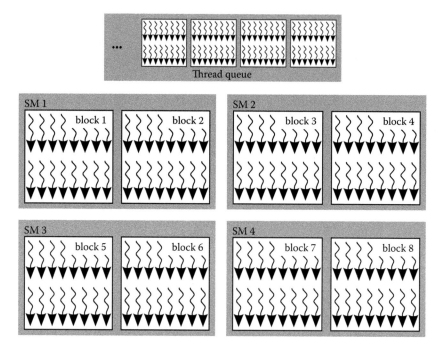

Figure 10.12 Parallel decomposition of computation in threads and thread blocks. Computation is decomposed in threads, which are grouped in thread blocks. Thread blocks are queued and scheduled on independent SMs. The threads within the same block are executed on the same SM for their entire lifetime.

One of the features that sets GPUs and CPUs apart is that GPUs can accommodate more cores on the same silicon real estate. GPU cores are simpler and require fewer transistors; they also pool certain resources to save transistors. For instance, the cores within an SM rely on a common instruction scheduler to decode instructions. On each clock cycle, the instruction scheduler decodes and broadcasts one instruction to a *thread warp*. The warp is a subdivision of the thread block and the basic unit of execution on the GPU; it typically contains 32 threads. The members of a thread warp must execute instructions in a lockstep fashion, also called *single-instruction multiple data* (SIMD). On a clock tick, the threads within a warp must either compute a common instruction or remain idle.

Although most efficient when all the threads within a warp issue the same instruction at the same time, GPU programming is still flexible with regard to conditional expressions (e.g., *if*, *for*, and *while*). Use of these expressions can cause threads to diverge, for instance, if a statement is true for some threads but false for others. In such cases, the instruction scheduler executes the diverging execution paths sequentially. For instance, in Figure 10.13, an "if" statement causes thread 2 to enter a different branch of the kernel. As a result, thread 2 is executed separately from the other threads. While overall efficiency is reduced—in the worst case by a factor equal to the warp size—the serialization of diverging threads ensures that the kernel always runs as intended by the programmer.

10.3.5 Allocating resources

To achieve optimal performance, the developer must carefully allocate hardware resources. As discussed in Section 10.3.1, the GPU is designed to prioritize throughput over latency: thousands of threads can reside on the GPU at any given time—many times more than the number of physical cores. Therefore, only a small number of thread warps actively execute instructions on each clock tick. This can be used to hide the latency of memory transactions: the scheduler can ignore thread warps that are waiting for memory transfers or arithmetic operations to complete. With a large number of thread warps residing on the same SM, the chance

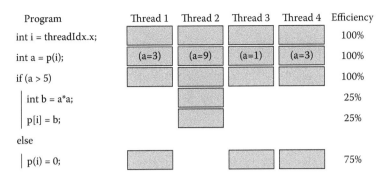

Figure 10.13 Example of thread divergence. A conditional statement causes thread 2 to follow an execution path different from the other threads. The execution of diverging execution paths is serialized, leading to a lower efficiency.

is high that some of these warps are ready to execute a new instruction. If all the warps are stalled, then no instruction can be issued, resulting in idle hardware and decreased performance.

A useful figure of merit to consider when optimizing GPU code is the *thread occupancy*, defined as the ratio of the number of threads residing on an SM to the SM's full capacity. Higher occupancy indicates higher *thread-level parallelism*, meaning that the scheduler has a higher chance of finding warps ready for new instructions. In practice, however, high thread occupancy is hard to achieve because of the limited availability of registers, which are split equally between threads, and shared memory, which is split between thread blocks. If the number of registers available on-chip is insufficient, the compiler may allocate temporary variables in global memory, leading to increased traffic between the GPU and the external memory. Likewise, the small amount of shared memory available puts a limit on the numbers of blocks that can reside on an SM at the same time, since this resource is divided among them. Because of the trade-off between thread occupancy and external memory usage, the developer should fine-tune register and shared memory usage to achieve good performance.

In addition, reducing the thread occupancy can sometimes increase efficiency due to *instruction-level parallelism*. SMs are able to schedule and execute at the same time consecutive instructions that have no data dependencies. (A data dependency exists when an instruction uses the result of a previous instruction.) With a lower thread occupancy, more registers are available for the threads to use and the compiler can remove data dependencies by reordering instructions and using these registers as temporary variables.

Because of all the aforementioned reasons, the number of thread blocks should also be chosen with care. Furthermore, with too few blocks, the code might not scale well to future GPU hardware, which is likely to have more SMs. For a given device, the number of blocks should also be a multiple of the number of SMs to ensure a balanced workload. For instance, if a GPU contains 4 SMs, and if each SM can accommodate 3 thread blocks, the total number of blocks should be a multiple of 12.

10.3.6 EFFICIENT MEMORY OPERATIONS

With thousands of cores processing data in parallel, memory bandwidth is very often the limiting factor for medical imaging computation on the GPU. For instance, the C1060 GPU can perform 933 billion FLOPS, but with a peak memory bandwidth of 408 GB/s, it can only read or write one floating-point value to memory for every 10 arithmetic operations. As a general rule, computation should be formulated to maximize the ratio of arithmetic to memory operations, a quantity called the *arithmetic intensity*. Memory latency can also limit performance, especially when thread occupancy is low. The best way to prevent memory latency from affecting performance is to ensure that the GPU has an ample supply of ready warps to keep its cores busy.

Reducing the amount of data transferred between the GPU and its external memory is key to achieving high performance. To avoid redundant transfers, threads can temporarily store data read from global memory in shared memory for other threads to reuse, a form of managed caching. These global memory accesses

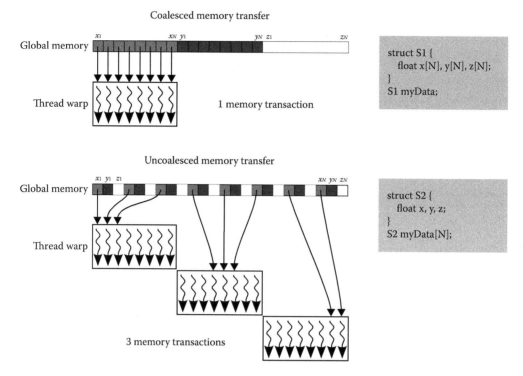

Figure 10.14 Example of coalesced and noncoalesced memory access. A list of (x, y, z) coordinates can be stored either as a structure of arrays (top) or an array of structures (bottom). The first scheme allows the GPU to access memory in a coalesced manner and is three times more efficient than the second scheme, which is only partially coalesced.

should be coalesced for optimal performance. A coalesced memory access is one where the hardware combines multiple memory requests from threads within a common warp into a single transaction. Full efficiency is achieved when a warp accesses a *contiguous* region of memory that is *aligned* to the size of the transaction. For instance, the 32 threads within a warp can each read one floating-point (4 bytes) value provided that those values are located within a 128-byte, aligned, contiguous region of memory. Reading noncontiguous memory locations (e.g., random access) would require 32 sequential memory transactions.

How data is organized in memory can affect how efficiently it can be accessed. Figure 10.14 shows two different data structures for storing a list of (x, y, z) coordinates, namely, a *structure of arrays* and an *array of structures*. In the first example, the threads within a warp can access the x component in a coalesced manner using a single memory transaction. However, the second structure requires three different memory transactions because noncontiguous memory accesses are serialized.

The GPU can also store certain data in two read-only memories called *constant* and *texture memory*. Constant memory is aggressively cached and most useful for broadcasting data to all the threads with minimum use of memory bandwidth. Texture memory can be allocated in external memory and may be 1D, 2D, or 3D. Texture elements can be accessed by a floating-point coordinate with hardware-accelerated interpolation (Figure 10.15). Texture reads are also cached such that threads within a warp achieve optimal performance when reading texture elements that are near one another in 1D, 2D, or 3D.

Recently developed devices also feature a unified L2 cache that services read and write requests from all threads to global memory. Each SM also includes a dedicated L1 cache. With these caches, the use of constant and texture memory has become less advantageous for performance. For instance, the L2 cache enables a single parameter to be efficiently broadcasted to all the threads in the kernel.

The GPU also provides special hardware for handling read–update–write operations—for instance, the operation a[i] = a[i] + c. On a parallel device such as the GPU, problems may occur if two or more threads attempt to increment the same memory address: one thread may, for instance, write a new value to a[i], while

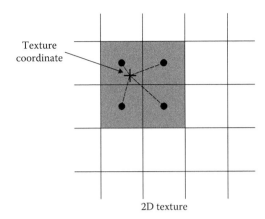

Figure 10.15 Example of 2D texture memory access. Texture memory can be accessed using floating-point coordinates, with optional linear interpolation.

another thread is computing the addition using the old value for a[i]. To solve this problem, the GPU provides special *atomic* functions that guarantee the correctness of read–update–write operations. The atomic equivalent of the example operation above is atomicAdd(&(a[i]), c). It should be noted that two atomic operations performed on the same memory address are executed serially, in arbitrary order. Hence, if thousands of threads attempt to update a few memory addresses (e.g., for a histogram), atomic operations can be very costly. A more efficient approach is to create local shared copies of the memory, which can be combined at the end using a reduce operation.

10.3.7 ADVANCED CONCEPTS

Before concluding this section, a few other topics are briefly mentioned. More details can be found on those topics in specialized resources (Sanders and Kandrot 2010; Farber 2011).

- *Streams*: We have previously seen that data can be transferred from GPU to CPU in a synchronous manner, with both GPU and CPU waiting for the transfer to complete to start other tasks. Streams offer a means to copy data asynchronously. A stream is a queue of memory transfers and kernels that are executed in order. By running multiple streams simultaneously, it is possible to run computation while copying data.
- *Zero-copy memory*: Zero-copy memory allows the device to read host memory directly. When data is only accessed once, it can be faster than copying the data to device memory, and then moving the data to the GPU chip. Zero-copy memory is also advantageous for avoiding duplicating data when using integrated GPUs, which allocate their memory directly on the host.
- *Warp vote*: Warp voting functions allow the GPU to execute a set of instructions only if a conditional statement is true for all (or any) threads within a warp.
- *Events*: Because the GPU runs code asynchronously, accurate timing performance can be challenging. Events can be used for precisely timing GPU functions.
- *Warp shuffle*: Warp shuffle functions are available to exchange data between threads in the same warp without accessing shared memory.

10.4 APPLICATIONS OF GPU COMPUTING

10.4.1 BACKPROJECTION USING TEXTURE MAPPING

In the following, we review a few applications of GPU computing in emission tomography. As discovered early on, backprojection can be reformulated using a graphics operation called texture mapping (Cabral et al.

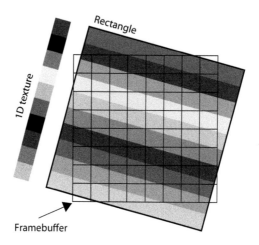

Figure 10.16 2D backprojection of a set of parallel line projections using texture mapping. The line projections are smeared at a given angle over the framebuffer. Additive blending is used to accumulate backprojected values in the framebuffer.

1994; Xu and Mueller 2005, 2007). There are many similarities between the graphics pipeline and the operations performed during backprojection, which makes backprojection particularly efficient on the GPU.

The basic idea behind texture mapping backprojection is to stretch a 1D texture (representing parallel line projections) such that the contribution of each sinogram element is smeared along parallel projective lines (Figure 10.16). More precisely, the entire 2D input sinogram is stored as a 2D texture in the GPU's external memory. For each projection angle, a rectangle is drawn parallel to the projection axis. One column of the sinogram, corresponding to a given projection angle, is mapped onto the rectangle as a texture. The texture is stretched to fill the rectangle entirely, with linear filtering enabled. Additive blending is enabled so that texture-mapped rectangles are accumulated into the GPU's framebuffer. The procedure is repeated for all sinogram angles, with each new rectangle rotated with respect to the previous one.

The aforementioned procedure can be implemented entirely in OpenGL, using the default pipeline and without writing any code for the GPU. The backprojection procedure can be improved slightly on a programmable GPU: instead of drawing multiple rectangles in the framebuffer, one can draw a single rectangle that covers the entire framebuffer. This will generate one fragment for each framebuffer pixel. A fragment shader (which runs on the GPU) can loop over the sinogram angles, fetching and accumulating the corresponding projection values. These fragment shaders are executed in parallel for each fragment created by the GPU.

10.4.2 BACK- AND FORWARD PROJECTION USING CUDA

A number of algorithms have also been developed for PET image reconstruction using modern GPU computing hardware (Herraiz et al. 2011; Kim and Ye 2011; Zhou and Qi 2011; Kinouchi et al. 2012; Nassiri et al. 2012). Backprojection can easily be implemented using CUDA or another high-level language by using concepts and ideas very similar to the example shown in Section 10.4.1. Rather than drawing a rectangle to create fragment shaders, one can use CUDA to create a grid of threads, with one thread assigned to each output pixel, and one thread block representing a 16×16 block in the image. Each thread runs a "for loop" over the sinogram angles to gather sinogram elements corresponding to all the projection angles. By storing the sinogram as a 2D texture, the GPU can linearly interpolate the sinogram values without increasing the computation time, and cache surrounding texture elements for faster access. The values read sequentially are accumulated locally in a register, and finally written back to global memory for transfer back to the host. Threads that are close to one another in image domain are more likely to access neighboring memory addresses and should be in a common block. The technique described here can be readily extended to 3D image reconstruction (e.g., cone-beam CT) by creating a 3D grid of threads.

Similar to backprojection, forward projection can be easily implemented with CUDA. In a gather formulation, threads are assigned to sinogram elements and gather image pixels along lines of response. To facilitate cooperation, threads are further grouped into blocks that work on parallel lines of response. Each thread runs a "for loop" that steps along a line of response, reading image samples at each location. Those image samples combine the four closest pixels via linear interpolation. Each thread keeps a private register in which it accumulates image samples as it moves along the line of response, and which gets written to global memory at the end.

This approach has several advantages. The use of a texture to store the input image provides free bilinear interpolation and data caching optimized for 2D locality. The final data write to global memory is fully coalesced because threads within a warp write to consecutive memory addresses. There is also no thread divergence because the threads are all following the same steps. The main bottleneck is memory bandwidth for accessing the texture memory, due to the low arithmetic intensity of the kernel. Indeed, for each memory element read from memory, there are only five additions.

10.4.3 MULTI-GPU RECONSTRUCTION

Reconstruction of emission tomography images can be greatly improved simply by dividing the workload to multiple processors within a GPU. However, if this strategy is generalized to a cluster of multiple GPUs, the processing speed does not improve linearly with the number of GPUs. This is because updating the image estimate requires large data transfers between the GPUs after each ordered subset expectation maximization (OSEM) iteration, effectively reducing the level of parallelism. Fortunately, the maximum-likelihood expectation maximization (MLEM) algorithm can be reformulated using the alternating direction method of multipliers (ADMM) to reduce the frequency of data exchange between GPUs (Cui et al. 2013). While being mathematically different, the distributed MLEM algorithm maximizes the same convex likelihood function as standard MLEM, and thus converges to the same solution. Experiments have shown that on the cluster of six GPUs, distributed MLEM can perform reconstruction five times faster than a single GPU, whereas standard MLEM is only three times faster.

10.4.4 LIST-MODE PROJECTION OPERATIONS

List-mode projection operations differ significantly from their sinogram counterparts. Early work used the graphics pipeline to perform list-mode reconstruction of PET data (Pratx et al. 2009), with time-of-flight information (Pratx et al. 2011), as well as spatially varying resolution recovery (Pratx and Levin 2011). These concepts were later adapted to modern GPU computing using CUDA (Cui et al. 2011).

One of the challenges of list-mode processing is that voxel-driven processing is nearly impossible because there is no simple mapping from image voxels to randomly oriented list-mode events. Hence, computation can only be partitioned over list-mode events. For backprojection, this means that computation must be carried in a scatter fashion. The use of atomics is essential here to avoid errors that could result from parallel threads writing to the same memory address.

The other issue with list-mode processing is that the GPU must access the large image volume along lines of integration that have no spatial organization. The resulting memory accesses are random and therefore very inefficient. Recall that the efficiency of a noncoalesced memory transfer can be as slow as 1/32 of the total memory bandwidth. The texture cache is unlikely to help improve performance because memory read requests have neither spatial nor temporal locality. Furthermore, because list-mode lines have different lengths and orientations, the computational load is heterogeneous and threads are prone to diverge, which can further reduce the overall efficiency.

A solution to all the aforementioned problems is to use shared memory as a managed cache. The idea is to partition computation—both in the list-mode domain *and* in the image domain. This approach—a hybrid between scatter and gather—is very powerful for list-mode processing. In this scheme, each thread performs computation that relates to a given slice in the image and a set of list-mode events. A thread block contains only threads that work on the same image slice, which they load in shared memory. Therefore, computation is partitioned in the image domain at the block level, and in the list-mode domain at the thread level (Figure 10.17, left).

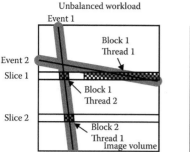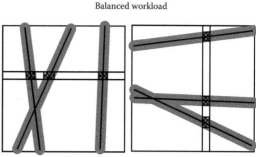

Figure 10.17 List-mode backprojection on a GPU (shown in 2D for simplicity). Each thread block stores one slice in its shared memory. The threads within that block perform all the computation relating to that slice, with individual threads working on different coincidence events. Left: Due to variations in line orientation, the workload is unbalanced. Right: Sorting the lines according to their main orientation helps ensure that workload is similar among threads.

We focus here on forward projection; backprojection can be implemented in a similar way. Threads within a block first collaboratively transfer an image slice from global memory, where the full image is stored, to shared memory. This transfer is fully coalesced and achieves peak bandwidth. Then, each thread receives a subset of the list-mode data to process. Threads read the data describing the assigned list-mode events from global memory in a coalesced manner, since these events are stored in a contiguous block of memory. The list-mode data is a long array that contains the position and orientation of each line. Then, each thread computes the contribution of the assigned slice to forward projection of the current list-mode event. This computation may include the use of a spatial resolution kernel to model the spatially varying response of the imaging system. The contribution is written back to the list-mode event in global memory, in a coalesced manner.

The last remaining issue is that the workload assigned to each thread is unbalanced, leading to thread divergence. For 3D reconstruction, each thread is responsible for computation relating to the intersection of a tube (representing the spatial extent of the line of response) and a slice. Based on the relative position of the tube and the slice, this intersection may be void, if both are parallel but away from each other; a disk, if they are orthogonal to each other; or an ellipse, in the most general case. Therefore, threads within a warp may have very different workloads and their execution could diverge (Figure 10.17, left). Fortunately, a simple partitioning of the list-mode events in three groups helps reduce thread divergence. The partitioning is made based on the dominant orientation of the line of response that corresponds to each list-mode event. Lines that are most orthogonal to the *coronal* and *sagittal* plane are separated into two groups (Figure 10.17, right). The third group—lines that are most orthogonal to the *axial* plane—is empty for conventional PET scanners with limited axial extent and can be ignored.

Line projection operations are performed separately for each group of lines. The volume is sliced in the dimension that is most orthogonal to the group orientation. This helps ensure that most lines intersect the current slice, and that the number of voxels in the intersection is strictly bounded. These two properties help ensure that threads have a balanced workload and do not diverge. For each intersection between a line and a slice, a thread processes the voxels contained in a square mask using a 2D "for loop" with constant bounds. The size of the mask is determined such as it always encloses the intersection of a tube and a slice.

Using all the aforementioned strategies, list-mode reconstruction was implemented on a single high-end GPU and ran 200 times faster than a reference single-threaded CPU version. Interestingly, the naïve GPU implementation, which was implemented by directly transposing C code into CUDA code, was only 17 times faster due to low global memory bandwidth and high thread divergence.

10.4.5 MONTE CARLO SIMULATION

A number of Monte Carlo packages have been developed for the GPU (Badal and Badano 2009; Jia et al. 2010; Hissoiny et al. 2011; Lippuner and Elbakri 2011; Jahnke et al. 2012). It needs to be emphasized that the theoretical simplicity of the map–reduce formulation presented in Section 10.2 can be misleading because efficient Monte Carlo simulation can be difficult to achieve on the GPU. In particular, data input, data output, and thread divergence can all degrade the performance of Monte Carlo computations.

The first challenge is that, in a distributed Monte Carlo simulation, the geometry of the simulated system must be shared among all the threads. For a simple geometry, this may be done efficiently using fast constant or shared memory, but for more complex cases (e.g., a CT-based discretized volume representing a patient model), the geometry must be stored in global memory and accessed in a pseudo-random manner. One possible solution is to store the CT volume in texture memory for fast interpolation and data caching, although data caching has limited usefulness because of the low chance of data reuse between parallel threads. As a result, memory access is a bottleneck for Monte Carlo simulation based on large CT patient models.

Handling the output of the simulation is another challenging issue. For a verbose output—logging all events and interactions—the size of the output can be larger than the available GPU memory; the GPU must therefore frequently dump data to the host's hard drive. For a more compact output (e.g., a dose distribution or a sinogram), data storage is easier to handle, but the programmer must still worry about the large number of threads trying to write to a small number of memory addresses. To circumvent the issue of memory conflicts, the output of the simulation (if not too large) can be stored temporarily in shared memory at the thread-block level, and be reconstituted at the end of the simulation. This strategy allows the GPU to perform multiple write operations in parallel with a lower probability of conflicts between threads.

One last challenge to consider is the issue of thread divergence. Recall that the GPU is composed of multiple SIMD-like processors. At the SM level, parallel processing occurs only if the threads within a warp all execute the same instruction at the same time. However, Monte Carlo simulation is by definition pseudo-stochastic. Different threads compute different particle histories, and these particles may be different in nature (electron, photon, or positron) and be undergoing different physical processes (e.g., Compton scatter for a photon and bremsstrahlung emission for an electron). To make matters worse, some particles may undergo a single event, while others may undergo a dozen sequential events. Different physical processes require the GPU to execute completely different sequences of instructions, which cause threads to diverge. The issue of thread divergence in Monte Carlo simulation is complex and has no ideal solution. A few strategies have been proposed to circumvent this issue: for instance, particles can be stored in a global queue, which is regularly updated. The GPU can remove particles that have been fully simulated (this is known as *stream compaction*). It can also add to the queue secondary particles created by primary particles (e.g., bremsstrahlung photons and photoelectrons). To better balance the workload, it is more efficient to add secondary particles to a global queue than to simulate those within the parent thread. Even with a global queue, it is difficult to guarantee that all the threads within a warp will calculate the same physical processes at the same time. For this reason, a significant fraction of the cores may be idle most of the time, considerably lowering the highest speedup achievable.

10.5 OTHER CONSIDERATIONS

The availability of GPU computing tools has enabled researchers to compute common imaging algorithms considerably faster. Owing to a rich collection of software packages, it is now relatively straightforward to port an existing code to the GPU. The first step is common to any distributed platform: the algorithm must be formulated as a set of independent tasks that can be executed in parallel. Basic building blocks such as map, reduce, and gather can be used to expose the parallelism within an algorithm. Often, this decomposition is not unique; the developer should carefully investigate which decomposition is best suited to the targeted computing platform. As seen in Section 10.2, gather operations are usually more efficient than equivalent scatter operations—although this is not true for every algorithm (e.g., list-mode backprojection). The next step is to select the right tools: either a high-level library such as CUFFT or a GPU-specific API such as CUDA. While writing the code, debugging and profiling tools should be used to optimize performance and identify bottlenecks. Last, the application can be deployed in a production environment, which can be a cluster, a virtual cloud, or a local workstation.

To conclude this chapter, a word should be said about speedup factors, which are often reported in the scientific literature. These factors are important to compare the performance of an algorithm on the GPU and the CPU, but they have been criticized for being inflated and unfair to CPUs. In a controversial article, Intel researchers reported that they had reduced the performance gap between GPUs and CPUs to, on average, 2.5× for a variety of applications (Lee et al. 2010), which they achieved using high-end CPUs and CPU-specific optimization (such as multicore processing, cache optimization, and SIMD streaming extensions). While various GPU experts have disputed this conclusion, speedups above 100× are often best-case estimates measured against unoptimized CPU codes, and therefore these numbers should not be taken literally. Furthermore, as stated by Amdahl's law, the highest speedup achievable is limited by the sequential fraction of the program. In the case of emission tomography, this includes loading data from the hard drive, computing data corrections (e.g., scatter, randoms, and sensitivity matrix), and writing image data back to a network storage system. After GPU acceleration, image reconstruction may no longer be the primary factor limiting the overall processing time, meaning that other sequential parts in the image workflow should be optimized as well.

While this chapter has focused on the highly successful GPU platform, we will mention that other manufacturers have proposed alternative parallel architectures. For instance, there is a trend toward the convergence of CPU and GPU with architectures such as the Heterogeneous System Architecture developed by AMD and the Many Integrated Core Architecture developed by Intel and commercialized under Xeon Phi. These platforms attempt to facilitate GPU computing by using the standard x86 instruction set and by improving GPU/CPU integration. Another platform is the Cell Broadband Engine, a custom processor developed by IBM that comprises one main processor and eight parallel cores. The Cell was commercialized in 2005 and found use mainly as the processor of the Playstation 3. Although the Cell was found useful for accelerating tasks such as backprojection, it has never enjoyed as much success as the GPU. Last, an emerging trend is the use of cloud computing for scientific applications. Cloud computing changes the way we think about computation. Computation no longer requires purchasing and maintaining a local computing infrastructure; rather, massive amounts of resources can be allocated on demand in a remote commercial location. Cloud computing is now used routinely for processing massive bioinformatics tasks (Gunarathne et al. 2011) and has been shown to be a viable option for Monte Carlo simulation (Wang et al. 2011). The use of cloud computing in emission tomography is a remote possibility that is worth exploring.

In the last 30 years, emission tomography technology has progressed at an astounding pace. This trend, which is likely to continue in the future, means that more powerful computing systems will need to be designed to accommodate these new needs. New interventional applications will require reconstructing and processing images in real time with a high level of numerical sophistication. The increasing use of PET and SPECT for quantitative imaging will require image corrections computed with the highest level of accuracy possible. Parallel computing on the GPU is our best bet for tackling these challenges. Because GPU computation is formulated in terms of independent computation blocks, GPU codes developed today should seamlessly scale to the massively parallel hardware of tomorrow. Ultimately, with video games growing ever more popular, scientists can rely on the fact that vast consumer demand for graphics accelerators will keep high-performance GPUs affordable for years to come.

REFERENCES

Asanovic, K., R. Bodik, B. C. Catanzaro, J. J. Gebis, P. Husbands, K. Keutzer, et al. 2006. The landscape of parallel computing research: A view from Berkeley. University of California, Berkeley.

Badal, A., and A. Badano. 2009. Accelerating Monte Carlo simulations of photon transport in a voxelized geometry using a massively parallel graphics processing unit. *Med Phys* 36:4878–4880.

Cabral, B., N. Cam, and J. Foran. 1994. Accelerated volume rendering and tomographic reconstruction using texture mapping hardware. In *Proceedings of the 1994 Symposium on Volume Visualization*, pp. 91–98. New York: ACM.

Cui, J., G. Pratx, B. Meng, and C. S. Levin. 2013. Distributed MLEM: An iterative tomographic image reconstruction algorithm for distributed memory architectures. *IEEE Trans Med Imaging* 32:957–967.

Cui, J., G. Pratx, S. Prevrhal, and C. S. Levin. 2011. Fully 3D list-mode time-of-flight PET image reconstruction on GPUs using CUDA. *Med. Phys.* 38:6775–6786.

Farber, R. 2011. *CUDA Application Design and Development*. Amsterdam: Elsevier Science.

Gunarathne, T., T. L. Wu, J. Y. Choi, S. H. Bae, and J. Qiu. 2011. Cloud computing paradigms for pleasingly parallel biomedical applications. *Concurr Comput* 23:2338–2354.

Herraiz, J., S. España, R. Cabido, A. Montemayor, M. Desco, J. J. Vaquero, et al. 2011. GPU-based fast iterative reconstruction of fully 3-D PET sinograms. *IEEE Trans Nucl Sci* 58:2257–2263.

Hissoiny, S., B. Ozell, H. Bouchard, and P. Despres. 2011. GPUMCD: A new GPU-oriented Monte Carlo dose calculation platform. *Med Phys* 38:754–764.

Jahnke, L., J. Fleckenstein, F. Wenz, and J. Hesser. 2012. GMC: A GPU implementation of a Monte Carlo dose calculation based on Geant4. *Phys Med Biol* 57:1217–1229.

Jia, X., X. Gu, J. Sempau, D. Choi, A. Majumdar, and S. B. Jiang. 2010. Development of a GPU-based Monte Carlo dose calculation code for coupled electron–photon transport. *Phys Med Biol* 55:3077–3086.

Kim, K. S., and J. C. Ye. 2011. Fully 3D iterative scatter-corrected OSEM for HRRT PET using a GPU. *Phys Med Biol* 56:4991–5009.

Kinouchi, S., T. Yamaya, E. Yoshida, H. Tashima, H. Kudo, H. Haneishi, et al. 2012. GPU-based PET image reconstruction using an accurate geometrical system model. *IEEE Trans Nucl Sci* 59:1977–1983.

Lee, V. W., C. Kim, J. Chhugani, M. Deisher, D. Kim, A. D. Nguyen, et al. 2010. Debunking the 100× GPU vs. CPU myth: An evaluation of throughput computing on CPU and GPU. *Comput Archit News* 38:451–460.

Lippuner, J., and I. A. Elbakri. 2011. A GPU implementation of EGSnrc's Monte Carlo photon transport for imaging applications. *Phys Med Biol* 56:7145–7162.

Martino, R. L., C. A. Johnson, E. B. Suh, B. L. Trus, and T. K. Yap. 1994. Parallel computing in biomedical research. *Science* 265:902–908.

Nassiri, M. A., S. Hissoiny, J.-F. Carrier, and P. Després. 2012. Fast GPU-based computation of the sensitivity matrix for a PET list-mode OSEM algorithm. *Phys Med Biol* 57:6279–6293.

Owens, J. D., M. Houston, D. Luebke, S. Green, J. E. Stone, and J. C. Phillips. 2008. GPU computing. *Proc IEEE* 96:879–899.

Owens, J. D., D. Luebke, N. Govindaraju, M. Harris, J. Krüger, A. E. Lefohn, et al. 2007. A survey of general-purpose computation on graphics hardware. *Comput Graph Forum* 26:80–113.

Phelps, M., E. Hoffman, S. Huang, and D. Kuhl. 1978. ECAT: A new computerized tomographic imaging system for positron-emitting radiopharmaceuticals. *J Nucl Med* 19:635–647.

Pratx, G., G. Chinn, P. D. Olcott, and C. S. Levin. 2009. Fast, accurate and shift-varying line projections for iterative reconstruction using the GPU. *IEEE Trans Med Imaging* 28:435–445.

Pratx, G., and C. Levin. 2011. Online detector response calculations for high-resolution pet image reconstruction. *Phys Med Biol* 56:4023–4040.

Pratx, G., S. Surti, and C. Levin. 2011. Fast list-mode reconstruction for time-of-flight PET using graphics hardware. *IEEE Trans Nucl Sci* 58:105–109.

Pratx, G., and L. Xing. 2011. GPU computing in medical physics: A review. *Med Phys* 38:2685–2697.

Rumpf, M., and R. Strzodka. 2001. Level set segmentation in graphics hardware. In *2001 International Conference on Image Processing*, pp. 1103–1106. Piscataway, NJ: IEEE.

Sanders, J., and E. Kandrot. 2010. *CUDA by Example: An Introduction to General-Purpose GPU Programming*. New York: Pearson Education.

Surti, S., A. Kuhn, M. E. Werner, A. E. Perkins, J. Kolthammer, and J. S. Karp. 2007. Performance of Philips Gemini TF PET/CT scanner with special consideration for its time-of-flight imaging capabilities. *J Nucl Med* 48:471–480.

Wang, H., Y. Ma, G. Pratx, and L. Xing. 2011. Toward real-time Monte Carlo simulation using a commercial cloud computing infrastructure. *Phys Med Biol* 56:N175–N181.

Xu, F., and K. Mueller. 2005. Accelerating popular tomographic reconstruction algorithms on commodity PC graphics hardware. *IEEE Trans Nucl Sci* 52:654–663.

Xu, F., and K. Mueller. 2007. Real-time 3D computed tomographic reconstruction using commodity graphics hardware. *Phys Med Biol* 52:3405–3419.

Zhou, J., and J. Qi. 2011. Fast and efficient fully 3D PET image reconstruction using sparse system matrix factorization with GPU acceleration. *Phys Med Biol* 56:6739–6757.

Methods and applications of dynamic SPECT imaging

ANNA M. CELLER, TROY H. FARNCOMBE, ALVIN IHSANI, ARKADIUSZ SITEK, AND R. GLENN WELLS

11.1	Introduction to dynamic SPECT	286
	11.1.1 Challenges of dynamic SPECT studies	286
	11.1.2 Clinical single-photon dynamic studies	286
11.2	Classification of dynamic SPECT methods	287
	11.2.1 Classification based on data acquisition methods	288
	11.2.1.1 Slow camera rotation methods	288
	11.2.1.2 Fast camera rotation methods	289
	11.2.1.3 Mixed planar–SPECT acquisitions	290
	11.2.1.4 Dynamic SPECT using stationary systems	290
	11.2.2 Classification based on data processing methods	291
	11.2.2.1 Image-based approaches	291
	11.2.2.2 Projection-based approaches	292
11.3	Detailed discussion of selected methods	293
	11.3.1 Imposing temporal constraints in image reconstruction: dynamic SPECT method	293
	11.3.2 Selection of alternative temporal basis functions	298
	11.3.2.1 Spatiotemporal modeling of dynamic image data	298
	11.3.2.2 Spatiotemporal data representation using splines	300
	11.3.2.3 Image reconstruction methods employing spatiotemporal basis functions	304
	11.3.3 Factor analysis of dynamic structures	306
	11.3.3.1 Mathematical formulation and nonuniqueness	307
	11.3.3.2 Algorithms for factor analysis and correction for nonuniqueness	308
	11.3.3.3 Clinical example of factor analysis	309
	11.3.4 Dynamic SPECT with stationary systems	309
	11.3.4.1 Dynamic SPECT measurements of myocardial blood flow	309
	11.3.4.2 Dynamic SPECT with the discovery NM530c	311
11.4	Conclusions	314
References		314

11.1 INTRODUCTION TO DYNAMIC SPECT

Physiological processes occurring in the human body are dynamic. Therefore, imaging techniques that have the ability to trace *in vivo* changing distributions of radiolabeled molecules can potentially provide important information about organ function, leading to more accurate diagnoses of various diseases with a positive impact on medical research. In particular, dynamic SPECT (dSPECT) studies that can measure temporal changes of three-dimensional (3D) radiotracer distributions can substantially increase the scope and capacity of nuclear medicine for a number of clinical applications.

This chapter deals with such *dynamic imaging* situations where the distribution of an administered radiotracer does not remain stationary during imaging, but rather, its concentration or localization changes relatively quickly over the duration of the study, and the information about this change has important clinical implications. The chapter begins with a discussion of challenges encountered when attempting dSPECT studies, followed by a short review of the dynamic imaging procedures that are currently performed in the clinical setting. In the following section, the difficult task of categorizing the different imaging techniques and methods that have been proposed for dSPECT is undertaken. In the final section, a discussion of the principles, advantages, and limitations of some of the techniques is presented. Each method is illustrated by examples of the results obtained when the method was applied to processing simulated and clinical patient data. Finally, an example of the dSPECT imaging study performed with one of the recently introduced stationary cardiac cameras is presented.

11.1.1 CHALLENGES OF DYNAMIC SPECT STUDIES

Typically, SPECT studies are performed using an Anger-type camera with one to three detector heads equipped with parallel-hole collimators. Projection data acquired while the camera detectors rotate over a half or full circle are used to reconstruct a 3D volume that reveals the distribution of the radiotracer in the imaged object. In cardiac studies, usually two detectors of a dual-head camera are positioned at right angles to each other, and hence each detector only has to rotate by 90° in order to collect a full 180° dataset. However, in the majority of noncardiac studies, the detectors are positioned at 180° to each other and each detector performs a 180° rotation, thus resulting in the collection of a full 360° dataset.

As mentioned, the purpose of SPECT imaging is to determine the 3D distribution of the radiotracer within the body. One of the central assumptions of conventional SPECT is that the radiotracer distribution remains constant over the duration of the scan. This is because standard tomographic reconstruction algorithms assume that all projections have been created by the same object. However, in dSPECT studies, when the radiotracer distribution changes during the data acquisition, resulting projections acquired at different times will measure seemingly different objects (i.e., the projections will be inconsistent). Reconstructions of such dynamic data with standard (static) reconstruction algorithms will typically result in image artifacts that can lead to serious errors in diagnosis. Such artifacts have been observed if the time over which the radiotracer changes (characteristic half-life of the radiotracer dynamics) is one-half or less of the scanning time (Oppenheim and Krepshaw 1987; Links et al. 1991; O'Connor and Cho 1992; Nakajima et al. 1992). Furthermore, since only a single static image is reconstructed with these methods, the time-dependent part of the physiological information is disregarded and not available to aid in the analysis.

11.1.2 CLINICAL SINGLE-PHOTON DYNAMIC STUDIES

In order to avoid the creation of image artifacts, the majority of clinically performed dynamic studies employ a planar acquisition mode (i.e., planar scintigraphy). The list of clinical applications is quite long, with the most common being renal studies where image-based evaluation of the glomerular filtration rate (GRF), renal clearance, tubular extraction rate, and renal plasma flow are being investigated using dynamic scintigraphic techniques (Mulligan et al. 1990; Sfakianakis and Georgiou 1997; Prigent 2008). Evaluation of the renal pathology, global or split renal clearance, and GRF is usually done with diethylenetriamine penta-acetic acid

(^{99m}Tc-DTPA); evaluation of the tubular extraction rate is done with mercapto-acetyltriglycerin (^{99m}Tc-MAG3), and evaluation of the renal plasma flow is done with ^{123}I-hippuran. Similarly, dynamic hepatobiliary (^{99m}Tc-HIDA) scans can be performed for the diagnosis of liver diseases and examination of gallbladder and bile ducts (Lambie et al. 2011). Other types of dynamic scintigraphy studies can provide information about esophagus transit and gastric emptying (McCallum 1990; Mariani et al. 2004) or can be used to localize sources of gastrointestinal bleed (Maurer and Parkman 2006). Less frequently performed dynamic imaging tests include cardiac first pass; dynamic lung ventilation and perfusion; and scintigraphy of the lacrymal glands (dacroscintigraphy), salivary glands, testes, and lymph nodes (MacDonald and Burrell 2008).

Owing primarily to their planar nature, these studies may suffer from poor site localization and low contrast, in addition to inaccurate quantification. This situation creates strong motivation for the development of tomographic dynamic imaging techniques. An obvious choice is to use PET, where the data for all projections are collected simultaneously, and therefore there is no problem with inconsistent data (Muzi et al. 2012). The discussion of dynamic PET methods is presented in Chapter 12. Although dynamic PET studies were first performed in the early 1970s, because of long and complicated acquisition protocols (often requiring the acquisition of blood samples) and subsequent complex data processing, dynamic PET is not used for routine clinical diagnosis, but rather has been limited to studies performed for research purposes. In addition, not all medical problems are easily investigated using PET due to various technical factors, higher costs, or lower clinical availability. For these reasons, a substantial effort has been directed toward the development of dSPECT imaging methods.

As already mentioned, if changes in the radiotracer distribution occur during SPECT acquisition, the resulting projection data are deemed "inconsistent." One option is to collect data while the camera is rotating fast enough so that activity changes related to the investigated physiology can be ignored during each rotation. Multidetector SPECT systems with three heads have higher sensitivity and are able to collect complete datasets more quickly than the more prevalent dual-head cameras, but use of both dual- and triple-head cameras has been investigated for dSPECT. Exploitation of these systems to perform fast-rotation dSPECT imaging has been proposed not only for myocardial perfusion imaging (MPI) (Nakajima et al. 1991; Chua et al. 1993; Smith et al. 1994), but also for renal (Akahira et al. 1999), pulmonary (Sakaji et al. 2001), and neurological (Onishi et al. 1996) applications. Typically, these studies focused on investigations of metabolism and perfusion of the heart using ^{201}Tl, ^{99m}Tc-teboroxime, or free ^{123}I-fatty acid imaging of the brain blood flow or dopamine receptors (using ^{123}I-labeled tracers such as iodoamphetamine [IMP], iodobenzamide [IBZM], and iodobenzofuran [IBF]), regional lung functions (^{133}Xe), or evaluation of renal plasma flow (^{99m}Tc-DTPA, ^{99m}Tc-MAG3, and ^{123}I-hippuran). More detailed discussion of the fast-rotation technique is provided in Section 11.2.1.2.

In parallel, dynamic brain studies have been performed using dedicated stationary multidetector ring scanners (Ogasawara et al. 2001; Iida et al. 1994). Because these scanners are able to simultaneously acquire all tomographic projections (similar to PET), they do not suffer from the problem of inconsistent data. However, due to their specialized use, ring cameras have limited adoption, with most systems being dedicated primarily to research of brain physiology.

More recently, a number of new-generation stationary SPECT cameras have been introduced, mostly serving cardiac applications (DePuey 2012). Their highly specialized detector and collimator designs enable rapid and simultaneous (or semisimultaneous) acquisition of all the projections required for image reconstruction. This property makes them ideally suited for dynamic applications. The use of one of these systems for dSPECT is presented in Section 11.3.4.

For a comprehensive review of different imaging systems used in dSPECT studies, a history of such studies, and a list of clinical applications, with a particular emphasis on cardiology, see the excellent review article by Gullberg et al. (2010).

11.2 CLASSIFICATION OF DYNAMIC SPECT METHODS

Several approaches have been proposed for dSPECT studies. They use a variety of often very sophisticated techniques to address the challenges outlined in Section 11.1 and to extract meaningful diagnostic functional information. As data acquisition and data reconstruction go hand in hand, it is sensible to discuss dSPECT methods in both of these contexts. Clear classification of the proposed methods is difficult, as there are substantial overlaps between different techniques. Here, we propose to group dSPECT methods into categories using two criteria based on (1) how the data are acquired and (2) how they are processed. Hence, in the next section, various approaches used for the acquisition of dSPECT data are discussed, and in the following section, various methods that are used to process dynamic data and extract the underlying functional information are presented.

11.2.1 CLASSIFICATION BASED ON DATA ACQUISITION METHODS

11.2.1.1 SLOW CAMERA ROTATION METHODS

As already mentioned, conventional SPECT is most often performed using a single, relatively slow rotation of a gamma camera equipped with one or more detectors and a parallel-hole collimator. Standard tomographic reconstruction theory demands that projection data be collected over a minimum of 180°, but more commonly, data are acquired over a full 360°. During a study, the camera will stop at multiple angular positions (typically 10–30 s per stop) acquiring projection data; thus, a typical SPECT scan takes from 10–15 min (cardiac) to 30–40 min (oncology) to perform. Additionally, as many modern cameras combine SPECT and computed tomography (CT), a separate CT image is often acquired to be used for improved localization and attenuation correction (Delbeke et al. 2006). We refer to this type of acquisition as slow rotation, as compared with fast rotation, which consists of multiple rapid acquisitions, often as fast as 10 s per rotation (cf. Smith et al. 1994). The latter technique is discussed in Section 11.2.1.2.

The projection data, when combined with the system matrix (describing the camera-object geometry and potentially including information regarding the distribution of attenuating media in the object), form a system of linear equations that are used for image reconstruction. In the case of a dynamic study, the purpose of image reconstruction is to provide information on both the 3D spatial activity distribution and the temporal behavior of this distribution. This can be thought of as constituting a four-dimensional (4D) image (3D spatial + temporal).

When activity changes in the object are rapid compared with the time needed for acquisition, each projection corresponds to a different activity distribution and a suitable dynamic reconstruction algorithm must be utilized that can account for these differences. As already mentioned, the data collected during a single slow camera rotation result in inconsistent projections that, when combined with the system matrix, form an underdetermined system of equations (i.e., more unknowns than equations). In order to solve such a system, additional information is required. Typically, this information comes in the form of educated assumptions or from measurements made using other modalities (e.g., CT for combined SPECT/CT systems). This additional information must restrict the scope of possible solutions and is usually provided as a set of constraints, which may take many different forms.

If one assumes that the temporal behavior of the tracer can be described by an underlying function (which may be derived from a pharmacokinetic model), then it is possible to reconstruct the kinetic parameters directly from the projection data. Such image reconstructions yield images representing spatial distributions of the parameters of interest and hence are called parametric images. This technique has been used previously (Limber et al. 1995; Hebber et al. 1997) in order to estimate washout parameters directly from projection data. The methods that were used in these studies made the assumption that the underlying temporal behavior is governed by the dilution principle in that the tracer concentration within each object voxel can be described by an exponential (or dual exponential) function. The reconstruction procedure then determines the initial activity and decay parameters within each object voxel.

Other techniques, such as the dSPECT method proposed by Farncombe et al. (1999) and Bauschke et al. (1999), take a different approach. Rather than incorporating an underlying kinetic model for each object voxel, this method imposes loose constraints on the temporal behavior of activity, assuming that activity changes in each voxel follow one of three scenarios: monotonically increasing, monotonically decreasing, or a combination of these two—increasing and then decreasing. However, no particular functional behavior for the time–activity curves (TACs) is assumed. This leads to a set of linear equations where the first derivative of every TAC may change sign at most once. These constraints are applied independently to every voxel so different regions of interest (ROIs) or even separate voxels may have different temporal behaviors. The 4D distribution of activity is then reconstructed iteratively using either a constrained least-squares (CLS) or dynamic expectation maximization (dEM) approach. Section 11.3.1 provides a detailed description of the dSPECT method.

A modification of the dSPECT approach imposes constraints on the second derivative of the TAC in every voxel, eliminating some nonphysical solutions by enforcing smooth TAC behavior (Humphries et al. 2011). Alternatively, a factor analysis (FA) approach has been proposed where the dynamic activity in every voxel is assumed to be a linear combination of a small number of time-dependent functions (factors) (Sitek et al. 2001). The functional form of these factors can be either described ahead of time (based on some physiological process) or determined as part of the reconstruction process, along with the factor coefficients for each voxel.

11.2.1.2 FAST CAMERA ROTATION METHODS

In contrast to the slow-rotation methods, in which the tracer changes are rapid with respect to the acquisition time, the fast-rotation methods increase temporal data sampling by acquiring projection data during multiple, fast rotations of the camera. Within each rotation, it is assumed that the tracer distribution changes slowly. Thus, the projection data are consistent over each rotation of the camera. A particular study is then comprised of several rotations, often more than a hundred, thus necessitating acquisition times as short as a few seconds per rotation (Smith et al. 1994; Chen et al. 2004). The result of such rapid-acquisition procedures is extremely low count levels in projections. However, since the projections are assumed to be consistent, standard reconstruction methods such as filtered backprojection (FBP) or standard iterative methods such as ordered subsets expectation maximization (OSEM) can be used to generate a dynamic series of 3D images (one image per rotation).

As triple-head cameras have higher sensitivity than single- or dual-head systems, the fast camera rotation method has been almost exclusively used with such cameras and predominantly with a continuous rotation protocol (Chua et al. 1993; Onishi et al. 1996). Unfortunately, triple-head cameras have currently become increasingly rare, with only a few older systems available in clinics and only a subset of those capable of performing multiple fast rotations.

With the fast-rotation approach, each reconstructed image provides information about the state of the object (or a certain region within this object) at the time when the dataset was acquired. Subsequently, the data extracted from the whole series of images are combined into a TAC that describes the dynamic behavior of the radiotracer within a region (Smith et al. 1996). For diagnosis, the determined temporal behavior can then be compared with that of normal physiology. For example, reductions in cardiac blood flow compared with normal levels may indicate areas of ischemia or infarct. Alternatively, the images reconstructed from fast-rotation acquisitions can be used in conjunction with a physiological model in order to extract kinetic parameters associated with specific metabolic processes (Smith et al. 1994; Onishi et al. 1996). Yet another approach proposes to completely omit the image reconstruction stage and calculate kinetic parameters directly from projection data without reconstructing images (Chiao et al. 1994; Reutter et al. 2000). Such a technique is directly comparable to parametric imaging methods used in PET imaging.

In spite of the fact that triple-head cameras are relatively rare and the images reconstructed from fast-rotation datasets suffer from low signal-to-noise ratio, this approach has been used in several clinical studies investigating myocardial perfusion with ^{99m}Tc-teboroxime (Smith et al. 1996; Chua et al. 1993), myocardial metabolism with ^{123}I-BMIPP (Okizaki et al. 2007), brain receptors (Onishi et al. 1996), and brain infection (Kataoka et al. 2007).

An ideal fast-rotation method would acquire projection data using a continuous camera rotation, a feat made possible only with slip-ring gantry systems. As most SPECT systems do not utilize this type of gantry, some studies thereby make use of a "fanning" acquisition technique where the camera rotates multiple times back and forth. This method has been proposed for myocardial perfusion studies with ^{99m}Tc-teboroxime, with a dual-head camera performing a series of rapid 36 s rotations with alternating clockwise and counterclockwise orbits (Chen et al. 2004). Another approach takes advantage of the fact that during a 360° rotation of a triple-head camera system, each detector moves through a total of 120°. Data from each rotation can be subdivided into two 180° rotation datasets (60° for each detector). This method allows for reconstruction of two images (instead of one when no data grouping is used) from each 360° camera rotation (Celler et al. 1997).

11.2.1.3 MIXED PLANAR–SPECT ACQUISITIONS

An approach that avoids the need for temporal constraints or high temporal sampling uses a combination of dynamic planar acquisitions and static SPECT acquisitions. This method may be helpful when the dynamics of the tracer have a rapid initial phase, followed by a slower washout or clearance phase, during which the tracer distribution is reasonably static and standard SPECT imaging is applicable. This is often the situation with biodistribution or dosimetry studies where the wash-in or uptake of the tracer is rapid, but its clearance from differing compartments is slow. In this case, a two-dimensional (2D) scan, acquired by a carefully positioned camera (at an angle that adequately separates the organs of interest), can provide the initial time information about fast tracer uptake, while the details of the 3D tracer distribution during the washout phase can be later obtained with a standard SPECT acquisition.

Measurement of myocardial blood flow (MBF) is one example of a clinical application in which this approach has been applied (Sugihara et al. 2001). ^{99m}Tc-labeled flow tracers typically have rapid uptake into the myocardium, followed by slow clearance. As discussed in Section 11.3.4.1, one of the objectives of dynamic cardiac blood flow measurement is to obtain the myocardial flow reserve (MFR), which is the ratio of the blood flow at stress to that at rest. As flow can be approximated by the final uptake of the tracer normalized by the integral of the arterial input function, the ratio of this measurement at stress and rest is a surrogate for the MFR. Sugihara et al. (2001) and later Storto et al. (2004) showed that the arterial input function could be estimated from an ROI drawn over the pulmonary artery on a dynamic planar image acquired during tracer injection, while the regional MBF could be established from a SPECT study acquired 30 min postinjection. This approach correlated well with intracoronary Doppler measures of flow (Storto et al. 2004) and showed incremental prognostic information over relative perfusion imaging alone (Daniele et al. 2011). A drawback of this approach is that accurate quantification of planar data is not possible, and so measurement of absolute myocardial flow cannot be done.

11.2.1.4 DYNAMIC SPECT USING STATIONARY SYSTEMS

dSPECT can also be performed using a stationary (or quasi-stationary) camera consisting of multiple detector elements. The basic requirement in this case is that the camera configuration must permit the acquisition of sufficient projection data such that tomographic image reconstruction can be performed. Such cameras are best suited for dSPECT because simultaneous acquisition of all projections removes the inconsistencies in the measured data that are always present in dynamic studies performed with rotating cameras.

Unfortunately, the geometry of stationary SPECT cameras, while allowing for simultaneous (or very fast) acquisition of multiple views, often imposes limits on the scope of studies that can be performed with these systems. Historically, stationary multiring systems have been available for brain imaging—CeraSPECT (Zito et al. 1993), FASTSPECT (Klein et al. 1995), Headtome (Kanno et al. 1981), and others (see Gullberg et al. 2010 for additional references). More recently, several stationary and quasi-stationary systems have been developed for cardiac imaging (DePuey 2012). They allow for simultaneous acquisition of all projection data, mostly through changes in philosophy of the camera design. Instead of using a small number of large detectors covering a large field of view (FOV), these cameras typically focus on a very small FOV and use multiple small detectors. The large number of detectors allows acquisition of all projection angles simultaneously, removing the need to rotate the gantry. The increased sensitivity of such multiprojection acquisition supports increases in temporal resolution. Additionally, if the data can be acquired using list mode, it can be partitioned in time as needed in order to capture the kinetics of the changing tracer distribution. This is the approach that has traditionally been taken with PET (Chapter 12), so in principle, the techniques that have been developed for dynamic PET kinetic analysis can also be applied to dSPECT. While designed and marketed only for cardiac imaging, there is also the potential that these or very similar systems might be applied to other relatively small organs, such as the brain (Park et al. 2013). The performance of these systems and their potential to improve the accuracy of cardiac dynamic studies is of great interest (Ben-Haim et al. 2013).

Because each time frame corresponds to a complete dataset required for a 3D SPECT reconstruction, modern methods of iterative reconstruction that include correction for attenuation, scatter, distance-dependent resolution losses, and partial volume effects can be applied, resulting in quantitatively accurate images at each time point. The challenge with this approach is that these new dedicated cardiac systems still have an order of magnitude less sensitivity than PET, and so the reconstructed images suffer from poor signal-to-noise ratio. This can degrade the accuracy and precision of kinetic analysis and the estimated kinetic parameters. For this reason, there may still be a benefit to applying dynamic reconstruction approaches developed for slow-rotating SPECT systems, as these can capitalize on the correlations between temporal frames to reduce image noise and further improve the quality of the reconstructions.

11.2.2 CLASSIFICATION BASED ON DATA PROCESSING METHODS

Following data acquisition using one of the techniques described above, many different approaches can be used for image reconstruction or data processing. In an effort to describe these methods, we have broadly grouped them into two general categories: (1) image-based approaches, whereby projection data are first reconstructed into a series of dynamic images depicting the 3D radiotracer distribution changes over time and then analyzed in order to obtain kinetic information concerning patient physiology, and (2) direct estimation approaches, where kinetic parameters are estimated directly from the measured projection data without first performing explicit image reconstruction.

11.2.2.1 IMAGE-BASED APPROACHES

The simplest image-based approach reconstructs a series of images from the datasets that were acquired during multiple fast rotations of the SPECT camera or were obtained from multiple acquisitions using a stationary system. Under the assumption that the radiotracer distribution remains constant during the acquisition of each dataset, each time frame (corresponding to a single camera rotation) is then processed separately using a standard (i.e., static) reconstruction algorithm to form a single 3D image representing the activity distribution averaged over the time when these data were acquired. Afterwards, these images can be combined into a 4D (3D + time) object and used to create TACs for subsequent analysis of radiotracer kinetics.

Because of limitations in spatial resolution and low signal to noise, the fast-rotation methods have been mostly used to determine TACs based on counts contained within user-determined ROIs rather than in individual voxels. In the simplest approach, these TACs can be used to extract basic temporal information regarding tissue physiology and can be compared with normal physiological behavior. This method has been used in a large number of clinical investigations (Nakajima et al. 1991; Ogasawara et al. 2001).

Alternatively, kinetic parameters of the underlying physiology can be extracted from TACs that were defined for ROIs or even for particular voxels (Okizaki et al. 2007; Bal et al. 2003; Chen et al. 2004; Ross et al. 1997; Kadrmas and Gullberg 2001; Di Bella et al. 2001). Some methods rely on relatively simple image reconstruction methods, such as FBP, without attenuation or scatter correction (Okizaki et al. 2007). The major advantages of using this approach are short reconstruction time. However, the limited quantitative accuracy and high image noise of FBP images may result in data that are difficult to interpret or produce large uncertainties in the fitted kinetic parameters. Alternatively, more advanced reconstruction methods, such as the 4D ordered subsets maximum *a posteriori* (OSMAP) method (Kadrmas and Gullberg 2001), have been proposed. This technique can include compensations for all image degradation factors (e.g., scatter, attenuation, and spatial response), as well as incorporate a compartmental model–based temporal *prior*.

In image-based approaches, subsequent ROI boundaries are most often drawn by hand, although additional information obtained from anatomical imaging (e.g., CT and MRI) may be used when delineating regions. In fact, it is not uncommon to threshold anatomical images when segmenting specific organs. Segmentation based on anatomy alone may prove problematic, so alternative methods that utilize the underlying dynamic behavior of the tracer may be used instead. Specific methods that segment SPECT images based on kinetic behavior rather than anatomy include a semiautomatic segmentation that uses a maximum-likelihood estimator (Chiao et al. 1994; Di Bella et al. 1997) or factor analysis of dynamic structures (FADS) methodology that is used to extract regions that share similar TACs from a series of dynamic images (Sitek et al. 2000, 2002b). A number of methods have been proposed to apply cluster analysis techniques to dSPECT image sequences in order to achieve image segmentation into various ROIs with different dynamic behaviors (Bal et al. 2003; Saad et al. 2008).

To a separate class belong studies that attempt to jointly process the series of images acquired during cardiac gated studies. Strong correlations between gated time frames have been exploited in the 4D image reconstructions using the Karhunen–Loeve (KL) transform (Narayanan et al. 1999). Extensions of this type of method into five-dimensional (5D) imaging combining dynamic changes of radiotracer distributions with cardiac motion have been investigated using dEM and temporal regularization (Jin et al. 2006; Feng et al. 2006). Other studies investigated the use of the modified block sequential regularized expectation maximization (BSREM) II or the one-step-late (OSL) algorithms to reconstruct the 5D data (Niu et al. 2010, 2012).

11.2.2.2 PROJECTION-BASED APPROACHES

Several different dSPECT techniques that bypass the image reconstruction step are able to extract kinetic parameters directly from projection data. In principle, projection-based approaches must include an accurate description of the data acquisition process (system matrix) and contain information regarding the tissue input function, and spatial and temporal behavior of the radiotracer in voxels or ROIs. In practice, such a description is difficult to achieve, as it requires *a priori* information regarding the location of each organ (or ROI), along with the underlying kinetic model. In addition, combining these two components would result in a rather complicated set of nonlinear equations that may prove difficult to solve. Therefore, in order to extract useful kinetic parameters, most methods in this category apply some simplifying assumptions.

For example, methods that attempt to estimate kinetic parameters directly from projections utilize compartmental modeling. This approach restricts the set of solutions by assuming that the data are represented by kinetic parameters that are tied to an underlying pharmacokinetic model (Shargel et al. 2005; Macheras and Iliadis 2006). These models are typically determined *a priori* based on known or assumed tracer behavior, and therefore these assumptions restrict the behavior of the TACs to a set of solutions that are deemed adequate or "meaningful."

Some methods, such as the integration-by-parts technique proposed by Zeng et al. (2012), determine kinetic parameters using wavelet functions and replacing differential equations into equations without any derivatives. Other methods first extract information about the temporal behavior of the radiotracer within an ROI from projection data and then determine kinetic parameters from these TACs (Maltz 2000).

In order to restrict possible solutions regarding temporal behavior, alternative temporal basis functions have also been proposed. For example, Reutter et al. (2000) described the temporal behavior of a radiotracer by a set of temporal B-splines. The overall tracer dynamics is then described as a linear combination of these assumed temporal functions. More information on this technique is provided in Section 11.3.2. Other alternative basis functions that have been investigated consist of a series of exponential (orthogonal) functions (Hebber et al. 1997; Maltz 2000) or discrete physical factors describing time changes of radiotracer concentration in organs obtained using principal component analysis (Barber 1980) and related techniques, such FADS (Sitek et al. 2000). Regardless of the basis function used, the underlying problem can be formulated as a linear set of equations to be solved using least-squares (LS), weighted least-squares (WLS), or statistical (Poisson or other) methods. Often, to simplify the problem, some additional conditions are applied. For example, the boundaries of regions with different dynamic behaviors are assumed to be known *a priori* (Reutter et al. 2000). In such a case, only a single compartmental model needs to be employed or the number of exponential functions or factors restricted (Maltz and Budinger 2000). Alternative techniques propose smoothing projection data using parabolic interpolation to reduce noise and artifacts (Lau et al. 1998), or using (regularized) Kalman filters for image reconstruction (Kervinen et al. 2004).

11.3 DETAILED DISCUSSION OF SELECTED METHODS

11.3.1 IMPOSING TEMPORAL CONSTRAINTS IN IMAGE RECONSTRUCTION: DYNAMIC SPECT METHOD

As mentioned, with slow-rotation dSPECT methods, temporal changes in the activity distribution can lead to inconsistent projections that do not permit an accurate image reconstruction when using conventional approaches. In addition, images obtained from conventional reconstruction algorithms of such data will not contain any information regarding the underlying changes in radiotracer distribution; thus, all potentially meaningful temporal information regarding organ function will be lost.

In this case, to reconstruct an accurate 4D radiotracer distribution, the procedure must include an additional mechanism that will allow the reconstruction algorithm to account for the dynamics and cope with inconsistent projections. The mechanism employed by the dSPECT method (Farncombe et al. 1999, 2000; Bauschke et al. 1999) uses temporal constraints on each object voxel to establish a temporal link from one projection to the next. In this approach, the radioactivity present within the investigated object is assumed to vary smoothly over time, and in each voxel, it may be independently decreasing, increasing, or increasing and then decreasing over time. Please note that the tracer dynamics in every voxel is independent of its neighbors.

In the case of decreasing activity (such as the case for physical decay or physiological excretion), the activity $f_i(t_k)$ in the ith voxel of the object at each kth time point can be described by the inequality

$$f_i(t_0) \ge f_i(t_1) \ge f_i(t_2) \ge \ldots f_i(t_k) \cdots \ge f_i(t_n) \ge 0 \tag{11.1}$$

The difference in voxel activity from one time point to the next is also positive:

$$f_i(t_0) - f_i(t_1) \ge 0, f_i(t_1) - f_i(t_2) \ge 0, \ldots f_i(t_{n-1}) - f_i(t_n) \ge 0, f_i(t_n) \ge 0 \tag{11.2}$$

Through a matrix–vector relation, we can now assign a new variable, $\tilde{f}$, to represent the difference in activity from one time point to the next.

$$\begin{bmatrix} f_i(t_0) - f_i(t_1) \\ f_i(t_1) - f_i(t_2) \\ \ldots \\ \ldots \\ f_i(t_n) - 0 \end{bmatrix} = \begin{bmatrix} 1 & -1 & 0 & \ldots & 0 \\ 0 & 1 & -1 & 0 & \vdots \\ \vdots & \vdots & \ddots & \ddots & \vdots \\ \vdots & \vdots & \vdots & 1 & -1 \\ 0 & \ldots & \ldots & \ldots & 1 \end{bmatrix} \begin{bmatrix} f_i(t_0) \\ f_i(t_1) \\ \ldots \\ \ldots \\ f_i(t_n) \end{bmatrix} = Af = \tilde{f} \tag{11.3}$$

This new variable can be incorporated into a standard reconstruction algorithm, such as expectation maximization, thus resulting in a dynamic reconstruction algorithm:

$$\tilde{f}^{new} = \frac{\tilde{f}^{old}}{\sum \left(\mathbf{HA}^{-1} \right)^T} \frac{\sum \left(\mathbf{HA}^{-1} \right)^T g}{\mathbf{HA}^{-1} \tilde{f}^{old}} \tag{11.4}$$

where $\mathbf{H}$ represents the system matrix that transforms a 3D activity distribution into a set of 2D projections g, and $\mathbf{A}$ is the aforementioned difference matrix. It should be noted that the original vector, f, can always be determined from the cumulative sum of $\tilde{f}$. That is, the matrix $\mathbf{A}$ is always invertible, as the determinant is 1 and is simply equal to

$$\mathbf{A}^{-1} = \begin{bmatrix} 1 & 1 & 1 & \ldots & 1 \\ 0 & 1 & 1 & \ldots & 1 \\ \vdots & \vdots & \ddots & \ddots & \vdots \\ \vdots & \ldots & \ldots & 1 & 1 \\ 0 & \ldots & \ldots & \ldots & 1 \end{bmatrix} \tag{11.5}$$

We can extend this method to the situation where the activity within each voxel increases over time (the case of radiotracer uptake) with the simple change of the above expression. That is, for an increasing activity, the difference matrix $\mathbf{A}$ becomes

$$\begin{bmatrix} f_i(t_0) \\ f_i(t_1) - f_i(t_0) \\ \ldots \\ \ldots \\ f_i(t_n) - f_i(t_{n-1}) \end{bmatrix} = \begin{bmatrix} 1 & 0 & \ldots & \ldots & 0 \\ -1 & 1 & 0 & \ldots & \vdots \\ 0 & -1 & \ddots & \ddots & \vdots \\ \vdots & \ldots & \ddots & \ddots & 0 \\ 0 & \ldots & \ldots & -1 & 1 \end{bmatrix} \begin{bmatrix} f_i(t_0) \\ f_i(t_1) \\ \ldots \\ \ldots \\ f_i(t_n) \end{bmatrix} = \mathbf{A}f = \tilde{f} \tag{11.6}$$

Again, these new variables can be inserted into any image reconstruction algorithm in order to obtain a temporal link within the object at different time frames. Note that this method of incorporating temporal constraints within the reconstruction framework makes no assumption as to the behavior of the temporal changes, but only requires that the changes in activity from one frame to the next be a positive quantity, a trait lending itself well to the use of iterative algorithms.

Combining the two inequality constraints, it is possible to model the case of both increasing and decreasing activity within a given object voxel, provided the time point corresponding to the peak activity is known. This type of behavior is more physiologically appropriate, as it accounts for uptake of the radiotracer into a voxel, followed by a subsequent washout phase.

$$0 \le f_i(t_0) \le \ldots \le f_i(t_p - 1) \le f_i(t_p) \ge f_i(t_p + 1) \ldots \ge f_i(t_n) \ge 0 \tag{11.7}$$

While providing a mechanism for activity uptake, the time point of maximum uptake must be known *a priori* and incorporated into the image reconstruction process. A further modification can be made to provide a more flexible peak definition:

$$f_i(t_{p-1}) \le 2f_i(t_p) \ge f_i(t_{p+1}) \quad \text{or} \quad 2f_i(t_p) \ge f_i(t_{p-1}) + f_i(t_{p+1}) \tag{11.8}$$

As can be seen in Figure 11.1, with this new definition, the peak position is allowed to vary within three time points, yet still satisfy these constraints. In this case, the difference matrix $\mathbf{A}$ becomes

$$\begin{bmatrix} f_i(t_0) \\ f_i(t_1) - f_i(t_0) \\ \ldots \\ f_i(t_p) \\ \ldots \\ f_i(t_{n-1}) - f_i(t_n) \\ f_i(t_n) \end{bmatrix} = \begin{bmatrix} 1 & 0 & \ldots & \ldots & \ldots & \ldots & 0 \\ -1 & 1 & 0 & \ldots & \ldots & \ldots & \vdots \\ 0 & \ddots & \ddots & \ldots & \ddots & 0 & \vdots \\ \vdots & \ldots & -1 & 2 & -1 & 0 & 0 \\ \vdots & \ldots & \ddots & 0 & 1 & -1 & 0 \\ 0 & \ldots & \ldots & \ldots & \ddots & \ddots & \ddots \\ 0 & \ldots & \ldots & \ldots & \ldots & \ldots & 1 \end{bmatrix} \begin{bmatrix} f_i(t_0) \\ f_i(t_1) \\ \ldots \\ f_i(t_p) \\ \ldots \\ f_i(t_n) \end{bmatrix} = \mathbf{A}f = \tilde{f} \tag{11.9}$$

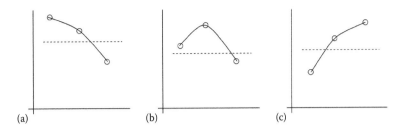

Figure 11.1 Diagram depicting the three cases considered by the dSPECT method. The dashed line represents the average activity, $f_i(t_{p-1}) + f_i(t_{p+1})/2$. In all three cases, the peak inequality condition is satisfied.

We have previously incorporated this type of constraint into the expectation maximization algorithm (Farncombe et al. 2001), choosing initially the mid–time frame to be the peak activity position for each voxel. In this approach, the peak is free to move (to a time point with the higher value) within one of three positions. After every iteration, the new peak location is determined for each voxel and the updated difference matrix determined prior to the next iteration. Keep in mind that each voxel will have its own difference matrix, and so each voxel is free to behave independently with its own peak activity location.

To test the feasibility of this approach, a simulation exercise was performed using a simple 2D annulus phantom. Projection data were simulated modeling various slow-rotation acquisition methods: (1) single head rotating over 180°; (2) dual-head camera with detectors positioned at 90° (L-mode), each rotating over 90°; and (3) triple-head camera with each detector rotating over 180°. The annulus was divided into four segments with differing kinetics within each segment. The total acquisition time was 20 min with a total of 64 projection angles. Results presented in Figure 11.2 show that those acquisitions that involve more detectors (i.e., two heads at 90° and three heads at 120°) yield improved image quality and improved TACs compared with the data acquired with a single detector. This is due to the increased number of simultaneous projection views, thus providing more consistent projection data. This simple experiment shows that the dSPECT method is able to provide useful temporal data from slow-rotation SPECT acquisitions comprised of inconsistent projection data.

The dSPECT method was initially developed for use with slow-rotation SPECT but has since been incorporated into fast-rotation acquisitions as well. While the slow-rotation dSPECT method imposes constraints from one projection to the next, the fast-rotation dSPECT incorporates these temporal constraints from one reconstructed time frame to the next and uses all the projection data from a single rotation to reconstruct the activity distribution at each time point.

The dSPECT method has been applied to various clinical applications, including renal imaging (Celler et al. 2001), MPI (Farncombe et al. 2003a; Feng et al. 2006), and bone imaging (Farncombe et al. 2003b; Wells et al. 2004). In fact, it has even been demonstrated that the dEM approach can be used to process both wall motion and tracer kinetics simultaneously during 5D cardiac studies (Farncombe et al. 2003a; Feng et al. 2006). This work used the NCAT cardiac-torso phantom (Segars et al. 1999), and simulated both cardiac wall motion and blood flow kinetics of [99mTc]-teboroxime (Stewart et al. 1990). Blood flow was simulated in two different regions of the myocardium corresponding to healthy and ischemic myocardium. Simulated gated SPECT projection data were obtained using a rapid-rotation method. For each cardiac gate interval, blood flow data are reconstructed as a set of temporal images representing the tracer distribution. The reconstruction used the dEM algorithm combined with simultaneous filtering across the cardiac phases using the KL transform (Narayanan et al. 1999). Results indicated that even in the case of very low-count projection data, the temporal link enforced between images with the dEM algorithm was able to significantly improve image quality compared with conventional iterative reconstructions (Figure 11.3).

Bone scans utilizing [99mTc]-phosphonate complexes such as methylene diphosphonate (MDP) are routinely used to assess bone remodeling as a result of skeletal fractures or cancer infiltration. While it is common to perform planar imaging to assess the extent of disease, in the regions of the pelvis, overlapping structures can make localization of tracer uptake difficult. In these cases, it is beneficial to perform 3D imaging using SPECT. However, changes in activity concentration within the bladder as a result of tracer washout during

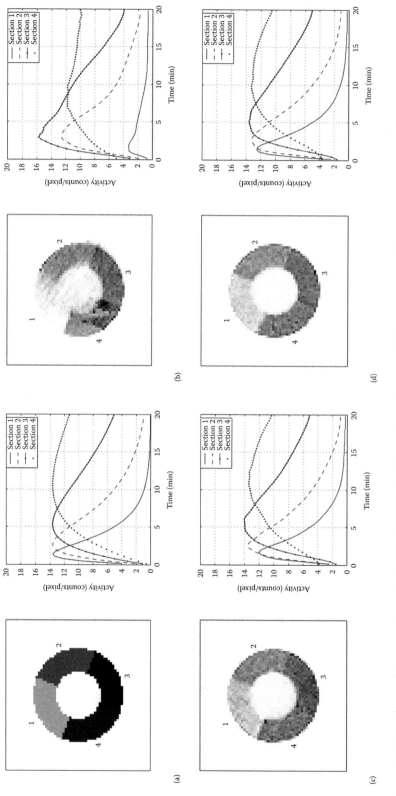

Figure 11.2 Simple simulation experiment to test the dSPECT algorithm using various acquisition geometries. The total scan time in each case was equal to 20 min. (a) True activity distribution in the object at time $t = 5$ min, along with the associated TACs for each segment. (b) Results from simulated data acquired with a single-head camera rotating over 64 angles. Note the streaking artifacts present in images and inaccuracies produced in the TACs. (c) Reconstructed data from a dual-head system with detectors positioned at 90° to each other and using data acquired over a 90° rotation of each detector (180° total). The reconstructed image quality is vastly improved, along with more accurate TACs. (d) Results from a triple-head SPECT camera yielded the best image quality and TAC accuracy.

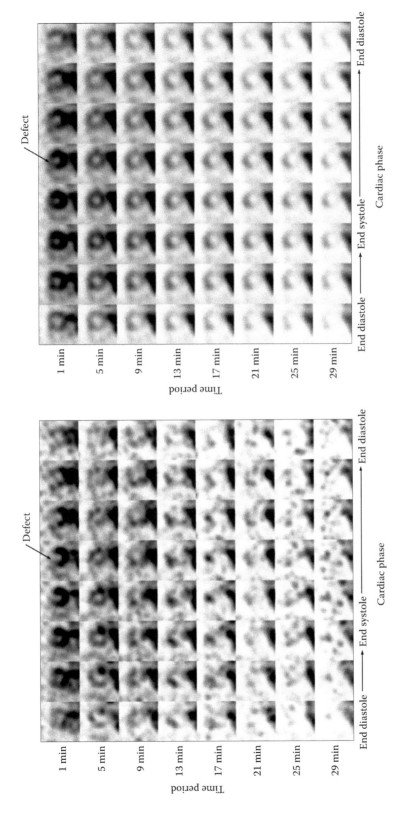

Figure 11.3 Comparison of 5D dynamic iterative reconstruction methods. Multiple, fast-rotation SPECT data were reconstructed using conventional OSEM and then spatially and temporally filtered (left). The image sequence on the right has been reconstructed using the dEM approach across time frames and filtered temporally across cardiac phases using the KL transform. It is apparent that in the presence of low-count data, the temporal constraints imposed via the dEM algorithm were able to provide significantly improved image quality, rendering the defect region visible even at later time frames. (Reproduced from Farncombe, T.H., et al., Toward 5 dimensional SPECT reconstruction: Determining myocardial blood flow and wall motion in a single study, presented at International Conference on Fully 3D Reconstruction in Radiology and Nuclear Medicine, Saint Malo, France, 2003.)

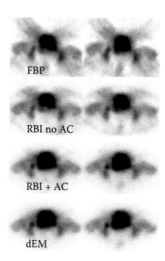

Figure 11.4 Transaxial slices showing a patient with metastatic bone disease where an 88% change in bladder activity occurred during acquisition of this scan. Each row corresponds to two consecutive slices of a different reconstruction. From top to bottom, the reconstruction methods are FBP, rescaled block iterative without attenuation correction (RBI no AC), RBI + AC, and dEM. Significant streak artifacts that are seen in the FBP image (and to some extent, the RBI image) and decrease visibility of the lesion are a result of attenuation and bladder filling effects. They disappear in the RBI + AC and dEM images, making the lesion much better visible. (Reproduced from Wells, R.G., et al., *J. Nucl. Med.*, 55, 1685–1691, 2004.)

data acquisition may result in inconsistent projection data. This will create streaking artifacts in the reconstructed SPECT images (Figure 11.4) (Farncombe et al. 2003b; Wells et al. 2004). Application of the dSPECT reconstruction method removes these artifacts.

11.3.2 SELECTION OF ALTERNATIVE TEMPORAL BASIS FUNCTIONS

11.3.2.1 SPATIOTEMPORAL MODELING OF DYNAMIC IMAGE DATA

An integral part of any image reconstruction process is the correct representation of the data. The selection of data representation is usually problem dependent and is typically used to restrict the solutions obtained from image reconstruction to a set of meaningful solutions. For example, image reconstruction methods that attempt to estimate kinetic parameters directly from projections (known as direct methods [Gullberg et al. 2010]) utilize compartmental modeling to restrict the set of solutions by assuming that the data are represented by kinetic parameters that are tied to a particular compartmental model (Shargel et al. 2005; Macheras and Iliadis 2006). The choice of the model is typically based on what is known about the behavior of the contrast agent or radiotracer.

While being an idealized model of tracer distribution, a compartmental model may not provide the best representation of the underlying processes under study. As a result, alternative data representation models have been developed that are not tied to any particular kinetic model and are known as semidirect methods of image reconstruction. While several of these representations exist, we focus on data representation that employs spatiotemporal spline interpolation (Reutter et al. 2000; Gullberg et al. 2010).

Here, we let the activity distribution be denoted by $f(\mathbf{x}, t)$, where $t \in \mathbb{R}$ represents time and $\mathbf{x} \in \Omega \subset \mathbb{R}^d$ represents a point in the image space Ω that is a subset of the spatial domain, with d as the spatial dimensionality of the object (typically $d = 2, 3$). The activity distribution is then represented as a sum of spatial and temporal basis functions:

$$f(\mathbf{x}, t) = \sum_{i,j} c_{ij} v_i(\mathbf{x}) u_{ij}(t)$$

(11.10)

where $v_i(\mathbf{x})$ are spatial basis functions (such as cubic voxels), $u_{ij}(t)$ are temporal basis functions, and $c_{ij} \in \mathbb{R}$ are the coefficients of the basis expansion. Note that in the representation shown in Equation 11.10, the temporal basis functions are allowed to vary based on the spatial spline coefficient. In other words, each spatiotemporal coefficient c_{ij} may represent a different set of temporal basis functions $u_{ij}(t)$, depending on the index i. Spatially varying temporal splines may be useful in cases where prior information is available about TACs based on spatial location, and therefore a different set of temporal basis functions may be used. When the set of temporal basis functions is assumed to be spatially invariant, then the activity distribution may be represented by

$$f(\mathbf{x},t) = \sum_{i,j} c_{ij} v_i(\mathbf{x}) u_j(t) \tag{11.11}$$

In the interest of simplicity, it will be assumed that the set of temporal basis functions, u_{ij}, does not vary in the spatial sense and will therefore be denoted by u_i

Let us denote a rotating detector surface of M pixels at time t by $\mathbf{y}(t) \in \mathbb{R}^M$. Then, the projections of the activity distribution $f(\mathbf{x}, t)$ are a function of the position of the detector surface y at a time t and can be written as

$$p(\mathbf{y}(t),t) = \int_\Omega H(\mathbf{x},\mathbf{y}(t)) f(\mathbf{x},t) d\mathbf{x} \tag{11.12}$$

where $p : \mathbb{R}^M \times \mathbb{R} \to \mathbb{R}^M$ is the map of projected values onto detector surface $\mathbf{y}(t)$ at time t, $\mathbf{x} \in \Omega$ is a location in the image space Ω, and $H(\mathbf{x},\mathbf{y}(t))$ is a function that maps the activity at $f(\mathbf{x}, t)$ to the projection $p(\mathbf{y}(t), t)$.

Substituting $f(\mathbf{x}, t)$ from Equation 11.11, the projections $p(\mathbf{y}(t), t)$ are written as

$$
\begin{aligned}
p(\mathbf{y}(t),t) &= \int_\Omega H(\mathbf{x},\mathbf{y}(t)) \sum_{i,j} c_{ij} v_i(\mathbf{x}) u_j(t) d\mathbf{x} \\
&= \sum_{i,j} c_{ij} u_j(t) \int_\Omega H(\mathbf{x},\mathbf{y}(t)) v_i(\mathbf{x}) d\mathbf{x} \\
&= \sum_{i,j} c_{ij} u_j(t) V_i(\mathbf{x})
\end{aligned}
\tag{11.13}
$$

where

$$V_i(\mathbf{x}) = \int_\Omega H(\mathbf{x},\mathbf{y}(t)) v_i(\mathbf{x}) d\mathbf{x} \tag{11.14}$$

is the projection of the ith spatial basis function onto the detector surface position $\mathbf{y}(t)$. Equations 11.13 and 11.14 provide a representation in terms of spatiotemporal basis functions of the instantaneous projection:

$$p_m(t) = p(y_m(t),t) = \sum_{i,j} c_{ij} u_j(t) V_i(y_m(t)) \tag{11.15}$$

with $y_m(t) \in \mathbb{R}$ representing a detector pixel location at time t, and $m = 1,\ldots,M$ is the detector pixel index.

Typically in SPECT, the projection data are recorded as a number of detected events collected over a time segment $[t_{s,k}, t_{e,k}]$, where $t_{s,k}$ is the start time and $t_{e,k}$ is the end time of the kth acquisition. Therefore, the kth projection is the cumulative activity over the kth time segment and is represented by

$$
\begin{aligned}
p_{mk} &= \int_{t_{s,k}}^{t_{e,k}} p_m(t)\,dt \\
&= \int_{t_{s,k}}^{t_{e,k}} \sum_{i,j} c_{ij} u_j(t) V_i\big(y_m(t)\big)\,dt \\
&= \sum_{i,j} c_{ij} \int_{t_{s,k}}^{t_{e,k}} u_j(t) V_i\big(y_m(t)\big)\,dt
\end{aligned}
\tag{11.16}
$$

where $k = 1,\ldots,K$ is the projection index with the total number of projections K.

In Equation 11.16, we denote

$$
B_{mk,ij} = \int_{t_{s,k}}^{t_{e,k}} u_j(t) V_i\big(y_m(t)\big)\,dt
\tag{11.17}
$$

and therefore

$$
p_{mk} = \sum_{i=1}^{I} \sum_{j=1}^{J} B_{mk,ij} c_{ij}
\tag{11.18}
$$

where I is the number of spatial basis functions and J is the number of temporal basis functions. This last equation can be written in matrix form as

$$
\mathbf{p} = \mathbf{Bc}
\tag{11.19}
$$

where $\mathbf{p} \in \mathbb{R}^{MK}$ is a MK-sized vector, $B \in \mathbb{R}^{MK \times IJ}$ is an $MN \times IJ$ matrix, and $\mathbf{c} \in \mathbb{R}^{IJ}$ is an IJ-sized vector with M as the number of pixels in the detector space, K the total number of projections, and IJ the total number of spatiotemporal basis functions.

The projection operator $\mathbf{B}$ is a linear operator that maps the basis function coefficients in image space $\mathbf{c}$ to the projection space with elements $\mathbf{p}$. The matrix $\mathbf{B}$, in addition to modeling data representation by spatiotemporal basis functions, also models the physical effects of the imaging system, which include attenuation, the geometric response of the collimator, scatter, and other system-dependent effects (Zaidi 2006).

11.3.2.2 SPATIOTEMPORAL DATA REPRESENTATION USING SPLINES

Splines are commonly used in many fields for data representation since they provide a simple, efficient, and accurate method of representing continuous functions from discrete samples. A large body of work exists related to data representation using splines. The reader may refer to Bartels et al. (1987), Pratt (2007), and Jain (1989) for a comprehensive and detailed explanation of the design and applications of splines.

In the context of dynamic data representation, splines can be employed to describe the object both spatially and temporally. In image reconstruction problems, spatial information about the image to be reconstructed is typically unavailable, and therefore the image is described by a spline basis that is spatially invariant, so standard methods of spline interpolation can be used. In the next few paragraphs, the discussion focuses on the design of temporal splines (splines used to represent TACs) for which some prior information is typically available.

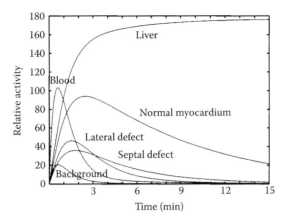

Figure 11.5 Simulated TACs. The variation of the TACs is rapid in the beginning of the acquisition and slower as time progresses. (From Reutter, B.W., et al., *IEEE Trans. Med. Imaging*, 19, 434–450, 2000.)

Generally, the behavior of TACs during a dynamic image acquisition is marked by a more rapid variation in activity at the beginning of an acquisition, followed by a slower variation at later times, as shown in Figure 11.5. This information about TACs can be exploited in order to reduce *a priori* the number of splines used to represent a TAC, thereby reducing the dimensionality of the problem and possibly regularizing an otherwise underdetermined problem by constraining the variation to an expected (or desired) set of solutions.

As an example, the TACs used in Reutter et al. (2000) (and shown in Figure 11.6) were designed with the aforementioned assumption. In this instance, the splines were used to span 15 time segments that had geometrically increasing support. The most rapid variation representable in a TAC using this spline basis covers a minimum of 10 s at the very beginning of the study, followed by geometrically slower variations as time progresses.

Careful design of a spline basis is important. The set of basis functions must not only accurately represent the expected TACs but also (ideally) be designed so that each TAC is uniquely determined by a set of spline coefficients. If these criteria are not met, then the reconstructed TACs may misrepresent the true curves and the image reconstruction problem may be ill-posed. The reader may refer to Chen et al. (1991) and Nichols et al. (1999) for examples of methodologies used to choose an appropriate temporal spline set based on prior information about the TACs.

TACs can be represented temporally by a set of splines that increase geometrically in support. The geometric scaling of the splines follows the predicted wash-in and washout phases of the radiotracer, where the wash-in phase has large variations over very short periods of time and the washout phase exhibits very small variations over large periods of time. That is, splines with relatively small support are required to accurately describe the wash-in phase, and splines with large support are more adequate to describe the washout phase.

The representation of the TACs by splines does more than just provide an interpolation scheme; it provides a "soft constraint" for the TACs to variations that are desirable or expected.

As an example, let us look at the spline set shown in Figure 11.7. This spline set assumes

1. The fastest variation happens at the very beginning of the time sequence (taking about 10 units of time).
2. The variations become geometrically slower as time progresses.

In other words, the assumption implied by the usage of these splines for temporal representation of the data is the geometric slowing of the TACs over the duration of the study.

Now let us consider the sample TACs shown in Figure 11.8. The TAC for the blood pool (blue line) was generated using

$$c_B(t) = a_1 e^{-b_1(t-d_1)} + a_2 e^{-b_2(t-d_2)}$$
$$c_T(t) = (1-f_v)k_1 c_b(t) * e^{-k_2 t} + f_v c_B(t) \tag{11.20}$$

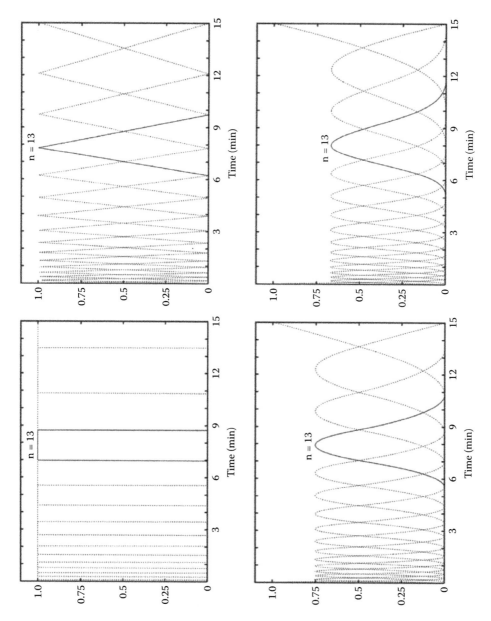

Figure 11.6 Examples of splines used as temporal basis functions: (a) piecewise constant, (b) linear, (c) quadratic, and (d) cubic B-spline basis functions. The TACs are to be represented by a spline set of 16 basis functions where the fastest decay of the TACs is determined by the spline with the narrowest support in the time axis, namely, 10 s. (From Reutter, B.W., et al., *IEEE Trans. Med. Imaging*, 19, 434–450.)

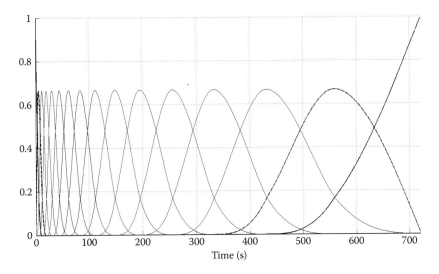

Figure 11.7 Geometrically increasing spline set consisting of 16 splines. Notice that the temporal behavior for the splines at the left and right temporal boundaries is different from that for the rest of the splines in order to account for extrapolated activity. The ordinate axis represents the value of the spline in arbitrary units.

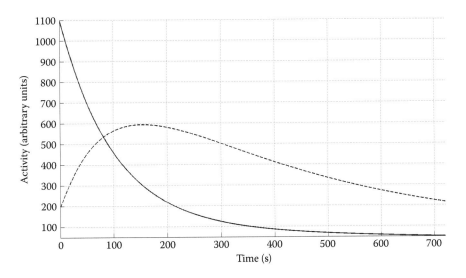

Figure 11.8 TACs generated from a reversible two-compartment model. The blue curve represents the activity in the blood pool, while the red curve represents the radioactivity contained within the tissue.

where the operator * denotes convolution, c_B is the time–activity function of the blood pool, f_v is the fractional volume ratio (i.e., the fraction of blood as opposed to tissue per unit volume), and k_1 and k_2 are the kinetic parameters of a reversible two-compartment model.

We can project the TACs generated by this model onto the spline basis of Figure 11.7 to obtain 16 coefficients whose linear combination provides an adequate description of the variation observed (Figure 11.9).

It must be noted that the basis chosen seems to be adequate since it captures the fastest and slowest variations in the TACs; however, if the TACs were to exhibit faster variations than the spline basis (i.e., no spline decays as fast as the TAC during a certain interval of time), then this information would not be representable by the spline basis and would be "lost." In other words, the temporal resolution of the spline basis is limited to the spline with the smallest support.

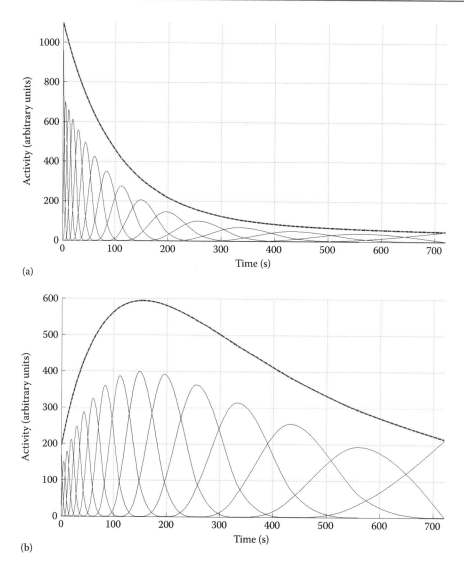

Figure 11.9 The original simulated TAC (thick red), the TAC as interpolated by the spline set (dashed thick blue), and the individual splines scaled according to the respective coefficients (thin blue) shown for (a) the time–activity function in the blood pool and (b) the time–activity function in the tissue. An almost complete overlap of the thick red and dashed blue curves implies high accuracy of the interpolation.

11.3.2.3 IMAGE RECONSTRUCTION METHODS EMPLOYING SPATIOTEMPORAL BASIS FUNCTIONS

The modeling of the image reconstruction method complements the selection of data representation since the latter makes assumptions about the image to be reconstructed, while the former makes assumptions about the underlying nature of the problem. This concept is more easily explained in the following example, which is based on the material presented in Reutter et al. (2000).

Recall the projection matrix **B** shown in Equations 11.18 and 11.19 with elements equal to

$$B_{mk,ij} = \int\limits_{t_{s,k}}^{t_{e,k}} u_j(t) V_i\big(y_m(t)\big)$$

which relates the estimated projections to the spatiotemporal coefficients,

$$\mathbf{p} = \mathbf{Bc}$$

where u_j are temporal basis functions and V_i are defined as in Equation 11.14. Let the set of measured projections be denoted by $\overline{\mathbf{P}}$. Furthermore, let us assume that the noise observed in the measured data $\overline{\mathbf{P}}$ is Gaussian, that is,

$$P\left(\overline{\mathbf{p}}|\mathbf{p};\Sigma\right) = \frac{1}{\sqrt{2\pi|\Sigma|}} \exp\left(-\frac{1}{2}\left(\mathbf{p} - \overline{\mathbf{p}}\right)^T \Sigma^{-1}\left(\mathbf{p} - \overline{\mathbf{p}}\right)\right) \tag{11.21}$$

where Σ is assumed to be a diagonal matrix that is known. Substituting Equation 11.17 into Equation 11.21, we obtain the likelihood:

$$P\left(\overline{\mathbf{p}}|\mathbf{c};\Sigma\right) = \frac{1}{\sqrt{2\pi|\Sigma|}} \exp\left(-\frac{1}{2}\left(\mathbf{Bc} - \overline{\mathbf{p}}\right)^T \Sigma^{-1}\left(\mathbf{Bc} - \overline{\mathbf{p}}\right)\right) \tag{11.22}$$

In this last equation, we have made two fundamental assumptions. The first assumption is due to the data representation, where it is assumed that the space spanned by $\mathbf{B}$ is adequate to map the estimated spatiotemporal coefficients $\mathbf{c}$ to the measurements $\overline{\mathbf{P}}$. The second assumption is due to the nature of the acquisition; that is, the noise in the projections can be modeled by a normal distribution.

In order to simplify the estimation of the spatiotemporal coefficients, $\mathbf{c}$, Equation 11.22 can be written as

$$\log \ P\left(\overline{\mathbf{p}}|\mathbf{c};\Sigma\right) = \log\left(\frac{1}{\sqrt{2\pi|\Sigma|}}\right)\left(-\frac{1}{2}\left(\mathbf{Bc} - \overline{\mathbf{p}}\right)^T \Sigma^{-1}\left(\mathbf{Bc} - \overline{\mathbf{p}}\right)\right) \tag{11.23}$$

Equation 11.23 is commonly known as the log-likelihood. The coefficients estimated through Equation 11.23 would be the same as the coefficients estimated from Equation 11.22 since the logarithm is a monotonically increasing function and achieves its maximum at the same argument points as the likelihood. The optimal coefficients $\mathbf{c}$ can then be estimated by solving

$$\mathbf{c}^* \in \arg\min_{\mathbf{c}}\left(\mathbf{Bc} - \overline{\mathbf{p}}\right)^T \Sigma^{-1}\left(\mathbf{Bc} - \overline{\mathbf{p}}\right) \tag{11.24}$$

where the log term in Equation 11.23 has been dropped since it is a constant and does not change the value of the argument minimizer. If $\boldsymbol{\mathcal{E}}$ is the identity matrix, then Equation 11.24 reduces to

$$\mathbf{c}^* \in \arg\min_{\mathbf{c}}\left\|\mathbf{Bc} - \overline{\mathbf{p}}\right\|^2 \tag{11.25}$$

In summary, from the assumptions made about the nature of the acquisition in Equations 11.21 and 22, where the noise in the measurements is assumed to be contaminated by Gaussian noise, a deterministic optimization problem was formulated, as shown in Equations 11.24 and 11.25.

It must be noted that even though the assumption of Gaussian noise is adequate for some imaging systems, it may not adequately approximate others. In fact, in SPECT imaging, it is more common to model the noise contribution as a Poisson process, and therefore the likelihood function would be better described by the Poisson distribution, with mean $\mathbf{p} = \mathbf{Bc}$ and measurements $\overline{\mathbf{P}}$. If the same derivation as above was followed with this new assumption, then the resulting optimization problem would be minimizing the Kullback–Leibler divergence (Kullback and Leibler 1951) instead of minimizing the Euclidean distance, as in Equation 11.25.

As a final remark, the optimization problem proposed in Equation 11.25 can be further augmented by adding a penalty term in order to further restrict the set of solutions. For instance, let us assume that the nature of the TACs for a certain radiotracer is unknown, yet we still wish to employ spatiotemporal basis functions for data representation. In this case, one alternative to solving for the spatiotemporal spline coefficients would be to use a larger number of temporal splines; however, our model may be prone to overfitting since the chosen basis does not restrict the set of solutions sufficiently to regularize the problem. To address this drawback, a penalty term to the formulation in Equation 11.24 can be added where "unwanted" solutions are penalized. For example, the problem can be written as

$$\mathbf{c}^* \in \arg \min_{\mathbf{c}} \left\| \mathbf{Bc} - \bar{\mathbf{p}} \right\|^2 + \beta \left| \mathbf{c} \right|_1 \tag{11.26}$$

where the second term penalizes the solutions that use a large number of spatiotemporal coefficients. In other words, the aim is to try to find the minimum number of coefficients that adequately describe the TACs given that $\mathbf{B}$ overrepresents the data. Here, $\beta > 0$ is a scalar parameter that emphasizes the data-fitting term (the first term in Equation 11.26) when small and the penalty term (the second term) when large. The formulation in Equation 11.26 originates from additional assumptions about the distribution of the spatiotemporal spline coefficients, which are commonly referred to as priors, and the model is known as a maximum *a posteriori* estimator. The reader is directed to Gullberg et al. (2010), Green (1990), and Levitan and Herman (1987) for instances of using maximum *a posteriori* estimation for dynamic image reconstruction.

11.3.3 FACTOR ANALYSIS OF DYNAMIC STRUCTURES

FA or FADS (Barber 1980; Buvat et al. 1993; Samal et al. 1989; Di Paola et al. 1982; Huston 1984; Sitek et al. 2000, 2002a, 2002b) is a semiautomatic technique used to estimate factors that correspond to TACs of distinct physiological regions and can be extracted from dynamic sequences of volumetric images. In addition, FA provides factor coefficient images that spatially define factors. The numbers of factors and factor coefficient images are the same. The method is considered to be semiautomatic because it requires that the user specify the following three conditions, which we refer to as preprocessing:

1. The number of factors has to be specified *a priori*. This number is usually small (up to four) and defines the number of physiological components that are present in the analyzed volume of interest (VOI).
2. A regularization approach has to be specified. The solution of the factor model is not mathematically unique, and therefore some constraint has to be specified in order to obtain a consistent answer.
3. The VOI for analysis must be specified.

The entire volume of the image will not be of interest in most of the cases. Typically, the VOI is restricted to a subregion of the entire image that is of interest, and the rest of the image is not analyzed. This is an important step, as analysis of the entire image would increase the number of physiological regions and, consequently, the number of factors required to describe them. Unfortunately, in the presence of noise, the number of factors used must often be limited to less than four due to severe problems with nonuniqueness when the number of factors increases.

To provide an example, suppose we consider a dynamic cardiac perfusion study. We expect to have three factors if the VOI is defined as encompassing the myocardium. These three factors include myocardial tissue, left ventricle, and right ventricle. In other words, each voxel in the volume will contain some contributions from these three factors. Note the important difference between FA and clustering methods. In the latter, voxels are assigned only to a single cluster, whereby FA permits voxels to belong to all groups.

After these three steps are specified, the FA is an automatic process that provides factors (curves) and factor coefficients (images of the weights of contribution of each factor to each voxel in the image).

There are several advantages of using FA. The most important is that once the preprocessing is done, the method automatically calculates the TACs corresponding to different physiological compartments in the VOI. The alternative to this approach would be to use manual determination of ROIs drawn on different physiological regions, which would be time-consuming and operator dependent. The FA method is able to separate the partially overlapped structures that are always present in SPECT imaging due to partial volume and finite-resolution effects. This again is an advantage over manual ROI delineation, in which the problems with overlap of different structures are difficult to overcome. Finally, the factor curves will exhibit much less noise than the ROI curves. The intuitional explanation of this feature is that in the FA process, all voxels in VOI are used to calculate the factor curve, whereas in ROI measurements, only selected voxels are used.

Obviously, the technique also has limitations that, in fact, are quite serious. The factor model assumes a fixed number of K factors in the VOI. In other words, it assumes that there are only K physiological components. In the real situation, the behavior of the tracer is never completely uniform over the physiological compartment, and many more components would be needed to accurately describe such behavior. As mentioned above, one obvious solution to this problem would be to use a higher number K, but this would make FA much more prone to the other limitation of the technique, which is nonuniqueness.

The nonuniqueness is an effect that must be addressed in some way when FA is used. Unfortunately, there is no general method to address this problem. The authors' experience suggests that different imaging situations require different and customized approaches to handle the nonuniqueness problem. The small and fixed number of factors and the nonuniqueness of the solutions seriously limit the use of FA and must be weighed against its benefits when considering each specific application.

11.3.3.1 MATHEMATICAL FORMULATION AND NONUNIQUENESS

Mathematically, the factor model can be expressed by the following:

$$\mathbf{A} = \sum_{k=1}^{K} C_k F_k + \varepsilon \tag{11.27}$$

where $\mathbf{A}$ is a data matrix with elements A_{it}, i indexes the voxels in the VOI, and t indicates the time frame. It is assumed that there is a total of N voxels in VOI and T time frames. Columns of matrix $\mathbf{A}$ can be considered vectors of size T corresponding to the dynamic data. These vectors are sometimes referred to in the literature as *dixels*. The C_k is a vector of size N of factor coefficients for the kth factor. This vector can be interpreted as an image of the physiological compartment where index k indicates the factor. As mentioned, the total number of factors is K. The row vector F_k of size T describes the temporal behavior of the factor k. All the above matrices and vectors are nonnegative because their values have physiological interpretation. For example, values of $\mathbf{A}$ represent the concentrations of radioactive tracer in the voxels. Finally, the matrix ε is an error that encompasses the systematic error due to mismatch between the data and the factor model, as well as the error coming from the random nature of data acquisition. The notation $C_k F_k$ indicates the outer product of column vector C_k and row vector F_k.

Because the factor model constitutes a multiplication of two vectors, it is insensitive to scaling. Multiplying C_k by number a and dividing F_k by the same constant provides the same model. Therefore, we often use a convention that all C_k's are normalized to 1; that is, the values are in the range 0–1.

To explain the nonuniqueness of the FA,* we consider a two-factor model with two factors such that C_1, C_2 are column vectors corresponding to factor coefficients and F_1 and F_2 are row vectors corresponding to factor curves. The factor model can be specified as $\mathbf{A} = C_1 F_1 + C_2 F_2$. Using this formulation, we have

$$\mathbf{A} = C_1 F_1 + C_2 F_2 - aC_1 F_2 + aC_1 F_2 = C_1 \left(F_1 - aF_2 \right) + \left(C_2 + aC_1 \right) F_2 \tag{11.28}$$

---

* Nonuniqueness of FA is not related to the freedom of scaling discussed above.

where a is some constant. We added and subtracted an identical term to the factor model and rearranged the terms. The result is a new factor model with new factors $F_1 - aF_2$ and F_2 and factor coefficients C_1 and $C_2 + aC_1$. If the new F's and C's are nonnegative, they provide a solution that is as equally valid as the original factors, and therefore an infinite number of solutions of the factor model corresponding to the observed data $\mathbf{A}$ can be found.

More generally, the solution to the factor model ($\mathbf{C}$ and $\mathbf{F}$), obtained when only nonnegativity constraints are used, is a linear combination of true factors and factor coefficients (Sitek et al. 2000). The particular linear combination (shown in Equation 11.27) that is obtained as a solution depends on the algorithms used for calculating the factors and factor coefficients. It follows that if the nonuniqueness of the factor model is not addressed, the results are incorrect and unpredictable regardless of the algorithm that is used.

11.3.3.2 ALGORITHMS FOR FACTOR ANALYSIS AND CORRECTION FOR NONUNIQUENESS

The basic computing task is to decompose the matrix of the observed data $\mathbf{A}$ into the nonnegative matrices $\mathbf{C}$ and $\mathbf{F}$, where $\mathbf{C}$ and $\mathbf{F}$ are built from k vectors C_k and F_k, respectively. In early applications of the FA in radiography (Barber 1980; Buvat et al. 1993; Di Paola et al. 1982; Huston 1984), a simple algorithm (so-called apex seeking) was used. With the availability of faster computers, more computationally intensive algorithms were used based on LS (Sitek et al. 2000, 2002b) or maximum likelihood (Su et al. 2007). In fact, the computational problem is identical to performing a nonnegative matrix factorization (NNMF), which is extensively used in machine learning (Seung and Lee 2001; Hoyer 2004). A schematic of the decomposition is presented in Figure 11.10a.

Regardless of the algorithm used to perform factorization, the solutions ($\mathbf{C}$ and $\mathbf{F}$) are not unique. An interesting observation can be made based on the fact that from the definition, the true factor coefficient images never completely overlap because they correspond to different physiological regions. Therefore, in the example given in the previous section, $C_2 + aC_1$ can be nonnegative at every voxel only if a is nonnegative. This can be generalized, and it implies that factor images (matrix $\mathbf{C}$) obtained by FA that are affected by the nonuniqueness effect will be the sums of all factor images. It follows that factors ($\mathbf{F}$) obtained by the FA algorithm will correspond to true factors with some fraction of other factors subtracted from them (see the figurative example of $F_1 - aF_2$ with a nonnegative). Thus, if the true factors are such that it is impossible to subtract one from another without violating nonnegativity, then the solution will be unique (Figure 11.10b). However, if such a subtraction is possible for at least one factor, then the solution will not be unique.

One approach that can be used to correct for nonuniqueness using the above consideration is to require that the factor images obtained during factorization have the least overlap between each other (Sitek et al. 2002b). This can be accomplished in the LS-FA formulation by adding a penalty term that penalizes the overlap (Sitek et al. 2002b). Another approach to implementing this correction is to first perform the factorization (estimating $\tilde{\mathbf{C}}$ and $\tilde{\mathbf{F}}$) using any of the standard algorithms (apex seeking, LS, or NNMF) and then find an $K \times K$ oblique rotation matrix $\mathbf{R}$ that minimizes the overlap between rotated factor images $\mathbf{C} = \tilde{\mathbf{C}}\mathbf{R}$. Once the

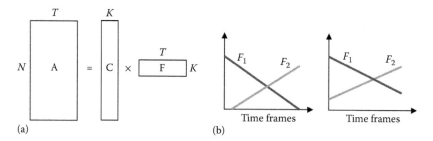

(a) (b)

Figure 11.10 (a) Schematics of factorization of matrix A into nonnegative matrices C and F. The boxes represent the size of the matrices denoted N, T, and K. Typically, in medical imaging $K \ll T$, and therefore the FA factorization can be considered a data compression technique. (b) Examples of factors in a two-factor model ($K = 2$). On the left are factors that would provide a unique solution to FA factorization, and on the right are factors that would cause the nonuniqueness factorization.

R is determined, the factors are obtained by $\mathbf{F} = \mathbf{R}^{-1}\tilde{\mathbf{F}}$ (note that $\mathbf{CF} = \tilde{\mathbf{C}}\tilde{\mathbf{F}}$). Recently, this approach was successfully used in an investigation of quantitative cardiac SPECT (Ben-Haim et al. 2013).

11.3.3.3 CLINICAL EXAMPLE OF FACTOR ANALYSIS

To demonstrate the performance of this method, the FADS algorithm was applied to the data obtained from a planar dynamic study of the renal function performed with ^{99m}Tc-MAG3. The patient was imaged using a dual-head camera for 1500 s with 3 s frames for a total of 300 frames. A region encompassing the right kidney was selected and analyzed by the simple LS-FA method (Sitek et al. 2000), where only the nonnegativity constraints were used, and by the penalized LS-FA (PLS-FA) algorithm, where a least-overlap constraint was used (Sitek et al. 2002b). The results are presented in Figure 11.11 and demonstrate that the application of constraints removes apparent artifacts caused by the nonuniqueness of FADS. For example, in Figure 11.11b (top row) corresponding to the background, images of other structures, such kidney cortex and renal pelvis, are clearly visible, which is due to the nonuniqueness. When nonuniqueness constraints are used (bottom row), the overlap of components is mostly removed. A similar effect can be appreciated in Figure 11.11c, where on the factor image of the renal pelvis the cortex can clearly be seen when no correction for nonuniqueness is used. The effect of nonuniqueness correction is quite dramatic on the factor curves as well (Figure 11.11a–c), where the corrected curves are in much better agreement with ROI measurements.

11.3.4 DYNAMIC SPECT WITH STATIONARY SYSTEMS

Traditional SPECT cameras rotate around the patient acquiring projections sequentially, which complicates the reconstruction of tomographic dynamic images. Stationary or quasi-stationary systems avoid this problem by simultaneously acquiring all the projections needed for such images. There are two widely available commercial systems that offer this capability for cardiac imaging.

The D-SPECT system (Spectrum Dynamics) (Erlandsson et al. 2009; Slomka et al. 2009) uses a set of nine 4×16 cm detectors with very high-sensitivity parallel-hole collimators. The detector gantry does not move, but each detector oscillates over the FOV, and they are programmed to spend more time directed at the heart, giving the system a sensitivity that is about eight times higher than that of a traditional dual-head gamma camera. The oscillation time can be as short as 3 s, which is faster than the rate at which the tracer distribution changes for common cardiac perfusion agents. The second system, the Discovery NM530c/570c camera (GE Healthcare), uses nineteen 8×8 cm detectors with pinhole collimators, all focused on the heart (Bocher et al. 2010). The system is completely stationary and has a four times increase in sensitivity over that of the traditional dual-head camera (Bocher et al. 2010). Thus, both of these systems are capable of acquiring high temporal resolution tomographic data of the heart at high sensitivity. The primary application of dynamic imaging of the heart is the measurement of absolute MBF.

11.3.4.1 DYNAMIC SPECT MEASUREMENTS OF MYOCARDIAL BLOOD FLOW

Cardiovascular disease continues to be a leading cause of morbidity and mortality in the modern world. MPI with nuclear medicine plays a crucial role in the assessment, prognosis, and follow-up of patients with suspected or known coronary artery disease (CAD). However, typical MPI studies only compare the uptake in the myocardium relative to other parts of the heart. No absolute measurement of blood flow to the tissue is done. PET imaging has paved the way in demonstrating that the measurements of absolute MBF and MFR provide important incremental value to the measurement of relative perfusion alone (Kajander et al. 2011; Camici and Rimoldi 2009; Valenta et al. 2013; Murthy et al. 2011). Correlated with many other risk factors for coronary disease, they may provide information regarding microvascular disease and may yield an earlier indication of perfusion abnormalities (Kaufmann and Camici 2005). Quantitative MBF has been shown to be an independent predictor of major cardiac events (cardiac death, myocardial infarction, revascularization, and cardiac hospitalization) in patients with both normal and abnormal relative perfusion (Herzog et al. 2009; Tio et al. 2009), therefore improving the accuracy of triaging patients for appropriate additional testing and management of their disease.

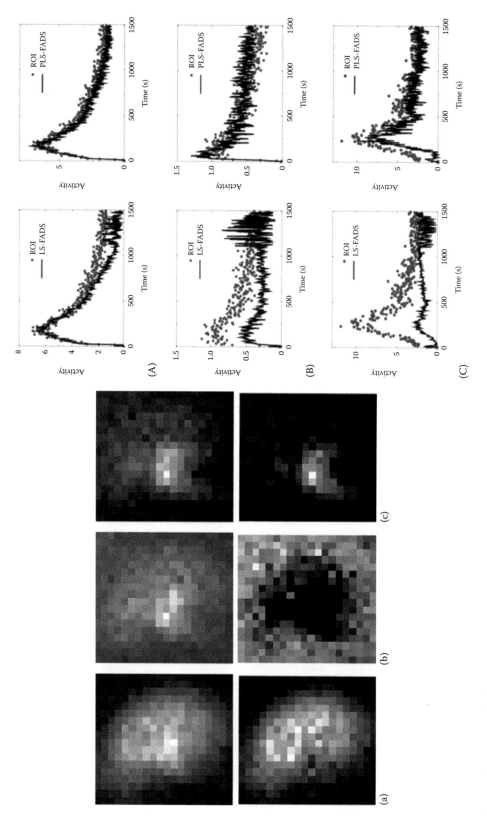

Figure 11.11 Figure 11. The results of LS FADS methods applied to a 99mTc-MAG3 patient renal study. The top row in the figure on the left corresponds to images of factor coefficients reconstructed by the LS-FADS for (a) kidney cortex, (b) background, and (c) pelvis and ureter components; while the bottom row presents images from the PLS-FADS. The same gray scale representing values from zero to one is used for each image. Plots (A), (B), and (C) on the right present the factor obtained by the PLS-FADS methods with comparison to curves obtained by ROI measurements (From Sitek, A., et al., *IEEE Trans Med Imaging* 21:216–225, 2002b.).

PET has a strong history in dynamic imaging, but access to cardiac PET is limited due to the relatively low numbers of PET scanners and the demand on these scanners for oncology. Furthermore, the short half-life of the tracers used in cardiac PET requires either an on-site cyclotron (^{13}N ammonia /^{15}O water) or generator (^{82}Rb rubidium chloride). This makes cardiac PET for most sites prohibitively expensive. On the other hand, SPECT is a widespread technology with a much larger number of cameras installed and a much larger percentage of cardiac studies being done. Recent developments in SPECT hardware, image reconstruction, and quantification make clinical dSPECT much more feasible. Implementation of dSPECT for cardiac imaging has the potential to significantly improve patient care.

11.3.4.2 DYNAMIC SPECT WITH THE DISCOVERY NM530C

An example dSPECT study performed on one such system is presented here. The accuracy of cardiac blood flow measurement with the Discovery NM530c camera was investigated using a porcine model of cardiac disease (Wells et al. 2014). Pigs weighed between 30 and 40 kg and had normal myocardial perfusion at rest. At stress, the left-anterior descending artery of the heart was transiently occluded, mimicking stress-induced ischemia in the anterior wall of the heart and producing a range of blood flows in the heart muscle. Similar to standard 1-day MPI protocols, tracer was injected at rest, stress was induced pharmacologically 1 h later, and then a second injection of the same tracer was performed at stress. For this study, the three standard SPECT cardiac perfusion tracers were considered: ^{99m}Tc-sestamibi, ^{99m}Tc-tetrofosmin, and ^{201}Tl. Microspheres were injected simultaneously with the tracer injections to provide a reference flow measurement. Images were acquired in list mode for 11 min, starting immediately with each injection.

One challenge for dynamic cardiac SPECT imaging is interference from the rest tracer during stress imaging. The tracers used in PET cardiac imaging (^{15}O water, ^{13}N ammonia, and ^{82}Rb) have half-lives of 10 min or less. With these tracers, there is enough time between rest and stress imaging that the rest tracer has decayed and has a negligible contribution to the stress images. The half-lives of ^{99m}Tc and ^{201}Tl are 6 h and 3 days, respectively, making it impractical, with a 1-day SPECT protocol, to wait until the rest tracer has decayed away. However, an additional resting image acquired just prior to stress provides an accurate means of compensating for the residual rest contribution. In this example, the residual resting signal is subtracted from the projection data prior to reconstruction.

The list-mode data were divided into time frames for reconstruction (Figure 11.12). The first 3 min was divided into 9×10 s and 6×15 s time frames to capture the rapid kinetics of the arterial input function. Thereafter, the tracer distribution changed much more slowly, and the last 8 min could be divided into 2 min frames. Each time frame was then reconstructed independently using standard iterative techniques that include CT-based attenuation correction, scatter correction, and collimator modeling. In the example slices shown in Figure 11.12, the CT was acquired on a separate camera and then manually coregistered for attenuation correction. This approach created a dynamic series of images that is in the same format as a dynamic PET study, and analysis developed for PET could be applied.

In this example, the data were processed using FlowQuant™ (Klein et al. 2010a), which is a software package designed for cardiac PET analysis. This software is semiautomated and has been demonstrated to have excellent reproducibility for quantifying flow in PET (Klein et al. 2010b). TACs are created by sampling the tracer uptake from each time frame at 864 locations throughout the heart. The TACs are then fit individually to a compartment model generating parametric maps.

A detailed discussion of kinetic modeling is beyond the scope of this chapter, but has been treated elsewhere (e.g., Gullberg et al. 2010). A requirement of kinetic modeling is that an arterial input function, a measure of the concentration of tracer in blood over the course of imaging, is provided. This input function is usually measured directly from the images using a VOI placed in the left ventricle or atrium. Like many other tracers, SPECT cardiac tracers can bind to the blood, reducing the availability of tracer for extraction by the heart muscle (Iida et al. 2008; Gullberg et al. 2010). This blood binding can be corrected for either by measurement of blood samples (which is not clinically practical) or by application of a population-derived correction curve.

Figure 11.13 shows a measurement of K1 compared with a microsphere measurement of absolute blood flow from the described pig experiment. The hearts were divided into a standard 17-segment heart model and

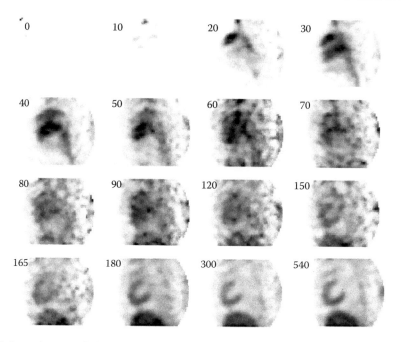

Figure 11.12 Example sagittal slice drawn from a dynamic cardiac pig study. The images show a sestamibi injection during rest with the starting time of the frame in seconds indicated in the top left. The activity is seen appearing first in the right ventricle (20 s) and then spreading into the left ventricle (30 s), dispersing out of the blood pool and accumulating in the myocardium over the later frames.

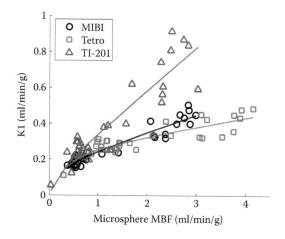

Figure 11.13 K1 parameters from a one-compartment model fit to dSPECT data. Data were acquired from a pig model of stress-induced ischemia using three common SPECT tracers: ^{99m}Tc-sestamibi (MIBI), ^{99m}Tc-tetrofosmin (Tetro), and Tl-201. K1 values are compared with MBF measured with microspheres. The fitted lines are based on assuming a Renkin–Crone model for the extraction fraction. The coefficients of determination (r^2) for the fits were 0.91, 0.77, and 0.85 for sestamibi, tetrofosmin, and Tl-201, respectively.

measurements compared at rest and stress for each segment. Although more complex compartmental models could be applied, one-tissue-compartment models have been shown to be adequate for ^{201}Tl (Iida et al. 2008) and some ^{99m}Tc-tracers (Gullberg et al. 2010; Ben-Haim et al. 2013), and this is what was used for this example. In this model, the K1 parameter is monotonically related to MBF (Klein et al 2010a.). The Spearman correlations (ρ) between K1 and microsphere MBF for the pigs shown in Figure 11.13 are $\rho = 0.86$, $\rho = 0.80$, and

$\rho = 0.79$ for ^{99m}Tc-sestamibi, ^{99m}Tc-tetrofosmin, and ^{201}Tl, respectively, demonstrating that quite reasonable flow estimates can be derived from the dSPECT images.

Figure 11.13 also highlights one of the difficulties of performing flow quantification with SPECT—the greatly reduced extraction fraction of ^{99m}Tc-tracers at high flow. The extraction fraction for tetrofosmin and sestamibi levels off at flows greater than ~2 ml/min/g. This limits the contrast between normal and abnormal tissues at stress, making it more difficult to distinguish between the two. While ^{201}Tl has much better pharmacokinetics, it also confers a much higher effective dose to the patient and produces much noisier images.

More advanced 4D reconstruction techniques, such as those described in the preceding sections and others (Gullberg et al. 2010; Feng et al. 2006; Jin et al. 2006; Kadrmas and Gullberg 2001; Niu et al. 2010), could provide higher signal-to-noise images and open the door to reducing the amount of activity needed for ^{201}Tl imaging, allowing us to take advantage of its superior extraction fraction properties, but this will require further assessment and validation. In particular, our preliminary tests suggest that simultaneous processing of all time frames with the dSPECT method creates images with much improved quality when compared with images reconstructed individually. Figure 11.14 compares TACs obtained from the images of the pig heart reconstructed using these two approaches. In particular, while the TACs for the entire heart are similar, those defined on a small ROI (with much lower statistics) have significantly less fluctuations when obtained from the dSPECT reconstructions.

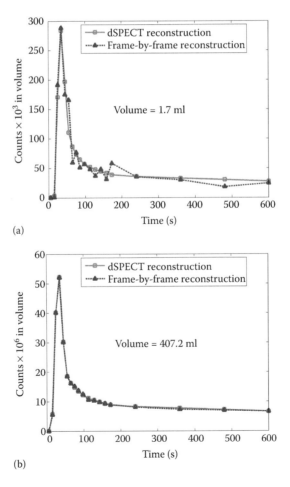

Figure 11.14 Comparison of TACs obtained from the images of the pig heart reconstructed using the dSPECT approach (which simultaneously processes all time frames) and from images where each time frame was reconstructed separately.

The main advantage of stationary or quasi-stationary SPECT cameras is that they permit clinically practical protocols for dynamic data acquisition by not requiring nonstandard modes, such as multiple rapid rotations. Additionally, the increased sensitivity of these systems also means that it is possible to obtain images of adequate visual quality without the need to implement more complicated 4D reconstruction approaches, although further research into the limitations of these systems still needs to be performed. However, it appears that the availability of dynamic data from standard acquisition modes and reconstruction algorithms greatly facilitates clinical implementation of dSPECT.

11.4 CONCLUSIONS

dSPECT is an imaging technique that captures the temporal behavior of radiotracers in the body from the data acquired using a single-photon emission technique. It has potential applications in the imaging of brain, liver, kidneys, and heart, where it can provide valuable information to clinicians and researchers. Additionally, in imaging studies where radiotracer distribution changes during acquisition, dynamic reconstructions may help to reduce image artifacts that are created when the data are processed using traditional static methods.

The 4D image reconstruction techniques that have been proposed for dSPECT use a wide range of data acquisition methods and different, often very sophisticated data processing algorithms that are designed to deal with problems due to projection data inconsistencies and can provide parameters related to the physiological function of studied organs. The uses of temporal constraints between time frames, a limited set of temporal basis functions, and FA are examples of 4D image reconstruction and analysis strategies that have been successful in extracting dynamic information from SPECT data. New advances in SPECT technology are simplifying the problem of dynamic data acquisition and processing by increasing sensitivity and improving temporal resolution. Although still primarily a research tool, recent advances in hardware, as well as the development of sophisticated methods for the processing of data acquired by dSPECT, bring this modality closer to becoming a clinical reality.

REFERENCES

Akahira H, Shirakawa H, Shimoyama H, Tsushima M, Arima H, Nigawara K, Funyu T, Sato M, Suzuki T. 1999. Dynamic SPECT evaluation of renal plasma flow using technetium-99m MAG3 in kidney transplant patients. *J Nucl Med Technol* 27:32–37.

Bal H, DiBella VR, Gullberg GT. 2003. Parametric image formation using clustering for dynamic cardiac SPECT. *IEEE Trans Nucl Sci* 50:1584–1589.

Barber DC. 1980. The use of principal components in the quantitative analysis of gamma camera dynamic studies. *Phys Med Biol* 25:283–292.

Bartels R, Beatty J, Barsky B. 1987. *An Introduction to Splines for Use in Computer Graphics and Geometric Modeling*. Burlington, MA: Morgan Kaufmann Publishers.

Bauschke HH, Noll D, Celler A, Borwein JM. 1999. An EM algorithm for dynamic SPECT. *IEEE Trans Med Imaging* 18:252–261.

Ben-Haim S, Murthy VL, Breault C, Allie R, Sitek A, Roth N, Fantony J, et al. 2013. Quantification of myocardial perfusion reserve using dynamic SPECT imaging in humans: A feasibility study. *J Nucl Med* 54:873–879.

Bocher M, Blevis IM, Tsukerman L, Shrem Y, Kovalski G, Volokh L. 2010. A fast cardiac gamma camera with dynamic SPECT capabilities: Design, system validation and future potential. *Eur J Nucl Med Mol Imaging* 37:1887–1902.

Buvat I, Benali H, Frouin F, Bazin JP, Di Paola R. 1993. Target apex-seeking in factor analysis on medical sequences. *Phys Med Biol* 38:123–128.

Camici PG, Rimoldi OE. 2009. The clinical value of myocardial blood flow measurement. *J Nucl Med* 50:1076–1087.

Celler A, Bong JK, Blinder CS, Attariwala R, Noll D, Hook L, Farncombe TH, Harrop R. 2001. Preliminary results of a clinical validation of the dSPECT method for determination of renal glomerular filtration rate (GFR). In *IEEE Nuclear Science Symposium and Medical Imaging Conference Record*. Piscataway, NJ: IEEE, pp. 1079–1082.

Celler A, Farncombe T, Harrop R, Lyster D. 1997. Three approaches to dynamic SPECT imaging. In *IEEE Nuclear Science Symposium and Medical Imaging Conference Record*. Piscataway, NJ: IEEE, pp. 1451–1455.

Chen J, Galt JR, Aarsvold JN, Krawczynska EG, Alazraki NP, Zafari AM, Faber TL, Garcia EV. 2004. Dynamic cardiac SPECT with Tc-99m teboroxime: Compensation for rapid myocardial washout and high liver uptake. *IEEE Trans Med Imaging* 51:2705–2712.

Chen K, Huang S, Yu D. 1991. The effects of measurement errors in the plasma radioactivity curve of parameter estimation on position emission tomography. *Phys Med Biol* 36:1183–1200.

Chiao PC, Rogers WL, Clinthorne NH, Fessler JA, Hero AO. 1994. Model-based estimation for dynamic cardiac studies using ECT. *IEEE Trans Med Imaging* 13:217–226.

Chua T, Kiat H, Germano G, Takemoto K, Fernandez G, Biasio Y, Friedman J, Berman D. 1993. Rapid back to back adenosine stress/rest technetium-99m teboroxime myocardial perfusion SPECT using a triple-detector camera. *J Nucl Med* 34:1485–1493.

Daniele S, Nappi C, Acampa W, Storto G, Pellegrino T, Ricci F, Xhoxhi E, Porcaro F, Petretta M, Cuocolo A. 2011. Incremental prognostic value of coronary flow reserve assessed with single-photon emission computed tomography. *J Nucl Cardiol* 18:612–619.

Delbeke D, Coleman RE, Guiberteau MJ, Brown ML, Royal HD, Siegel BA, Townsend DW, Berland LL, Parker JA, Zubal G, Cronin V. 2006. Procedure guideline for SPECT/CT imaging 1.0°. *J Nucl Med* 47:1227–1234.

DePuey EG. 2012. Advances in SPECT camera software and hardware: Currently available and new on the horizon. *J Nucl Cardiol* 19:551–581.

Di Bella EVR, Gullberg GT, Barclay AB, Eisner RL. 1997. Automated region selection for analysis of dynamic cardiac SPECT data. *IEEE Trans Nucl Sci* 44:1355–1361.

Di Bella EVR, Ross S, Kadrmas DJ, Khare HS, Christian PE, McJames S, Gullberg GT. 2001. Compartmental modeling of technetium-99m labeled teboroxime with dynamic single-photon emission computed tomography. *Invest Radiol* 36:178–185.

Di Paola R, Bazin JP, Aubry F, Aurengo A, Cavailloles F, Herry Y, Kahn E. 1982. Handling of dynamic sequences in nuclear medicine. *IEEE Trans Nucl Sci* 29:1310–1321.

Erlandsson K, Kacperski K, van Gramberg D, Hutton BF. 2009. Performance evaluation of D-SPECT: A novel SPECT system for nuclear cardiology. *Phys Med Biol* 54:2635–2649.

Farncombe T, Celler A, Bevert C, Noli D, Maeghty J, Harrop R. 2001. The incorporation of organ uptake into dynamic SPECT (dSPECT) image reconstruction. *IEEE Trans Nucl Sci* 48:3–9.

Farncombe TH, Blinder S, Celler AM, Noll D, Maeght J, Harrop R. 2000. A dynamic expectation maximization algorithm for single camera rotation dynamic SPECT (dSPECT). In *IEEE Medical Imaging Conference Record*. Piscataway, NJ: IEEE, pp. 15/31–15/35.

Farncombe TH, Celler AM, Noll D, Maeght J, Harrop R. 1999. Dynamic SPECT imaging using a single camera rotation (dSPECT). *IEEE Trans Nucl Sci* 46:1055–1061.

Farncombe TH, Feng B, Narayanan MV, Wernick MN, Celler AM, King MA, Leppo JA. 2003a. Towards 5 dimensional SPECT reconstruction: Determining myocardial blood flow and wall motion in a single study. Presented at International Conference on Fully 3D Reconstruction in Radiology and Nuclear Medicine, Saint Malo, France.

Farncombe TH, Gifford HC, King MA. 2003b. Reducing artifacts in pelvic bone SPECT: An assessment of lesion detectability using numerical and human observers. In *IEEE Nuclear Science Symposium and Medical Imaging Conference Record*. Piscataway, NJ: IEEE, pp. 2686–2689.

Feng B, Pretorius PH, Farncombe TH, Dahlberg ST, Narayanan MV, Wernick MN, Celler AM, Leppo JA, King MA. 2006. Simultaneous assessment of cardiac perfusion and function using 5-dimensional imaging with Tc-99m teboroxime. *J Nucl Cardiol* 13:354–361.

Green PJ. 1990. Bayesian reconstruction from emission tomography data using a modified EM algorithm. *IEEE Trans Med Imaging* 9:84–93.

Gullberg GT, Reutter BW, Sitek A, Maltz JS, Budinger TF. 2010. Dynamic single photon emission computed tomography—Basic principles and cardiac applications. *Phys Med Biol* 55:R111–R191.

Hebber E, Oldenburg D, Farncombe T, Celler A. 1997. Direct estimation of dynamic parameters in SPECT tomography. *IEEE Trans Nucl Sci* 44:2425–2430.

Herzog BA, Husmann L, Valenta I, Gaemperli O, Siegrist PT, Tay FM, Burkhard N, Wyss CA, Kaufmann PA. 2009. Long-term prognostic value of 13N-ammonia myocardial perfusion positron emission tomography added value of coronary flow reserve. *J Am Coll Cardiol* 54:150–156.

Hoyer PO. 2004. Non-negative matrix factorization with sparseness constraints. *J Mach Learn Res* 5:1457–1469.

Humphries T, Celler A, Trummer M. 2011. Slow-rotation dynamic SPECT with a temporal second derivative constraint. *Med Phys* 38:4489–4497.

Huston AS. 1984. The effect of apex-finding errors on factor images obtained from factor analysis and oblique transformation. *Phys Med Biol* 29:1109–1116.

Iida H, Eberl S, Kim KM, Tamura Y, Ono Y, Nakazawa M, Sohlberg A, Zeniya T, Hayashi T, Watabe H. 2008. Absolute quantitation of myocardial blood flow with (201)Tl and dynamic SPECT in canine: Optimisation and validation of kinetic modelling. *Eur J Nucl Med Mol Imaging* 35:896–905.

Iida H, Itoh H, Nakazawa M, Hatazawa J, Nishimura H, Onishi Y, Uemura K. 1994. Quantitative mapping of regional cerebral blood flow using iodine-123-IMP and SPECT. *J Nucl Med* 35:2019–2030.

Jain AK. 1989. *Fundamentals of Digital Image Processing.* Englewood Cliffs, NJ: Prentice-Hall.

Jin M, Yang Y, King M. 2006. Reconstruction of dynamic gated cardiac SPECT. *Med Phys* 33:4384–4394.

Kadrmas DJ, Gullberg GT. 2001. 4D maximum a posteriori reconstruction in dynamic SPECT using a compartmental model based prior. *Phys Med Biol* 46:1553–1574.

Kajander SA, Joutsiniemi E, Saraste M, Pietilä M, Ukkonen H, Saraste A, Sipilä HT, et al. 2011. Clinical value of absolute quantification of myocardial perfusion with (15)O-water in coronary artery disease. *Circ Cardiovasc Imaging* 4:678–684.

Kanno I, Uemura K, Miura S, Miura Y. 1981. Headtome: A hybrid emission tomography for single photon and positron emission imaging of the brain. *J Comput Assist Tomogr* 5:216–226.

Kataoka H, Inoue M, Shinkai T, Ueno S. 2007. Early dynamic SPECT imaging in acute viral encephalitis. *J Neuroimaging* 17:304–310.

Kaufmann PA, Camici PG. 2005. Myocardial blood flow measurement by PET: Technical aspects and clinical applications. *J Nucl Med* 46:75–88.

Kervinen M, Vauhkonen M, Kaipio JP, Karjalainen PA. 2004. Time-varying reconstruction in single photon emission computed tomography. *Int J Imaging Systems Technol* 14:186–197.

Klein R, Beanlands RS, deKemp RA. 2010a. Quantification of myocardial blood flow and flow reserve: Technical aspects. *J Nucl Cardiol* 17:555–570.

Klein R, Renaud JM, Zaidi MC, Thorn SL, Adler A, Beanlands RS, deKemp RS. 2010b. Intra- and inter-operator repeatability of myocardial blood flow and myocardial flow reserve measurements using rubidium-82 PET and a highly automated analysis program. *J Nucl Cardiol* 17:600–616.

Klein WP, Barrett HH, Pang IW, Patton DD, Rogulski MM, Sain JD, Smith WE. 1995. FASTSPECT: Electrical and mechanical design of a high-resolution dynamic SPECT imager. In *IEEE Nuclear Science Symposium and Medical Imaging Conference Record*, pp. 931–933. Piscataway, NJ: IEEE.

Kullback S, Leibler R. 1951. On information and sufficiency. *Ann Math Stat* 22:79–86.

Lambie H, Cook AM, Scarsbrook AF, Lodge JPA, Robinson PJ, Chowdhury FU. 2011. Tc[99m]- hepatobiliary iminodiacetic acid (HIDA) scintigraphy in clinical practice. *Clin Radiol* 66:1094–1105.

Lau CH, Feng D, Hutton BF, Pak-Kong Lun D, Siu WC. 1998. Dynamic imaging and tracer kinetic modeling for emission tomography using rotating detectors. *IEEE Trans Med Imaging* 17:986–994.

Levitan E, Herman G. 1987. A maximum a posteriori probability expectation maximization algorithm for image reconstruction in emission tomography. *IEEE Trans Med Imaging* 6:185–192.

Limber MA, Limber MN, Celler A, Barney JS, Borwein JM. 1995. Direct reconstruction of functional parameters for dynamic SPECT. *IEEE Trans Nucl Sci* 42:1249–1256.

Links J, Frank T, Becker L. 1991. Effect of differential tracer washout during SPECT acquisition. *J Nucl Med* 32:2253–2257.

MacDonald A, Burrell S. 2008. Infrequently performed studies in nuclear medicine: Part 1. *J Nucl Med Technol* 36:132–143.

Macheras P, Iliadis A. 2006. *Modeling in Biopharmaceutics, Pharmacokinetics, and Pharmacodynamics: Homogeneous and Heterogeneous Approaches.* Berlin: Springer Science and Business Media.

Maltz JS. 2000. Direct recovery of regional tracer kinetics from temporally inconsistent dynamic ECT projections using dimension-reduced time-activity basis. *Phys Med Biol* 45:3413–3429.

Maltz JS, Budinger TF. 2000. Multiresolution constrained least-squares algorithm for direct estimation of time activity curves from dynamic ECT projection data. *Proc SPIE* 3979:586–598.

Mariani G, Boni G, Barreca M, Bellini M, Fattori B, AlSharif A, Grosso M, et al. 2004. Radionuclide gastro-esophageal motor studies. *J Nucl Med* 45:1004–1028.

Maurer AH, Parkman HP. 2006. Update on gastrointestinal scintigraphy. *Semin Nucl Med* 36:110–118.

McCallum RW. 1990. Diagnosis of gastric motility disorders. In McCallum RW, Champion MC, eds., *Gastrointestinal Motility Disorders: Diagnosis and Treatment*, pp. 61–80. Baltimore: Williams & Wilkins.

Mulligan JS, Blue PW, Hasbargemn JA. 1990. Methods for measuring GFR with technetium-99m-DTPA: An analysis of several common methods. *J Nucl Med* 31:1211–1219.

Murthy VL, Naya M, Foster CR, Hainer J, Gaber M, Di Carli G, Blankstein R, Dorbala S, Sitek A, Pencina MJ, Di Carli MF. 2011. Improved cardiac risk assessment with noninvasive measures of coronary flow reserve. *Circulation* 124:2215–2224.

Muzi M, O'Sullivan F, Mankoff DA, Doot RK, Pierce LA, Kurland BF, Linden HM, Kinahan PE. 2012. Quantitative assessment of dynamic PET imaging data in cancer imaging. *Magn Res Imaging* 30:1203–1215.

Nakajima K, Shuke N, Taki J, Ichihara T, Motomura N, Bunko H, Hisada K. 1992. A simulation of dynamic SPECT using radiopharmaceuticals with rapid clearance. *J Nucl Med* 33:1200–1206.

Nakajima K, Taki J, Bunko H, Matsudaira M, Muramori A, Matsunari I, Hisada K, Ichihara T. 1991. Dynamic acquisition with a three-headed SPECT system: Application to technetium 99m-SQ30217 myocardial imaging. *J Nucl Med* 32:1273–1277.

Narayanan MV, King MA, Soares EJ, Byme CL, Pretorius PH, Wernick MN. 1999. Application of the Karhunen-Loeve transform to 4D reconstruction of cardiac gated SPECT images. *IEEE Trans Nucl Sci* 46:1001–1008.

Nichols T, Qi J, Leahy R. 1999. Continuous time dynamic PET imaging using list mode data. In A. Kuba et al. ed., *Information Processing in Medical Imaging: Proceedings of the 16th International Conference*, pp. 98–111. Berlin: Springer.

Niu X, Yang Y, King MA. 2010. Regularized fully 5D reconstruction of cardiac gated dynamic SPECT. *IEEE Trans Nucl Sci* 57:1085–1095.

Niu X, Yang Y, King MA. 2012. Comparison study of temporal regularization methods for fully 5D reconstruction of cardiac gated dynamic SPECT. *Phys Med Biol* 57:5523–5542.

O'Connor M, Cho D. 1992. Rapid radiotracer washout from the heart: Effect on image quality in SPECT performed with a single-headed gamma camera system. *J Nucl Med* 33:1146–1151.

Ogasawara K, Ogawa A, Ezura M, Konno H, Doi M, Kuroda K, Yoshimoto T. 2001. Dynamic and static ^{99m}Tc-ECD SPECT imaging of subacute cerebral infarction: Comparison with ^{133}Xe SPECT. *J Nucl Med* 42:543–547.

Okizaki A, Shukea N, Satoa J, Sasakia T, Hasebeb N, Kikuchib K, Aburanoa T. 2007. A compartment model analysis for investigation of myocardial fatty acid metabolism in patients with hypertrophic cardiomyopathy. *Nucl Med Commun* 28:726–735.

Onishi Y, Yonekura Y, Nishizawa S, Tanaka F, Okazawa H, Ishizu K, Fujita T, Konishi J, Mukai T. 1996. Noninvasive quantification of iodine-123-iomazenil SPECT. *J Nucl Med* 37:374–378.

Oppenheim BE, Krepshaw JD. 1987. Dynamic hepatobilary SPECT: A method for tomography of a changing radioactivity distribution. *J Nucl Med* 29:98–102.

Park MA, Moore SC, Müller SP, McQuaid SJ, Kijewski MF. 2013. Performance of a high-sensitivity dedicated cardiac SPECT scanner for striatal uptake quantification in the brain based on analysis of projection data. *Med Phys* 40:042504.

Pratt WK. 2007. *Digital Image Processing.* 4th ed. Hoboken, NJ: Wiley.

Prigent A. 2008. Monitoring renal function and limitations of renal function tests. *Semin Nucl Med* 38:32–46.

Reutter BW, Gullberg GT, Huesman RH. 2000. Direct least-squares estimation of spatiotemporal distributions from dynamic SPECT projections using a spatial segmentation and temporal B-splines. *IEEE Trans Med Imaging* 19:434–450.

Ross SG, Welch A, Gullberg GT, Huesman RH. 1997. An investigation into the effect of input function shape and image acquisition interval on estimates of washin for dynamic cardiac SPECT. *Phys Med Biol* 42:2193–2213.

Saad A, Hamarneh G, Möller T, Smith B. 2008. Kinetic modeling based probabilistic segmentation for molecular images. In *Medical Image Computing and Computer-Assisted Intervention—MICCAI 2008*, pp. 244–252. Lecture Notes in Computer Science 5241. Berlin: Springer.

Sakaji K, Akiyama M, Umeda H, Nakazawa Y, Takenaka H, Shinozuka A. 2001. Lung function assessment using Xe-133 dynamic SPECT in dual-camera system. *Jpn J Radiol Technol* 57:1138–1144.

Samal M, Karny M, Surova H, Penicka P, Marikova E, Dienstbier Z. 1989. On the existence of an unambiguous solution in factor analysis of dynamic studies. *Phys Med Biol* 34:223–229.

Segars WP, Lalush DS, Tsui BMW. 1999. A realistic spline-based dynamic heart phantom. *IEEE Trans Nucl Sci* 46:503–506.

Seung D, Lee L. 2001. Algorithms for non-negative matrix factorization. *Adv Neural Inf Process Syst* 13:556–562.

Sfakianakis GN, Georgiou MF. 1997. MAG3 SPECT: A rapid procedure to evaluate the renal parenchyma. *J Nucl Med* 38:478–483.

Shargel L, Wu-Pong S, Yu A. 2005. *Applied Biopharmaceutics and Pharmacokinetics.* 5th ed. New York: McGraw-Hill.

Sitek A, Di Bella EVR, Gullberg GT. 2000. Factor analysis with a priori knowledge—Application in dynamic cardiac SPECT. *Phys Med Biol* 45:2619–2638.

Sitek A, Di Bella EVR, Gullberg GT, Huesman RH. 2002a. Removal of liver activity contamination in teboroxime dynamic cardiac SPECT imaging using factor analysis. *J Nucl Cardiol* 9:197–205.

Sitek A, Gullberg GT, DeBella EVR, Celler A. 2001. Reconstruction of dynamic renal tomographic data acquired by slow rotation. *J Nucl Med* 42:1704–1712.

Sitek A, Gullberg, GT, Huesman RH. 2002b. Correction for ambiguous solutions in factor analysis using a penalized least squares objective. *IEEE Trans Med Imaging* 21:216–225.

Slomka PJ, Patton JA, Berman DS, Germano G. 2009. Advances in technical aspects of myocardial perfusion SPECT imaging. *J Nucl Cardiol* 16:255–276.

Smith A, Gullberg G, Christian P. 1996. Experimental verification of technetium 99m-labeled teboroxime kinetic parameters in the myocardium with dynamic single-photon emission computed tomography: Reproducibility, correlation to flow, and susceptibility to extravascular contamination. *J Nucl Cardiol* 3:130–142.

Smith A, Gullberg G, Christian P, Datz F. 1994. Kinetic modeling of teboroxime using dynamic SPECT imaging of a canine model. *J Nucl Med* 35:484–495.

Stewart RE, Schwaiger M, Hutchins GD, Chiao PC, Gallagher KP, Nguyen N, Petry NA, Rogers WL. 1990. Myocardial clearance kinetics of technetium-99m-SQ30217: A marker of regional myocardial blood flow. *J Nucl Med* 31:1183–1190.

Storto G, Cirillo P, Vicario ML, Pellegrino T, Sorrentino AR, Petretta M, Galasso G, De Sanctis V, Piscione F, Cuocolo A. 2004. Estimation of coronary flow reserve by Tc-99m sestamibi imaging in patients with coronary artery disease: Comparison with the results of intracoronary Doppler technique. *J Nucl Cardiol* 11:682–688.

Su Y, Welch MJ, Shoghi KI. 2007. The application of maximum likelihood factor analysis (MLFA) with uniqueness constraints on dynamic cardiac microPET data. *Phys Med Biol* 52:2313–2334.

Sugihara H, Yonekura Y, Kataoka K, Fukai D, Kitamura N, Taniguchi Y. 2001. Estimation of coronary flow reserve with the use of dynamic planar and SPECT images of Tc-99m tetrofosmin. *J Nucl Cardiol* 8:575–579.

Tio RA, Dabeshlim A, Siebelink HM, de Sutter J, Hillege HL, Zeebregts CJ, Dierckx RA, van Veldhuisen DJ, Zijlstra F, Slart RH. 2009. Comparison between the prognostic value of left ventricular function and myocardial perfusion reserve in patients with ischemic heart disease. *J Nucl Med* 50:214–219.

Valenta I, Dilsizian V, Quercioli A, Ruddy TD, Schindler TH. 2013. Quantitative PET/CT measures of myocardial flow reserve and atherosclerosis for cardiac risk assessment and predicting adverse patient outcomes. *Curr Cardiol Rep* 15:344–353.

Wells RG, Farncombe T, Chang E, Nicholson RL. 2004. Reducing bladder artifacts in clinical pelvic SPECT images. *J Nucl Med* 45:1309–1314.

Wells RG, Timmins R, Klein R, Lockwood J, Marvin B, deKemp RA, Wei L, Ruddy TD. 2014. Dynamic SPECT measurement of absolute myocardial blood flow in a porcine model. *J Nucl Med* 55:1685–1691.

Zaidi H. 2006. *A Qualitative Analysis of Nuclear Medicine Imaging*. Berlin: Springer.

Zeng GL, Hernandez A, Kadrmas DJ, Gullberg GT. 2012. Kinetic parameter estimation using a closed-form expression via integration by parts. *Phys Med Biol* 57:5809–5821.

Zito F, Savi A, Fazio F. 1993. CERASPECT: A brain-dedicated SPECT system. Performance evaluation and comparison with the rotating gamma camera. *Phys Med Biol* 38:1433–1442.

Dynamic PET imaging

SUNG-CHENG (HENRY) HUANG AND KOON-PONG WONG

12.1 Introduction	321
12.2 Dynamic PET imaging procedure	323
12.2.1 Scan time of dynamic PET imaging	323
12.2.2 Injected dose	324
12.2.3 Framing rate	324
12.2.4 Extraction of tracer time–activity curve in regional tissue	325
12.2.4.1 Image reconstruction	325
12.2.4.2 Movement correction	325
12.2.4.3 ROI definition	326
12.2.4.4 ROI value calculation and time–activity curve extraction	327
12.3 Tracer kinetic modeling	327
12.3.1 Validation of a tracer model for a specific tracer	327
12.3.2 Application of validated tracer kinetic model for determining the rates of biological processes from dynamic PET measured kinetics	328
12.3.3 Parametric imaging	330
12.4 Additional topics and issues of concern	330
12.5 Conclusion	332
References	332

12.1 INTRODUCTION

PET can be used to provide a variety of biological functions in regional tissues *in vivo*, using positron-emitting tracers that trace different biological pathways. Common positron emitters include F-18, C-11, N-13, and O-15, which are isotopes of elements that form the organic compounds in the body. Thus, these positron emitters can be incorporated radiochemically into a natural molecule or its analog in the body. This characteristic implies that positron-emitting tracers can be made to follow an almost unlimited number of biological processes in the body, thus enabling PET as a very versatile imaging technique. By using different tracers, completely different biological functions can be obtained with the same PET scanner.

However, for each new PET tracer, the biological behavior of the tracer in the body needs to be examined and characterized to validate that the tracer follows the expected biological process and has the desirable properties that allow the biological information to be easily obtained, since not every positron-emitting tracer synthesized satisfies the many requirements to become useful. Dynamic PET imaging is a critical procedure commonly used in evaluating and verifying new tracers for their intended uses. Frequently coupled

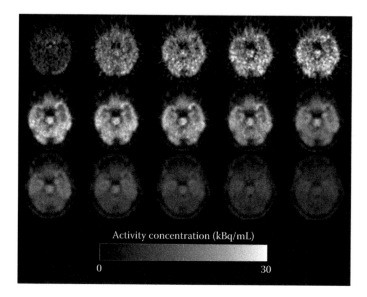

Figure 12.1 Image sequence in a transaxial section of the brain of a patient with Alzheimer's disease. The tracer used, FDDNP, has been shown to have strong binding to beta-amyloid plaques and neurofibrillary tangles (NFTs) in the brain tissue. The midtimes of the images, from left to right and top to bottom, were, respectively, 45, 75, 105, 135, 165, 270, 450, 630, 810, 1200, 1800, 2400, 3000, 3600, and 4500 s post–tracer injection. Qualitatively, the early images showed the amount of tracer delivery to tissue, thus reflecting the blood perfusion pattern in the transaxial section; the later images (e.g., at 1800 and 2400 s) showed the distribution of beta-amyloid plaques and NFTs (note the high activity levels in the medial and inferior temporal lobe) to which the tracer bound. (Images were obtained from a study performed at the University of California, Los Angeles in collaboration with Drs. Jorge Barrio, Vladimir Kepe, and Gary Small.)

with tracer kinetic modeling methods, dynamic PET imaging is also used to investigate the biological processes that an endogenous compound goes through in local tissues *in vivo*.

After the behavior of a tracer has been well understood, dynamic PET imaging can help determine the appropriate procedure that one should use to reliably extract the biological information from the PET images. Since PET is a quantitative imaging technique, the relevant biological information can be extracted in terms of its absolute units (e.g., ml/min/g for blood perfusion, mg/min/g for substrate utilization rates, ml/g for distribution volumes [DVs], and nmole/g for receptor densities). In such evaluations or quantitation, if the desired biological information is not revealed directly in a single static image taken at specific time point post–tracer administration, a dynamic PET imaging procedure could be developed for the particular tracer to help reveal the desired biological information. In some cases with specially tailored procedures, it is even possible to have a multiplicity of biological information obtained from a single dynamic PET imaging study (using either a single tracer or multiple tracers). In Figure 12.1, a set of dynamic PET images is shown that reveal different tissue tracer distributions at different times postinjection of a PET tracer 2-(1-{6-[(2-[^{18}F]fluoroethyl)(methyl)amino]-2-naphthyl}ethylidene)malononitrile (FDDNP). The different distributions reflect the different biological and physiological information in tissues being imaged.

As this introduction indicates, dynamic PET is an important imaging procedure for many critical applications. However, regardless of its application, dynamic PET imaging has some special requirements or limitations that one should consider before performing the study, analyzing the acquired images, or interpreting the results. Figure 12.2 shows a sketch of the procedure employed in general dynamic PET imaging. Many issues involved are separately addressed in this chapter.

Before starting on those issues, readers should be reminded of some basic assumptions underlying tracer kinetic techniques, and thus the use of dynamic imaging. First, in terms of biology, tissue biology in the body being studied is assumed to be in a steady state during the imaging time of a tracer kinetic study.

In terms of the labeled tracer used, the mass amount of tracer introduced is assumed not to affect the steady state of the body biology. In terms of measurement instrumentation, a linear relationship is assumed

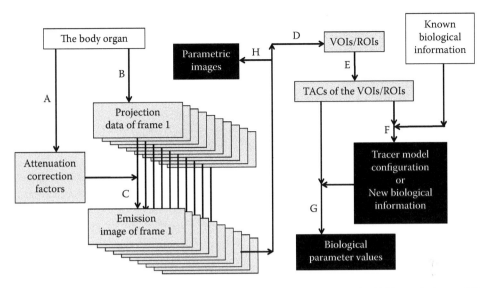

Figure 12.2 Sketch of the procedure of a general dynamic PET imaging study. (a) Transmission or CT scan of the body. (b) Dynamic emission scan of the body. (c) Movement correction and image reconstruction that incorporated proper attenuation correction factors. (d) Manual or template-based definition of VOI/ROI. (e) Projection of VOI/ROI to dynamic images to give tracer TACs. (f) Configuration of tracer model based on known biological information or generation of new biological information or understanding. (g) Generation of biological information based on previously validated kinetic models. (h) Generation of parametric images from a set of dynamic images.

between the obtained image value and the true radioactivity concentration. PET scanners used for dynamic PET imaging usually also need to have the following capabilities: (1) high temporal resolution scanning ability (i.e., can have serial short scan frames), (2) large data volume handling ability, and (3) fast processing power. The importance of each of these factors can vary, depending on the tracer kinetics, the organ tissue of interest, and the specific applications. Although the body being imaged in a dynamic PET imaging study is also assumed not to have any movement during the imaging, some body movement can be corrected (Wardak et al. 2010); this will be addressed in Section 12.2.4.2.

12.2 DYNAMIC PET IMAGING PROCEDURE

The procedure of dynamic PET imaging usually involves taking a transmission scan (e.g., a computed tomography [CT] scan), followed by an intravenous (IV) injection of a PET tracer and collection of coincidence counts using a framing sequence of emission scans (Figure 12.2). The transmission scan is performed to provide the photon attenuation information, with which the collected data from the emission scans can be corrected to give accurate distribution of the positron activity in the body (see Chapters 8 and 9 on PET corrections and image reconstructions). The labeled tracer is usually injected IV. Although other administrative routes (like oral ingestion of fluorodeoxyglucose [FDG]) can also be used, they are rarely used in a clinical setting. In this section, we address a few general procedural issues involved in the collection of positron radioactivity of the labeled tracer (i.e., the emission scans).

12.2.1 Scan time of dynamic PET imaging

One of the first things to determine for dynamic PET imaging is the total length of the imaging and the framing sequence of the emission scans to be used. Clearly, the total length of a dynamic scan is upper limited by the decay half-life of the positron-emitting isotope used, since after the positron radioactivity has decayed substantially, the PET image obtained would not provide any useful information anymore. Therefore, the dynamic PET imaging of O-15 (2 min half-life) and Rb-82 (76 s half-life) labeled tracers cannot be longer than four or five times their half-lives (usually much shorter). The total scan length is also related to biological parameters, such as the biological half-life of the tracer in the body tissue, the time interval the tracer kinetics is sensitive to the desired biological information, and the practical consideration of the length that a patient or subject can stay lying without much body movement in the scanner. For example, the perfusion information contained in the kinetics of a highly extracted tracer in tissue (e.g., F-18 flurpiridaz in myocardium) is mostly within the first few minutes after a bolus injection of the tracer, and the total scan length for obtaining the tissue perfusion information does not need to be much longer than that. However, for assay of the tissue glucose utilization rate (MRG) (e.g., with F-18 FDG), the tracer has a blood clearance time of longer than 10 min, and it needs to cross the capillary and cellular wall before it is involved in the key reaction of glucose utilization in tissue. The information in the tracer kinetics that is related to the tissue MRG is mainly in the time interval after 30 min post–tracer injection. So, a dynamic FDG PET scan usually takes about 60 min, which is also a reasonable procedural length required for a patient or subject to stay in the field of view of a PET scanner.

12.2.2 INJECTED DOSE

The amount of injected dose is also a consideration. Since most positron isotopes commonly used have rather short decay half-lives, a large fraction of the decayed activity is collected by the scanner for constructing the activity distribution of the tracer, leaving only a small amount for residual activity in the body after the imaging study is over. However, the detection sensitivity of the scanner, the image reconstruction algorithm used, the distribution of the tracer and the background activity level in the body, the target tissue volume size, the spatial resolution, and the rate of temporal change of the tracer activity in tissue could influence the selection of an adequate injected dose. While too low a dosage will give an inadequate signal-to-noise ratio, a dose much higher than what is required is equally undesirable.

12.2.3 FRAMING RATE

With the availability of list-mode data acquisition of most PET scanners, the framing rate of a dynamic scanning sequence can be altered after the scan data acquisition. Although one might want to have a framing rate as high as possible, the PET image is count limited (see Chapters 1, 6, and 8), and counting statistics would post an upper limit on the framing rate one could use. This issue is the same for dynamic SPECT as well (see Chapter 11). Since the number of collected coincidence counts is finite over a fixed time interval, a higher framing rate (shorter frame duration) would imply fewer total counts per frame. In general, frame duration should be inversely proportional to the radioactivity level in tissue and to the rate of change of the tracer activity. Since the tracer activity in body tissue is usually not constant over time, nor is the changing rate of activity in the tissues, the framing rates (or frame durations) commonly used are variable during a dynamic scan. The actual frame duration to be used would depend on many factors, including the decay half-life of the isotope, the detection sensitivity of the scanner, the injected dose, the dose administration schedule, the tracer kinetics in the body, body size, body movement, the image reconstruction algorithm used, the size of the regions of interest (ROIs), the image's spatial resolution desired, and the size of the resulting data volume (see Chapter 8 for the relationships among various parameters).

The framing rate can be greatly reduced if the tissue kinetics is known to follow what is predictable by some verified model for a particular tracer. In such cases, the full tracer kinetics in tissue can be determined by a small number (four or five) of parameters and the number of frames can be minimized to a comparable number. The lengths of the frame durations could also be adjusted to optimize the reliability of the information one wants to obtain (Li et al. 2001; Liao et al. 2002) and are dependent on the specific model and the kinetics of the tracer in tissues of interest.

A chosen framing sequence usually could be verified using computer simulations to ensure the desired temporal information is retained and the quality of the images is adequate.

12.2.4 Extraction of tracer time–activity curve in regional tissue

After the dynamic scanning, the next set of issues to consider is related to obtaining the tracer kinetics in regional body tissues. The main issues are (1) image reconstruction, (2) movement correction, and (3) ROI determination.

12.2.4.1 IMAGE RECONSTRUCTION

There are two major categories of image reconstruction algorithms—filtered backprojection (FBPJ) (Kak and Slaney 1987) and iterative (Herman 1980) reconstruction. The former one is a direct method based on Fourier theory (Bracewell 1978). FBPJ reconstruction does not specifically consider the statistical noise in the projection measurements, and would generate annoying streak artifacts when the measurements have a high noise level (i.e., low counts). Iterative reconstruction has many variations. The most popular one is the ordered subset expectation and maximization (OSEM) algorithm (Hudson and Larkin 1994). It specifically accounts for the Poisson statistics of photon counting in the measurements (Shepp and Vardi 1982; Lange and Carson 1984), and uses a row-action type of algorithm to speed up the convergence (Browne and De Pierro 1996; Censor 1981). Images reconstructed with OSEM do not have streak artifacts, and are visually more pleasing. However, the spatial resolution of the reconstructed image is not guaranteed to be uniform. Usually, a postreconstruction smoothing is performed to ensure the near uniformity of the spatial resolution. (See Chapter 9 for a full discussion of various image reconstruction methods.)

Sometimes, the scan durations of different frames can range from a few seconds to a few minutes, since the temporal changing rate of activity in tissue can vary by a large amount during a dynamic imaging procedure. The noise levels of the measurements in different frames can be very different. It would seem like the use of different reconstruction algorithms for different scan frames would be the right approach. However, the mixed use of different reconstruction algorithms for different frames in a single dynamic imaging study is seldom adopted. The concern is that different characteristics, such as the spatial resolution and noise level of the images reconstructed with different algorithms, could potentially create features in the kinetic data that are not easy to handle or interpret (see later subsections). In practice, either the FBPJ or OSEM algorithm is used for reconstruction images of all frames. The former one is more straightforward to use. The latter algorithm has more variable parameters to choose from, and one should ensure that the spatial resolution of the images is uniform spatially over the field of view and temporally for all frames.

12.2.4.2 MOVEMENT CORRECTION

As mentioned earlier, dynamic imaging takes a little bit of time that ranges from a few minutes to more than an hour. It is impossible to keep an awake subject completely stationary during the entire imaging time. Various approaches have been developed to deal with this patient movement problem. One type of method employs optical monitoring (or other sensing methods) to continuously record the subject movement during a dynamic imaging study, and the movement information is used to correct the projection measurements properly before image reconstruction. The method described by Buhler et al. (2004) represents this type. This type of method, although conceptually accurate and ideal, requires elaborate correction operations, and its performance is also dependent on the accuracy of the monitoring (or sensing) devices, the time synchronization, and the spatial calibrations.

A different type of method to deal with the movement problem is exemplified by the approach published by Wardak et al. (2010) and Ye et al. (2014). This type of approach first derives the movement information from the reconstructed images, and the derived information is then used to make the necessary corrections to generate the properly corrected set of dynamic images that are nearly movement-free. This type of movement correction does not need any special movement sensing or monitoring devices and can be applied *post hoc*. It is ideal for body organs (like the head) that only have rigid-body movements (Figure 12.3). This method is not expected to work well for images of high noise levels. The correction algorithms could get very complicated if the body movement is not rigid. Formally, this type of method appears to be able to correct only movements occurring

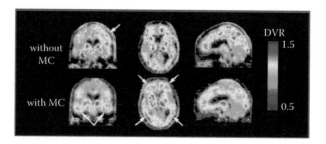

Figure 12.3 Example of movement correction (MC) results. Without MC, the FDDNP DVR image of an Alzheimer's disease subject with considerable head movement was subject to image artifacts (i.e., abnormally high scalp uptake and asymmetric left–right image values). With MC, the quality of the DVR image was improved. (Images adapted from Wardak, M., et al., *J. Nucl. Med.*, 51, 210–218, 2010.)

between image frames. However, if the list-mode data are acquired, statistical methods that detect extra data inconsistency (beyond counting noise) are available to determine if there existed significant intraframe movement (Huang et al. 2011b), and one can then reframe the data to minimize the intraframe movements.

12.2.4.3 ROI DEFINITION

Once the image data are well adjusted, the next procedure is to extract the tracer kinetics of the volume of interest (VOI) or ROI from the dynamic images. The first step is to define the VOI or ROI, within which the tracer kinetics is obtained. There are various VOI/ROI definition methods that are implemented in many general image analysis software packages (Janus, ImageJ, Vinci, Osirix, Amide, etc.) (Loening and Gambhir 2003; Rosset et al. 2004; www.idoimaging.com/program/334).

In general, there are different VOI/ROI definition methods. The first and simplest one is the use of geometric shapes (e.g., rectangular boxes, cylinders, spheres, and ellipsoids). One can select the center and dimensions of the geometric shape. The limitation of this type of method is that the shape of very few organ tissues in the body can only be defined geometrically.

The second type is to use a threshold image value to define a close contour on the image, such that the voxels or regions within the contour would be considered the VOI/ROI (Wong et al. 2013). The user can adjust the threshold value to shrink or expand the VOI/ROI. Variants of this method include the use of threshold on image gradients instead of image values (Sha et al. 2010).

The third type of method for VOI/ROI definition is manual tracing, which can give a contour that one desires. However, the task is a very time-consuming. The difficulty level is further elevated for tracing 3D surfaces. Besides, the subjectivity involved in defining VOI/ROI this way could be a serious problem, and could yield a large intersubject variability. So, this type of method is not generally used except for preliminary investigations.

Another type of method is the use of standard VOI/ROI templates. The templates are usually defined on a set of reference images that have high anatomical details (like MRI). For the brain, many templates have been constructed and are available on the Internet or by request from the original investigators. One can then use image warping methods (e.g., ANTS [Avants et al. 2008] and SPM8 [www.fil.ion.ucl.ac.uk/spm/software/spm8]) to align the reference images to the images of the individual that are of the same imaging modality (Wilks et al. 2012). Afterward, one can use rigid-body coregistration methods for cross-modality images to help place the VOI/ROI templates on the corresponding PET images. For myocardial studies, a polar map approach (like the one for SPECT images) is generally used and the heart is divided into a few standard territories or regions. Methods of this type, although they involve many sophisticated image processing steps, can be streamlined and automated to accomplish the task objectively without much user intervention.

The different types of methods presented above are not exhaustive. For example, one could use a combination of the different methods mentioned to obtain the volume or region that one desires. Another variation people have used is application of the threshold method to factor coefficient images after a factor analysis (Schiepers et al. 2007; Wardak et al. 2011). Usually, one of the decisions that one needs to make before determining the VOI/ROI is the image among all the dynamic PET images to use to guide the definition of the VOIs/ROIs. Generally, one uses the image with the most distinguished features. The image can be from a single frame, a sum of multiple frames, a factor image (mentioned above), or a parametric image (see Section 12.3.3).

One of the most challenging organs in which to define the VOI/ROI is the urinary bladder. For each time frame, one could use any of the above methods. However, since the size of the urinary bladder is usually expanding over the time period of dynamic PET imaging, a unique VOI/ROI needs to be defined for each frame (Wong et al. 2013). The changing contrast ratio to the background level over time further complicates the task involved.

12.2.4.4 ROI VALUE CALCULATION AND TIME–ACTIVITY CURVE EXTRACTION

In addition to the size and shape of the VOI/ROI, the image values within the VOI/ROI contain important information about the biological processes in tissue. There are a few different ways to calculate the VOI/ROI values. The most common one calculates the average value of all the voxels within the VOI/ROI. When there are apparent outliers among the voxel values, the median value is more reliable. When there are large spatially related variations, the maximum value is also frequently used. Since the maximum is a biased measure that can be affected by the noise level of the voxel values, some people use the average of the top 5% (or 10%) of the voxel values, and this is sometimes referred to as the peak value.

Since the spatial resolution of PET images is finite, there are always partial volume and spillover effects on the VOI/ROI values (Hoffman et al. 1979; Henze et al. 1983). The amounts of these effects are dependent on the radioactivity distribution and the VOI/ROI calculation method used. The corrections would thus also be different. When the tissue and true radioactivity within the VOI/ROI is heterogeneous, the accurate corrections can be quite challenging, and active investigations are still being pursued by many (Zheng et al. 2011; Zhou et al. 1997).

12.3 TRACER KINETIC MODELING

Tracer kinetic modeling is a method to incorporate prior information one has to help extract unknown information from the measured kinetics of a labeled tracer. This is a topic area that has been addressed extensively in the literature in the past (Huang and Phelps 1985; Huang 2008). In this section, we give brief discussions on the use of tracer kinetic modeling and its limitations. Some practical examples of the use of dynamic PET imaging are also shown.

With its mathematical tractability, a compartmental model is commonly used to describe the kinetics of tracers in biological systems. Although the assumption of uniform tracer concentration in a compartmental pool is seldom completely satisfied in tissues or organs, it is generally a reasonable approximation, especially in the presence of the noise in the measurement of the kinetics. Thus, the use of compartmental models represents a compromise between biological realism, statistical measurement noise, and mathematical tractability.

For dynamic PET imaging, there are generally two types of application of tracer kinetic models—one is to determine the biological pathways of a particular tracer to establish and validate an appropriate model configuration (Section 12.3.1); the other is to use a developed and validated model of a tracer to determine the rates of the biological processes that the tracer follows, as well as the proper protocol for dynamic PET imaging of the particular tracer (Section 12.3.2).

12.3.1 VALIDATION OF A TRACER MODEL FOR A SPECIFIC TRACER

For this application, the general question one tries to answer is whether the tracer goes through some particular transports or reactions in tissue (i.e., whether a particular model is appropriate to describe the tracer behavior in tissue).

Usually, based on *in vitro* assays or autoradiographic studies with a particular tracer in question, one can speculate a rough configuration of a compartment model for the tracer. However, the speculation needs to be validated or modified before the model can be used for determining the rates of related biological processes. The first step in the validation process is to evaluate whether the kinetics generated by the proposed model is consistent with what is measured (e.g., with dynamic PET imaging). If not, the model configuration will need to be modified. Modifications of the model configuration are based on biological information about the possible transport and reaction pathways of the tracer being considered, so each parameter in the model would correspond to some biological process in tissue. The modified model will again need to be checked to see if the generated kinetics is consistent with the measurement.

The kinetics consistency is usually done using model-fitting or regression analysis (Huang 2008; Huang and Phelps 1985; Bates and Watts 1988; Press et al. 2007), which automatically finds the model-generated kinetics that best fits the measured kinetics (e.g., obtained from the procedures described in Section 12.2). Model fitting usually requires that one has measured the input function, either taken from sequential blood samples or derived from the dynamic images (Ferl et al. 2007; Weinberg et al. 1988), since the model-generated kinetics in tissue is the convolution of the impulse response function of the model configuration and the input function (Huang and Phelps 1985; Huang et al. 1980). The input function is the time function of the tracer concentration in arterial blood or plasma that directly affects the rate of tracer transport in local tissue (Carson et al. 1993; Huang and Phelps 1985). Statistical methods will be applied to assess whether the model-fitting result is adequate (Box and Draper 1987; Landaw and DiStefano 1984). Statistical criteria are also available to prevent overfitting the measurements contaminated by noise (Akaike 1974; Box and Draper 1987; Landaw and DiStefano 1984).

The second level of validation is to check to see if the subcomponents of the labeled tracer or metabolites predicted by the best-fitted model match those determined by *in vitro* assay procedures. For example, for the FDG model that fits a measured FDG kinetics in tissue, the fractions of the phosphorylated FDG (i.e., FDG-6-P) can be calculated from the best-fitted model with the accompanying model parameters as a function of time. This fraction at any particular time can also be obtained by direct tissue assay procedures, although multiple assays are needed to overcome the variability of the assay results and obtain results at multiple time points. Again, the model-predicted results should be in agreement with the direct assayed results, if the model is to be regarded appropriate for describing the tracer kinetics in the tissue under consideration.

Due to the invasiveness required for determining the labeled metabolites in tissues with *in vitro* assay methodologies, the validation is usually done first in animals (Melega et al. 1991; Barrio et al. 1996), and is verified in a limited number of human or patient studies. Since the biological conditions in different tissues or different states (i.e., normal and disease) could be different, the validation needs to be performed for all the tissues and all the states in which the model is intended to be used.

In the determination of the appropriate model configuration for a tracer, some iterative steps are needed. During this iteration process, the strategy for modifying the model configuration at each step requires some practical experience, and any proposed alternative configurations should be guided by the known biological and physiological knowledge of the biochemical processes in the target tissue of interest.

Factors that could affect the tracer kinetics, uptake, or clearance in tissue need to be determined, and it could take a long time to test the many physiological or biological factors involved, but this should not preclude the possible translation of tracer use to the clinical environment even before all factors are completely understood. They could go in parallel. The involvement of some factors may not be known until after extensive clinical use. In other words, clinical use could help indicate the areas or factors that may need to be investigated further.

After the model configuration of a tracer in a particular target tissue has been determined, the characteristics of the model in terms of the sensitivity of the kinetics to model parameters can be determined and help the use of the tracer for extracting the biological information, as addressed in Section 12.3.2.

12.3.2 APPLICATION OF VALIDATED TRACER KINETIC MODEL FOR DETERMINING THE RATES OF BIOLOGICAL PROCESSES FROM DYNAMIC PET MEASURED KINETICS

After a model has been validated for a particular tracer in a target organ tissue, the model can then be used to help determine the relevant biological information noninvasively from PET images. The most straightforward approach to accomplish this is to perform dynamic PET imaging to obtain the tissue kinetics, and to model fit the measured kinetics to give the estimated biological parameter values of the tissue being studied using KIS (Huang et al. 2005), COMKAT (Muzic and Cornelius 2001), or PMOD (www.pmod.com).

This approach has the advantage that it is applicable for various shapes of the input function and can provide a multiplicity of biological information, since there are usually multiple model parameters, each of which corresponds to a separate biological process. However, the approach also has some limitations. Since the model-fitting procedure requires one to have dynamic scanning on the subject and the input function measured, the experimental procedure is relatively complicated and lengthy. The model fitting is also sensitive to body movement, and the parameter estimates could have large variability if the image noise level is high. The model-fitting approach is not generally preferred for routine studies.

To avoid the complicated procedure of model fitting, people have developed many different simplified approaches that have various degrees of procedural simplicities. The graphical methods, reference tissue methods, reference tissue graphical methods, and standardized uptake values (SUVs) (Keyes 1995) are representative of the ones in common use today, and are briefly introduced below.

There are two primary graphical methods—one for tracers that follow an irreversible uptake process, and the other for reversible tracers. The Patlak graphical method (Patlak et al. 1983) represents the first kind. Through a special transformation of the time axis, the kinetics of a tracer that is sequestered in tissue approaches a straight line after some time and the slope of the asymptotic line is equal to the uptake constant of the tracer from blood to tissue. The Logan graphical method (Logan et al. 1990) is representative of the second kind. Through a different transformation of the time axis, the kinetics of a tracer of zero sequestration in tissue approaches a straight line, with its slope equal to the DV of the tracer in tissue (relative to that in blood). There is no need to perform nonlinear regression for these graphical methods, and the results are much less sensitive to measurement noise. However, the methods still require the input function.

When the input function is replaced by a time–activity curve (TAC) of a reference tissue region that is obtained from the dynamic images, the resulting slope from the Logan method gives the DV ratio (DVR) value (Logan et al. 1996), which is the DV value relative to that of the reference tissue. Since the reference tissue is usually chosen to be similar to the target tissue of interest, except that its DV value is different and is subject-independent, one does not need to measure any labeled metabolites in blood that are not taken up by the tissues. An example of the application of this method to FDDNP, a tracer that binds to beta-amyloid and tau protein in brain tissues (Barrio et al. 1999; Agdeppa et al. 2001), is shown in Figure 12.4.

Simplified reference tissue modeling (SRTM) is a reference tissue method that is applicable to reversible tracers and uses the TAC of the reference tissue as a surrogate input function. The method uses nonlinear regression (instead of linear regression) and can provide estimates for the binding potential (BP, or DVR), k2, which is the efflux rate constant from the free compartment to the plasma compartment, and R1, which is the transport rate of the tracer in the target tissue of interest relative to that in the reference tissue (Lammertsma

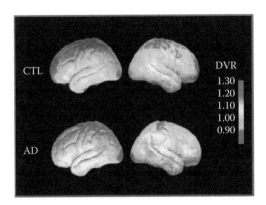

Figure 12.4 Average FDDNP DVR values of control subjects (CTL) and patients with Alzheimer's disease (AD) shown on the hemispheric cortical surface. (Images adapted from Protas, H., et al., *Neuroimage*, 49, 240–248, 2010.)

and Hume 1996; Gunn et al. 2002). Unlike the graphical methods, which provide only one or two parameter values at a time, SRTM, like general model fitting, yields a multiplicity of biological information (transport to and efflux from the free compartment, and BP) at the same time. Although nonlinear regression is used, the method only estimates three parameters and is not very sensitive to measurement noise as the general model-fitting approach. Since it fits the whole tissue kinetics (i.e., from time zero on), the method does not require *a priori* knowledge of the equilibrium time of the tracer in tissue that is needed for the application of the graphical methods.

SUV is the simplest of all quantitative methods. One does not even need to perform dynamic imaging to obtain the SUV. It is almost equivalent to the C-11 deoxyglucose (DG) autoradiographic method (Sokoloff et al. 1977; Huang 2000). In calculating the SUV, the variations in the injected dose and the body weight are accounted for by normalizing the measured tissue radioactivity concentration by the injected dose and the body weight of the subject. The method is widely used in tumor screening with FDG PET to determine the aggressiveness of the detected lesions. The validity of the SUV depends on the assumption that the input function for the tracer used is similar in all cases and in different subjects (Huang 2000). If this assumption is not valid (like the use of N-13 ammonia for myocardial blood perfusion measurement [Schelbert et al. 1979]), the SUV is of little value (Choi et al. 1999). The time of PET imaging for SUV calculation is also tracer dependent and needs to be determined and validated against the values obtained with full dynamic PET imaging studies.

The characteristics of a tracer kinetic model, which are dependent on the model configuration, the model parameter values, and the number of variable parameters used, and on the shape of the input function, can be investigated using either analytical methods or computer simulations. Many software packages are available to perform this type of investigation (e.g., KIS [Huang et al. 2005], COMKAT [Muzic and Cornelius 2001], and PMOD). The kinetic characteristics obtained could be very useful in determining the right simplified procedures to use for a particular tracer. With the availability of a valid tracer kinetic model, the reliability of a chosen simplified procedure or method could also be validated using computer simulation.

12.3.3 PARAMETRIC IMAGING

The procedure of the extraction of biological information discussed so far is focused on the TACs of a defined VOI/ROI. However, with the development of less noise-sensitive and computationally efficient methods (like the ones discussed in previous sections and others [Zhou et al. 2003; Huang and Zhou 1998; Zhou et al. 2009]), it is feasible to extract reliable biological information from TACs of a single voxel. Thus, images with their voxel value representing the biological parameters in their absolute units can be constructed. These images are generally called parametric images.

With this approach, one does not need to define the VOI/ROI in advance, and the spatial distribution of the tissue biological information could be more clearly conveyed to the viewer and investigators. Such parametric images can be more easily correlated with images of other modalities that show high anatomical information (e.g., MRI and CT), and are expected to have a more significant role in dual-modality imaging, like PET/CT and PET/MRI. Examples of parametric images are shown in Figures 12.3 and 12.4.

Since the reference tissue methods discussed above can use the TAC of a reference tissue as the input function, obviating the need to take serial blood samples, they are commonly used for generating the parametric images. One exception is the use of dynamic PET imaging for the combined measurement of cerebral blood flow (CBF) and cerebral metabolic rate of oxygen (CMRO), as shown in Figure 12.5. When combined with the measurement of the cerebral MRG and MRI/CT images, very valuable information about the regional tissue biology can be obtained in the brain posttraumatic brain injury (Wu et al. 2004, 2013).

12.4 ADDITIONAL TOPICS AND ISSUES OF CONCERN

For many applications of dynamic PET imaging, the procedures involve measurements from a number of devices, such as well counters for blood sample radioactivity concentration, and radioactivity dosimeter for

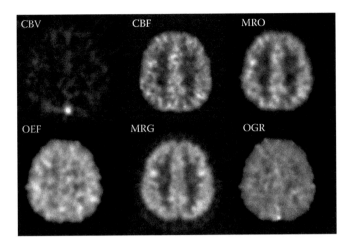

Figure 12.5 Parametric images from four brain PET scans of a normal subject with four different tracers, O-15 CO, O-15 water, O-15 oxygen, and FDG. The images correspond to the same transaxial cross section of the brain. The gray scales of the images were scaled to the maximal value on each image. Lighter shade is for higher values. Multiple biological functions for tissues in the same brain regions were shown: cerebral blood volume (CBV) from O-15 CO scan; CBF from O-15 water; metabolic rate of oxygen (MRO) and oxygen extraction fraction (OEF) from O-15 oxygen, along with the images of CBV and CBF; MRG from FDG; and oxygen to glucose molar ratio (OGR) of MRO and MRG. (Images were obtained from a study performed at the University of California, Los Angeles [UCLA] in collaboration with Drs. Marvin Bergsneider, H.M. Wu, Paul Vespa, David Hovda, et al., at UCLA Brain Injury Research Center.)

injected doses, in addition to the PET scanner. The absolute and cross-calibrations of these devices need to be performed correctly and their stability checked. Furthermore, since dynamic imaging utilizes not only the spatial distribution but also the temporal information of the imaged radioactivity, the performance demand of the imaging PET scanner is higher than that of regular static PET imaging. For example, the scanner needs to handle a wide dynamic range of count rates with accurate dead-time corrections. In addition to regular image quality checks, a quality control procedure for performing dynamic imaging on a phantom is highly recommended. In this quality control procedure, the image values (after decay correction) over all image frames (i.e., over time) should be constant. Otherwise, the measured tissue kinetics from dynamic PET imaging could contain serious errors.

As discussed earlier, in many applications, the input function is required. For the development of tracer kinetic models and for the investigation of biological pathways, the input function needs to be obtained by taking serial blood samples. One needs to assay not only the blood or plasma radioactivity concentrations, but also the fractions of labeled metabolites in blood or plasma as a function of time. For the applications to assess the biological activity in tissue with a validated tracer and model, the input function can sometimes be substituted with the TAC of a reference tissue region. However, the biological state of the reference tissue needs to be well understood beforehand. For some tracers, the time functions of the total blood concentrations can be derived from large blood pool regions on the dynamic images (Henze et al. 1983; Ferl et al. 2007; Weinberg et al. 1988; Schiepers et al. 2007; Chen et al. 1992; Huang et al. 2011a; Chen et al. 1998). In many cases, some kinds of partial volume and spillover corrections are involved in the derivation of the input function from dynamic images (Ferl et al. 2007; Schiepers et al. 2007; Huang et al. 2011a; Chen et al. 1998).

Although the partial volume effect has been extensively studied and is well known, the quantitative effect is quite complicated, especially for tissue structures that have irregular shapes, are not uniform in radioactivity level, or consist of large biological heterogeneity. The correction of the partial volume effect and the spillover activities are not straightforward. In such cases, the interpretation of the results should be done with care. Many assumptions of the physical and tracer models involved in the extraction of biological information may not be valid any more.

There are numerous biological factors that could affect the uptake or kinetics of a tracer in local tissue. While many of them are still unknown to us, it is likely that these confounding factors are more similar for the same individual over time than for different individuals. Therefore, monitoring the change of the extract biological information from dynamic PET imaging over time in a patient is more reliable than comparing the difference between patients or individuals. The ability to separate intrasubject from intersubject variability of dynamic PET imaging (e.g., using time series analysis methods in statistics) could thus be very useful to help in the interpretation of the extracted biological information (Sha et al. 2013), especially for treatment monitoring and assessment of treatment efficacy (Wardak et al. 2011).

12.5 CONCLUSION

Dynamic PET imaging has many applications, including the research and development of new PET tracers, the investigation of biological pathways and kinetics, and the extraction of regional tissue biological information noninvasively. In many cases, close collaborations with biologists, biochemists, physicists, and physicians are essential. In addition, dynamic PET imaging is used to help determine the appropriate protocols for static PET imaging. The reliability and limitation of such protocols can also be obtained by comparison with results of dynamic PET imaging studies. When performed with a multimodality imaging scanner (e.g., PET/CT or PET/MR), dynamic PET imaging can be used to provide a multiplicity of biological information in the body tissues, along with anatomical information, in a single study session. Therefore, dynamic PET imaging is a unique and very powerful tool in biology and medicine.

REFERENCES

Agdeppa, E.D., V. Kepe, J. Liu, S. Samuel Flores-Torres, N. Satyamurthy, A. Petric, G.M. Cole, G.W. Small, S.-C. Huang, and J.R. Barrio. 2001. Binding characteristics of radiofluorinated 6-dialkylamino-2-naphthylethylidene derivatives as positron emission tomography imaging probes for b-amyloid plaques in Alzheimer's disease. *J. Neurosci.* 21:RC189(1–5).

Akaike, H. 1974. A new look at the statistical model identification. *IEEE Trans. Automat. Contr.* 19:716–723.

Avants, B.B., C.L. Epstein, M. Grossman, and J.C. Gee. 2008. Symmetric diffeomorphic image registration with cross-correlation: Evaluating automated labeling of elderly and neurodegenerative brain. *Med. Image Anal.* 12:26–41.

Barrio, J.R., S.-C. Huang, G. Cole, N. Satyamurthy, A. Petric, M.E. Phelps, and G. Small. 1999. PET imaging of tangles and plaques in Alzheimer disease with a highly hydrophobic probe. *J. Labelled Comp. Radiopharm.* 42(Suppl. 1):S194–S195.

Barrio, J.R., S.C. Huang, D.C. Yu, W.P. Melega, J. Quintana, S.R. Cherry, A. Jacobson, M. Namavari, N. Satyamurthy, and M.E. Phelps. 1996. Radiofluorinated L-m-tyrosines: New in-vivo probes for central dopamine biochemistry. *J. Cereb. Blood Flow Metab.* 16:667–678.

Bates, D.M., and D.G. Watts. 1988. *Nonlinear Regression Analysis and Its Applications.* Wiley Series in Probability and Mathematical Statistics. New York: John Wiley & Sons.

Box, G.E.P., and N.R. Draper. 1987. *Empirical Model-Building and Response Surfaces.* New York: John Wiley & Sons.

Bracewell, R.N. 1978. *The Fourier Transform and Its Applications.* New York: McGraw-Hill Book Company.

Browne, J.A., and A.R. De Pierro. 1996. A row-action alternative to the EM algorithm for maximizing likelihoods in emission tomography. *IEEE Trans. Med. Imaging* 15:687–699.

Buhler, P., U. Just, E. Will, J. Kotzerke, and J. van den Hoff. 2004. An accurate method for correction of head movement in PET. *IEEE Trans. Med. Imaging* 23(9):1176–1185.

Carson, R.E., M.A. Channing, R.G. Blasberg, B.B. Dunn, R.M. Cohen, K.C. Rice, and P. Herscovitch. 1993. Comparison of bolus and infusion methods for receptor quantitation: Application to [^{18}F]cyclofoxy and positron emission tomography. *J. Cereb. Blood Flow Metab.* 13(1):24–42.

Censor, Y. 1981. Row-action methods for huge and sparse systems and their applications. *SIAM Rev.* 23:444–466.

Chen, B.C., G. Germano, S.C. Huang, R.A. Hawkins, H. Hansen, M.J. Robert, D. Buxton, H.R. Schelbert, I. Kurtz, and M.E. Phelps. 1992. A new noninvasive method for quantification of renal blood flow with N-13 ammonia, dynamic positron emission tomography and a two-compartmental model. *J. Am. Soc. Nephrol.* 3:1295–1306.

Chen, K., D. Bandy, E. Reiman, S.C. Huang, M. Lawson, D. Feng, L. Yun, and A. Palant. 1998. Non-invasive quantification of the cerebral metabolic rate for glucose using positron emission tomography, F-18-fluoro-2-deoxyglucose, the Patlak method, and an image-derived input function. *J. Cereb. Blood Flow Metab.* 18:716–723.

Choi, Y, S.C. Huang, R.A. Hawkins, J.Y. Kim, B.T. Kim, C.K. Hoh, K. Chen, M.E. Phelps, and H.R. Schelbert. 1999. Quantification of myocardial blood flow using N-13 ammonia and PET: Comparison of tracer methods. *J. Nucl. Med.* 40:1045–1055.

Ferl, G.Z., H.M. Wu, X. Zhang, and S.C. Huang. 2007. Estimation of the ^{18}F-FDG input function in mice using dynamic microPET and minimal blood sample data. *J. Nucl. Med.* 48:2037–2045.

Gunn, R.N., S.R. Gunn, F.E. Turkheimer, J.A. Aston, and V.J. Cunningham. 2002. Positron emission tomography compartmental models: A basis pursuit strategy for kinetic modeling. *J. Cereb. Blood Flow Metab.* 22:1425–1439.

Henze, E., S.C. Huang, O. Ratib, E.J. Hoffman, M.E. Phelps, and H.R. Schelbert. 1983. Measurements of regional tissue and blood pool indicator concentrations from serial tomographic images of the heart. *J. Nucl. Med.* 24:987–996.

Herman, G.T. 1980. *Image Reconstruction from Projections.* New York: Academic Press.

Hoffman, E.J., S.C. Huang, and M.E. Phelps. 1979. Quantitation in positron emission computed tomography. 1. Effect of object size. *J. Comput. Assist. Tomogr.* 3:299–308.

Huang, S.C. 2000. Anatomy of SUV. *Nucl. Med. Biol.* 27:643–646.

Huang, S.C. 2008. Role of kinetic modeling in biomedical imaging. *J. Med. Sci.* 28(2):57–63.

Huang, S.C., M. Dahlbom, J. Maddahi, D. Truong, J. Lazewatsky, D. Washburn, H. Schelbert, J. Czernin, and M. Phelps. 2011a. Streamlined quantification of absolute MBF at rest and stress with flurpiridaz F-18 injection PET in normal subjects and patients with coronary artery disease (CAD) [abstract]. *J. Nucl. Med.* 52(Suppl.):1114.

Huang, S.C., and M.E. Phelps. 1985. Principles of tracer kinetic modeling in positron emission tomography and autoradiography. In *Positron Emission Tomography and Autoradiography,* ed. J. Mazziotta M.E. Phelps, and H.R. Schelbert, 287–346. Philadelphia: Raven Press.

Huang, S.C., M.E. Phelps, E.J. Hoffman, K. Sideris, C.J. Selin, and D.E. Kuhl. 1980. Noninvasive determination of local cerebral metabolic rate of glucose in man. *Am. J. Physiol.* 238:E69–E82.

Huang, S.C., D. Truong, H.M. Wu, A.F. Chatziioannou, W. Shao, A.M. Wu, and M.E. Phelps. 2005. An Internet-based "kinetic imaging system" (KIS) for MicroPET. *Mol. Imaging Biol.* 7:330–341.

Huang, S.C., H. Ye, M. Wardak, K.-P. Wong, M. Dahlbom, W. Shao, G.W. Small, and J.R. Barrio. 2011b. A bootstrap method for identifying image regions affected by intra-scan body movement during a PET/CT scan. In *Conference Record of IEEE Medical Imaging,* Valencia, Spain, MIC12.M-51, 2905–2908.

Huang, S.C., and Y. Zhou. 1998. Spatially-coordinated regression for image-wise model fitting to dynamic PET data for generating parametric images. *IEEE Trans. Nucl. Sci.* 45:1194–1199.

Hudson, H.M., and R.S. Larkin. 1994. Accelerated image reconstruction using ordered subsets of projection data. *IEEE Trans. Med. Imaging* 13:601–609.

Kak, A.C., and M. Slaney. 1987. *Principles of Computerized Tomgraphic Imaging.* New York: IEEE Press.

Keyes, J.W. 1995. Standard uptake value or silly useless value. *J. Nucl. Med.* 36:1836–1839.

Lammertsma, A.A., and S.P. Hume. 1996. Simplified reference tissue model for PET receptor studies. *Neuroimage* 4:153–158.

Landaw, E.M., and J.J. DiStefano III. 1984. Multiexponential, multicompartmental, and noncompartmental modeling. II. Data analysis and statistical considerations. *Am. J. Physiol.* 246:R665–R677.

Lange, K., and R.E. Carson. 1984. EM reconstruction algorithms for emission and transmission tomography. *J. Comput. Assist. Tomogr.* 8:306–316.

Li, X., D. Feng, and K.-P. Wong. 2001. A general algorithm for optimal sampling schedule design in nuclear medicine imaging. *Comput. Method Programs Biomed.* 65:45–59.

Liao, W.-H., K. Lange, M. Bergsneider, and S.C. Huang. 2002. Optimal design in PET data acquisition: A new approach using simulated annealing and component-wise Metropolis updating. *IEEE Trans. Nucl. Sci.* 49:2291–2296.

Loening, A.M., and S.S. Gambhir. 2003. AMIDE: A free software tool for multimodality medical image analysis. *Mol. Imaging* 2(3):131–137.

Logan, J., J. Fowler, N. Volkow, A. Wolf, D. Dewey, D. Schlyer, R. MacGregor, R. Hitzmann, B. Bendriem, S. Gatley, and D. Christman. 1990. Graphical analysis of reversible radioligand binding from time-activity measurements applied to [N-11C-methyl]-(−)-cocaine PET studies in human subjects. *J. Cereb. Blood Flow Metab.* 10:740–747.

Logan, J., J.S. Fowler, N.D. Volkow, G.J. Wang, Y.S. Ding, and D.L. Alexoff. 1996. Distribution volume ratios without blood sampling from graphical analysis of PET data. *J. Cereb. Blood Flow Metab.* 16:834–840.

Melega, W.P., S.T. Grafton, Huang, S.C., N. Satyamurthy, M. Phelps, and J.R. Barrio. 1991. 6-[F-18]Fluoro-L-DOPA metabolism in monkeys and humans: Biochemical parameters for the formulation of tracer kinetic models with positron emission tomography. *J. Cereb. Blood Flow Metab.* 11:890–897.

Muzic, R.F., and S. Cornelius. 2001. COMKAT: Compartment model kinetic analysis tool. *J. Nucl. Med.* 42:636–645.

Patlak, C.S., R.G. Blasberg, and J. Fenstermacher. 1983. Graphical evaluation of blood-to-brain transfer constants from multiple-time uptake data. *J. Cereb. Blood Flow Metab.* 3:1–7.

Press, W.H., S.A. Teukolsky, W.T. Vetterling, and B.P. Flannery. 2007. *Numerical Recipes: The Art of Scientific Computing.* 3rd ed. New York: Cambridge University Press.

Protas, H., S.C. Huang, V. Kepe, K. Hayashi, A. Klunder, M.N. Braskie, L. Ercoli, S. Bookheimer, P.M Thompson, G.W. Small, and J.R. Barrio. 2010. FDDNP binding using MR derived cortical surface maps. *Neuroimage* 49:240–248.

Rosset, A., L. Spadola, and O. Ratib. 2004. OsiriX: An open-source software for navigating in multidimensional DICOM images. *J. Digit. Imaging* 17(3):205–216.

Schelbert, H.R., M.E. Phelps, E.J. Hoffman, S.C. Huang, C.E. Selin, and D.E. Kuhl. 1979. Regional myocardial perfusion assessed by N-13 labeled ammonia and positron emission computerized axial tomography. *Am. J. Cardiol.* 43:209–218.

Schiepers, C., W. Chen, M. Dahlbom, T. Cloughesy, C.K. Hoh, and S.C. Huang. 2007. 18F–fluoro-thymidine kinetics of malignant brain tumors. *Eur. J. Nucl. Med. Mol. Imaging* 34(7):1003–1011.

Sha, W., K.-P. Wong, C.L. Yu, and S.C. Huang. 2010. A new automated method to derive total bladder activity accumulation curve in dynamic mouse FDG PET studies. *J. Nucl. Med.* 51(Suppl.).

Sha, W., H. Ye, K.S. Iwamoto, K.-P. Wong, M.Q. Wilks, D. Stout, W. McBride, and S.C. Huang. 2013. Factors affecting tumor FDG uptake in longitudinal mouse PET studies. *Eur. J. Nucl. Med. Mol. Imaging Res.* 3:51.

Shepp, L.A., and Y. Vardi. 1982. Maximum likelihood reconstruction for emission tomography. *IEEE Trans. Med. Imaging* 1:113–121.

Sokoloff, L., M. Reivich, C. Kennedy, M.H. Des Rosiers, C.S. Patlak, K.D. Pettigrew, O. Sakurada, and M. Shinohara. 1977. The [14C]deoxyglucose method for the measurement of local cerebral glucose utilization: Theory, procedure, and normal values in the conscious and anesthetized albino rat. *J. Neurochem.* 28(5):897–916.

Wardak, M., C. Schiepers, M. Dahlbom, T. Cloughesy, W. Chen, N. Satyamurthy, J. Czernin, M.E. Phelps, and S.C. Huang. 2011. Discriminant analysis of 18F-fluorothymidine kinetic parameters to predict survival in patients with recurrent high-grade glioma. *Clin. Cancer Res.* 17(20):6553–6562.

Wardak, M., K.-P. Wong, W. Shao, M. Dahlbom, V. Kepe, N. Satyamurthy, G.W. Small, J.R. Barrio, and S.C. Huang. 2010. Movement correction for improving quantitative analysis of dynamic brain 18F-FDDNP PET images. *J. Nucl. Med.* 51:210–218.

Weinberg, I.N., S.C. Huang, E.J. Hoffman, L. Araujo, C. Nienaber, M. Grover-McKay, M. Dahlbom, and H. Schelbert. 1988. Validation of PET-acquired input functions for cardiac studies. *J. Nucl. Med.* 29:241–247.

Wilks, M., H. Protas, M. Wardak, V. Kepe, G.W. Small, J.R. Barrio, and S.C. Huang. 2012. Automated VOI analysis in FDDNP PET using structural warping: Validation through classification of Alzheimer's disease patients. *Int. J. Alzheimers Dis.* 2012:512069.

Wong, K.-P., X. Zhang, and S.C. Huang. 2013. Improved derivation of input function in dynamic mouse [^{18}F] FDG PET using bladder radioactivity kinetics. *Mol. Imaging Biol.* 15:486–496.

Wu, H.M., S.C. Huang, N. Hattori, T.C. Glenn, P. Vespa, C.L. Yu, D.A. Hovda, M.E. Phelps, and M. Bergsneider. 2004. Selective metabolic reduction in gray matter acutely following human traumatic brain injury. *J. Neurotrauma* 21(2):149–161.

Wu, H.M., S.C. Huang, P. Vespa, D.A. Hovda, and M. Bergsneider. 2013. Redefining the pericontusional penumbra following traumatic brain injury—Evidence of deteriorating metabolic derangements based on positron emission tomography. *J. Neurotrauma* 30(5):352–360.

Ye, H., K.-P. Wong, M. Wardak, M. Dahlbom, V. Kepe, J.R. Barrio, L. Nelson, G.W. Small, and S.C. Huang. 2014. Automated movement correction for dynamic PET/CT images: Evaluation with phantom and patient data. *PLoS ONE* 9(8):e103745.

Zheng, X., G. Tian, S.C. Huang, and D. Feng. 2011. A hybrid clustering method for the ROI delineation in small animal dynamic PET images: Application to automatic estimation of FDG input function. *IEEE Trans. Inform. Technol. Biomed.* 15(2):195–205.

Zhou, Y., C.J. Endres, J.R. Brasic, S.C. Huang, and D.F. Wong. 2003. Linear regression with spatial constraint to generate parametric images of ligand-receptor dynamic PET studies with a simplified reference tissue model. *Neuroimage* 18:975–989.

Zhou, Y., S.C. Huang, T. Cloughesy, C.K. Hoh, K. Black, and M. Phelps. 1997. A modeling-based factor extraction method for determining spatial heterogeneity of Ga-68 EDTA kinetics in brain tumors. *IEEE Trans. Nucl. Sci.* 44(6):2522–2527.

Zhou, Y., W. Ye, J.R. Brašić, A.H. Crabb, J. Hilton, and D.F. Wong. 2009. A consistent and efficient graphical analysis method to improve the quantification of reversible tracer binding in radioligand receptor dynamic PET studies. *Neuroimage* 44:661–670.

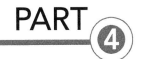
MULTIMODALITY IMAGING

13 PET/CT   339
     Søren Holm, Osama Mawlawi, and Thomas Beyer
14 SPECT/CT   369
     Yothin Rakvongthai, Jinsong Ouyang, and Georges El Fakhri
15 PET/MRI   379
     Ciprian Catana

13

PET/CT

SØREN HOLM, OSAMA MAWLAWI, AND THOMAS BEYER

13.1	PET/CT basics	340
	13.1.1 Anatometabolic imaging	340
	13.1.2 Dual-modality PET/CT	341
	13.1.3 PET/CT applications	343
13.2	PET/CT design and system parameters	345
	13.2.1 System architecture/models	345
	13.2.2 System characteristic performance	348
	13.2.3 Quality assurance	350
13.3	CT-based attenuation correction	352
	13.3.1 Basics	352
	13.3.2 Models for AC calculation from CT data	353
	13.3.3 Effect of the various CT parameters	356
	13.3.4 Artifacts and bias from CT-based AC	356
	13.3.4.1 Metal implants	356
	13.3.4.2 CT contrast agents	358
	13.3.4.3 Patient motion	358
13.4	Recent technical advances	359
	13.4.1 Extended FOV	360
	13.4.1.1 Axial FOV	360
	13.4.1.2 Transverse FOV, truncation, and wide gantry	360
	13.4.2 Continuous table motion	361
	13.4.3 TOF	362
	13.4.4 Iterative reconstruction and PSF	364
	13.4.5 Motion correction and gating	364
13.5	Summary	365
References		366

13.1 PET/CT BASICS

13.1.1 ANATOMETABOLIC IMAGING

Diagnostic tests are essential in cases of a suspected malignancy and subsequent treatment planning and follow-up. Typically, diagnostic tests entail a single imaging test or a series of complementary imaging examinations. Each imaging test, be it anatomical or functional, provides a wealth of information. Anatomical information, such as obtained from computed tomography (CT) or ultrasound (US), is represented by a set of submillimeter-resolution images that depict gross anatomy for organ and tissue delineation. Malignant disease is typically detected on these images by means of locally altered image contrast or abnormal deviations from standard human anatomy. Malignant diseases, however, are expressed as abnormal alterations of signaling or metabolic pathways that may not necessarily lead to detectable anatomical changes. Therefore, anatomical imaging alone may miss diseases frequently or diagnose diseases at an advanced stage only.

PET, as a representative of functional imaging, has been shown to support accurate diagnosis of malignant disease (Gambhir et al. 2001), as well as providing essential information for early diagnosis of neurodegenerative diseases (Herholz and Heiss 2004) and malfunctions of the cardiovascular system (Knuuti 2004). Nonetheless, more than 90% of all PET examinations are performed for oncology patients. PET is based on the use of trace amounts of radioactively labeled biomolecules that are injected into the patient whereby the distribution of the tracer is followed by detecting the annihilation photons resulting from the emission and annihilation of the positrons (Chapters 1 and 9).

In most cases of malignant diseases, early diagnosis is key, and therefore, imaging the anatomy of a patient may not suffice in making a correct and timely diagnosis. Thus, medical doctors typically employ a combination of imaging techniques during the course of diagnosis and subsequent treatment to monitor their patients. Henceforth, both functional and anatomical information is essential in state-of-the-art patient management.

The usefulness of combining anatomical and functional planar images was evident to physicians as early as the 1960s (Figure 13.1). Sophisticated image coregistration and fusion software was developed from the late 1980s onward (Pietrzyk 2005; Pietrzyk and Herzog 2013). For relatively rigid objects such as the brain, software can successfully align images from MR, CT, and PET. In general, software-based coregistration for brain applications assumes a rigid transformation with six parameters (three Cartesian coordinates and three

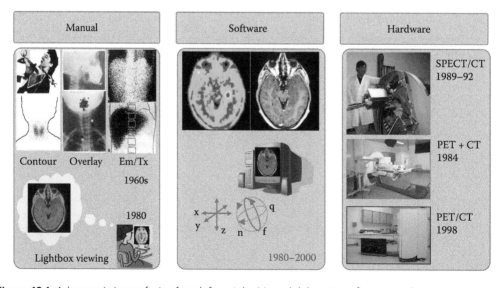

Figure 13.1 Advances in image fusion from left to right: Manual delineation of anatomical contours on scintigraphy images and basic image alignment using fiducial markers and lightbox display (Manual), computer-supported software-based image fusion (Software), and hardware-based image fusion (Hardware). Em, emission; Tx, transmission.

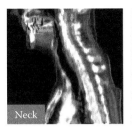
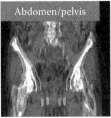
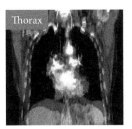
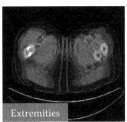

Figure 13.2 Simulated patient misalignment in PET/CT by means of repeat CT scans acquired within 1 h of the patient getting off the bed in between scans. (Data courtesy of University of Essen, Germany.)

angles) that are modified in order to align the two corresponding image volumes by means of mutual information principles, for example. Outside the brain, accurate spatial alignment of image volumes is difficult owing to the large number of possible degrees of freedom. Hence, the assumption of rigid transformations breaks down and more complex, nonlinear methods (e.g., warping) must be employed. For studies of the abdomen, movement of organs between two examinations, performed at different times and at different modalities, may even exclude a meaningful fusion of the two image volumes acquired separately (Figure 13.2).

Alternatives to software-based fusion have now become available through instrumentation that combines two complementary imaging modalities within a single system, an approach that has since been termed hardware fusion. An appreciation for this type of combined information is best illustrated with the introduction of the term *anatometabolic imaging* (Wahl et al. 1993), in reference to an ideal imaging modality that gathers both anatomical and functional information, preferably within the same examination.

13.1.2 DUAL-MODALITY PET/CT

A combined, or hybrid, tomograph such as PET/CT can acquire coregistered structural and functional information within a single study. The data are complementary, allowing CT to accurately localize functional abnormalities and PET to highlight areas of abnormal metabolism. As early as 1984, a research team at Gunma University in Japan had proposed a combination of a full-ring PET and a CT (Figure 13.3a). In their design, the two tomographs were placed next to each other with a patient handling system traversing between the two units. However, these developments were not widely known, and were not further developed toward a commercial product.

In an attempt to overcome the problems of missing anatomical reference and time-consuming quantification mentioned above, a proposal to combine PET with CT was made by Townsend and coworkers in the early 1990s (Townsend et al. 1998). In addition to the primary goal of intrinsic image alignment, the anticipated benefit of PET/CT hardware combination was to use the CT images to derive the PET attenuation correction (AC) factors (Kinahan et al. 1998). The first prototype PET/CT (Figure 13.4) became operational in 1998 (Beyer et al. 2000), designed and built by CTI PET Systems in Knoxville, Tennessee (now Siemens Molecular Imaging) and clinically evaluated at the University of Pittsburgh.

The design combined a single-slice helical CT (Somatom AR.SP; Siemens Medical Solutions, Forchheim, Germany) with a rotating ECAT ART PET system (CTI PET Systems). Torso imaging using the prototype PET/CT still took 1 h, or more, due to the partial PET ring of the ART (Townsend et al. 1999a,b). The results from the prototype, however, demonstrated the viability of the concept, and the importance of high-resolution anatomy accurately coregistered to functional data (Charron et al. 2000) (Figure 13.3b). It was shown to help localize functional abnormalities and clarify equivocal situations, thus improving the accuracy and confidence of the data interpretation. The use of rapidly acquired, low-noise CT data in place of a lengthy conventional PET transmission acquisition reduced the overall duration of the exam. The prototype PET/CT served as a key impulse to the subsequent development and commercialization of PET/CT instruments (Figure 13.5).

The advantages of integrated, anatometabolic imaging are manifold (Townsend 2008). A single imaging examination provides comprehensive information on the state of a disease. Consequently, functional information is gathered and displayed in an anatomical context. Patients are invited for only one exam, instead of multiple ones. The combination of complementary imaging modalities can yield synergy effects for the

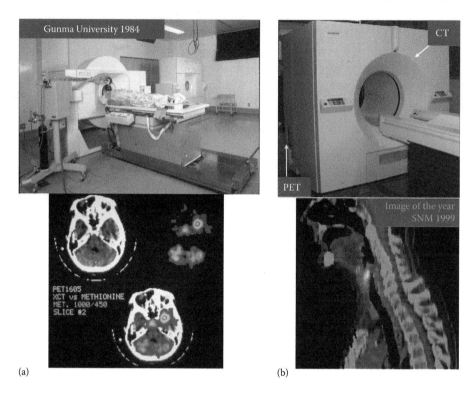

(a) (b)

Figure 13.3 (a) PET/CT prototype at Gunma University (Japan) first employed in 1984 (top) and a case study of patient with glioblastoma imaged with ¹¹C-methionine PET and CT (below). (b) Pittsburgh-based prototype PET/CT combining a single-slice CT and a rotating BGO-based PET tomograph within a single gantry (top) and an early case study of a patient with ear, nose, and throat cancer undergoing a FDG-PET/CT examination (bottom). (Panel a image courtesy of Professor Y. Sasaki.)

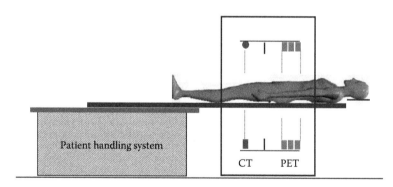

Figure 13.4 Conceptual drawing of the Pittsburgh prototype PET/CT (SMART) comprising a single-slice CT (Somatom AR CT system) and CTI Advanced Rotating Tomograph (ECAT ART) mounted onto the same rotating support system and housed within a single gantry.

acquisition and processing of image data (von Schulthess 2000; Czernin et al. 2007). And finally, experts in radiology and nuclear medicine are forced to discuss and integrate their knowledge in one report, which will perhaps be more appreciated and considered a benefit in the years to come.

The first commercial PET/CT to be announced was the *Discovery LS* (GE Healthcare, Milwaukee, WI, USA) in late 2000. This was followed a few months later by the *Biograph* (Siemens Medical Solutions), and then somewhat later by the *Gemini* (Philips Medical Systems, Cleveland, OH, USA). In the past years, PET/CT designs from all vendors have evolved following the advances in CT and PET instrumentation. All PET/CT systems offer multi-bed-position, whole-body imaging within a single examination and use the CT for

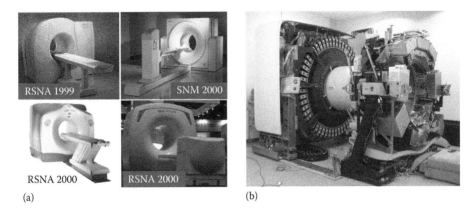

Figure 13.5 (a) Early design concepts of commercial PET/CT systems (1999 and later). (b) Example of a PET/CT (GE Discovery LS) opened for service inspection: The CT (GE Lightspeed) is shown in front with the x-ray tube below and the detector bow at the top of the ring; behind is the PET (GE Advance). The 3000 kg PET unit was moved on rails to allow access to PET detector modules and CT slip rings.

attenuation and scatter correction of the PET data, as a prerequisite to quantitative metabolic imaging. Today, four major vendors offer markedly revised PET/CT system series with increased performance over previous generations of PET/CT (see Section 13.2).

13.1.3 PET/CT APPLICATIONS

Over the past years, PET/CT imaging has rapidly emerged as an important imaging tool mainly in oncology (Fletcher et al. 2008) (Figure 13.6). The success of PET/CT imaging is based on several features. First, patients benefit from a comprehensive diagnostic anatomical and functional whole-body survey in a single session. Second, PET/CT provides more accurate diagnostic information than PET or CT alone. Third, PET/CT

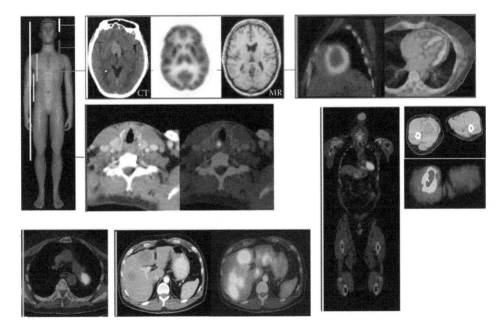

Figure 13.6 Range of applications of PET/CT imaging in clinical routine. The majority of examinations are performed on oncology patients, with only about 5%–10% of examinations being performed for indications in cardiology and neurology, the latter being preferred indications for MR (or PET/MR) imaging.

permits the routinely fast use of transmission images (CT) for the purpose of attenuation and scatter correction. Fourth, PET/CT imaging allows radiation oncologists to use the functional information provided by PET scans for radiation treatment planning. Several technological advances of the PET and CT components that are not available on PET-only systems also support the clinical success of PET/CT.

There is, mainly for oncology, a growing body of literature that supports the increased accuracy of staging and restaging with PET/CT compared with either CT or PET acquired separately (Czernin et al. 2007). These improvements are incremental when compared with PET, which alone demonstrates high levels of sensitivity and specificity for a wide range of disease states. However, improvement in the accuracy of PET/CT compared with PET or CT for staging and restaging is statistically significant and averages 10%–15% over all cancers (Czernin et al. 2007).

A typical PET/CT whole-body examination in oncology consists of (Figure 13.7)

1. A fast x-ray projection scan in one or two orthogonal planes, for overview and planning of the scan session. This is known as a scout scan (GE), topogram (Siemens), or surview (Philips).
2. A CT scan for AC, anatomic reference, or diagnostic use.
3. A multistep emission examination.

This sequence can be followed by a second CT scan for diagnostic use, including intravenous (IV) and oral contrast media, if this is not accepted as a part of the CT for AC. This is discussed in more detail in Section 13.3.

This standard protocol is applied, with minor variations, in a number of PET/CT examinations for oncology staging and follow-up (Krause et al. 2007). PET/CT, primarily with fluorodeoxyglucose (FDG), has been shown to yield improved diagnostic accuracy in the primary diagnosis, staging, and restaging for a variety of cancers, including head and neck, thyroid, lung, breast, esophageal, colorectal, lymphoma, sarcoma, gastrointestinal stroma tumor (GIST), carcinoma of unknown primary, and melanoma (Czernin et al. 2007; Facey et al. 2007; Hellwig et al. 2009; Ben-Haim and Ell 2009; Poeppel et al. 2009). An application for which PET/CT also has an impact is that of radiotherapy treatment planning.

Combined PET/CT gains importance for individualized treatment planning prior to radionuclide therapy that is increasingly used as a treatment modality for a range of cancers, for example, with radiolabeled peptides (Cremonesi et al. 2006). PET is the most accurate imaging method for the determination of activity concentrations *in vivo*. PET imaging can be considered for pretherapeutic treatment planning but ideally requires the use of a radioisotope from the same element as that used for treatment (e.g., I-124 for I-131 and Y-86 for Y-90). Furthermore, the combination of CT angiography together with a measurement of myocardial

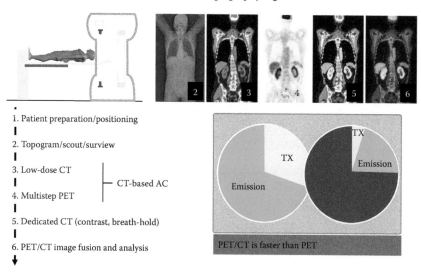

Figure 13.7 Sequence of whole-body PET/CT imaging: Patient positioning, topogram scan, helical CT acquisition, multistep emission acquisition, and series of contrast-enhanced CT scans. Tx, transmission.

perfusion using a PET tracer such as ^{82}Rb-chloride or ^{13}N-ammonia could, in a single exam, assess both the integrity of the cardiac arteries and the metabolic consequences to the myocardium (Menezes et al. 2009). These applications illustrate that after more than a decade of clinical evaluation, PET/CT continues to make a significant impact in patient management, mainly in the area of oncology diseases.

13.2 PET/CT DESIGN AND SYSTEM PARAMETERS

13.2.1 SYSTEM ARCHITECTURE/MODELS

Today (2016), four major vendors distribute numerous series of PET/CT systems (Figure 13.8). These vendors are General Electric (GE), Mediso, Philips Healthcare, and Siemens Healthcare. However, since Mediso is a much smaller vendor than the others, this section focuses on current commercially available systems from GE, Siemens, and Philips, with the exclusion of legacy systems that are still in the marketplace. The PET/CT systems from each of the three main vendors can be grouped into three tiers (entry, intermediate, and flagship models). GE systems are all grouped under the Discovery label and are the D-560 (entry), D-610 (intermediate), and D-710 (flagship). By mid-2014, GE had introduced a new PET/CT platform under the Discovery label, called the Discovery IQ. This system comes in different tiers depending on the number of full detector rings (two to five). More recently (summer of 2016) GE introduced their first digital PET/CT platform also under the Discovery label, called Discovery MI. This system also comes in different tiers (2-5 rings) although the 4 ring version is the one that GE is currently providing commercially. This system boast silicon PM tubes and a timing resolution of 385 ps. The Siemens systems are grouped under the Biograph label and are the Biograph TruePoint (entry), Biograph mCT 20 Excel (intermediate), and Biograph mCT, which also comes in a continuous bed motion option known as mCT flow (flagship). The Philips systems have a different naming system: Trueflight select (entry); Gemini TF (intermediate), which also comes in a big bore model; and Ingenuity TF (flagship). The differences in the Gemini and the Ingenuity systems are mainly in the CT component (ingenuity vs. Brilliance CT platform) of the tomograph. Philips has also just introduced the Vereos PET/CT system. This is the first commercial PET/CT system with digital detectors. Table 13.1 summarizes the main design and performance features of state-of-the-art PET/CT systems as of end 2016.

GEHC
Series: Discovery

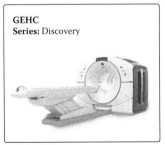

Philips
Series: Ingenuity

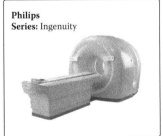

Siemens
Series: mCT

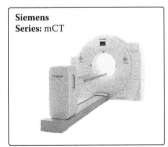

Mediso
Series: Anyscan

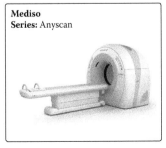

Figure 13.8 Images of various commercially available PET/CT systems from different vendors: (a) GE Healthcare (GEHC) D-710, (b) Philips Healthcare Ingenuity (c) Siemens Medical Solutions mCT, and (d) Mediso Anyscan.

Table 13.1 Design parameters of major commercial PET/CT systems

Model	GE Optima PET/CT 560	GE Discovery PET/CT 610	GE Discovery PET/CT 710	GE Discovery IQ	GE Discovery MI - 4 Rings
Gantry dimensions (H x W x D, cm)		193 x 225 x 146		193 x 225 x 162	193 x 224 x 156
Weight, kg (lb)	4,916 (10,834)	4,996 (11,014)	4,996 (11,014)	5262 (11597)	4661 (10254)
Gantry cooling		Air cooled			Water
Patient port		70 cm			
Patient scan range, cm		Standard: 170; option: 200			
Maximum patient weight, kg (lb)		227 (500)			
Number of detector blocks		256		144, 216, 288, or 360	544
Number of image planes		47		23, 35, 47, or 59	71
Plane spacing, mm		3.27			
Number of crystals	12,288	12,288	13,824	5,184 or 7,776 or 10,368 or 12,960	19,584
Ring diameter		88.6 cm		74 cm	
Number of PMTs		1,024 (256 quad-anode)		288, 432, 576, or 720	9792 (1632 Hex Anode) SiPM
Physical axial FOV, cm		15.7		10.3, 15.5, 20.8, or 26.0	20
Detector material	BGO	BGO	LBS	BGO	LBS
Crystal size, mm	4.7 x 6.3 x 30	4.7 x 6.3 x 30	4.2 x 6.3 x 25	6.3 x 6.3 x 30	3.95 x 5.3 x 25
Time of Flight (TOF) Capable	No	No	Yes	No	Yes
Timing resolution (ps)			550		385
System sensitivity - 3D, (NEMA 2001)	6.5 cps/kBq	10 cps/kBq	7.5 cps/kBq	3.5, 8, 14, or 22 cps/kBq	13.5 cps/kBq
Transverse resolution @ 1 cm, mm (NEMA 2001)	NEMA performance standards: 5; VUE Point HD: 4	NEMA performance standards: 5; VUE Point HD: 4	NEMA performance standards: 4.9; VUE Point HD: 4	VUE Point HD: 5.1	VUE Point HD: 4.0
Transverse resolution @ 10 cm, mm (NEMA 2001)	NEMA performance standards: 5.6; VUE Point HD: 4.5	NEMA performance standards: 5.6; VUE Point HD: 4.5	NEMA performance standards: 6.3; VUE Point HD: 4.5	VUE Point HD: 5.5	VUE Point HD: 4.5
Axial resolution @ 1 cm, mm (NEMA 2001)	NEMA performance standards: 5.6; VUE Point HD: 5			VUE Point HD: 4.9	VUE Point HD: 4.8
Axial resolution @ 10 cm, mm (NEMA 2001)	NEMA performance standards: 6.3; VUE Point HD: 5			VUE Point HD: 5.5	VUE Point HD: 4.7
Peak noise equivalent count rate, kcps (NEMA 2001)	54 kcps @ 15 kBq/ml	76 kcps @ 15 kBq/ml	130 kcps @ 29.5 kBq/ml	17, 36, 70, or 120 kcps @ 9 kBq/ml	180 kcps @ 20 kBq/ml
Scatter fraction - 3D (NEMA 2001)	38%	38%	37%	38%	41%
Number of CT slices	8 or 16	16, 64, 128	16, 64, 128	16	64, 128
CT Slice thickness, mm	8 slice: 1.25; 16 slice: 0.625	0.625	0.625	0.625	0.625
CT Rotation speed (sec)	0.5, 0.6, 0.7, 0.8, 0.9, 1	0.35 - 4	0.35 - 4	0.5-4	0.35-2

Philips Ingenuity TF (PET/CT)	Philips TruFlight Select (PET/CT)	Philips GEMINI TF Big Bore (PET/CT)	Vereos PET/CT	Siemens Biograph TruePoint 16 PET/CT	Siemens Biograph mCT 20 Excel	Siemens Biograph mCT	Mediso AnyScan SPECT-CT-PET
213 x 225 x 549		219 x 239 x 548	206 x 220 x 485	197 x 234 x 156	204 x 234 x 136		194.8 x 211.6 x 400
4,201 (9,262)	4,141 (9,130)	3,863 (8,500)	4,211 (9,284)	3,212 (7,079)	3,867 (8,505)	3,980 (8,755), w/ TrueV	3,850 (8,488)
Air cooled					water		NS
OpenView gantry (70 cm for PET/CT)			70 cm for PET & CT	70 cm	78 cm		70 cm
		190		185, w/ TrueV	186	198, w/ TrueV	360
195 (430)		227 (500)	195 (430)		227 (500)		229 (505)
28 pixelar modules			N/A	144 standard, 192, w/ TrueV (optional)	144	144 standard, 192, w/ TrueV (optional)	24
45 or 90	NS	45 or 90	N/A	81 standard, 109, w/ TrueV (optional)	81	81 standard, 109, w/ TrueV (optional)	NS
2 or 4	NS	2 or 4	1, 2, or 4		2		NS
28,336	NS	28,336	23,040	24,336 standard, 32,448, w/ TrueV (optional)	24,336	24,336 standard, 32,448, w/ TrueV (optional)	26,448 pixels (basic); 39,672 (extended)
90 cm	NS	90 cm	76 cm		842 mm		902 cm
420	NS	420	23,040 Digital photon counting detectors		4 per block		288 (basic); 432 (extended)
18	18	18	16.3	16.2 (standard); 21.6 w/ TrueV (optional)	16.2 (standard)	16.2 (standard); 21.6 w/ TrueV (optional)	15 (basic); 23 (extended)
LYSO					LSO		LYSO
	4 x 4 x 22				4 x 4 x 20		3.9 x 3.9 x 20
Yes	Yes	Yes	Yes		Yes	Yes	
						555	
7.4 cps/kBq @ 10 cm	4.55 cps/kBq @ 10 cm	6.7 cps/kBq @ 10 cm	21 cps/KBq @ 10 cm	7.6 @ 435 keV w/ TrueV	5.3 cps/kBq @ 435 keV	9.5 @ 435 keV w/ TrueV	5.8 cps/kBq (basic); 9.1 cps/kBq (extended)
4.7	4.7	4.7	4	4.2	4.4	4.4	4.1
5.2	5.2	5.1	4.5	4.8	4.9	4.9	4.9
4.7	4.7	4.7	4		4.5		4.2
5.2	5.2	5.2	4.5	5.7	5.9	5.9	5.1
120 kcps @ 19 kBq/ml	65 kcps @ 20 kBq/ml	90 kcps @ 14 kBq/ml	170 kcps @ 50 Kbq/cc	165 kcps @ 32 kBq/cc w True V	100 kcps @ 30 kBq/cc	175 kcps @ 28 kBq/cc w True V	77 kcps (basic); 150 kcps (extended)
30%	30%	26%	30%	< 36%	< 34%	< 34%	NS
64 or 128	16	16	64 or 128	16	20	40, 64, 128	16
0.5 – 12.5	0.6 – 12	0.65 – 12	0.5 –12.5	0.5 – 14.4	0.4 – 10	0.4 – 10	0.625 –10
0.4 – 2	0.4 (optional), 0.5, 0.75, 1, 1.5, 2	0.4, 0.5, 0.75, 1, 1.5, 2	0.4-2	0.33 – 1.5	0.33 – 1	0.3 – 1	0.4 (optional), 0.5, 0.7, 1, 1.5, 2

General to all PET/CT designs is that the two gantries are mounted with a common center axis (z-axis) and the patient is moved between the imaging positions for CT and PET on a common bed. It is very important for the principle of automatic coregistration and fusion of images that the position of the bed is controlled with great precision. The attenuation of the bed is important, and even with the use of carbon fiber constructions, only a limited amount of material can be allowed inside the gantry. A heavy patient makes the bed sag slightly, and if the unsupported length of the bed varies between CT and PET positions, this might induce a vertical shift in the images. This problem is minimized either by moving the whole support system continuously through the gantry (Siemens), by moving the bed support between two positions corresponding to the CT and PET center planes (GE), or by having additional support pillars between and behind the gantry (Philips and Mediso). PET/CT systems from Siemens, GE, and Mediso are designed such that the PET and CT components of the system are bolted together, resulting in a fixed distance between the CT and PET gantries. Philips systems, on the other hand, are unlocked, allowing varying distances between the PET and CT gantries, which facilitates access to the patient between the two systems. Their most recent PET/CT system (Vereos), however, is a fixed design similar to that of other manufacturers.

Currently, all commercially available PET/CT systems are three-dimensional (3D) mode only. They do not have septa, and hence allow the detection of annihilation events across the axial extent of the field of view (FOV), which improves the overall system sensitivity.

All current system configurations use circular designs with varying detector ring diameters. Detector material is either bismuth germanate (BGO) or lutetium oxyorthosilicate (LSO) (lutetium-yttrium oxyorthosilicate [LYSO]), and detectors are designed as blocks (GE, Siemens, and Mediso) of different sizes and number of elements per block, except for Philips, who uses pixelated detector modules. The number of detector blocks per ring is dependent on the detector ring diameter, while the total number of detector blocks depends also on the axial extent of the FOV (see Section 13.4.1.1).

All systems use photomultiplier tubes (PMTs) to transform the scintillation light to a corresponding electrical signal except for the Philips Vereos tomograph and GE Discovery MI, where the amplification is performed by digital silicon photomultiplier (SiPM). The CT component of a PET/CT also comes in different versions. Currently, 16-, 40-, 64-, and 128-slice CTs are available. Cooling of the x-ray tube is accomplished by either chilled water (Siemens) or cold air (GE). Quality assurance of these systems is performed by built-in Ge-68 rod sources (GE), prefilled Ge-68 phantoms (Siemens), or Na-22 point sources (Philips); see Section 13.2.3 on quality assurance of PET/CT scanners for further details.

PET/CT systems from all vendors have front and back (optional) control panels to move or release the patient couch, as well as perform basic operations, such as starting or stopping an examination. In addition, all systems have digital display panels that show various scan parameters, such as scan time, bed elevation and transverse position, detected count rate, and various physiological triggers, such as heart rate.

All systems include a console with the associated electronic or data processing cabinet to operate the PET/CT system. These consoles are used to perform various data processing tasks, such as image reconstructions and display, data transfer and archive, and system management and troubleshooting.

Whole-body PET imaging on all these systems is performed in a step-and-shoot fashion, except for the latest generation of Siemens PET/CT systems (Biograph mCT Flow), which use a continuous bed motion option with either a fixed or varying amount of bed overlap (see Section 13.4.2). In addition, all vendors allow changing the duration of different bed positions during a whole-body acquisition.

13.2.2 System Characteristic Performance

PET system performance characterization is done according to the National Electrical Manufacturers Association (NEMA) NU 2 standard. The NEMA NU 2 standard includes tests for PET spatial resolution, sensitivity, scatter fraction and count rate, image quality, and accuracy of corrections. The results of these tests should be compared with those that are provided by the manufacturer or are published in the public domain by other investigators. The most recent NU 2 standard is that of 2012; however, most manufacturers report their scanner performance characterization based on the 2007 standard. There is little difference

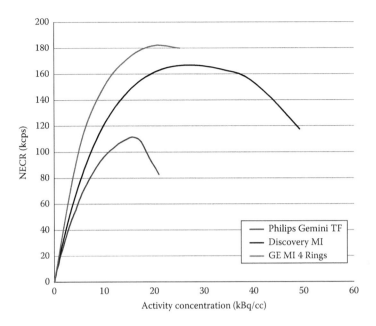

Figure 13.9 Noise equivalent count rate (NECR) performance of three different PET/CT systems. Overall, these curves are similar, demonstrating a rise to a peak NECR value and a decline caused by an excess randoms rate and system deadtime. Clinical operation is typically in the lower-activity concentration region covering the early rise of the NECR curves.

between the 2012 and 2007 standards except for source location when measuring the scanner resolution. The NU 2 performance characterizations of scanners from three vendors are shown in Figures 13.9 and 13.10 for the noise equivalent count (NEC) and image quality test, respectively. The following is a brief description of the NEMA NU 2 performance characterization tests:

- *Spatial resolution*: The spatial resolution of a system represents its ability to distinguish between two points after image reconstruction. The measurement is performed by imaging point sources in air, and then reconstructing the corresponding images with no smoothing or apodization. The location of the point sources should be at 1, 10, and 20 cm from the center of the FOV, along either the *x*- or *y*-axes. Spatial resolution is then determined by measuring the full width at half maximum (FWHM) amplitude and the full width at tenth maximum (FWTM) amplitude of a profile through the point source images. The measurement is repeated for both isocenter and three-eighths of the axial FOV.
- *System sensitivity*: The purpose of this test is to measure the coincidence count rate capability in the absence of confounding factors such as dead time, attenuation, randoms, and scatter. The test is performed by the repeated measurement of the coincidence count rate from a small amount of radioactivity placed in a series of concentric tubes of increasing attenuation. The sensitivity of the PET system with no attenuating material inside the FOV can then be determined by back extrapolation of the results of these measurements. The sensitivity measurement is performed at the central axis, as well as at 10 cm off-axis. PET systems with larger axial extents have a higher volume sensitivity, primarily due to their ability to detect more of the annihilation photons along the axial direction (see Section 13.4.1.1).
- *Scatter fraction and count rate*: The purpose of this test is to evaluate the scatter fraction and count rate (trues, randoms, and NECR) at varying amounts of activity concentration. The test is performed by repetitively imaging a large amount of radioactivity placed in a 70 cm long phantom (simulating a patient) positioned centrally in the FOV of the PET system as the radioactivity decays. Plots of scatter fraction, randoms rate, trues rate, prompt (total) rate, and NEC rate are then generated from the

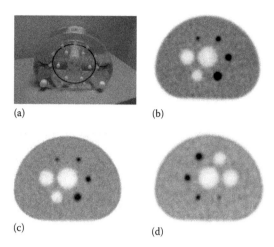

Figure 13.10 PET images of the standard image quality phantom (a) acquired on different PET/CT systems: Philips Gemini TF (b), GE Discovery 710 (c), and Siemens mCT (d). The phantom contains six spherical lesions of 11–37 mm with a lesion-to-background value of 6, immersed in a hot background with a cold cylindrical insert.

measured data (Figure 13.9). This test requires a long time (about 14–18 h) to perform since data are acquired throughout the decay of the radioactivity (usually ^{18}F) placed in the phantom.

- *Accuracy of corrections*: The purpose of this procedure is to measure the accuracy of corrections for dead time, count losses, and random event counts under widely varying amounts of radioactivity. Such information can be determined by first reconstructing the acquired data in the count rate performance test described above, with all corrections applied (except for decay). The error in the corrections is then calculated by measuring the ratio of the trues count rate in a region of interest drawn on the reconstructed phantom images to the actual trues count rate at different decay times. Plots of this error are then generated for different activities (as the activity decays).
- *Image quality*: The purpose of this measurement is to evaluate the quality of images produced from a phantom that simulates a total body imaging study with both hot and cold lesions. A thorax-shaped phantom with a lung insert (nonuniform attenuation) and spheres of different diameters is used for this purpose (Figure 13.10). In addition, a radioactive source placed in a scattering medium and positioned outside the FOV of the scanner is also used to represent scattered events in a total body imaging study. Image quality is determined by calculating the contrast and background variability ratios for both hot and cold spheres in the phantom. In addition, the accuracy of the attenuation and scatter corrections is determined from the uniform background and cold lung insert regions.

13.2.3 QUALITY ASSURANCE

The complexity of a combined PET/CT system needs to be balanced with rigorous quality control (QC) procedures. Likewise, the new information provided by combined PET/CT examinations must be complemented with a thorough understanding of potential pitfalls and artifacts arising from the combined imaging procedure. PET/CT, as any other imaging modality, is acceptable for routine clinical and research applications only if technical pitfalls can be avoided prospectively; if artifacts from incorrect or suboptimal acquisition procedures can be recognized and, if possible, corrected retrospectively; and if the resulting image information can be interpreted correctly, which entails an appreciation of variants of the represented image information.

The quality assurance for PET and CT in a combined PET/CT is not different from what is required for the stand-alone PET or CT systems (Busemann Sokole et al. 2010). PET or PET/CT systems should be tested on a daily basis to ensure that all detector modules and associated electronic signal processing boards are operational. This is usually performed by placing a source (point, line, or cylinder) of radioactivity in the FOV of the scanner and exposing the detectors to annihilation events for a preset count density or time interval. Detector performance is then evaluated by qualitative and quantitative assessment of the corresponding sinogram; detector block or module efficiency; singles, coincidence, and dead-time rates and variances; and timing and energy offsets. On some systems, such as the Biograph mCT, scanner calibration is also performed daily by using a prefilled Ge-68 cylindrical phantom, while on other PET/CT systems, such as all the GE scanners, this procedure is performed using a F-18 water-filled phantom and should be conducted as frequently as possible to ensure proper scanner calibration.

Additional quality assurance tests include weekly or quarterly PMT gain and position map updates, uniformity assessment, and normalization. On an annual basis, a scanner performance evaluation is recommended (ACR-AAPM) to assess resolution, sensitivity, count rate, image quality, image uniformity, and accuracy. There is, however, no current criteria on how these parameters should be tested. The American College of Radiology (ACR) Committee on Nuclear Medicine/PET Accreditation Program currently recommends that PET scanners be tested on a quarterly basis using the ACR PET phantom. Parameters to be tested according to the ACR committee on PET accreditation include qualitative assessment of image resolution, contrast, and uniformity, in addition to quantitative assessment of standardized uptake value (SUV) measurement accuracy in the different cylindrical inserts and background. The International Atomic Energy Agency (IAEA) publication on quality assurance for PET and PET/CT systems (IAEA 2009) also has recommendations on the frequency of QC tests for PET systems that are similar to those presented above. These recommendations can be found in table 8 of that publication.

Additional quality assurance tests of the PET/CT scanner include testing the CT component of the system. On a daily basis, these tests include CT number uniformity, linearity, and CT image artifact (ring) assessment. Additional tests are done on an as-needed basis, depending on service requirements. Finally, annual system performance testing is recommended for all CT systems. The recommended annual tests are described in the ACR–American Association of Physicists in Medicine (AAPM) technical standard on CT imaging and include many parameters covering different aspects of CT imaging, such as laser light alignment, bed travel, beam collimation, slice thickness, dosimetry, CT number accuracy, display, protocol reviews, and safety parameters.

The lack of QC testing of PET scanners can result in several image artifacts. Figure 13.11 shows artifacts due to a bad detector module on the reconstructed PET image.

The only added complexity in a hybrid PET/CT system over dedicated PET and CT systems is the necessary check of alignment between PET and CT images. Once installed, the PET and CT gantries in the GE and Siemens systems are moved apart for service only, and frequent controls in addition to these events are not supposed to be necessary. In contrast, the Philips Gemini can be run with PET and CT at different positions. The different vendors apply different strategies to measure and correct alignment. GE uses a body size (in cross section) styrene foam phantom with five embedded glass spheres to coregister between CT and a PET transmission scan with ^{68}Ge line sources. Siemens calculates the alignment correction from the acquisition

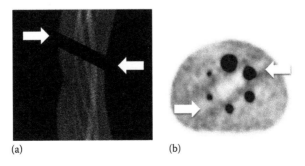

(a)   (b)

Figure 13.11 Effects of malfunctioning detector module on sinogram (a) and corresponding reconstructed PET image (b).

of two noncoplanar ^{68}Ge line sources (mounted in a plastic box) that are visible on both PET and CT, while Philips applies the images of six ^{22}Na point sources in a well-defined support structure. Once the transformation matrix between the PET and CT systems coordinate frames is calculated, it can be applied to align all subsequent image sets. The accuracy of these measurements is in the order of 1 mm. Deviations of a few millimeters in, for example, a brain study, are clearly visible on careful inspection.

13.3 CT-BASED ATTENUATION CORRECTION

It was long debated whether AC in whole-body emission imaging should be performed at all, due to the quite long acquisition times needed, or if quantification should be refrained from (Zasadny et al. 1996). Even without a need for quantification, however, the relations between observed activities in tissues at different depths and of different densities in the body are strongly influenced by attenuation and the inherent inconsistency of noncorrected projections (Figure 13.12). AC based on transmission sources (lines or points, annihilation or single photons) requires almost as much time as the emission acquisition itself in order to optimize the noise in the corrected images, and yet the noise contribution is significant. The advent of segmented attenuation maps and accelerated iterative reconstruction (ordered subset expectation maximization [OSEM]) in commercial software improved the situation, but still, measuring transmission counts in the presence of an injected tracer in general requires a correction for this, since the emission counts may constitute a significant and spatially varying fraction of the observed sum of counts. This correction in turn presumes that the tracer distribution is stable over, or at least predictable at, the time of the measurements.

13.3.1 BASICS

The information provided in a CT measurement is basically that of tissue attenuation. The reconstructed CT image contrast owes its anatomical information to the fact that different tissues have slightly different compositions and densities, and therefore different (linear) attenuation coefficients. The standard Hounsfield unit (HU) of the CT image is calculated from a linear scaling of the reconstructed attenuation coefficients,

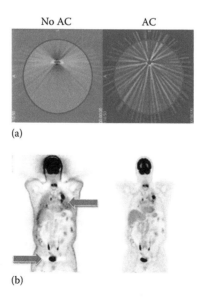

Figure 13.12 Effects of AC: (a) A line source in an attenuating medium, reconstructed with filtered back-projection. Due to the inconsistency in the observed projections, a point source may appear deformed and suppressed in activity. (b) In a patient image, the lack of AC is easily recognized from the skin flare, the "hot" lungs, and the bladder "halo" (arrows). Activity values in the center are severely suppressed, and foci may be distorted.

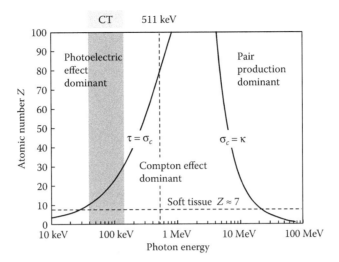

Figure 13.13 Curtain diagram. The two "curtain edges" are formed by curves representing the points in a (E, Z) diagram, where two of the interaction cross sections τ, σ, and κ are equal. The horizontal dashed line $(Z \approx 7)$ shows that for soft tissue, Compton scattering is dominating between 20 keV and 25 MeV, while the vertical dashed line illustrates that at the PET photon energy, Compton scattering is the more important interaction for $Z < 78$.

assigning the values –1000 to air and 0 to water (Kalender 2005). However, photon attenuation is strongly dependent on the photon energy.

The energy dependency of (mass) attenuation coefficients for all elements is different but well known (Hubbell 1999; NIST XAAMDI; NIST XCOM), and the mass attenuation of a compound material or mixture is determined by its elemental composition alone. Overall, the mass attenuation cross section at the energies relevant to CT and PET is dominated by the sum of Compton scattering σ_c and photo absorption τ, while pair production κ in general cannot occur (Figure 13.13). Compton scattering is almost independent of Z (for $Z > 1$) and has a low dependency on E, while photo absorption depends strongly on both Z (power of 3–4) and E (power of –3). At effective CT energies of 50–80 keV and for the soft tissue components (mainly consisting of hydrogen, $Z = 1$; carbon, $Z = 6$; nitrogen, $Z = 7$; and oxygen, $Z = 8$), only Compton scattering is of significance, while for bone (with phosphorus [10%], $Z = 15$, and calcium [23%], $Z = 20$), the photoabsorption is important too (Figure 13.14). In CT contrast materials (iodine, $Z = 53$, and barium, $Z = 56$) and in metallic implants or dental work (e.g., iron, $Z = 26$, and gold, $Z = 79$), photoabsorption is dominant for CT. At 511 keV, the scattering process dominates except at very high Z, leading to similar mass attenuation coefficients. The two contributions of absorption and scatter equal each other at Z 78.

13.3.2 MODELS FOR AC CALCULATION FROM CT DATA

Since each pixel of a CT image represents a mixture of elements, and the same composite value (in HU) in principle may result from different underlying mixtures of unknown elements and densities, the problem of translation to 511 keV does not have a strictly unique mathematical solution free of assumptions. This has led to a number of empirical approaches.

It is evident from the description above that a simple scaling with one common HU-to-μ-value factor cannot account for the difference in *materials* even among homogeneous pixels. A segmentation of the CT volume into bone and nonbone (soft tissue), assigning a single 511 keV μ value to each of the two domains, on the other hand, cannot reflect the fact that both types of tissues can still have very different *densities*; for example, in the lung volume the density is only ~0.3 g/cm³. A combined CT segmentation with a threshold based on Hounsfield units and subsequent pixel-wise scaling of the segmented parts' HU values with two separate factors (hybrid method) was shown to work reasonably well (Kinahan et al. 1998). This is equivalent to

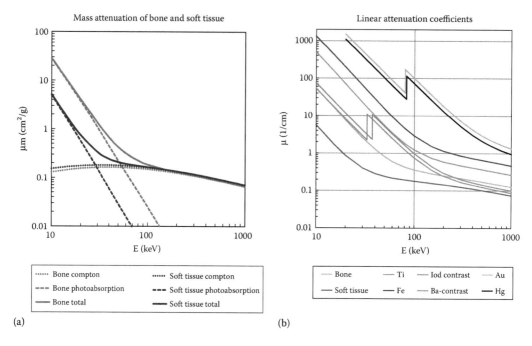

Figure 13.14 Attenuation coefficients for materials of interest in PET/CT. (a) Components of mass attenuation coefficients (in cm²/g) for compact bone and soft tissue (ICRU 1989). At low energy (photo absorption), the two tissues differ due to differences in Z; at higher energies (Compton scattering), they are almost identical. (b) Linear attenuation coefficients (cm⁻¹). Here, bone and soft tissue are seen to also differ at high energy, due to differences in density. In addition, two contrast media (iodine and barium), two typical metals for prostheses (titanium and iron), and elements for dental work (mercury and gold) are shown (see also Table 13.2).

an assumption that pixels within a certain range of HU (set by the segmentation threshold) have homogenous elemental composition, but differ in density (Figure 13.15a). The linear attenuation coefficient as a function of HU is a piecewise linear function with a discontinuity at the threshold. Note that this implies that the same PET μ value may occur in pixels with different HU values, belonging to either segment.

An alternative to the hybrid method that is essentially equivalent over a wide range of values is the simpler pixel-wise scaling via a bilinear function (Figure 13.15a). It differs from the hybrid method by being a continuous and unique function of HU, and therefore does not require image segmentation per se. The method assumes the presence only of air, water and soft tissue, and bone. The lower part of the curve (line) intercepts at zero attenuation and, therefore, still represents a simple scaling, corresponding to the density of a mixture of air and soft tissue. The upper curve (line) represents a mixture of soft tissue and bone. The separation point corresponds to pure soft tissue of density ~1 g/cm³, and the slope accounts for an increasing amount of compact bone (~1.9 g/cm³) in the mixture. Originally proposed only for use with the highest available CT energy, 140 kV$_p$, to minimize the scaling factors and the effects of their potential uncertainties, Carney et al. (2006) extended the bilinear method to a wider range of CT energies (from 80 to 140 kV$_p$) and demonstrated that almost identical values could be obtained for the 511 keV attenuation map independent of the kV$_p$ applied in the CT scan. An example is shown in Figure 13.15b.

Once the 511 keV attenuation map is known, it can be resampled along lines of response (LORs) to provide a correction sinogram matrix for direct multiplication of the emission data, or included as part of the system matrix in the loop of an attenuation weighted (AW) iterative reconstruction algorithm (AW-OSEM). Violation of the assumptions by the presence of other materials (contrast agents or metal) may result in image artifacts that are shown and discussed below. The different vendors have introduced various proprietary extensions of the conversion methods in order to reduce these effects. Table 13.2 shows linear attenuation values at a CT effective energy of 80 keV and at 511 keV, as well as their ratio, the "downscaling factor," for some tissues and materials of interest.

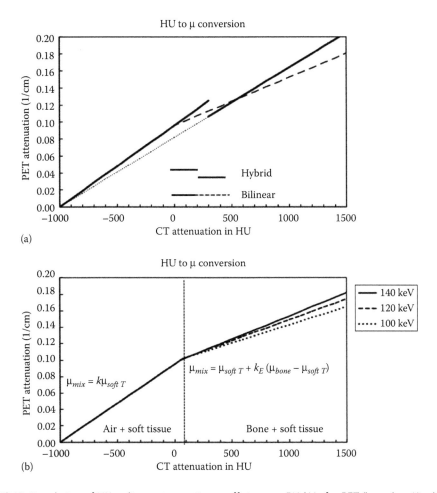

Figure 13.15 Translation of HU to linear attenuation coefficients at 511 kVp for PET (based on Kinahan et al. 1998). (a) Comparison of hybrid and bilinear method (see text). (b) Example of an implementation of the bilinear method for three CT energies (given as kV_p).

Table 13.2 Density, linear attenuation coefficients at 80 keV (average CT energy) and 511 keV (PET energy), and ratio between these (downscaling factor)

Material	Density (g/cm³)	μ (80 keV) cm⁻¹	μ (511 keV) cm⁻¹	Ratio CT/PET
Soft tissue	1.06	0.193	0.101	1.91
Compact bone	1.92	0.428	0.172	2.49
Ti (Z = 22)	4.5	1.83	0.366	5.00
Fe (Z = 26)	7.8	4.64	0.649	7.15
Iodine contrast	1.3	1.23	0.123	10.0
BaSO₄ contrast	1.5	1.61	0.142	11.3
Au (Z = 79)	19.3	107	2.86	37
Hg (Z = 80)	13.6	71.5	2.05	35

Note: Mass attenuation values are calculated using XCOM. The composition and density of soft tissue and bone are from ICRU 44 (ICRU 1989). Values for the four elements shown (Ti, Fe, Au, and Hg) are for pure elemental material. The μ values at 80 keV for Au and Hg are calculated as a mean of the values above and below the K-edge. The values for the contrast agents are for the material before administration and dilution in the patient: the iodine contrast is an aqueous solution of 300 mg/ml of I, while barium contrast is a suspension containing 600 mg/ml of BaSO₄.

13.3.3 Effect of the various CT parameters

The quality of the correction naturally depends on the quality of the CT scan and its parameters. Any dependency on exposure (milliampere-seconds or mAs) works through its effect on image noise only. A CT scan in diagnostic quality is essentially noiseless. In general, also "low-dose" CT provides sufficient signal for AC after resampling to PET pixel size, even if these images have comparatively little diagnostic value (Figure 13.16). Modulation of tube current to reduce patient dose is now standard in CT, and does not give any problems in the calculation.

As mentioned above, the first implementations of the bilinear methods assumed that the CT scan was run at a fixed 140 kV_p to minimize the size of correction to 511 keV. Today, however, any kV_p available in CT is also allowed by the PET reconstruction software, applying different scalings for each. Recent attempts toward the reduction of patient CT doses by automated or guided suggestions on the selection of kV_p have not influenced AC quality per se, because the kV_p is selected on a per-scan basis, and unlike the current, it is not modulated during scan. New reconstruction methods in CT applying iterative methods may reduce noise, or maintain the noise level at lower dose. As long as the result is unbiased in HU, this will not change the AC values for PET.

13.3.4 Artifacts and bias from CT-based AC

While the benefits of CT-based attenuation are now well known and documented, a number of challenges have emerged as the technique has become more widely adopted for PET/CT. There are two main reasons for possible artifacts that propagate into PET through the use of a CT-generated attenuation map for reconstruction: (1) the presence of materials in the patient containing elements with high atomic numbers that do not conform to the basic assumptions in the bilinear transformation model and (2) spatial misalignment between the CT and PET due to external movement, patient respiration, cardiac motion, and bowel movement (Beyer 2006, IAEA 2014). Since the first commercial PET/CT installation in 2001, these issues have received considerable attention. In most cases, associated artifacts can be limited or avoided by adopting disease-specific and optimized imaging protocols (Beyer et al. 2004). One important means to identify artifacts created in the AC process is to compare the final images with a set of noncorrected images.

13.3.4.1 METAL IMPLANTS

High-density implants, such as dental fillings, prostheses, chemotherapy infusion ports, or pacemakers, may impact PET image quality in two steps. First, they may seriously distort the CT images themselves by creating the

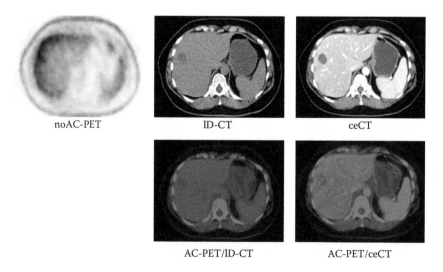

noAC-PET   lD-CT   ceCT

AC-PET/lD-CT   AC-PET/ceCT

Figure 13.16 Transaxial views of PET images without AC (noAC-PET), CT images acquired at low-dose settings (lD-CT) and with CT contrast (ceCT), and corresponding fused PET/CT images using lD-CT and ceCT for the purpose of CT-based AC.

characteristic streak artifacts associated with beam hardening and filtered backprojection. Second, CT artifacts, or just high local CT values, have been shown to propagate through CT-based AC into the corrected PET emission images, where artificially increased tracer uptake patterns may then be generated. Even if the CT artifact itself were corrected to represent the correct picture of CT values, a local high CT value exceeding that of compact bone may create a local PET artifact. The high end of the bilinear transformation from HU to PET attenuation values is valid only for a mixture of soft tissue and bone. In the presence of higher-Z-density implants, this bilinear algorithm may overestimate the attenuation of the implants, and thus lead to an overestimated tracer concentration in the vicinity of these implants. The underlying physics for this is that for high-Z materials, the photoelectric effect continues to have importance for much higher energies than for bone. Therefore, the ratio of the attenuation values at, for example, 80 and 511 keV is much higher for these materials than that for bone (Table 13.2); hence, the effective downscaling is underestimated—that is, the estimated attenuation coefficient will be too high. The local overcorrection of all LORs through a point can thereby create a hot spot in the PET image, even if there is no local activity present at all. However, whether this effect actually appears may depend on the implementation of CT corrections and the representation of the values in the CT image. If very high attenuation values in CT are clipped at, for example, 3000 HU, the calculated AC for PET may still be very much *below* the real value at 511 keV. In this case, the PET image at this point remains a "cold" spot.

Of the different types of metal artifacts, dental fillings (often gold, $Z = 79$, or amalgame containing mercury, $Z = 80$) are by far the most common in patients (Figure 13.17). In imaging of the head and neck region, increased FDG uptake frequently results in the vicinity of such fillings, even if the fillings themselves are negative (cold spots). These artifact uptake patterns are more pronounced when patients move between the CT and the PET since this necessarily increases the volume of mismatch between assumed and true attenuation.

Less frequent than patients with dental implants are patients with hip prostheses or orthopedic fixation (Figure 13.18). These implants are more often made from stainless steel or titanium alloys, with the major part of the material having Z in the range of 22–27 and densities of 4–8 g/cm^3. Their linear dimensions are much larger than those of dental work, and they most often remain photopenic on PET images. The patterns of image distortion are similar. As in the case of imaging in the head and neck region, the magnitude of the artifacts increases when the patient has moved between the CT and PET scan, and viewing the uncorrected emission images may help in the discrimination of artifactual and true tracer uptake patterns.

Some oncology patients who are referred for a PET/CT scan during therapy present with chemotherapy ports (Figure 13.18a). These ports are small and most often made of stainless steel or titanium alloys, leading to a focal overestimation of the attenuation properties, which in turn may introduce a focal hot spot of tracer activity. The presence of a cardiac pacemaker may also create a hot spot in the image (Figure 13.18b). Pacemakers are generally made from titanium alloys, but also contain a small battery that may have higher Z (e.g., Li-I$_2$ with $Z = 53$ for I).

Metal implants can easily be identified on the localizer scan prior to the PET/CT acquisition, thus allowing the operator to define, if possible, a coaxial imaging range that does not cover these implants. The reconstruction of the images should include both the corrected and uncorrected emission images.

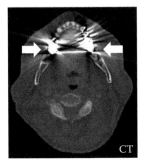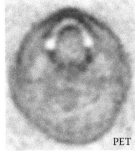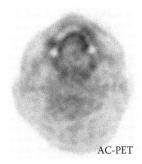

CT   PET   AC-PET

Figure 13.17 Metal artifacts from dental work. CT shows a severe "star artifact" around each of the two pieces of dental work (arrows). These artifacts do not directly propagate into the AC-PET image, but comparison of corrected and uncorrected PET indicates that the apparent uptake next to the teeth is biased.

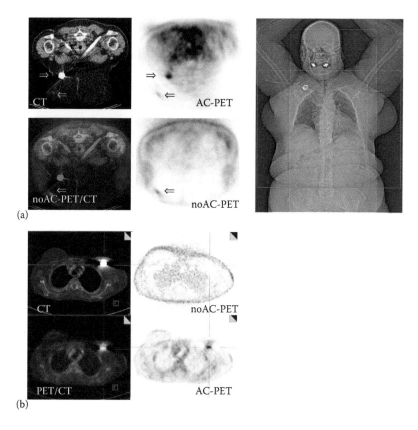

Figure 13.18 Dense implants: (a) Chemo port and (b) pacemaker, both resulting in a false hot spot on AC-PET that is clearly absent on the noncorrected PET.

13.3.4.2 CT CONTRAST AGENTS

Clinical CT and PET/CT scans are acquired with IV contrast or oral contrast to enhance the visualization of structures. Typically, contrast media are based on substances with high Z values, such as iodine ($Z = 53$) or barium ($Z = 56$), to increase the attenuation of the vessels, bowel, and intestines. At 511 keV, however, these two elements have approximately the same mass attenuation coefficients as soft tissue and do not add significantly to the total attenuation. In the case of IV contrast, soft tissue enhancement in CT of up to 2000 HU can be observed routinely. While the use of positive oral contrast leads to an average enhancement of no more than 1000 HU, it is potentially more problematic, as it collects in larger-volume structures (e.g., intestines) and in a wider range of concentrations. Like the metal artifacts, the CT-based AC algorithm may incorrectly scale the enhanced structures, thus resulting in a bias in the attenuation factors. Such biases could potentially generate artifacts in the corrected PET images. The use of CT contrast in PET/CT imaging was, and still is, a subject of debate (Antoch et al. 2004), primarily because of the potential image distortions associated with its use for AC. However, since most of these distortions relate to contrast administration protocols that were adopted without modification from standard radiology practice, careful revision and optimization of these protocols may help to reduce the likelihood and magnitude of associated image distortion while maintaining diagnostic quality (Brechtel et al. 2006).

13.3.4.3 PATIENT MOTION

Any change in body position between CT and PET will lead to some error in the reconstructed AC-PET. Larger movements could be, for example, a repositioning of the arms. The risk of movements in general increases with the duration of the time interval between CT and PET. In examinations of extended coaxial

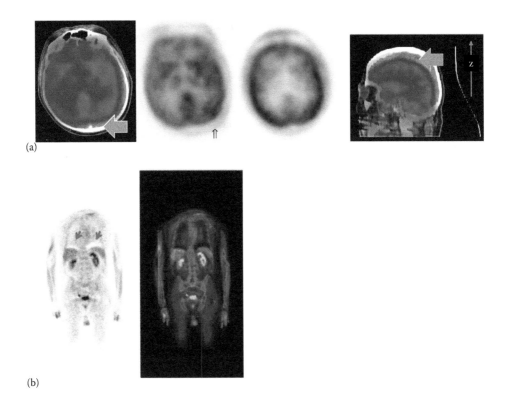

Figure 13.19 Patient motion: (a) Example of a head motion between CT and PET acquisition. The error is easily recognized on the fused images. Looking at the AC-PET alone, one might have the impression of an asymmetric tracer uptake (arrow), but the uncorrected image is symmetric, clearly indicating that the asymmetry is induced by the AC. (b) Banana artifact (photopenic area above the dome of the liver, red arrows) synonymous for a mismatch of PET and CT data from respiratory motion.

imaging ranges, the time difference between acquiring the CT and the emission data of the head can be significant (up to 30 min) since the CT is acquired head first, whereas the multibed emission scan is acquired feet first in order to limit artifacts in the pelvic region (bladder uptake). Given the rather lengthy delays in imaging the head and neck regions, involuntary patient motion in that area is not uncommon. This relates to relaxation of the neck muscles causing a misalignment of that anatomical region during the CT and PET scan (Figure 13.19a).

Cardiac motion has long been addressed by gating the acquisition with electrocardiogram (ECG). Respiratory motion constitutes a separate problem. PET data acquisition requires a longer scan time than its corresponding CT scans, which may even be taken during a single breath-hold. Such a temporal difference could result in a mismatch between the PET and CT images. This mismatch may result in a photopenic or photoenhanced area at the diaphragm location, colloquially known as the "banana" artifact (Figure 13.19b). Also, bowel motion, shifting the position of bowel contents, and gas may create local artifacts by the mechanism described above for contrast (Rosenbaum et al. 2006).

13.4 RECENT TECHNICAL ADVANCES

Major technical advances include the extension of the axial FOV of the PET (Jakoby et al. 2011; MacDonald et al. 2011), the incorporation of time-of-flight (TOF) PET acquisition mode (Karp et al. 2008), and the incorporation of system information, such as the variability of the point-spread function (PSF) across the FOV, into the reconstruction process (Panin et al. 2006; Jakoby et al. 2009).

13.4.1 EXTENDED FOV

13.4.1.1 AXIAL FOV

Extending the axial FOV of a PET system comes at the (financial) expense of more PET detectors added in the axial direction. However, for a given injected activity, more annihilation photons can be detected, thus increasing the system sensitivity by 80% for an additional 33% axial coverage. This gain in sensitivity can be used for reduced emission scan times or activities injected (Figure 13.20). Despite the required increase in axial bed position overlap, the number of contiguous bed positions required to cover a given coaxial imaging range is reduced in the case of PET imaging systems with an extended axial FOV because of the given increase in system sensitivity per bed position. Currently, axial FOVs of PET components in commercially available PET/CT systems range between 10.3 and 26 cm (Table 13.2), with the Discovery IQ (five-axial-ring option) having the longest axial FOV today.

13.4.1.2 TRANSVERSE FOV, TRUNCATION, AND WIDE GANTRY

Early PET/CT systems were designed with a typical transverse gantry opening of about 60 cm, thus supporting the same patient setup scenarios as in standard PET. The corresponding transverse FOV of the PET components in the first PET/CT systems was less than 60 cm, such as 55 cm for the Discovery LS. The measured transverse FOV of the CT, however, was even smaller, at 50 cm. The limitations in transverse FOV had two effects. First, some patients would feel uncomfortable during extended imaging times of 45 min, and frequently would not tolerate holding their arms above their head for the duration of the examination, thus giving rise to increased PET noise, beam hardening, and truncation artifacts. Truncation artifacts arise from part of the patient anatomy extending beyond the measured FOV of the CT, or PET. With the transverse CT FOV being markedly smaller than the PET, truncation artifacts would be observed in large patients or patients positioned with their arms resting along their body (Figure 13.20).

Recent PET/CT technology was modified in order to overcome the limitations of the small gantry diameter and discrepancies in the transverse FOV. First, the gantry diameter was increased to 70 cm, and larger, by reducing the side shielding of the front and rear end of the axial FOV, this accommodating a wider tunnel.

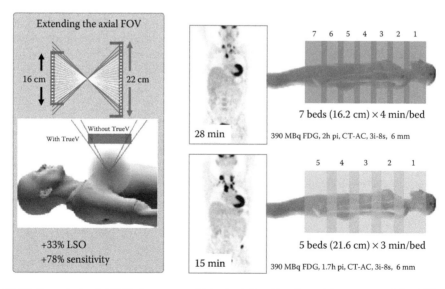

Figure 13.20 Extended axial FOV: System sensitivity is defined by the axial coverage of the PET detector system—the larger the axial FOV, the higher the system sensitivity. By increasing the axial coverage of the PET (through 33% more detector materials), the volume sensitivity can be increased by 78%. This increased sensitivity may be used for shortening the emission scan time per bed position while maintaining SNR. (Courtesy of Siemens and David Townsend, Singapore.)

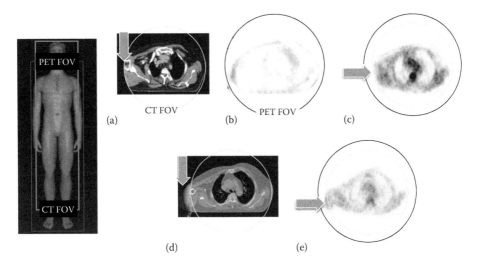

Figure 13.21 For large patients, and for most patients scanned with arms down, part of the body will fall outside the CT FOV (a), while the PET FOV often covers most of the patient opening (b). When AC-PET is performed from the truncated data, severe artifacts will occur in the regions of missing CT data (c), and quantitation inside the FOV will be affected too. Using extended CT reconstruction (d) improves the situation considerably (e) (arrows).

Reducing the side shielding comes at the expense of an increased fraction of random and scattered events from activities outside the FOV without clinically significant deterioration of the image quality. Second, modern PET/CT provides an "extended CT reconstruction" mode whereby the measured 50 cm FOV is extended to 70 cm by estimating the missing anatomy from applying consistency conditions to the measured and truncated projections during the CT acquisition. The anatomy of the patient that extends beyond the measured FOV can be estimated for the purpose of calculating the AC factors. Selected PET/CT systems have been proposed with gantry diameters of up to 85 cm (reduced side shielding) to accommodate patients in treatment planning position for radiation treatment (Figure 13.21).

13.4.2 CONTINUOUS TABLE MOTION

Fast CT scanning of the whole body is performed with helical CT, where the x-ray tube is rotating while the patient bed is moved in a continuous linear motion through the gantry. Traditionally, in PET, whole-body imaging has been performed as a step-and-shoot operation. Dahlbom et al. (1992) suggested replacing the discrete PET acquisition by a continuous axial sampling similar to the CT scan, originally as a one-slice step movement, though.

As a result, better image uniformity and sensitivity were achieved, together with a reduction in noise compared with standard multibed acquisition modes. Further refinements of the continuous acquisition mode for PET were suggested by the same authors (Dahlbom et al. 2001). However, the improvements in clinical image quality were less obvious than in simulation studies. Nonetheless, continuous bed motion based on modern hardware and highly accurate bed positioning and position tracing might yield an improvement in whole-body PET image quality. Finally, continuous bed motion supports the free definition of coaxial imaging ranges that otherwise would be limited by an integer number of PET bed positions, and thus lead to an overexposure of the patients (by CT) in the coaxial imaging range (Figure 13.22). To avoid the problem of the reduced edge sensitivity, it will, however, still be necessary to cover a certain additional distance, including CT for AC.

The mCT flow motion from Siemens is the first commercial PET/CT system with continuous bed motion. This system allows continuous bed travel over a wide range of speeds from 0.1 to 10 mm/s during the data acquisition period. The system also allows the flexibility of defining multiple zones (up to four) that have different speeds, which is similar to prescribing different durations per bed position in the conventional

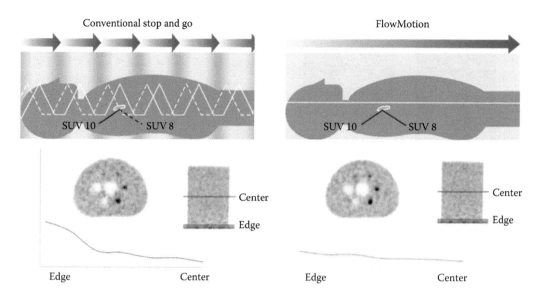

Figure 13.22 Conventional PET (and PET/CT) is performed in step-and-shoot emission mode with slightly overlapping bed positions to account for the axial sensitivity profile of the PET (left). This bed overlap can be noticed through reduced SNR in the overlap region. By acquiring emission data through continuous bed motion, noise in the overlap regions can be reduced and volume sensitivity can be made constant across the coaxial imaging range (right). (Adapted from Siemens, Forchheim, Germany.)

step-and-shoot approach. For example, one can prescribe a speed of 2 mm/s over the head and neck region, 1 mm/s over the chest region, and 1.5 mm/s over the abdominal and legs region. One additional potential advantage of continuous bed motion is an improvement in patient comfort during the imaging session. This is primarily due to the patient perception that continuous bed motion results in faster imaging than the step-and-shoot approach. Improved patient comfort can result in better image quality due to a reduction in patient motion during scan time.

13.4.3 TOF

One of the recent developments of PET imaging is the introduction of TOF data acquisition. TOF PET was first suggested in the late 1960s as a novel data acquisition approach to improve the signal-to-noise ratio (SNR) in PET (Tomitani 1981; Budinger 1983). However, TOF PET was discontinued in commercial PET equipment since the mid-1980s primarily because these scanners were based on BGO crystals, which are characterized by a very slow scintillation light output. The emergence of faster-response-time LSO and LYSO detectors in the mid-1990s revitalized the interest in TOF PET imaging, leading to the introduction of the Gemini TF in 2006 (Surti et al. 2007) by Philips—the first successful commercial TOF PET system.

With TOF imaging, information about the arrival time of an annihilation gamma ray at the corresponding detector pair is recorded. This information can be used to help better identify the location of the origin of an annihilation event within the PET FOV, which ultimately results in a superior reconstructed image SNR (Budinger 1983). For example, Figure 13.23a shows that with conventional (non-TOF) PET imaging, no information is available about the origin of the annihilation event. Consequently, during image reconstruction, the origin of the event is given an equal probability to all voxels along the LOR between the two detectors that detected the annihilation photons. With TOF imaging, on the other hand, information about the arrival time of annihilation photons helps in restricting this probability to a smaller number of voxels along the LOR and results in better SNR images.

The extent of restriction is determined by the accuracy of the arrival time measurements, which is currently on the order of 385–625ps, depending on the manufacturer and the system model, and translates to a positional accuracy (FWHM) of about 5.8–9.4 cm along the LOR. Improving the timing resolution

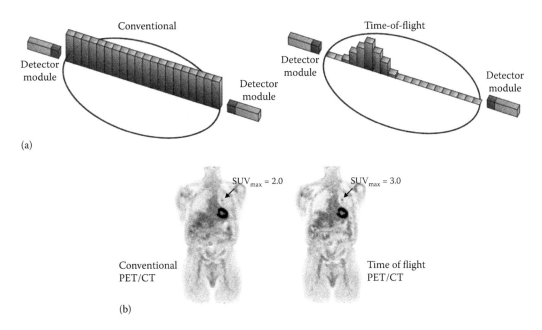

(a)

(b)

Figure 13.23 Principle of conventional (a, left) and TOF (a, right) PET imaging. Bottom panel showing a patient with conventional (b, left), and with TOF (b, right) imaging displaying an improvement in lesion conspicuity and increased SUV measurement. (Adapted from Erasmus, J.J., et al., *Semin. Respir. Crit. Care Med.*, 35, 145-56, 2014.)

measurement further tightens this restriction but requires very fast detectors and associated electronics. Ultimately, if the arrival time of the annihilation photons can be exactly determined, image reconstruction will no longer be needed since we can accurately determine the location of each annihilation event. Currently, TOF PET imaging is performed using LSO or LYSO detectors, which are characterized by very fast response compared with BGO detectors. The improvement in SNR in TOF compared with non-TOF imaging has been shown to be dependent on the positional accuracy of the annihilation event, as well as the size of the object being imaged according to (Budinger 1983)

$$SNR_{TOF} \cong \sqrt{\frac{D}{\Delta x}} \cdot SNR_{conv}$$

where D is the object diameter and Δx is the positional accuracy. For current TOF systems, this theoretically translates to an SNR improvement on the order of 1.6–1.9 times for a 25 cm diameter object, such as a patient head, or 2.3–2.6 times for a 50 cm diameter object, such as a patient torso. In reality, however, improvements ranging between 15% and 30% have only been reported in clinical studies (Schaefferkoetter et al. 2013). This is primarily due to confounding factors encountered during image generation, such as image reconstruction and image smoothing. One important aspect of TOF imaging is that both TOF and non-TOF images can be generated from the same acquired data set as long as TOF information is included during the acquisition stage.

Improvements in SNR with TOF imaging have been shown to lead to increased lesion detectability, particularly in large patients whose image quality is usually degraded due to increased photon attenuation. Furthermore, it has been suggested that improvements in lesion detectability with TOF imaging can potentially be traded off for a decrease in scan duration. In this case, TOF images would have similar lesion detectability as non-TOF images, except for a shorter scan duration, which could potentially have the advantage of reduced patient anxiety, decreased patient voluntary motion during data acquisition, and increased scanner throughput. Figure 13.23b shows PET images of a patient with (right) and without (left) TOF processing, showing the improvement in lesion conspicuity with TOF imaging.

The increase in SNR with TOF imaging should be taken into consideration when evaluating PET images quantitatively, particularly in longitudinal studies. Changes in SUV due to TOF imaging could mask or enhance the activity concentration in areas of interest, leading to biased patient management. For such studies, standardized processing either with or without TOF should be used for all time points.

Currently, most new PET/CT systems from different manufacturers have a TOF option. However, as of this writing, the majority of studies evaluating the performance of TOF to non-TOF PET imaging have been based on phantoms or small patient studies. Only one relatively large clinical study by Schaefferkoetter et al. (2013) has evaluated the advantages of TOF over non-TOF PET imaging on lesion detectability. However, subsequent effects on oncology patient management in general, or thoracic patients in particular, are still under investigation.

The incorporation of TOF information during image reconstruction results in increased reconstruction time primarily due to the added complexity of the reconstruction algorithm. In this regard, faster reconstruction engines are necessary for TOF tomographs, particularly if such images are to be generated at the end of a patient imaging session. This drawback, however, is balanced by the faster convergence of TOF versus non-TOF reconstruction (Lois et al. 2010). Nevertheless, some sites generate non-TOF-reconstructed images prior to releasing the patient and later produce the TOF images for physicians' interpretation as a method to overcome the potential delay in TOF reconstruction.

13.4.4 ITERATIVE RECONSTRUCTION AND PSF

The spatial resolution of the PET image is variable across the FOV. While the tangential resolution remains rather constant, the radial and axial resolution both deteriorate with the distance from the axis. A full description of the resolution, beyond the concept of the frequently quoted value of FWHM, is contained in the PSF that is derived from a full 3D image set of a point source. An algorithm for reconstruction in SPECT using information on collimator geometry was suggested as early as 1989 (Formiconi et al. 1989). By measuring the PSF in a large number of points between center and edge and incorporating this information into the system matrix for the iteration loop of, for example, the standard AW-OSEM algorithm, the image resolution is improved and becomes much more uniform (Panin et al. 2006; Alessio et al. 2010; Jakoby et al. 2011). Such algorithms have been developed and described by all major vendors: TrueX (Siemens), SharpIR (GE), and Astonish TF (Philips). The reduced partial volume effect that is a consequence of the reduced FWHM leads to considerably increased values of activity concentration or SUV of small lesions and may increase the detection rate of metastases in oncology patients (Andersen et al. 2013) (Figure 13.24).

In the study by Akamatsu et al. (2012), it was shown that the combination of OSEM with both TOF and PSF showed better image quality (by several measures) than OSEM alone, or OSEM with either TOF or PET.

13.4.5 MOTION CORRECTION AND GATING

Motion suppression is another novel tool in PET/CT imaging. It is well known that PET requires relatively long imaging times ranging to about 30 min to cover the length from the eyes to thighs (with an average time per bed position of 3 min). In this regard, lesions that are affected by involuntary motion, such as breathing or cardiac motion, will be blurred and consequently will have an underestimated SUV measurement. Motion suppression reduces this blurring and increases the SUV measurement 30%–60%, depending on the extent of motion and lesion size (Boellaard et al. 2009). Several approaches have been proposed and implemented on commercial PET/CT scanners to suppress motion blur (Nehmeh et al. 2004, 2007; Nehmeh and Erdi, 2008; Chang et al. 2010; Liu et al. 2010). These techniques include four-dimensional (4D) PET/CT data acquisition, which could also be followed by deformable image registration to improve the resultant image statistics. With 4D PET/CT, the PET data are acquired into multiple bins using gated acquisition mode, depending on different phases or amplitudes of the breathing cycle. A corresponding CT is also acquired for each phase or amplitude and is used for AC. The result is a series of PET/CT images at different parts of the breathing cycle, which can then be registered to one another to improve the resultant image statistics. Other motion suppression techniques acquire PET data only during the quiescent state of the breathing cycle (usually end

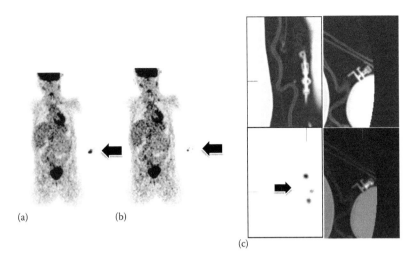

Figure 13.24 PET image reconstruction with resolution recovery: (a) Coronal PET with standard OSEM reconstruction demonstrating hot spot in left arm of this patient. (b) Coronal PET following OSEM reconstruction with PSF recovery demonstrating resolution of the blurred focal activity into individual foci corresponding to residual activity foci in the catheter system used for tracer injection (c).

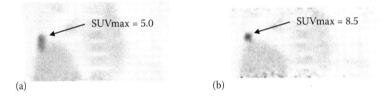

Figure 13.25 PET image of a patient with a lung lesion before (a) and after (b) motion suppression. (Adapted from Erasmus, J.J., et al., *Semin. Respir. Crit. Care Med.*, 35, 145–56, 2014.)

expiration). In this case, a corresponding CT attenuation map should also be acquired during this part of the breathing cycle for proper AC. In either case, a motion tracking device is necessary to record the motion and synchronize the PET and CT data acquisitions. Figure 13.25 shows a PET image of a patient with a lung lesion before (left) and after (right) motion suppression using 4D PET/CT. The figure clearly shows that with motion, the lesion is blurred and has a low SUV, while with motion suppression (4D PET/CT), the lesion is more conspicuous and has a higher SUV measurement.

13.5 SUMMARY

PET has evolved from a proof of concept in the 1970s to a clinical concept in the late 1990s. Since then, this technology has been driven primarily by physics and methodological advances, elevating PET from a single-slice imaging modality to a quantitative, volumetric molecular imaging concept that is applied in clinical routine and research alike. The addition of helical, multislice CT has further excelled the adoption of PET, namely, in oncology applications. PET/CT was once coined a technical evolution that led to a medical revolution. Clearly, the introduction of 3D, septa-less system designs, combined with TOF acquisition schemes employing faster scintillator-based detectors with improved detector electronics, has fostered the establishment of PET/CT as a state-of-the-art imaging modality in the management of patients with malignant diseases (Boellaard et al. 2010). This progress on the hardware side was matched with progress made in data handling and image reconstruction. While most of these advances were technical in nature, they do benefit patients and medical professionals alike. However, it is now time to utilize the potential of PET/CT imaging methodology in all facets of its clinical adoption.

REFERENCES

ACR-AAPM [American College of Radiology–American Association of Physicists in Medicine]. ACR-AAPM technical standard for medical physics performance monitoring of PET/CT imaging equipment. http://www.acr.org/~/media/ACR/Documents/PGTS/standards/MonitorPETCTEquipment.pdf (accessed October 16, 2014).

Akamatsu G., Ishikawa K., Mitsumoto K., et al. 2012. Improvement in PET/CT image quality with a combination of point-spread function and time-of-flight in relation to reconstruction parameters. *J Nucl Med* 53:1716–22.

Alessio A., Stearns C., Tong S., et al. 2010. Application and evaluation of a measured spatially variant system model for PET image reconstruction. *IEEE Trans Med Imaging* 29:938–49.

Andersen F.L., Klausen T.L., Loft A., Beyer T., Holm S. 2013. Clinical evaluation of PET image reconstruction using a spatial resolution model. *Eur J Radiol* 82:862–69.

Antoch G., Freudenberg L.S., Beyer T., Bockisch A., Debatin J.F. 2004. To enhance or not to enhance? 18F-FDG and CT contrast agents in dual-modality 18F-FDG PET/CT. *J Nucl Med* 45(Suppl. 1):56S–65S.

Ben-Haim S., Ell P. 2009. 18F-FDG PET and PET/CT in the evaluation of cancer treatment response. *J Nucl Med* 50:88–99.

Beyer T. 2006. Technical artifacts in PET/CT imaging. In *Clinical PET-CT*, ed. P. Shreve, D.W. Townsend, chap. 5. New York: Springer.

Beyer T., Antoch G., Müller S., et al. 2004. Acquisition protocol considerations for combined PET/CT imaging. *J Nucl Med* 45(Suppl. 1):25S–35S.

Beyer T., Townsend D.W., Brun T., et al. 2000. A combined PET/CT scanner for clinical oncology. *J Nucl Med* 41:1369–79.

Boellaard R.J. 2009. Standards for PET image acquisition and quantitative data analysis. *Nucl Med* 50(Suppl. 1):11S–20S.

Boellaard R., O'Doherty M.J., Weber W.A., et al. 2010. FDG PET and PET/CT: EANM procedure guidelines for tumour PET imaging: Version 1.0. *Eur J Nucl Med Mol Imaging* 37:181–200.

Brechtel K., Klein M., Vogel M., et al. 2006. Optimized contrast-enhanced CT protocols for diagnostic whole-body 18F-FDG PET/CT: Technical aspects of single-phase versus multiphase CT imaging. *J Nucl Med* 47:470–76.

Budinger T.F. 1983. Time-of-flight positron emission tomography: Status relative to conventional PET. *J Nucl Med* 24:73–76.

Busemann Sokole E., Płachcínska A., Britten A; EANM Physics Committee. 2010. Acceptance testing for nuclear medicine instrumentation. *Eur J Nucl Med Mol Imaging* 37:672–81.

Carney J.P., Townsend D.W., Rappoport V., Bendriem B. 2006. Method for transforming CT images for attenuation correction in PET/CT imaging. *Med Phys* 33:976–83.

Chang G., Chang T., Pan T., Clark J.W. Jr., Mawlawi O.R. 2010. Implementation of an automated respiratory amplitude gating technique for PET/CT: Clinical evaluation. *J Nucl Med* 51:16–24.

Charron M., Beyer T., Bohnen N.N., et al. 2000. Image analysis in patients with cancer studied with a combined PET and CT scanner. *Clin Nucl Med* 25:905–10.

Cremonesi M., Ferrari M., Bodei L., Tosi G., Paganelli G. 2006. Dosimetry in peptide radionuclide receptor therapy: A review. *J Nucl Med* 47:1467–75.

Czernin J., Allen-Auerbach M., Schelbert H.R. 2007. Improvements in cancer staging with PET/CT: Literature-based evidence as of September 2006. *J Nucl Med* 48(Suppl. 1):78S–88S.

Dahlbom M., Hoffman E.J., Hoh C.K., et al. 1992. Whole-body positron emission tomography. Part I. Methods and performance characteristics. *J Nucl Med* 33:1191–99.

Dahlbom M., Reed J., Young J. 2001. Implementation of true continuous bed motion in 2-D and 3-D whole-body PET scanning. *IEEE Trans Nucl Sci* 44:1465–69.

Erasmus J.J., Mawlawi O., Howard B., Patz E.F. Jr. 2014. PET/CT: Current applications and new applications in thorax. *Semin Respir Crit Care Med* 35:145–56.

Facey K., Bradbury I., Laking G., Payne E. 2007. Overview of the clinical effectiveness of positron emission tomography imaging in selected cancers. *Health Technol Assess* 11:iii–iv, xi–267.

Fletcher J.W., Djulbegovic B., Soares H.P., et al. 2008. Recommendations on the use of 18F-FDG PET in oncology. *J Nucl Med* 49:480–508.

Formiconi A.R., Pupi A., Passeri A. 1989. Compensation of spatial system response in SPECT with conjugate gradient reconstruction technique. *Phys Med Biol* 34:69–84.

Gambhir S.S., Czernin J., Schwimmer J., Silverman D.H., Coleman R.E., Phelps M.E. 2001. A tabulated summary of the FDG PET literature. *J Nucl Med* 42(5 Suppl.):1S–93S.

Hellwig D., Baum R., Kirsch C. 2009. FDG-PET, PET/CT and conventional nuclear medicine procedures in the evaluation of lung cancer: A systematic review. *Nuklearmedizin* 48:59–69.

Herholz K., Heiss W.D. 2004. Positron emission tomography in clinical neurology. *Mol Imaging Biol* 6:239–69.

Hubbell J.H. 1999. Review of photon interaction cross section data in the medical and biological context. *Phys Med Biol* 44:R1–22.

IAEA [International Atomic Energy Agency]. 2009. *Quality Assurance for PET and PET/CT Systems.* IAEA Human Health Series No. 1. Vienna, IAEA. http://www-pub.iaea.org/MTCD/Publications/PDF/Pub1393_web.pdf (accessed October 16, 2014).

IAEA [International Atomic Energy Agency]. 2014. *PET/CT Atlas on Quality Control and Image Artefacts.* STI/PUB/1642. http://www-pub.iaea.org/MTCD/Publications/PDF/Pub1642web-16821314.pdf (accessed October 16, 2014).

ICRU [International Commission on Radiation Units and Measurements]. 1989. Tissue substitutes in radiation dosimetry and measurement. Report 44 of the International Commission on Radiation Units and Measurements. Bethesda, MD: ICRU.

Jakoby B.W., Bercier Y., Conti M., Casey M.E., Bendriem B., Townsend D.W. 2011. Physical and clinical performance of the mCT time-of-flight PET/CT scanner. *Phys Med Biol* 56:2375–89.

Jakoby B., Bercier Y., Watson C., Bendriem B., Townsend D. 2009. Performance characteristics of a new LSO PET/CT scanner with extended axial field-of-view and PSF reconstruction. *IEEE Trans Nucl Sci* 56: 633–39.

Kalender W. 2005. *Computed Tomography.* 2nd ed. Erlangen, Germany: Publicis Corporate Publishing.

Karp J.S., Surti S., Daube-Witherspoon M.E., Muehllehner G. 2008. Benefit of time-of-flight in PET: Experimental and clinical results. *J Nucl Med* 49:462–70.

Kinahan P.E., Townsend D.W., Beyer T., Sashin D. 1998. Attenuation correction for a combined 3D PET/CT scanner. *Med Phys* 25:2046–53.

Knuuti J. 2004. Clinical cardiac PET in the future. *Eur J Nucl Med Mol Imaging* 31:467–68.

Krause B.J., Beyer T., Bockisch A., et al. 2007. FDG-PET/CT in oncology. German guideline [in German]. *Nuklearmedizin* 46:291–301.

Liu C., Alessio A., Pierce L. 2010. Quiescent period respiratory gating for PET/CT. *Med Phys* 37:5037–43.

Lois C., Jakoby B.W., Long M.J., et al. 2010. An assessment of the impact of incorporating time-of-flight information into clinical PET/CT imaging. *J Nucl Med* 51:237–45.

MacDonald L.R., Harrison R.L., Alessio A.M., Hunter W.C., Lewellen T.K., Kinahan P.E. 2011. Effective count rates for PET scanners with reduced and extended axial field of view. *Phys Med Biol* 56:3629–43.

Menezes L.J., Groves A.M., Prvulovich E., et al. 2009. Assessment of left ventricular function at rest using rubidium-82 myocardial perfusion PET: Comparison of four software algorithms with simultaneous 64-slice coronary CT angiography. *Nucl Med Commun* 30:918–25.

Nehmeh S.A., Erdi Y.E. 2008. Respiratory motion in positron emission tomography/computed tomography: A review. *Semin Nucl Med* 38:167–76.

Nehmeh S.A., Erdi Y.E., Meirelles G.S.P., et al. 2007. Deep-inspiration breath-hold PET/CT of the thorax. *J Nucl Med* 48:22–26.

Nehmeh S.A., Erdi Y.E., Pan T. 2004. Four-dimensional (4D) PET/CT imaging of the thorax. *Med Phys* 31:3179–86.

NEMA [National Electrical Manufacturers Association]. Performance measurements of positron emission tomographs. NEMA Standards Publication NU 2. Arlington, VA: NEMA. http://www.nema.org/stds/nu2.cfm.

NIST [National Institute of Standards and Technology]. Tables of x-ray mass attenuation coefficients and mass energy—Absorption coefficients from 1 keV to 20 MeV for elements Z = 1 to 92 and 48 additional substances of dosimetric interest. X-Ray Attenuation and Absorption for Materials of Dosimetric Interest Database (XAAMDI). Gaithersburg, MD: NIST. http://www.nist.gov/pml/data/xraycoef/ (accessed October 16, 2014).

NIST [National Institute of Standards and Technology]. XCOM: Photon cross sections database. http://www.nist.gov/pml/data/xcom/index.cfm (accessed October 16, 2014).

Panin V., Kehren F., Michel C., Casey M. 2006. Fully 3-D PET reconstruction with system matrix derived from point source measurements. *IEEE Trans Med Imaging* 25:907–21.

Pietrzyk U. 2005. Does PET/CT render software registration obsolete? Nuklearmedizin 2005(Suppl. 1):S13–17.

Pietrzyk U., Herzog H. 2013. Does PET/MR in human brain imaging provide optimal co-registration? A critical reflection. *MAGMA* 26:137–47.

Poeppel T.D., Krause B.J., Heusner T.A., Boy C., Bockisch A., Antoch G. 2009. PET/CT for the staging and follow-up of patients with malignancies. *Eur J Radiol* 70:382–92.

Rosenbaum S.J., Stergar H., Antoch G., Veit P., Bockisch A., Kühl H. 2006. Staging and follow-up of gastrointestinal tumors with PET/CT. *Abdom Imaging* 31:25–35.

Schaefferkoetter J., Casey M., Townsend D., El Fakhri G. 2013. Clinical impact of time-of-flight and point response modeling in PET reconstructions: A lesion detection study. *Phys Med Biol* 58:1465–78.

Surti S., Kuhn A., Werner M.E., Perkins A.E., Kolthammer J., Karp J.S. 2007. Performance of Philips Gemini TF PET/CT scanner with special consideration for its time-of-flight imaging capabilities. *J Nucl Med* 48:471–80.

Tomitani T. 1981. Image-reconstruction and noise evaluation in photon time-of-flight assisted positron emission tomography. *IEEE Trans Nucl Sci* 28:4581–89.

Townsend., D.W. 2008. Multimodality imaging of structure and function. *Phys Med Biol* 53: R1–39.

Townsend D.W., Beyer T., Jerin J., Watson C.C., Young J., Nutt R. 1999a. The ECAT ART scanner for positron emission tomography. 1. Improvements in performance characteristics. *Clin Positron Imaging* 2:5–15.

Townsend D.W., Beyer T., Kinahan P.E., et al. 1998. The SMART scanner: A combined PET/CT tomograph for clinical oncology. *Radiology* 209P:169–70.

Townsend D.W., Beyer T., Meltzer C.C., et al. 1999b. The ECAT ART scanner for positron emission tomography. 2. Research and clinical applications. *Clin Positron Imaging* 2:17–30.

von Schulthess G.K. 2000. Cost considerations regarding an integrated CT-PET system. *Eur Radiol* 10(Suppl. 3):S377–80.

Wahl R.L., Quint L.E., Cieslak R.D., Aisen A.M., Koeppe R.A., Meyer C.R. 1993. "Anatometabolic" tumor imaging: Fusion of FDG PET with CT or MRI to localize foci of increased activity. *J Nucl Med* 34:1190–97.

Weber W., Grosu A., Czernin J. 2008. Technology insight: Advances in molecular imaging and an appraisal of PET/CT scanning. *Nat Clin Pract Oncol* 5:160–70.

Zasadny K.R., Kison P.V., Quint L.E., Wahl R.L. 1996. Untreated lung cancer: Quantification of systematic distortion of tumor size and shape on non-attenuation-corrected 2-[fluorine-18]fluoro-2-deoxy-D-glucose PET scans. *Radiology* 201:873–76.

SPECT/CT

YOTHIN RAKVONGTHAI, JINSONG OUYANG, AND GEORGES EL FAKHRI

14.1	Introduction	369
14.2	Instrumentation	370
	14.2.1 Instrument	370
	14.2.2 CT component	370
14.3	Data corrections and image reconstruction in SPECT/CT	371
	14.3.1 CT reconstruction	371
	14.3.2 Use of CT for corrections in SPECT image reconstruction	371
	14.3.2.1 Attenuation correction	371
	14.3.2.2 Scatter correction	373
	14.3.3 Quantitative SPECT	374
14.4	Clinical Applications	374
	14.4.1 SPECT/CT in cardiology	374
	14.4.2 SPECT/CT in oncology	375
	14.4.3 SPECT/CT in bone scans	375
14.5	Future developments and applications of SPECT/CT	375
	References	376

14.1 INTRODUCTION

SPECT–computed tomography (CT) is a medical imaging technique integrating both SPECT and CT into one unit that generates both functional (SPECT) and anatomical (CT) images in the same imaging session. Coregistered multimodality images allow anatomical referencing and accurate patient-specific attenuation correction, which increase both the sensitivity and the specificity in the diagnosis and improve patient management.

SPECT/CT has recently gained widespread acceptance in clinical practice, even though the idea of the integration of SPECT and CT was mentioned several years ago (Mirshanov 1987; Kaplan 1989; Hasegawa et al. 1989, 1990). At the outset, the integration of SPECT and CT was for attenuation correction in SPECT reconstruction, in which a radioisotope external beam, such as ^{153}Gd, was used initially to derive an attenuation map. However, there are limitations for this approach in terms of low radiation output and maintenance cost when the sources decayed and needed replacement. The acquisition of SPECT and CT data can be performed on separate machines in different locations or on the machines in a single unit. The former approach was not successful since it has some drawbacks, including difficulties in combining data acquired from different machines, or even on different dates due to poor scheduling. This leads to the misalignment between the SPECT and CT data, which is difficult to correct.

The early commercial SPECT/CT system had the CT component consisting of a prefixed low-dosed x-ray tube, which provided sufficient CT image quality for attenuation correction purposes. There has been substantial development in the CT component in later SPECT/CT systems, where it can offer comparable image quality to stand-alone diagnostic CT machines and can adjust imaging parameters. In terms of applications, CT information in SPECT/CT systems has been utilized for other purposes rather than merely for attenuation correction, as in the early days. The acquisition flexibility available in recent developments improves the cost-effectiveness (i.e., value for money) of the hybrid systems in that it serves as a backup diagnostic CT machine when a stand-alone x-ray CT scanner is not available. Moreover, the integration of diagnostic CT with SPECT makes a new imaging workflow possible since it can benefit patients, especially in enabling those who were previously required to have several scans to possibly have only one imaging scan in one hospital visit instead of multiple scans in multiple visits.

Compared with PET/CT, which is another hybrid imaging system that was discussed in Chapter 13, SPECT/CT is less expansive, especially when the cost and maintenance of cyclotron and PET radiopharmaceuticals are also considered, thus opening an opportunity for smaller institutions to have hybrid imaging capability at a fraction of the cost of PET/CT. The widespread use in clinical routines of SPECT modality indicates that SPECT/CT could be complementary to PET/CT. Nowadays, the number of studies demonstrating the value of a hybrid SPECT/CT modality in comparison with single imaging modalities is increasing rapidly, and the trend is expected to continue in the future.

14.2 INSTRUMENTATION

14.2.1 INSTRUMENT

A typical state-of-art SPECT/CT system consists of SPECT and CT subsystems that are placed side by side and integrated with a patient table and a computer system. Figure 14.1 shows an example of a clinical SPECT/CT system (Siemens Symbia T6).

SPECT/CT acquires SPECT and CT data sequentially. The CT data are reconstructed for anatomical display. The reconstructed CT map is also used for attenuation correction for SPECT reconstruction. Three displays are generated at the end: the reconstructed CT image, the SPECT image reconstructed with the attenuation map, and the fused image with the SPECT image in color scale and the CT image in gray scale.

14.2.2 CT COMPONENT

Currently, the CT component of the SPECT/CT is the x-ray CT scanner, which uses an x-ray tube that generates a relatively high flux of x-rays. This high flux results in the high statistics of the acquisition being achieved quickly, which means that the CT acquisition could be finished in a matter of seconds.

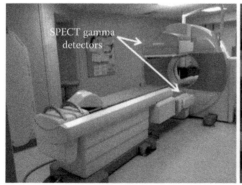 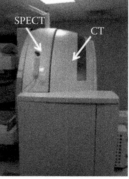

Figure 14.1 Clinical SPECT/CT scanner (Siemens Symbia T6).

The x-ray CT scanner is comprised of the x-ray tube and the detector mounted on a rotating gantry. The x-ray tube is a vacuum tube inside which there is a cathode consisting of a tungsten wire, called a filament. As the current passes through and heats up the filament, electrons are generated that later produce bremsstrahlung radiation. At the detectors, the photons arrive at very high rates, which makes detection of individual photons impossible. Therefore, the x-ray detectors operate in an integration mode; that is, the output current is proportional to the photon flux. The CT data are acquired as the patient moves through the gantry rotating, usually in a spiral trajectory, at a speed of about three rounds per second.

14.3 DATA CORRECTIONS AND IMAGE RECONSTRUCTION IN SPECT/CT

14.3.1 CT RECONSTRUCTION

For CT, the acquired projection data are the transmission of x-rays through the object (i.e., patient's body). Considering one ray, the measured intensity I is given by

$$I = I_0 e^{-\sum_j \mu_j \Delta x_j} \tag{14.1}$$

where I_0 is the measured intensity without an object (i.e., the blank-scan intensity), Δx_j is the interception length of the ray inside voxel j, and μ_j is the attenuation coefficient in that voxel. The log-attenuation projection is computed using

$$P = -\log\left(\frac{I_0}{I}\right) = \sum_j \mu_j \Delta x_j \tag{14.2}$$

The log-attenuation projections for all rays are reconstructed to obtain the attenuation map.

The filtered back projection (FBP) algorithm is widely used for CT reconstruction, while recently there have been rapid advancements for CT reconstruction using iterative methods (Fessler 2000).

Once the values of μ_j have been reconstructed, it is conventional in CT that these values are normalized to compensate for different parameters and instruments using the expression of the CT number in Hounsfield units (HU):

$$CT_j = 1000 \times \frac{\mu_j - \mu_{\text{water}}}{\mu_{\text{water}}} \tag{14.3}$$

where μ_{water} is the attenuation coefficient of water. The CT numbers are 0, –1000, and 300 HU for water, lungs, and bone, respectively.

14.3.2 USE OF CT FOR CORRECTIONS IN SPECT IMAGE RECONSTRUCTION

14.3.2.1 ATTENUATION CORRECTION

One of the critical components for SPECT image reconstruction is attenuation correction. Obtaining an accurate and patient-dependent attenuation map is key to performing attenuation correction. A SPECT-alone system typically assumes a uniform μ-map, which can lead to severe artifacts in the reconstructed images, especially in body images. SPECT/CT makes it possible to perform attenuation correction using a measured μ-map. The acquired CT images are converted to a μ-map for the energy of the corresponding gamma particles used for SPECT, which is in turn used for attenuation correction (King et al. 1995). One of the most popular attenuation correction methods in SPECT is Chang's (Chang 1978). The key idea of this method is to compensate for attenuation by multiplying each voxel value of the reconstructed image with FBP by a correction factor that is the reciprocal of the average probability that a photon that is emitted from the voxel transmits and is detected by the detector, and if necessary, in an iterative fashion. Specifically, this correction factor, $CF(x, y)$, at each (x, y) in the slice of interest can be determined as follows:

$$CF(x, y) = \frac{1}{\dfrac{1}{N_\Theta} \displaystyle\sum_{k=1}^{N_\Theta} e^{-\int_{L_k(x,y)} \mu(\vec{r}) d\vec{r}}} \tag{14.4}$$

where N_Θ is the number of projection angles, $L_k(x, y)$ is the ray from the point (x, y) to the detector at angle index k, and $\mu(\vec{r})$ is the attenuation coefficient at point $\vec{r}$ in the polar coordinate system. To perform the iterative attenuation correction, at initialization, the corrected image is obtained by multiplying each voxel value of the (uncorrected) original reconstructed image by the corresponding correction factor. In each iterative step, projection data of the corrected image are calculated, and the error projections are then obtained by subtracting the measured projection data by these computed projection data. The updated corrected image is obtained by summing the corrected image with the error image, which is reconstructed (using FBP) from the error projection data, and then each of its voxels is multiplied with the corresponding correction factor.

In practice, we need merely one iteration to have a reasonable corrected image. Nevertheless, this method has a pitfall in that it does not guarantee convergence (Lalush and Tsui 1994); that is, if we perform the iterative process at higher iterations, the noise is amplified, especially in the case of low count projections (King et al. 1996). As a result, we have to terminate the iterative process with only a few iterations, although the correction is not achieved.

The other approach for attenuation correction is based on the statistical framework. The statistical image reconstruction framework formulates the problem from noise modeling in data acquisition, and estimating the activity distribution. These methods can conveniently incorporate physical effects, including attenuation, into the model. The maximum-likelihood expectation maximization (ML-EM) (Shepp and Vardi 1982; Carson and Lange 1985) models the noise as Poisson and derives the estimate based on the maximum-likelihood criterion. Its algorithm is given by

$$\lambda_j^{[n+1]} = \frac{\lambda_j^{[n]}}{\displaystyle\sum_i a_{ij}} \sum_i a_{ij} \frac{Y_i}{\displaystyle\sum_k a_{ik} \lambda_k^{[n]}} \tag{14.5}$$

where $\lambda_j^{[n]}$ is the estimate of activity in voxel j at iteration n, Y_i is the measured projection at detector bin i, and a_{ij} is the (i, j)th element of the system matrix, which is the probability of a photon emitted from voxel j to be detected in detector bin i. The physical effects are modeled via the system matrix. Specifically, to include attenuation in the model, the element a_{ij} would be computed as the product between the fractional contribution of voxel j to detector bin i and the line integral of the attenuation map from that voxel to the detector bin. This calculation is usually performed on the fly because of the large dimensions of the system matrix.

The reconstruction can be accelerated with the ordered subset version of the ML-EM algorithm (OSEM) (Hudson and Larkin 1994). In this OSEM, the projection data are partitioned into subsets and only data from one subset are used for projections and back projections at each subiteration. The OSEM algorithm with N_s subsets ($S_l, l = 1, \ldots, N_s$) at iteration n, subiteration l is given by

$$\lambda_j^{[n+1, l]} = \frac{\lambda_j^{[n,l]}}{\displaystyle\sum_{i' \in S_l} a_{i'j}} \sum_{i \in S_l} a_{ij} \frac{Y_i}{\displaystyle\sum_k a_{ik} \lambda_k^{[n,l]}} \quad \text{and} \quad \lambda_j^{[n, N_s+1]} = \lambda_j^{[n+1,1]} \tag{14.6}$$

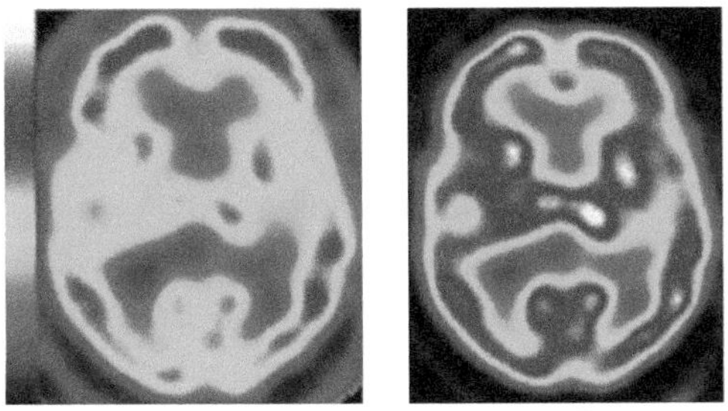

(a)   No AC   (b)   AC

Figure 14.2 Brain SPECT images reconstructed (a) without and (b) with attenuation correction (AC) from CT.

The OSEM algorithm has great success in speeding up the reconstruction process, and therefore is being employed routinely for several clinical applications. Figure 14.2 illustrates the impact of attenuation correction using the μ-map obtained from SPECT/CT on brain SPECT imaging.

14.3.2.2 SCATTER CORRECTION

Scattered photons degrade the image quality in SPECT imaging. Typically, 30%–40% of total counts are from scattered photons for SPECT (Hutton et al. 2011).

Several methods have been proposed for scatter correction for SPECT-alone imaging. A simple approach for scatter correction would be subtracting the estimated scatter contribution from the counts acquired within the photopeak window for each detector bin. Using the fact that scattered photons have less energy than primary photons, energy window approaches estimate the scattered photon contribution by acquiring projection data with one or two scatter energy windows. For example, one of the earliest approaches acquires data with two energy windows (Jaszczak et al. 1984), the main photopeak energy window and a consecutive window with a small energy width. A scaled version of the counts in the scatter window are assumed to be from scatter events; therefore, the counts from primary photons in each detector bin can be computed by subtracting this scatter portion from the counts in the photopeak energy window in the corresponding bin. The triple energy window (TEW) method (Ogawa et al. 1994) uses three energy windows, where data are acquired with three windows: the main photopeak window, and the higher and lower scatter windows. The scatter is estimated from the area of the trapezoid formed by the two bracketing windows. Scatter windows used in TEW should be narrow so that the scatter contribution can be estimated accurately. This in turn results in few counts and noisy estimate.

With the SPECT/CT, we can estimate the scatter contribution accurately from the attenuation map with the aid of Monte Carlo (MC) simulation. However, full MC simulation for scatter estimation for each individual patient was thought to be computationally expensive, and thus not practical in clinical use. There are some recent developments (Beekman et al. 2002; Ouyang et al. 2007) on fast MC simulation for scatter estimation for practical use.

The approach for scatter correction by subtracting of the scatter estimate directly from the counts within the photopeak energy window increases noise, and may introduce negative values in detector bins, especially in the case of low counts. Alternatively, including the scatter correction into the statistical-based reconstruction would be more optimal. The ML-EM reconstruction iterative algorithm with scatter correction is given by

$$\lambda_j^{[n+1]} = \frac{\lambda_j^{[n]}}{\sum_i a_{ij}} \sum_i a_{ij} \frac{Y_i}{\sum_k a_{ik}\lambda_k^{[n]} + S_j} \tag{14.7}$$

where S_j is the scatter estimate in detector bin j, and other variables are defined as in Equation 14.5, with the emphasis that a_{ij} is the probability of a primary photon emitted from voxel j to be detected in detector bin i

without any interaction inside the object. Another way to include the scatter correction into the reconstruction is to model the system matrix such that a_{ij} accounts for primary and scattered photons, but would in turn come with high computational complexity, especially in the case of three-dimensional (3D) implementation.

14.3.3 QUANTITATIVE SPECT

Conventionally, PET has been exclusively perceived as the quantitative radionuclide emission tomography, while SPECT has often been deemed nonquantitative owing to numerous physical factors (Seo et al. 2008). Quantitative radionuclide imaging via PET/CT has been proven to be greatly useful and is widely used in clinical practice. On the other hand, the feasibility of quantitative SPECT imaging has recently gained wider interest, primarily because of the advent of the combined SPECT and CT (Bailey and Willowson 2014).

SPECT/CT, which provides coregistered SPECT and CT data, has made data corrections such as attenuation, scatter, and partial volume corrections more accurate. Furthermore, the advancement in reconstruction algorithms, which can incorporate these corrections, yields significantly improved image quality and the accuracy of tracer concentration quantitation. As a result, the SPECT standardized uptake value (SUV) can be obtained accordingly.

It has been reported in phantom studies that quantitative SPECT imaging using SPECT/CT yields a concentration accuracy within 5% for ^{99m}Tc (Bailey and Willowson 2013), while studies for other radionuclides, such as ^{111}In, ^{123}I, ^{131}I, ^{177}Lu, and ^{201}Tl, have also been documented (Bailey and Willowson 2014). Quantitative SPECT in clinics has also been investigated in several other studies (Cachovan et al. 2013; Zeintl et al. 2010; Iida et al. 2010). SPECT manufacturers have begun to introduce new SPECT/CT systems with quantitative capabilities. In 2013, Siemens received Food and Drug Administration (FDA) approval for their quantitative xSPECT SPECT/CT system. It is expected that quantitative SPECT will be gradually integrated into clinical practice in the future.

14.4 CLINICAL APPLICATIONS

SPECT/CT has been used in a broad range of clinical applications. It is superior to SPECT or CT alone since it provides sequentially functional information from SPECT and anatomic information from CT in a single imaging session. Moreover, SPECT/CT provides anatomical data to localize radiotracer uptake, and thus improves diagnostic capability, especially in the case where SPECT images alone do not obviously provide the regional anatomy. Finally, CT is used for accurate attenuation correction in SPECT image reconstruction.

Following the commercial success of PET/CT scanners, there has been rising interest in SPECT/CT systems even though stand-alone SPECT systems are available at lower cost. It is estimated that one-fourth of the worldwide SPECT market sales belong to the hybrid systems (Leitha and Staudenherz 2012), with continuing growth in terms of both market sales and developments (Buck et al. 2008).

14.4.1 SPECT/CT IN CARDIOLOGY

Cardiac imaging with SPECT, especially myocardial perfusion imaging, is the most important SPECT clinical application. According to the American Society of Nuclear Cardiology (Heller et al. 2004), the use of CT in SPECT reconstruction can reduce false positives when imaging myocardial defects. In addition, SPECT/CT has potential in other cardiac applications in which myocardial SPECT could be fused with CT angiography for betterment of clinic standard practice.

Figure 14.3 shows an example of myocardial perfusion SPECT images without attenuation correction and PET images reconstructed with CT-based attenuation correction for the same subject. The one without attenuation correction demonstrates a false-positive inferior-wall defect, which implies coronary artery disease (CAD). The images with attenuation correction were reconstructed using a CT attenuation map obtained from a PET/CT scanner, where the inferior wall appeared to be normal. This demonstrates the importance of the attenuation correction for myocardial perfusion studies.

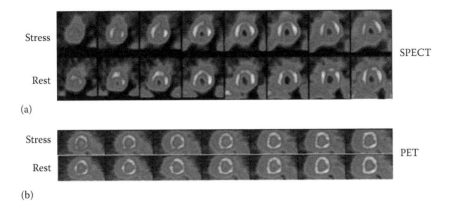

Stress — SPECT
Rest

(a)

Stress — PET
Rest

(b)

Figure 14.3 Short-axis myocardial perfusion images. (a) ^{99m}Tc-MIBI SPECT images reconstructed without attenuation correction. (b) ^{82}Rb PET images reconstructed with CT-based attenuation correction. This study shows that a false-positive myocardial perfusion defect may present if attenuation is not corrected.

14.4.2 SPECT/CT IN ONCOLOGY

SPECT/CT has been proven to play a vital role for oncologic imaging in terms of improving anatomical localization of disease, helping to define the extent of disease, and improving differentiation of physiological and pathological uptake (Keidar et al. 2003; Chowdhury and Scarsbrook 2008). Its clinical importance follows the same trend as ^{18}F-FDG PET/CT imaging.

Many neuroendocrine tumors (NETs) express somatostatin receptors. Planar imaging with somatostatin analogues such as ^{111}In-DTPA-octreotide has been in clinical use for more than a decade with high sensitivity. Nevertheless, this imaging technique is limited owing to small tumor size, the normal biodistribution of radiolabeled octreotide, and the lack of precise anatomical reference. SPECT/CT improves the detectability of primary or metastatic tumors, yields better tumor delineation, and allows differentiation between physiological and pathological uptake (Even-Sapir et al. 2001).

Planar ^{131}I imaging has been used for the detection of thyroid cancer, but its image interpretation is impeded because of many factors, such as low count density and poor anatomical reference. This would be improved by image fusion from the SPECT/CT. The improvement would significantly improve differentiation of focal uptake between benign and malignant causes, leading to the betterment of clinical management (Tharp et al. 2004; Yamamoto et al. 2003).

14.4.3 SPECT/CT IN BONE SCANS

Bone scintigraphy (with widely used ^{99m}Tc-MDP) has been a main battery for bone imaging. SPECT alone improves the performance in evaluating uptake abnormalities compared with bone scintigraphy because of the nonoverlap of structures, but still lacks ideal localization. The hybrid SPECT/CT has incremental value in improved anatomical localization and characterization of bone lesions, which results in better specificity (Horger and Bares 2006).

14.5 FUTURE DEVELOPMENTS AND APPLICATIONS OF SPECT/CT

There are several possible developments and potential applications of SPECT/CT imaging in the future (Seo et al. 2008).

New technologies on gamma-ray detection are emerging. These new technologies will likely improve both spatial resolution and sensitivity of SPECT/CT in the future. Given the fact that SPECT/CT has been widely accepted in clinical practice, new clinical applications are also under development. One of the evolving advancements in SPECT and SPECT/CT is the use of silicon photodiode or solid-state materials in detectors, which provides better spatial and energy resolution than conventional photomultiplier tube technology (Seo et al. 2008). It has been shown that this use of new detector materials has potential in cardiac (Kubo et al. 2002) and breast (Hruska et al. 2005) imaging. Many new designs of collimator materials and geometries have been proposed to improve the detection efficiency. The use of high-sensitivity detectors reduces imaging time, and thus increases patient throughput in myocardial perfusion studies. A compact SPECT/CT system (Brzymialkiewicz et al. 2005; Tornai et al. 2003; McKinley et al. 2004) has been designed for dedicated breast imaging as well. It consists of a cadmium-zinc-telluride (CZT)–based gamma camera for SPECT and a CsI flat detector for a cone-beam quasi-monochromatic CT on the same rotation gantry. Despite cross-modality contamination from SPECT to CT owing to simultaneous acquisition, this could simplify data acquisition, dual-modality registration, and corrections.

In clinical settings, SPECT/CT has many potential applications. There has been growing use of radionuclides in treatments such as ^{90}Y or ^{177}Lu for peptide receptor radionuclide therapy (Al-Nahhas and Fanti 2012) or ^{90}Y microsphere therapy of nonresectable colorectal liver metastases (Dezarn et al. 2011). This leads to the need for accurate imaging to confirm localization or radiation dose calculation. Using the anatomical information acquired by CT has potential to improve quantitative accuracy of radiation dosimetry in radionuclide therapy. The conventional approach for dosimetry in radionuclide treatment is to image via planar scintigraphy of a low dose of the therapeutic radionuclide or the therapeutic compound labeled with ^{111}In or [123]I. To improve the accuracy from using two-dimensional (2D) assessment, information from CT can be utilized by means of organ volumes or appropriate attenuation and scatter corrections to obtain 3D dosimetry (Thierens et al. 2005). Integration of the data from SPECT/CT imaging into the MC simulation offers the possibility to improve regional dosimetry for the spatial distribution of the absorbed dose (Prideaux et al. 2007). In a situation that the assessment of two physiological functions under identical conditions is desirable, simultaneous dual-radionuclide (DR) SPECT imaging, which produces two radionuclide SPECT images, has been proposed for several applications, including brain (El Fakhri et al. 2001; Du et al. 2007), cardiac (Ouyang et al. 2009), and oncologic (Rakvongthai et al. 2013) imaging. The simultaneous imaging allows imaging of two functions under identical physiological conditions, perfectly registered dual-tracer images, reduced imaging time, and better patient management. Several reports show that it has great potential for image quality comparable to that of sequential imaging while reducing cost and increasing patient throughput. Due to downscatter from one radionuclide to another in DR imaging, scatter correction, which requires an accurate attenuation map acquired by CT, is essential. Therefore, we may see simultaneous DR using SPECT/CT introduced into the clinical settings.

REFERENCES

Al-Nahhas, A., and S. Fanti. 2012. Radiolabelled peptides in diagnosis and therapy: An introduction. *Eur J Nucl Med Mol Imaging* 39(Suppl. 1):S1–3.

Bailey, D. L., and K. P. Willowson. 2013. An evidence-based review of quantitative SPECT imaging and potential clinical applications. *J Nucl Med* 54(1):83–89.

Bailey, D. L., and K. P. Willowson. 2014. Quantitative SPECT/CT: SPECT joins PET as a quantitative imaging modality. *Eur J Nucl Med Mol Imaging* 41(Suppl. 1):S17–25.

Beekman, F. J., H. W. de Jong, and S. van Geloven. 2002. Efficient fully 3-D iterative SPECT reconstruction with Monte Carlo-based scatter compensation. *IEEE Trans Med Imaging* 21(8):867–77.

Brzymialkiewicz, C. N., M. P. Tornai, R. L. McKinley, and J. E. Bowsher. 2005. Evaluation of fully 3-D emission mammotomography with a compact cadmium zinc telluride detector. *IEEE Trans Med Imaging* 24(7):868–77.

Buck, A. K., S. Nekolla, S. Ziegler, A. Beer, B. J. Krause, K. Herrmann, K. Scheidhauer, et al. 2008. SPECT/CT. *J Nucl Med* 49(8):1305–19.

Cachovan, M., A. H. Vija, J. Hornegger, and T. Kuwert. 2013. Quantification of 99mTc-DPD concentration in the lumbar spine with SPECT/CT. *EJNMMI Res* 3(1):1–8.

Carson, R. E., and K. Lange. 1985. The EM parametric image reconstruction algorithms. *J Am Stat Assoc* 80(389):20–22.

Chang, L. T. 1978. A method for attenuation correction in radionuclide computed tomography. *IEEE Trans Nucl Sci* 25(1):638–43.

Chowdhury, F. U., and A. F. Scarsbrook. 2008. The role of hybrid SPECT-CT in oncology: Current and emerging clinical applications. *Clin Radiol* 63(3):241–51.

Dezarn, W. A., J. T. Cessna, L. A. DeWerd, W. Feng, V. L. Gates, J. Halama, A. S. Kennedy, et al. 2011. Recommendations of the American Association of Physicists in Medicine on dosimetry, imaging, and quality assurance procedures for 90Y microsphere brachytherapy in the treatment of hepatic malignancies. *Med Phys* 38(8):4824–45.

Du, Y., B. M. Tsui, and E. C. Frey. 2007. Model-based crosstalk compensation for simultaneous 99mTc/123I dual-isotope brain SPECT imaging. *Med Phys* 34(9):3530–43.

El Fakhri, G., S. C. Moore, P. Maksud, A. Aurengo, and M. F. Kijewski. 2001. Absolute activity quantitation in simultaneous 123I/99mTc brain SPECT. *J Nucl Med* 42(2):300–8.

Even-Sapir, E., Z. Keidar, J. Sachs, A. Engel, L. Bettman, D. Gaitini, L. Guralnik, N. Werbin, G. Iosilevsky, and O. Israel. 2001. The new technology of combined transmission and emission tomography in evaluation of endocrine neoplasms. *J Nucl Med* 42(7):998–1004.

Fessler, J. A. 2000. Statistical image reconstruction methods for transmission tomography. In *Medical Image Processing and Analysis*, ed. M. Sonka and J. M. Fitzpatric, 1–70. Bellingham, WA: SPIE Press.

Hasegawa, B. H., E. L. Gingold, S. M. Reilly, S.-C. Liew, and C. E. Cann. 1990. Description of a simultaneous emission-transmission CT system. Presented at the Proceedings of SPIE Medical Imaging, Newport Beach, CA.

Hasegawa, B. H., S. M. Reilly, E. L. Gingold, and C. E. Cann. 1989. Design considerations for simultaneous emission transmission CT scanner. Presented at the Proceedings of the 75th Anniversary Scientific Assembly and Annual Meeting of the Radiological Society of North America, Chicago.

Heller, G. V., J. Links, T. M. Bateman, J. A. Ziffer, E. Ficaro, M. C. Cohen, and R. C. Hendel. 2004. American Society of Nuclear Cardiology and Society of Nuclear Medicine joint position statement: Attenuation correction of myocardial perfusion SPECT scintigraphy. *J Nucl Cardiol* 11(2):229–30.

Horger, M., and R. Bares. 2006. The role of single-photon emission computed tomography/computed tomography in benign and malignant bone disease. *Semin Nucl Med* 36(4):286–94.

Hruska, C. B., M. K. O'Connor, and D. A. Collins. 2005. Comparison of small field of view gamma camera systems for scintimammography. *Nucl Med Commun* 26(5):441–45.

Hudson, H. M., and R. S. Larkin. 1994. Accelerated image reconstruction using ordered subsets of projection data. *IEEE Trans Med Imaging* 13(4):601–9.

Hutton, B. F., I. Buvat, and F. J. Beekman. 2011. Review and current status of SPECT scatter correction. *Phys Med Biol* 56(14):R85–112.

Iida, H., J. Nakagawara, K. Hayashida, K. Fukushima, H. Watabe, K. Koshino, T. Zeniya, and S. Eberl. 2010. Multicenter evaluation of a standardized protocol for rest and acetazolamide cerebral blood flow assessment using a quantitative SPECT reconstruction program and split-dose 123I-iodoamphetamine. *J Nucl Med* 51(10):1624–31.

Jaszczak, R. J., K. L. Greer, C. E. Floyd Jr., C. C. Harris, and R. E. Coleman. 1984. Improved SPECT quantification using compensation for scattered photons. *J Nucl Med* 25(8):893–900.

Kaplan, C. H. 1989. Transmission/emission registered image (TERI) computed tomography scanners. International Patient Application No. PCT/US90/03722.

Keidar, Z., O. Israel, and Y. Krausz. 2003. SPECT/CT in tumor imaging: Technical aspects and clinical applications. *Semin Nucl Med* 33(3):205–18.

King, M. A., B. M. Tsui, and T. S. Pan. 1995. Attenuation compensation for cardiac single-photon emission computed tomographic imaging. Part 1. Impact of attenuation and methods of estimating attenuation maps. *J Nucl Cardiol* 2(6):513–24.

King, M. A., B. M. Tsui, T. S. Pan, S. J. Glick, and E. J. Soares. 1996. Attenuation compensation for cardiac single-photon emission computed tomographic imaging. Part 2. Attenuation compensation algorithms. *J Nucl Cardiol* 3(1):55–64.

Kubo, N., M. Mabuchi, C. Katoh, H. Arai, K. Morita, E. Tsukamoto, Y. Morita, and N. Tamaki. 2002. Validation of left ventricular function from gated single photon computed emission tomography by using a scintillator-photodiode camera: A dynamic myocardial phantom study. *Nucl Med Commun* 23(7):639–43.

Lalush, D. S., and B. M. Tsui. 1994. Improving the convergence of iterative filtered backprojection algorithms. *Med Phys* 21(8):1283–86.

Leitha, T., and A. Staudenherz. 2012. Hybrid PET/CT and SPECT/CT imaging. In *Computed Tomography— Clinical Applications*, ed. L. Saba, 269–92. Rijeka, Croatia: InTech.

McKinley, R. L., M. P. Tornai, E. Samei, and M. L. Bradshaw. 2004. Simulation study of a quasi-monochromatic beam for x-ray computed mammotomography. *Med Phys* 31(4):800–13.

Mirshanov, D. M. 1987. Transmission-emission computer tomograph. Moscow: All-Union Research Surgery Center, USSR Academy of Medical Science.

Ogawa, K., T. Ichihara, and A. Kubo. 1994. Accurate scatter correction in single photon emission CT. *Ann Nucl Med Sci* 7:145–50.

Ouyang, J., G. El Fakhri, and S. C. Moore. 2007. Fast Monte Carlo based joint iterative reconstruction for simultaneous Tc-99m/I-123 SPECT imaging. *Med Phys* 34(8):3263–72.

Ouyang, J., X. Zhu, C. M. Trott, and G. El Fakhri. 2009. Quantitative simultaneous 99mTc/123I cardiac SPECT using MC-JOSEM. *Med Phys* 36(2):602–11.

Prideaux, A. R., H. Song, R. F. Hobbs, B. He, E. C. Frey, P. W. Ladenson, R. L. Wahl, and G. Sgouros. 2007. Three-dimensional radiobiologic dosimetry: Application of radiobiologic modeling to patient-specific 3-dimensional imaging-based internal dosimetry. *J Nucl Med* 48(6):1008–16.

Rakvongthai, Y., G. El Fakhri, R. Lim, A. A. Bonab, and J. Ouyang. 2013. Simultaneous 99mTc-MDP/123I-MIBG tumor imaging using SPECT-CT: Phantom and constructed patient studies. *Med Phys* 40(10):102506.

Seo, Y., C. Mari, and B. H. Hasegawa. 2008. Technological development and advances in single-photon emission computed tomography/computed tomography. *Semin Nucl Med* 38(3):177–98.

Shepp, L. A., and Y. Vardi. 1982. Maximum likelihood reconstruction for emission tomography. *IEEE Trans Med Imaging* 1(2):113–22.

Tharp, K., O. Israel, J. Hausmann, L. Bettman, W. H. Martin, M. Daitzchman, M. P. Sandler, and D. Delbeke. 2004. Impact of 131I-SPECT/CT images obtained with an integrated system in the follow-up of patients with thyroid carcinoma. *Eur J Nucl Med Mol Imaging* 31(10):1435–42.

Thierens, H. M., M. A. Monsieurs, and K. Bacher. 2005. Patient dosimetry in radionuclide therapy: The whys and the wherefores. *Nucl Med Commun* 26(7):593–99.

Tornai, M. P., J. E. Bowsher, R. J. Jaszczak, B. C. Pieper, K. L. Greer, P. H. Hardenbergh, and R. E. Coleman. 2003. Mammotomography with pinhole incomplete circular orbit SPECT. *J Nucl Med* 44(4):583–93.

Yamamoto, Y., Y. Nishiyama, T. Monden, Y. Matsumura, K. Satoh, and M. Ohkawa. 2003. Clinical usefulness of fusion of 131I SPECT and CT images in patients with differentiated thyroid carcinoma. *J Nucl Med* 44(12):1905–10.

Zeintl, J., A. H. Vija, A. Yahil, J. Hornegger, and T. Kuwert. 2010. Quantitative accuracy of clinical 99mTc SPECT/CT using ordered-subset expectation maximization with 3-dimensional resolution recovery, attenuation, and scatter correction. *J Nucl Med* 51(6):921–28.

15

PET/MRI

CIPRIAN CATANA

15.1 Introduction   380
15.2 Challenges in combining PET and MRI   380
    15.2.1 Considerations on the PET side   380
        15.2.1.1 Magnetic field sensitivity of PET photon detectors   380
        15.2.1.2 Electromagnetic interference   380
        15.2.1.3 Temperature effects   381
    15.2.2 Considerations on the MR side   381
        15.2.2.1 Main magnetic field homogeneity   381
        15.2.2.2 Electromagnetic interference   381
        15.2.2.3 RF coils' PET compatibility   381
        15.2.2.4 Space limitations inside the MR bore   382
15.3 Approaches to combining PET and MRI   382
    15.3.1 Simultaneous data acquisition   382
        15.3.1.1 PMT-based systems   382
        15.3.1.2 APD-based systems   383
        15.3.1.3 SiPM-based systems   385
    15.3.2 Sequential data acquisition   386
    15.3.3 PET data corrections in an integrated PET/MR scanner   387
        15.3.3.1 MR-based photon attenuation correction   387
        15.3.3.2 Tissue attenuation correction   388
        15.3.3.3 Hardware attenuation correction   393
    15.3.4 MR-assisted PET motion correction   394
        15.3.4.1 Rigid-body motion correction   394
        15.3.4.2 Non-rigid-body motion correction   396
    15.3.5 Other methods for improving the PET data quantification using the
        MR information   398
        15.3.5.1 Partial volume effects correction   398
        15.3.5.2 Image-based radiotracer arterial input function estimation   399
15.4 Promising research and clinical applications   400
References   402

15.1 INTRODUCTION

PET and MRI provide complementary data that are routinely analyzed concurrently in research and clinical applications. Recognizing the potential to combine the strengths of the two modalities while mitigating some of their limitations, approaches to combine PET and MRI in a single scanner have been proposed even before the first integrated PET–computed tomography (CT) scanners were developed. In recent years, there has been renewed and sustained interest in combining PET with MRI, perhaps as a result of the success and widespread clinical adoption of PET/CT. Given the completely different physical principles underlying these two imaging modalities, development of PET/MRI has faced even bigger technological and methodological hurdles than those PET/CT had to overcome in the first years after it was introduced. Just to give two examples, avoiding the mutual electromagnetic interference and the need for developing MR-based attenuation correction methods have been particularly difficult to address.

In this chapter, the challenges in integrating PET and MRI are first discussed, with a focus on the ways the two modalities can interfere and interact with each other. Next, the approaches that have been investigated for overcoming these challenges and the integrated scanners for sequential or simultaneous data acquisition developed using these approaches are described. Methodological aspects relevant to PET/MRI are then introduced, particularly focusing on MR-based photon attenuation correction for both brain and whole-body applications and on rigid- and non-rigid-body MR-assisted PET motion correction, a unique and very exciting opportunity opened up by the simultaneous acquisition. Other methods that could lead to an improvement in PET data quantification in integrated PET/MRI scanners, such as partial volume effects correction and MR-assisted image-based radiotracer arterial input function estimation, are also briefly discussed. Finally, examples of promising applications are given to highlight the tremendous potential of this novel imaging modality.

15.2 CHALLENGES IN COMBINING PET AND MRI

15.2.1 CONSIDERATIONS ON THE PET SIDE

15.2.1.1 MAGNETIC FIELD SENSITIVITY OF PET PHOTON DETECTORS

The major obstacle to PET in or near an MRI scanner is the presence of the strong magnetic field. Photomultiplier tubes (PMTs), historically the photon detector of choice for PET scanners, have the significant disadvantage of being very sensitive to magnetic fields. Even fields as weak as the earth's (0.5 G) can cause changes in their gain. Magnetic influence is greatest in the space between the cathode and first dynode, where electron trajectories are longest. Although some PMT designs have better magnetic field immunity than others, PMTs cannot be used within the bore or even in the close vicinity of a high-field magnet. Depending on the orientation of the magnetic field with respect to the tube axis, the maximum vicinity field that is tolerated by a PMT, with acceptable performance (less than 10% loss in gain), is approximately 100 G (Shao et al. 1997c). Although the PMTs could be shielded from low-frequency magnetic fields using mu-metal, this is not a solution for higher field magnets, as the material saturates at approximately 2 T.

On the other hand, solid-state photon detectors, such as avalanche photodiodes (APDs) and Geiger-mode APDs (also called solid-state photomultipliers [SSPMs], silicon photomultipliers [SiPMs], or multiphoton pixel counters [MPPCs] by different vendors), are magnetic field insensitive.

15.2.1.2 ELECTROMAGNETIC INTERFERENCE

In an integrated system, the electromagnetic radiation emitted by one device can interfere with the other. The PET electronics can also easily pick up the strong radiofrequency (RF) signals generated by the MRI's RF transmit and gradient coils. Although decoupling components can be used in some cases, very careful shielding is generally necessary and is realized by placing the PET detectors in conductive enclosures (Faraday cages). These enclosures have to be designed considering the specific requirements, which include knowing exactly which frequencies need to be shielded.

In the case of APD-based detectors, a charge-sensitive preamplifier needs to be placed as close as possible to the detector to minimize the capacitance and ensure lower noise and better signal quality (Pichler et al. 2001). Fortunately, MR-compatible preamplifiers are already available as part of the MR RF systems.

15.2.1.3 TEMPERATURE EFFECTS

The performance of semiconductor detectors is a strong function of temperature, which affects their gain, breakdown voltage, and capacitance (Conradi 1974). For example, a gain change of up to 5%/°C due to changes in breakdown voltage has been reported (Kolb et al. 2010). In an integrated PET/MRI scanner, there are at least two aspects that have to be considered in this context. First, the heat produced by the PET electronics (e.g., charge-sensitive preamplifiers) can lead to substantial increases in temperature. Second, the eddy currents that are induced by the switching gradients in conductive shielding material, such as the materials used in the PET scanner components, can also induce an increase in the temperature of the shielding material and, consequently, inside the detector enclosure.

15.2.2 CONSIDERATIONS ON THE MR SIDE

15.2.2.1 MAIN MAGNETIC FIELD HOMOGENEITY

The magnetic field homogeneity is affected by the magnetic susceptibility (χ) of the materials placed inside the bore. Based on their susceptibility, materials are classified as diamagnetic ($-1 < \chi < 0$), paramagnetic ($0 < \chi < 0.01$), or ferromagnetic ($\chi > 0.01$). The main magnetic field (B_0) homogeneity must not be significantly degraded by the introduction of dia- or paramagnetic materials or asymmetrically placed components. Ideally, any object located within the region of MRI should not perturb the preexisting field. Materials with $|\chi| < 20 \times 10^{-6}$ are considered MRI compatible. For example, water susceptibility at 37°C is -9.05×10^{-6}, and most body tissues have values in the range of -7.0×10^{-6} to -11×10^{-6} (Schenck 1996). Due to their high susceptibility, ferromagnetic materials are not normally useful or even tolerable in MRI and consequently are to be avoided.

The magnetic susceptibility of several scintillators used in PET detectors has been evaluated. Bismuth germanium oxide (BGO) and lutetium oxyorthosilicate (LSO) showed susceptibility similar to that of human tissue (-19.0×10^{-6} and -21.7×10^{-6}, respectively) and only produced small artifacts on the MR images. In contrast, lutetium gadolinium oxyorthosilicate (LGSO) showed much greater susceptibility (790×10^{-6}) than human tissue, and produced significant artifacts and distortion in the MR images due to the presence of gadolinium (Gd) in this scintillator (Yamamoto et al. 2003).

15.2.2.2 ELECTROMAGNETIC INTERFERENCE

Any electromagnetic interference in the RF part of the spectrum where the MR system operates will lead to artifacts or decreased signal-to-noise ratio (SNR). The photon detectors and associated electronics commonly used in PET contain conducting and RF-radiating components that have the potential to interfere with the MR system if not properly shielded.

The eddy currents are of special concern on the MR side as well. These small, time-varying currents create magnetic fields that oppose the change in the magnetic field that created them, producing image artifacts and spatial distortions. Breaks or slits in the material are sometimes used to reduce the eddy currents, but this could lead to degradation in the shielding efficiency of the enclosure. A more efficient solution is to precompensate for the loss by adjusting the gradients' driving current so that the desired magnetic field is obtained.

15.2.2.3 RF COILS' PET COMPATIBILITY

Since the performance of the receive RF coils is substantially improved when located very close to the area of interest, they are usually positioned between the subject and the PET detectors in an integrated PET/MRI scanner. This means, however, that the annihilation photons can interact in the coils, leading to a loss of counts. Consequently, the RF coils have to be carefully designed to fulfill minimum attenuation requirements.

For example, in the case of the RF coil currently used with the integrated PET/MRI scanners (discussed in Section 15.3), most of the highly attenuating components (i.e., capacitors and preamplifiers) had to be positioned outside the PET field of view (FOV). Furthermore, when a fully shielded PET insert is introduced in the MR bore, the standard body transmit coil cannot be used and a local transmit coil has to be integrated into the system and could further contribute to photon attenuation.

15.2.2.4 SPACE LIMITATIONS INSIDE THE MR BORE

Perhaps the most significant challenge on the MR side is the limited space available inside the bore of standard small-animal and human MR systems. For example, the 30 mm space between the standard gradient coils and the RF coil on the 7 T Bruker small-animal MR scanner poses significant constraints on the MR-compatible PET detector design. In the case of human MR scanners, gradient systems pay a steep price or performance penalty from increased size, as power requirements go up with radius, and manufacturing tolerance for gradient shielding becomes much more demanding. For many years, the widest-bore human MRI systems were no larger than 60 cm in diameter, providing no additional space for integrating key PET components. Recently, new gradient designs have been proposed by all three major medical equipment manufacturers (i.e., Siemens, General Electric, and Philips) that allow peak performance with larger 70 cm bore diameters, providing enough space for the PET detectors.

15.3 APPROACHES TO COMBINING PET AND MRI

While PET/CT scanners have quickly become well-established clinical tools (Townsend et al. 2004), development of combined PET and MRI has been much slower. In this section, the history of this field is presented, highlighting especially those efforts that lead to complete integrated PET/MRI systems.

15.3.1 SIMULTANEOUS DATA ACQUISITION

The initial motivation for simultaneous PET and MRI, at least from a technical perspective, was the potential improvement in PET spatial resolution due to the reduction of the positron range in a magnetic field. Since the positron is an electrical charge, it was hypothesized (Iida et al. 1986) and later demonstrated that when moving in a magnetic field, the component of its motion in the plane perpendicular to the field becomes helical instead of approximately rectilinear, leading to annihilation closer to the place of emission (Raylman 1991). To confirm this effect, measurements of the positron range at various magnetic fields were performed using pairs of opposing PET detector modules based on APDs (Hammer and Christensen 1995) and PMTs (Christensen et al. 1995), two of the photon detectors that would eventually be used for building MR-compatible PET scanners, as discussed in more detail later in this section. Monte Carlo simulations were used to further characterize the potential benefit in more realistic situations and for clinically relevant positron emitters (Raylman et al. 1996; Wirrwar et al. 1997). To summarize these results, high magnetic fields (e.g., more than 7 T), high-energy positron emitters (e.g., ^{15}O and ^{82}Rb), and scanners with small diameter (to minimize the contribution of the noncollinearity effect) and submillimeter-scintillation crystals (so that the spatial resolution is not dominated by the crystal size) are needed for this effect to be relevant.

15.3.1.1 PMT-BASED SYSTEMS

Since PMTs were the photon detectors of choice in PET when the first attempts to combine it with MRI were made in the 1990s, methods to overcome the PMT's magnetic field sensitivity had to be investigated and implemented. A first approach was to use 4 m long optical fibers to couple LSO scintillator elements placed inside the magnet to multichannel PMTs and electronics placed outside a 0.2 T open-magnet MRI system. The prototype scanner, called McPET I (MRI compatible PET I) had a 38 mm detector ring diameter that, although too small for scanning animals, allowed the simultaneous acquisition of PET and MRI phantom images for the first time (Shao et al. 1997a). The second-generation prototype, called McPET II, had a 54 mm diameter detector ring and several modifications that slightly improved the PET performance. However, the axial FOV was still limited to 2 mm (Shao et al. 1997b). Nevertheless, this scanner was used for simultaneously acquiring for the first time PET images and ^{31}P nuclear magnetic resonance (NMR) spectra from isolated, perfused hearts (Garlick et al. 1997) and performing *in vivo* rat brain studies. A multilayered single-ring PET insert based on this approach, which significantly improves the sensitivity and spatial resolution uniformity compared with the first prototypes, was subsequently developed and tested in a Philips Achieva whole-body 3 T MRI scanner (Mackewn et al. 2005, 2010).

While important first steps, there were several drawbacks to this approach, such as the limited axial coverage and the less than optimal PET performance due to the light loss in the long fibers.

To increase the axial FOV, bent optical fiber bundles (2.5 m long) were proposed to couple the 20×20 LSO arrays of $2.5 \times 2.5 \times 15$ mm^3 crystals to position-sensitive PMTs (Raylman et al. 2006). Although a full system was not built using this approach, two prototype MR-compatible PET detector modules were used for performing simultaneous PET/MRI and PET–magnetic resonance spectroscopy (MRS) studies in a GE 3 T MRI scanner (Raylman et al. 2007).

Similarly, slanted light guides connected to 75 cm long optical fibers were used to couple multiple rings of LGSO crystals to position-sensitive PMTs located right outside a 0.3 T permanent magnet in the integrated iPET/MRI prototype (Yamamoto et al. 2010). By using LGSO arrays with different decay times (i.e., 33 and 43 ns), depth-of-interaction information could also be obtained with this scanner. With a relatively large transaxial FOV (i.e., 80 mm), this prototype was used for performing proof-of-principle whole-body studies in rats using various radiotracers (Tatsumi et al. 2012).

An alternative approach to address the aforementioned limitations (Lucas et al. 2006) was to use a split magnet that allowed a relatively large number of PET detectors to be placed inside the gap of the 1 T MR system and also reduced the fiber length. One advantage of this approach was that PET detectors very similar to those available in the state-of-the-art preclinical PET scanners were used, and hence the PET scanner performance was only minimally degraded and the axial FOV was maintained. In another approach involving a "nonconventional" MR design, commercially available PMT-based detectors were integrated into a field-cycled MRI (fcMRI) system (Bindseil et al. 2011; Peng et al. 2010). The fcMRI system consists of two independent magnets, a stronger one (e.g., 0.3 T) that produces the initial magnetization and a lower-strength one (e.g., 94 mT) used during the readout. Because the magnetic field can be quickly cycled on and off, PET data can be acquired during the off state when the effect of the weaker magnetic field on the PMTs is minimal. Although it allows only interleaved acquisition of PET and MRI data, this might suffice when changes in the observed processes occur relatively slowly compared with the imaging time. Although innovative in design, such systems compromise modern MR performance to a degree that is likely suboptimal for clinical use.

15.3.1.2 APD-BASED SYSTEMS

The fundamental technical advance that has allowed the PET/MRI field to significantly move forward and transition from the preclinical to the clinical arena was the emergence of APDs, which maintain PMT's light sensitivity while remaining insensitive to magnetic fields. APDs have been demonstrated to work inside MRI scanners at fields as high as 9.4 T (Pichler et al. 1997), and integrated small-animal scanners using this technology have been used to simultaneously acquire good-quality PET and MRI data *in vivo* (Catana et al. 2008; Judenhofer et al. 2008; Maramraju et al. 2011).

The first APD-based PET/MRI scanner that was used for *in vivo* small-animal studies was developed at University of California, Davis (Catana et al. 2006, 2008). Each of the 16 PET detector modules consisted of an 8×8 LSO array with individual crystals measuring $1.43 \times 1.43 \times 6$ mm^3 coupled through a short optical fiber bundle to 14×14 mm^2 position-sensitive APDs (RMD, Watertown, Massachusetts) and charge-sensitive preamplifiers (Cremat, Newton, Massachusetts). The optical fiber bundle consisted of 6×6 square-section double-clad optical fibers bent 90°, with the straight portion measuring 10 cm. These short fibers were preferred instead of direct coupling to minimize the interference between the two scanners by placing all the PET electronics just outside the MR FOV. The modules were arranged in ring geometry with a 60 mm detector ring diameter and 12 mm axial coverage (Figure 15.1). The temperature inside each of the two shielding enclosures that made up the scanner was maintained at –10°C by passing dried and cooled air. Using this

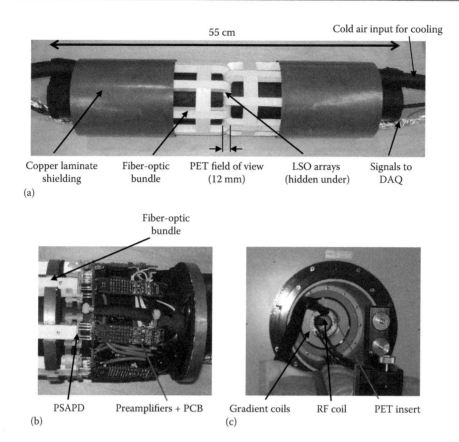

Figure 15.1 MR-compatible small-animal position-sensitive APD (PSAPD)–based PET scanner. (a) Photograph of the PET insert. (b) Close-up view showing the PSAPDs and associated electronics that reside under the high-frequency copper laminate. (c) PET insert in place within a 7 T Bruker BioSpin preclinical MRI system. PCB, printed circuit board; DAQ, data acquisition. (Originally published in Catana, C., et al., *Proc. Natl. Acad. Sci. U.S.A.*, 105(10), 3705–3710, 2008.)

scanner, detailed experiments to assess the mutual interference between the two devices and *in vivo* small-animal studies were performed (Catana et al. 2008).

In parallel, another APD-based insert for a 7 T small-animal MR scanner (ClinScan, Bruker, Germany) was built at the University of Tubingen (Judenhofer et al. 2007). No optical fibers were used in this case, and the photon detectors were coupled to the scintillator arrays using a 3 mm thick light guide. The PET detector module consisted of a 12×12 array of LSO crystals measuring $1.5 \times 1.5 \times 4.5$ mm^3 coupled to a 3×3 APD array (Hamamatsu Photonics, Hamamatsu, Japan). The complete system had 10 modules arranged in a ring with an axial FOV of 19 mm and a transaxial FOV of 40 mm. *In vivo* brain and tumor imaging studies in mice were performed using this scanner (Judenhofer et al. 2008).

Using a similar approach, researchers from Brookhaven National Laboratory built a PET insert for a Bruker 9.4 T MRI scanner. The PET detector was based on the RatCAP design and used APDs read out by custom-designed application-specific integrated circuits (ASICs). Each of the 12 detectors that made up the 4 cm diameter ring consisted of a 4×8 array of $2.3 \times 2.3 \times 5$ mm^3 LSO crystals read out by a 4×8 array of APDs (Woody et al. 2007). The scanner was used for performing rat brain and gated mouse heart simultaneous PET and MRI studies (Maramraju et al. 2011).

The first integrated PET/MRI scanner for human use was designed and built by Siemens (Schlemmer et al. 2008). This prototype device, called BrainPET (Figure 15.2a), is a head-only PET insert that fits into the standard 3 T MRI commercially available scanner (Magnetom Trio, Siemens, Erlangen, Germany). The PET detector module consists of a 12×12 array of $2.5 \times 2.5 \times 20$ mm^3 LSO crystals read out by a 3×3 array of APDs (Hamamatsu Photonics). Electromagnetic interference was minimized by individually shielding each

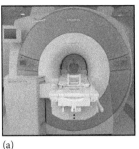 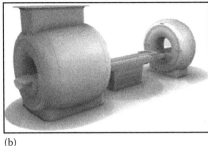 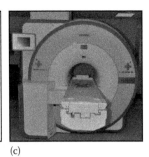

(a) (b) (c)

Figure 15.2 Integrated PET/MR scanners currently available for human use: (a) Siemens MR-BrainPET proto-type, (b) Philips sequential PET/MR whole-body scanner, and (c) Siemens Biograph mMR whole-body scanner. (Originally published in Catana, C., et al., *J. Nucl. Med.*, 54(5), 815–824, 2013.)

of the 32 detector cassettes (each consisting of 6 detector modules) that make up the PET gantry. The inner diameter of the gantry is 35 cm, and the axial FOV is 19.125 cm. The temperature in this scanner is controlled using two mechanisms. The hardware mechanism consists of an air compressor and a water chiller controlled through a negative feedback mechanism to maintain constant the mean global temperature inside the detector cassettes. When the chiller is activated, the temperature of the air flowing through the heat exchanger (located in the vicinity of the gantry) is changed. The software mechanism, called photopeak tracking, adjusts the position of the 511 keV photopeak for each detector block to compensate for more rapid changes in the cassettes' temperature (i.e., those induced by the running MR sequences).

The first BrainPET scanner was installed in 2007, and 8 years later, three of these prototype devices were still in use, one at the A. A. Martinos Center, Massachusetts General Hospital, and two in Juelich, Germany (one of them installed in a 9.4 T magnet). These scanners have been used in a variety of studies, including those aimed at investigating the mutual interference between the two devices and investigating the performance of the PET camera (Kolb et al. 2012; Chonde et al. 2013), developing methods to use the information obtained from one device to improve the other modality (Catana et al. 2010, 2011), and demonstrating the tremendous potential of this novel technology through proof-of-principle studies in small-animal, nonhuman primates and humans (Catana et al. 2012, 2013; Sander et al. 2013; Frullano et al. 2010; Uppal et al. 2011). Attesting to the remarkable stability of the BrainPET scanner (and implicitly of APD technology), all the original detectors are still in working condition in the device installed at the A. A. Martinos Center.

The experience gained from the BrainPET prototype allowed Siemens to introduce in 2010 the first fully integrated whole-body MR/PET scanner, called Biograph mMR (Figure 15.2c). This scanner also uses APD technology, but the PET and MRI hardware and software are now fully integrated. The PET detectors have been placed between the body RF coil and the gradient set, and the two scanners share the same gantry. Each PET detector block consists of an 8×8 array of $4 \times 4 \times 20$ mm^3 LSO crystals read out by an array of 3×3 APDs. They are arranged in eight rings with 56 detectors each, providing a transaxial FOV of 59.4 cm and an axial FOV of 25.8 cm. Water cooling is used to control the temperature of the detectors and associated electronics. The MR system is based on the 70 cm diameter bore Magnetom 3T Verio MR scanner (Siemens, Erlangen, Germany). A complete characterization of the PET scanner performance according to the National Electrical Manufacturers Association (NEMA) NU 2-2007 protocol was performed and revealed that the PET component of the mMR is similar to the commercially available PET/CT scanner (Siemens mCT) in terms of spatial resolution, peak noise-equivalent count rate, and scatter fraction, while its sensitivity is ~50% better (15 kcps MBq^{-1} at the center of the FOV) (Delso et al. 2011). The Biograph mMR received 510k clearance from the Food and Drug Administration (FDA), and at least 40 units have been sold at the time of this writing.

15.3.1.3 SIPM-BASED SYSTEMS

More recently, Geiger-mode APDs (aka SiPMs) have been proposed and tested for PET applications (Kolb et al. 2010; Roncali and Cherry 2011). Their very good performance and magnetic field insensitivity make them very promising candidates for replacing APDs as the photon detector of choice for simultaneous PET and MRI. In one of the first studies investigating the potential of these devices for this application, LYSO-SSPM detector modules were tested inside a 3 T GE MRI scanner. An energy resolution of 16% full width at half maximum (FWHM) and coincidence time resolution of ~1.3 ns were measured outside the magnet, and no performance degradation was reported inside the magnet (Seong Jong et al. 2008).

Building on previous experience with PMT-based scanners, a SiPM-based PET scanner for a 0.15 T permanent magnet was designed (Yamamoto et al. 2011, 2012). Sixteen dual-layer phoswich LGSO arrays coupled to 4 × 4 SiPM arrays (Hamamatsu Photonics) were used to build a PET scanner with a ring diameter of 68 cm and an axial FOV of 20 mm. Although the integrated scanner was successfully used for simultaneously acquiring PET and MRI data in phantoms and small animals, interference between the two scanners was reported, especially on the MRI side.

In a similar approach, PET detector modules were built by coupling a 4 × 4 array of $3 \times 3 \times 10$ mm³ LYSO crystals to a Geiger-mode APD array (SensL, Cork, Ireland) (Kang et al. 2011). Particular to this scanner, 3 m long flexible flat cables were used to couple the Geiger-mode APDs to amplifiers located outside the 5 G line of the 7 T MRI scanner (Bruker BioSpec, Ettlingen, Germany). In this way, the amount of PET electronics located in the MR FOV was reduced, minimizing the potential for electromagnetic interference and the shielding requirements. A complete scanner was built using 16 such detector modules arranged in a 70 mm diameter ring with an axial FOV of 13 mm. The mean energy resolution measured was 17.6%, and the time resolution was 1.5 ns. No performance degradation was observed inside the magnet, and successful acquisition of simultaneous PET and MRI images in phantoms and live animals was reported (Kang et al. 2011).

In an approach that reminds us of the early PMT-based prototypes, a SiPM-based integrated PET/MR scanner was built using short optical fiber bundles (Hong et al. 2012). However, the 31 mm long fibers were not used to allow the PET detectors to be positioned outside the MR FOV, but to introduce gaps between the modules so that the body transmit coil of the 3 T MRI scanner (Siemens Magnetom Trio, Erlangen, Germany) could be used.

Another SiPM MR-compatible PET scanner developed has 12 detector modules with a ring diameter of 13.6 cm and an axial FOV of 3.2 cm (Yoon et al. 2012). Each module consists of a 20 × 18 array of $1.5 \times 1.5 \times 7$ mm³ LGSO crystals coupled to four 4 × 4 SiPM arrays and was individually shielded, thus minimizing the interference with the Siemens 3 T MR scanner (Magnetom Trio, Erlangen, Germany). Furthermore, a mechanism for retrospectively compensating the gain fluctuations due to temperature changes was implemented. Interference-free PET and MRI data were acquired simultaneously using this scanner.

At the RSNA meeting in December 2013, General Electric introduced a SiPM-based whole-body integrated PET/MRI scanner, and several of these devices are currently being tested around the world. The PET detector gantry (with transaxial and axial FOVs of 60 and 25 cm, respectively) was designed to fit between the body RF coil and the MR gradient set of the GE 750w 3 T MR scanner, and it consists of five rings of 112 detector blocks (LYSO coupled to arrays of SiPMs). A preliminary test demonstrated interference-free operation on both the MR and PET side. More importantly, a per-crystal timing resolution of ~400 ps was reported, making this scanner the first time-of-flight integrated PET/MR scanner for human use (Levin et al. 2013).

15.3.2 SEQUENTIAL DATA ACQUISITION

While most of the efforts in the field have focused on developing scanners capable of simultaneous acquisition, there are numerous applications that would benefit even from the sequential acquisition of PET and MRI data, similar to PET/CT scanning. This approach is more straightforward to implement from a technical perspective.

With the aim of allowing sequential human brain imaging, two high-end commercially available scanners—the high-resolution research tomograph (HRRT) PET (Siemens, Knoxville, Tennessee) and the ultra-high-field 7 T MRI (Siemens, Erlangen, Germany)—were coupled using a shuttle bed built using MR-compatible materials that transfers the subject between the two scanners located in adjacent rooms. Since the benefit of using these advanced scanners for acquiring high-resolution morphological and metabolic data would be offset by hardware misregistration, the shuttle system was very carefully calibrated to allow near-perfect coregistration of the imaged volumes (Cho et al. 2008). This system was successfully used for a number of studies focusing on small brain structures that are very difficult to assess using standard devices (Cho et al. 2011, 2013).

The hybrid system introduced by Philips, the Ingenuity TF PET/MRI (Figure 15.2b), combines the Gemini TF PET and Achieva 3T X-Series MRI scanners, placed at 4.2 m from each other (center-to-center distance) with a common rotating patient table that moves the subject between the two scanners. Although the manufacturer's goal was to build a scanner capable of whole-body PET and MR data acquisition using existing state-of-the-art devices, significant modifications of the PET scanner were still required to minimize the RF interference (Zaidi et al. 2011). For example, although shielding materials were placed at the side of the PET scanner closer to the MR scanner and in multiple layers around the PMTs, the detectors had to also be reoriented and recalibrated to minimize magnetic field effects; in turn, to reduce the effects on the MR side, most of the front-end PET electronics were moved from the standard PET gantry outside the Faraday cage. Additionally, the PMT bias voltage had to be reduced while acquiring MR data to minimize the MR background floor caused by the signal associated with the detection of the LYSO scintillator background. In spite of these modifications, the performance of the PET component was similar to that of the PET scanner on which it is based in terms of spatial resolution (~5 mm FWHM), sensitivity (7000 cps MBq^{-1} at the center of the FOV), scatter fraction, count rate capabilities, and image quality. These scanners installed at a limited number of sites were used for successfully performing hundreds of studies, mainly in oncological patients, as well as for exploring the remaining methodological challenges (e.g., MR-based attenuation correction) (Kalemis et al. 2013).

General Electric proposed an approach similar to that of Cho et al. (2008) as an initial solution to the integration of PET and MRI for whole-body imaging using minimally modified state-of-the-art devices. As opposed to the Philips approach, no hardware modifications were required, as the two scanners were placed in adjacent rooms and an MR- and PET-compatible patient shuttle system was used to transfer the subject between the two scanners (Veit-Haibach et al. 2013). This trimodality PET/CT-MR system consists of the 3 T MRI scanner (Discovery 750w 3T, GE Healthcare, Waukesha, Wisconsin) and the time-of-flight PET/CT scanner (Discovery 690, GE Healthcare). Although the shuttle system minimizes the hardware-related image misregistration, errors could still occur because of patient motion between the two scans, and they could be particularly difficult to address in the case of the nonrigid deformation of different body regions. One advantage of the trimodality approach is that CT-based attenuation correction obviates the need for not yet validated MR-based methods. Another obvious advantage is that two scanners could be used separately, which could maximize the scanners' utilization except for those clinical situations in which both examinations are required.

Although most of the efforts in the preclinical arena have focused on simultaneous PET and MRI, devices that allow sequential acquisition have also been developed. In the simplest approach, an MR- and PET-compatible animal holder (that includes the devices required for anesthesia, physiological monitoring, etc.) can be used to transport the animal between the two scanners. If conventional small-animal MR scanners (e.g., 7 T) are used for this purpose, the two scanners have to be located in separate rooms, given the more stringent shielding requirements. On the other hand, lower field magnets (e.g., 1 T) that have a minimal external stray field could be placed in the vicinity of a preclinical PET scanner without any performance degradation. Interestingly, it has been recently demonstrated that one of these 1 T MR scanners provides excellent-quality morphological images, comparable to those obtained with the 7 T device, and these data can be successfully combined with PET images for studying animal models of neurology, cardiovascular, or oncology diseases (Schmid et al. 2013). A fully integrated hybrid system (i.e., the PET and MR scanners share the same gantry) is now commercially available (nanoScan PET/MRI, Mediso, Budapest, Hungary). This scanner combines a 1 T permanent magnet with a PMT-based PET scanner capable of achieving 700 μm resolution using a state-of-the-art image reconstruction engine (Mediso).

15.3.3 PET DATA CORRECTIONS IN AN INTEGRATED PET/MR SCANNER

15.3.3.1 MR-BASED PHOTON ATTENUATION CORRECTION

The absorption of the 511 keV annihilation photons before they reach the PET detectors by interactions with the subject and other materials placed in the PET FOV leads to a reduction in the number of detected photons, affecting the PET data quantification. To compensate, methods to measure the attenuation along all lines of response have initially been proposed. They were based on using either external gamma-ray-emitting sources rotated in the FOV or the information provided by the CT in integrated PET/CT scanners. However, these methods cannot be used in integrated PET/MRI scanners because these systems are not equipped with a transmission source or a CT scanner. Instead, approaches for deriving similar information from the MR images had to be developed. This is not straightforward because the MR signal does not directly reflect tissue linear attenuation coefficients, being related to proton density and tissue relation times rather than electron density. Furthermore, other aspects have to be considered in an integrated PET/MR scanner, such as the challenging task of imaging bone or lung tissue with conventional MR sequences, the limited FOV of MR that leads to truncation artifacts in larger patients, the interaction of the 511 keV photons with the RF MR coils located in the PET FOV, and the mismatch between the MR-derived attenuation map and the emission data caused by motion.

15.3.3.2 TISSUE ATTENUATION CORRECTION

15.3.3.2.1 Methods to generate discrete-valued attenuation maps

Identifying bone is particularly relevant for accurate attenuation correction in neurological PET studies, as this tissue class has the highest linear attenuation coefficient, and inaccuracies in its estimation can introduce large biases in the adjacently located cortical structures (Catana et al. 2010). Additionally, a spatial gradient in the radial direction was reported in patient and phantom studies when bone tissue was misclassified as soft tissue (Andersen et al. 2014).

Segmenting the head MR images into different tissue classes was initially proposed as an alternative to transmission scanning even before integrated PET/MR human scanners were developed (Zaidi et al. 2003). In this first approach that required some manual intervention, a fuzzy clustering technique was used to segment the MR images into air, skull, brain tissue, and nasal cavities. Although good correlation was observed when comparing the PET images reconstructed using the MR- and the transmission-based attenuation correction methods, an overall overestimation of the activity was reported using the former.

Since using conventional MRI pulse sequences bone tissue and air-filled cavities are very difficult to distinguish, novel sequences have been developed to address this challenge. These ultrashort echo time (UTE) sequences can be used to image tissues with very short T2 relaxation times, such as bone (Reichert et al. 2005; Robson and Bydder 2006), and several methods for generating segmented head attenuation maps from these data have been implemented. The first methods proposed focused on segmenting the head into three compartments (i.e., bone and soft tissue and air cavities) based on the relationship between the two echoes on a voxel-by-voxel basis (Catana et al. 2010; Keereman et al. 2008). The contrast between the different compartments was enhanced using simple mathematical operations to postprocess the data. A triple-echo UTE (UTILE) MRI sequence was then proposed to also segment fat tissue using a 3-point Dixon-like decomposition (Berker et al. 2012). Although good overall agreement between the UTE-derived attenuation maps and those obtained by segmenting the corresponding CT images was reported, there were still misclassified voxels, particularly at the air-soft tissue and bone-soft tissue interfaces, and the skull tissue was overestimated, likely due to the partial volume effects inherent in segmentation-based approaches. Significantly improved attenuation maps were obtained by incorporating dual-echo UTE and T1-weighted MRI data and a probabilistic atlas. The Dice similarity coefficients quantifying agreement between the Atlas-T1w-DUTE and segmented CT-based attenuation maps for the 13 glioblastoma patients included in the study were 0.81, 0.96, and 0.69 for bone, soft tissue, and air, respectively. In terms of PET data quantification, the mean of the absolute relative change values was 1.75% (Poynton et al. 2014).

For whole-body imaging, the first approach utilized for attenuation correction was to segment the body into three components (i.e., water, lung, and air) as on the Philips Ingenuity TF PET/MRI scanner (Schulz et al. 2011), or four compartments (i.e., water, fat, lung, and air), as on the Siemens Biograph mMR scanner (Martinez-Moller et al. 2009), and to neglect the bone (Figure 15.3). Not surprisingly, the largest changes in SUV estimation using this attenuation correction method were observed in the bone (up to 13%), followed by lung and neck lesions, but the clinical interpretation was not affected in 52 of the lesions examined.

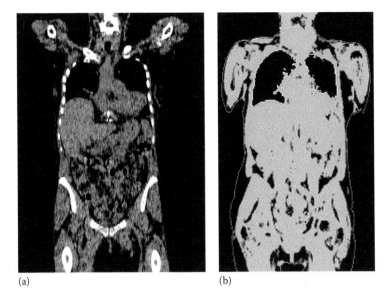

(a)   (b)

Figure 15.3 Whole-body MR-based attenuation correction: (a) CT- and (b) segmented VIBE-based attenuation maps. The patient was positioned arms up and arms down for the PET/CT and PET/MR exams, respectively. Note that only four tissue classes (i.e., water, fat, lung, and air) are present in the MR-based attenuation map.

Nevertheless, even these relatively small changes could be significant for patient follow-up when comparable SUV changes are expected in response to therapy (Martinez-Moller et al. 2009). Equally concerning is the variability in the performance of the segmentation procedure between subjects, particularly in the lung region (Schramm et al. 2013).

Simulation studies were also performed to investigate these effects (Akbarzadeh et al. 2013; Keereman et al. 2011). For example, the effect of using a limited set of segments, instead of the seven classes that could be discriminated by clustering the CT values (i.e., air, lung, adipose tissue, soft tissue, liver, and spongious and cortical bone), and the errors introduced by tissue misclassification have been investigated (Keereman et al. 2011). Errors below 5% were reported when liver and adipose tissue were treated as soft tissue and only five tissue classes were included in the attenuation map. The largest errors were introduced when a linear attenuation coefficient corresponding to air was assigned to the lung tissue (i.e., up to 45% in lung tissue and 17% in the thoracic spine). The second largest source of errors (up to 20%) was caused by the removal of cortical bone from the segmentation. A similar study using simulated phantom and clinical data confirmed the importance of segmenting the bone and reported errors of up to 30% in bone and adjacent tissue otherwise (Akbarzadeh et al. 2013). As expected, the errors introduced by tissue misclassification depended on the proportion of voxels incorrectly identified and the differences between the linear attenuation coefficients of the tissue classes involved (i.e., more significant errors are introduced when bone is classified as air or vice versa).

Interestingly, a lower systematic bias was observed using the three-class than the four-class segmentation method, except for the lung region, where the latter was superior (Arabi et al. 2015). On the other hand, including the bone tissue class was shown to reduce the SUV underestimation in spine and liver lesions (Kim et al. 2012). Furthermore, the magnitude of the error introduced by the misclassification of bone tissue seemed to depend on the composition of the lesions involved, ranging on average from 15.9% to 7.2% for sclerotic and osteolytic spine lesions, respectively (Samarin et al. 2012). When bone segmentation is possible, assigning an attenuation value corresponding to spongious bone (i.e., 350 HU) reduces the bias in bone lesions (Aznar et al. 2014).

One very important issue when scanning the patients with their arms down (as is typically done in MRI) or in the case of very large patients is the truncation artifact caused by the limited FOV of the MR compared with that of the PET (Delso et al. 2010). In these cases, parts of the arms are actually missing from the

MR-derived attenuation map, which leads to 10%–20% bias in the resulting PET images. The first solution proposed to address this issue was to use the non-attenuation-corrected PET images to guide the placement of a pair of cylinders that approximated the missing arms, which was shown to reduce the bias to ±2% in simulation studies (Delso et al. 2010). A similar solution was proposed for the Philips scanner, except that a more advanced algorithm was used to estimate the contour of the body from the non-attenuation-corrected PET images (Kalemis et al. 2013). In both cases, linear attenuation coefficients corresponding to soft tissue were assigned to the missing voxels, including those corresponding to bone tissue. A more advanced method for addressing the truncation issue is discussed later in this chapter.

To assess the performance of the attenuation correction procedure in realistic clinical situations, several initial PET/MRI studies have focused on comparing the SUVs obtained from PET/CT and PET/MRI (Drzezga et al. 2012; Heusch et al. 2013; Kershah et al. 2013; Partovi et al. 2013; Bini et al. 2013). Although the correlation reported was variable but overall good, the consensus was that the PET/MRI data could be used for routine clinical studies. These comparisons are intrinsically difficult to perform because the datasets are acquired sequentially on the two scanners, and thus changes in SUVs could also occur due to biological factors given the substantial delay between the two acquisitions.

15.3.3.2.2 Methods to generate continuous-valued attenuation maps

Atlas- or template-based methods have been proposed for obtaining continuous-valued attenuation maps. The atlas or template can be obtained after anatomic standardization either from transmission or CT images (Montandon and Zaidi 2005; Rota Kops and Herzog 2008). In one of the first attempts (Montandon and Zaidi 2005), a fluorodeoxyglucose (FDG)–PET template was coregistered to the subject's PET volume reconstructed with an approximate attenuation correction, and the same transformation matrix was then applied to the transmission template. Although the emission data corrected using this method were deemed qualitatively acceptable and suitable for routine research and clinical applications, the quantitative voxel-based analysis demonstrated under- and overestimation of the activity in various brain structures.

As atlas-based methods are particularly susceptible to errors in the image registration procedure, local pattern recognition combined with atlas registration was proposed to reduce these errors (Hofmann et al. 2008). The idea was that knowledge of the properties of the voxels in the neighborhood of the voxel of interest (i.e., the patch) could improve the estimation of a pseudo-CT value directly from the MR data. The information in the atlas allowed the selection of the patch that most likely matched the patch of interest by restricting the search to a specific anatomical region where the voxel of interest is located. Using this method, the reported mean error in PET quantification in predefined regions of interest was 3.2%. Although this method was specifically developed and tested for brain imaging, the authors claimed that it could also be applied to other regions based on initial results obtained using one MRI/CT rabbit dataset (Hofmann et al. 2008).

Another common limitation of atlas-based methods is that they can potentially fail in the case of subjects with modified anatomy (e.g., postsurgery) or in regions with variable anatomy (e.g., abdomen). CT-similar images could in principle be obtained from the MR data without using an atlas. Johansson et al. (2011) proposed a method to derive substitute CTs from the MR data acquired using two dual-echo UTE sequences with different flip angles and a T2-weighted SPACE sequence. Using a Gaussian mixture regression model, the intensities in the MR images were linked to the Hounsfield units in the corresponding CT images for the five patients enrolled in the study. The two echo times (0.07 and 3.76 ms) and two flip angles (10° and 60°) for the UTE sequences allowed the discrimination of voxels with short versus long T2* and of voxels with short T2* but different T1, respectively. The T2-weighted SPACE was initially included to facilitate the separation of voxels with long T1 (e.g., cerebrospinal fluid) from air, but these data were later found redundant (Johansson et al. 2012). Acknowledging the difficulty in generating CT-equivalent images from MR data due to the differences in the physical principles underlying the two modalities, the same authors also proposed a method to evaluate the uncertainty in their estimation of the substitute CT values (Johansson et al. 2012).

In another method that uses MR data exclusively, an air mask was first generated from the UTE1, in- and opposed-phase 2-point Dixon–volume-interpolated breath-hold examination (VIBE) images. Subsequently, a support vector regression technique was used to derive pseudo-CT values from MR data. The method was developed and tested using the CT/MR/PET brain datasets available from five subjects, and a mean absolute

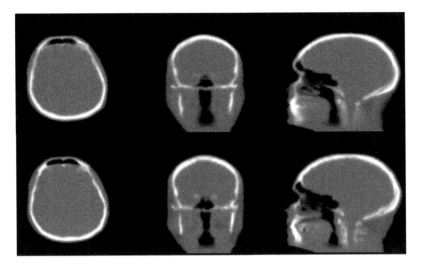

Figure 15.4 Head MR-based attenuation correction: (a) Continuous-valued attenuation maps derived from the MR data acquired with an MPRAGE sequence using a hybrid atlas–segmentation-based approach and (b) the corresponding scaled CT-based attenuation map, demonstrating very good overall agreement. (Images courtesy of Dr. David Izquierdo, A. A. Martinos Center, Massachusetts General Hospital, Boston.)

error of 2.4% was reported for the regions investigated. Initial results also suggested that this method could be extended to other body regions where accurate registration between the MR and CT images used for training can be achieved (e.g., pelvis) (Navalpakkam et al. 2013).

A patch-based method was also proposed to generate synthetic CT images from the UTE images (Roy et al. 2014). Instead of performing registration of segmentation, this approach relies on the identification of similar patterns of intensities (patches) between the subject of interest and the reference patches from the database.

An SPM8-based method for generating a head attenuation map from a single morphological MR dataset was recently proposed (Figure 15.4). The MR images are first segmented into six tissue classes using the "New Segment" SPM8 tool, and are then coregistered to a previously created template using a diffeomorphic nonrigid image registration algorithm (SPM8 DARTEL). The inverse transformation is finally applied to obtain the pseudo-CT in the subject space. The quantitative analysis showed small errors in brain linear attenuation coefficient estimation ($1.86 \pm 4.06\%$ relative change) compared with the scaled CT method. The voxel- and ROI-based analysis of the corresponding reconstructed PET images revealed quantification errors of $3.87 \pm 5.0\%$ and $2.74 \pm 2.28\%$, respectively (Izquierdo-Garcia et al. 2014).

For whole-body applications, a registration-based approach was suggested for adding bone tissue to the segmented pseudo-CT obtained from the MR data by deriving the missing information from a CT database. The most similar CT from the database was selected based on 19 similarity metrics (e.g., sex, height, age, body-normed superior–inferior center of mass, and lung volume) and nonrigidly coregistered to the subject's MRI. Finally, the structures with Hounsfield units greater than 80 were added to the pseudo-CTs, and the standard scaling procedure was used to generate the PET attenuation maps. The relative errors observed in the subjects investigated were significantly reduced using this procedure (from –37% to –8% to –3% to 4%), especially in volumes of interest containing bone. However, several limitations have been identified, including the need for operator intervention for several of the metrics proposed (e.g., to specify the profile of the spine and the shape of the pelvis) (Marshall et al. 2013).

15.3.3.2.3 Methods using the emission data to iteratively improve the attenuation map

All the MR-based attenuation correction methods discussed above share the same limitation—using only the MR data and atlases or templates of linear attenuation coefficients, it is impossible to account for large inter-subject variability. Additional data are required to overcome this limitation, and an interesting approach is to incorporate the information inherently present in the PET emission data (Censor et al. 1979). This class of methods, which was initially proposed for deriving attenuation maps even before the introduction of transmission-based approaches, has regained popularity in recent years after the advent of integrated PET/MR and time-of-flight PET (Mollet et al. 2012; Panin et al. 2013; Rezaei et al. 2012; Salomon et al. 2011; Censor et al. 1979). This is because the anatomical information provided by the MR or the time-of-flight minimizes the attenuation emission estimation "cross talk" that limited the usefulness of the early approaches (i.e., any errors in the estimation of the emission image lead to compensatory errors in the estimation of the attenuation image). In the context of attenuation correction for PET/MRI, this class of methods can be used in a number of ways. For example, a modified version of the previously proposed maximum-likelihood reconstruction of attenuation and activity (MLAA) algorithm (Nuyts et al. 1999) has been implemented for addressing the truncation artifact described above. The missing data can be recovered using the emission data as currently implemented on the Siemens Biograph mMR scanner. This method was shown to reduce the error in the SUV estimation from 15%–50% (Delso et al. 2010) to less than 5% (Nuyts et al. 2010). As another example, a similar method and the time-of-flight information were used to improve the estimation of the linear attenuation coefficients assigned to the different regions segmented from the MR data (Salomon et al. 2011). In principle, starting from a continuous-valued attenuation map, this technique could be used to further refine the linear attenuation coefficients in the regions where their estimation is uncertain.

15.3.3.2.4 Additional considerations for whole-body attenuation correction

In addition to correctly estimating the attenuation of bone tissue, which is arguably not as critical outside the brain except for certain applications and in specific body regions (e.g., head and neck, spine, and pelvis), other aspects have to be considered for implementing an accurate whole-body MR-based attenuation correction method.

Imaging the lungs with conventional MR sequences is very challenging, but this is an organ in which large variability in attenuation has been reported (Martinez-Moller et al. 2009; Schulz et al. 2011). Additionally, the lung attenuation properties change during the different phases of the respiratory cycle, and even more so in diseased versus normal conditions (Marshall et al. 2012). At least in the near future, estimating the lung attenuation maps will continue to be one of the most challenging aspects in PET/MRI. Accurate quantification will likely be clinically relevant in the thorax, for both oncology and cardiovascular applications, and progress in this area will require development of advanced fast MR sequences for improved lung imaging.

Any implants that cause susceptibility artifacts in the MR images will lead to errors in the attenuation map. These effects were initially reported in brain PET/MRI studies when dental fillings and implants were observed to affect the attenuation maps generated from DUTE data (Catana et al. 2010). Endoprostheses of the hips are causing beam-hardening effects in CT and severely bias the CT-derived attenuation maps. Although the majority of these devices are considered MR-safe, the susceptibility artifacts cause signal voids on the MR images, and thus linear attenuation coefficients corresponding to air are assigned to the voxels affected, leading to inaccurate PET quantification. A simple semiautomated method that allows for the assignment of linear attenuation coefficients corresponding to titanium alloy to these voxels has already been suggested for addressing this issue (Ladefoged et al. 2013). Alternatively, MR sequences that are less sensitive to susceptibility artifacts (Ai et al. 2012; Sutter et al. 2012) have been proposed to minimize these effects and could likely be applied to PET/MRI.

The effect of oral and intravenous CT contrast agents on PET attenuation correction in PET/CT scanners has been extensively investigated (Ahmadian et al. 2008; Antoch et al. 2003, 2004; Cohade et al. 2003; Dizendorf et al. 2003; Nehmeh et al. 2003). The presence of these iodinated agents leads to an increase in the Hounsfield units in the CT images without a proportional increase in the linear attenuation coefficients at 511 keV, which means the PET attenuation maps derived from these CT images are biased. As MR contrast agents are also routinely used for MRI, the potential effects of MR contrast agents on the PET attenuation maps generated from these data have to be understood. In an initial study, it was shown that ferumoxil (an oral contrast agent that contains iron oxide particles) and gadobutrol (a gadolinium-based intravenous agent) at clinically relevant concentrations have attenuation properties similar to those of water and, in general, do not bias the attenuation maps (Lois et al. 2012). An exception reported in this study is the accumulation of iron oxide–based contrast agent in the stomach, which leads to the assignment of lung attenuation coefficient to these voxels, an issue that can be relatively easily corrected using a more advanced method for generating the attenuation map. In another study, it was reported that ferumoxytol (an ultrasmall supramagnetic iron oxide–based intravenous contrast agent) has the potential to significantly alter the attenuation map, particularly in the liver, where the effect can persist for more than 5 weeks (Borra et al. 2013).

Finally, a common source of errors for all attenuation correction methods is the misregistration between the emission volume and the attenuation map, usually caused by subject motion. These effects can be reduced on an integrated PET/MR scanner. First, the hardware coregistration is likely to be at least as accurate as the software coregistration of the separately acquired datasets. More importantly, the temporal correlation of the PET and MR signals allows simultaneous acquisition systems to use the MR signal for tracking the motion of the subject dynamically *during* the PET acquisition and for correcting the PET data retrospectively, as discussed later in this chapter.

In a recent study aimed at assessing the impact of time-of-flight PET data on the errors introduced by some of these factors, it was shown that the bias introduced by implants and motion can be significantly reduced. Similarly, the time-of-flight MR-based attenuation correction method helped reduce the errors in lesions in or near lung and bone tissue (Mehranian and Zaidi 2015).

15.3.3.3 HARDWARE ATTENUATION CORRECTION

The MR coils used in integrated PET/MRI scanners have to be redesigned to minimize photon attenuation and trade-offs between PET compatibility, MR performance and practical considerations have to be made. For example, although the smallest loop wire provides the least photon attenuation, the SNR also decreases with the wire diameter. Since the preamplifiers are the most attenuating components, they have to be placed outside of the PET FOV and connected to the loops using longer coaxial cables. Fortunately, the SNR loss is minimal when 10 cm long or shorter coaxial cables are used (Sander et al. 2015).

In the case of the manufacturer-provided one-channel transmit/eight-channel receive coil that was delivered with the BrainPET prototype, it was demonstrated that large bias could be introduced if the coil attenuation correction was ignored (Catana et al. 2010; Tellmann et al. 2011).

For the commercially available scanners, the major manufacturers provide the attenuation maps for the standard RF coils. For example, for the Biograph mMR scanner, Siemens provides the attenuation maps for the head and neck and spine coils and for the patient table. The body flexible arrays have been redesigned and built using low-attenuation materials, which can then be ignored for routine applications. For more advanced whole-body studies where accurate quantification is required, fiducial markers (e.g., cod liver capsules) can be used for determining the position of the coil in the PET FOV so that the coil attenuation map can be included in the attenuation correction procedure. Without this correction, deviations of up to 15% were observed in the regions close to the phantom and the results were also confirmed in patient scans (Paulus et al. 2012). In a different study, it was shown that when removing the surface coil, the mean SUV increased by 6% in the liver and by more than 20% in some of the tumor lesions analyzed. Furthermore, the number of recorded true coincidences decreased by 19% due to the presence of the patient table. The authors concluded that the PET/MR scan duration would have to be increased compared with PET/CT examinations to achieve similar statistics (Furst et al. 2014). For specific applications, such as dedicated breast imaging, a commercially available MR-only four-channel receive array was carefully evaluated. Although an 11% loss in true counts was reported in the presence of the coil, the signal attenuation was successfully accounted for using the previously generated CT-based coil attenuation map (Aklan et al. 2013).

Similarly, attenuation maps for the head, neurovascular, cardiac, spine, and breast coils, as well as for the patient table, are provided by Philips for its integrated scanner (Kalemis et al. 2013). Furthermore, given the sequential nature of the acquisition, some of these coils can be removed between the MR and PET exams with minimal patient repositioning. When MR coils that were not specifically designed to be "PET friendly" are needed, MR markers can be used to position the coil attenuation map previously derived from CT. For example, a V-spline registration algorithm gave the best results in the case of the flexible anterior part of the cardiac coil used with the Philips scanner. Using such a method, minimal local overestimation of the activity was reported in phantom and patient studies (Eldib et al. 2014).

In the case of the GE sequential approach (i.e., scanners located in adjacent rooms), the patient's head holder actually slides inside the RF coil and the torso coils are removed before the patient goes inside the PET/

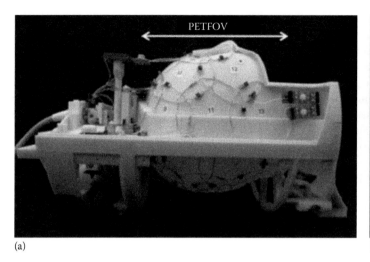
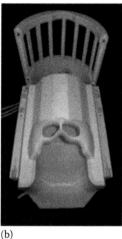

(a)   (b)

Figure 15.5 MR-compatible 31-channel coil for the BrainPET prototype: (a) Side view without the cover showing the placement of the components to minimize photon attenuation. (b) Placement inside the local transmit coil. (Originally published in Sander, C. Y., et al., *Magn. Reson. Med.*, 73(6), 2363–2375, 2015.)

CT scanner, obviating the need to redesign the RF coils for PET compatibility. Without these modifications, severe underestimation of the activity concentration (e.g., 20%) and image artifacts would be introduced by the head and surface coils (MacDonald et al. 2011). In the case of whole-body imaging, 6% bias was reported for the GE GEM anterior array coil. Furthermore, the bias when ignoring the coil was only slightly reduced when using the time-of-flight information (Wollenweber et al. 2014).

In addition to these coils that were redesigned by the scanner manufacturer to be PET compatible, organ-dedicated coils have also been developed for the brain (Figure 15.5) (Sander et al. 2015) and breast (Dregely et al. 2015) PET/MRI. In both cases, this was motivated by the need to improve MR performance to match that of stand-alone devices. For example, the 8-channel receive array delivered with the BrainPET prototype was inferior to the 32-channel array that was routinely used at the time. Similarly, using a 4-channel coil or the standard body array for breast imaging was deemed unacceptable when compared with the 16-channel version.

15.3.4 MR-ASSISTED PET MOTION CORRECTION

PET studies are usually long, and subject motion (voluntary and involuntary) is difficult to avoid, leading to degradation (blurring) of the images and severe artifacts when motion has large amplitude, often offsetting the benefit of using a high-resolution scanner. In a combined PET/MRI scanner, the MR data acquired simultaneously with the PET data can be used to derive high temporal resolution motion estimates. In general, motion correction is a twofold problem: first, motion has to be characterized, and then the motion estimates have to be integrated into the PET reconstruction. There are two distinct cases that have to be considered—rigid-body and non-rigid-body motion—each with distinct solutions for tracking the motion and applying the correction.

15.3.4.1 RIGID-BODY MOTION CORRECTION

In the case of rigid-body motion, the displacements of just three points completely characterize the motion of the whole volume, but no assumptions can be made about the amplitude, direction, or periodicity of the motion during the scan. This means a method to derive three-dimensional (3D) rigid-body transformations (i.e., three rotations, three translations) with high temporal resolution is required to accurately characterize the motion of the head throughout the PET data acquisition. MR could provide such information, and the potential of MR-assisted motion correction to improve the PET data quantification in brain studies was first demonstrated using the BrainPET prototype (Catana et al. 2011). In these proof-of-principle studies, motion estimates were derived from echo-planar imaging series or from embedded cloverleaf navigators (van der Kouwe et al. 2006). A data processing and motion compensation algorithm for PET data at full line of response resolution in frame mode was developed for applying these MR-derived transformers to the PET data. The list-mode dataset was first divided into frames of progressively longer duration according to the desired dynamic protocol. Each of these frames was subsequently divided into subframes based on the available motion estimates. After the reference position was selected (e.g., corresponding to the initial position of the head), the rigid-body transformation matrices for all the subsequent subframes were obtained from the MR data. These list-mode data from each subframe were histogrammed, generating prompt and random events line of response files. The motion was accounted for in the line of response space by "moving" the coordinates of all crystals based on the transformer. For each frame, prompt and random events sinograms were generated from these data. Since the RF coil is stationary with respect to the scanner, its attenuation cannot simply be combined with the head attenuation, and it was instead combined with the sensitivity. The sensitivity sinogram for each frame was then obtained by transforming the coil-corrected sensitivity line of response data. The rebinning dwell that accounts for the variable number of lines of response in each sinogram bin was also calculated in a similar way. The normalization sinogram was obtained from the summed time-weighted transformed sensitivity and dwell sinograms. The emission data from all the subframes were added in the sinogram space to obtain the corrected prompt and random coincidences files. Head attenuation and the scatter correction sinogram were estimated only for the reference frame. The motion-corrected PET volume was reconstructed from these summed sinograms using the standard reconstruction algorithm.

As opposed to applying the motion correction postreconstruction, combining the corrected data in the line of response space has the advantage of reducing the noise in the final images. Furthermore, this method allows the proper handling of the regions that are not inside the PET FOV during the whole scan.

The proof-of-principle studies in healthy volunteers performed using this method demonstrated substantial improvement in image quality (Figure 15.6) (e.g., cortical structures are more clearly visible after correction) and data quantification (e.g., more accurate time–activity curves) after applying the correction.

In principle, motion estimates could be derived from the MR data with a frequency of anywhere from 0.1 to 50 Hz. However, generating PET frames shorter than 1 s is likely not necessary for the majority of PET applications. Furthermore, processing thousands of very short frames would be very time-consuming, and a

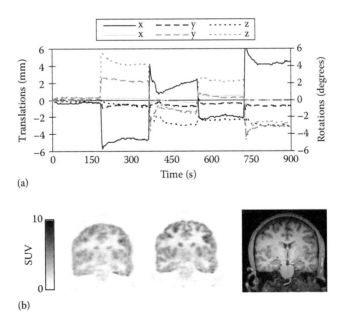

Figure 15.6 MR-assisted rigid-body motion correction in a healthy volunteer using EPI-derived motion estimates: (a) Plot of the motion estimates: Translations along (black) and rotations about (gray) the three orthogonal axes are shown. (b) PET data reconstructed before (first column) and after (second column) MC. Note the substantial improvement in the PET image quality after MC. The corresponding MR images are provided as a reference (third column). (Originally published in Catana, C., et al., *J. Nucl. Med.*, 52(1), 154–161, 2011.)

method to use the MR information to guide the framing of the PET data has been recently proposed (Ullisch et al. 2012). A new frame could be started when the mean voxel displacement of the brain relative to the reference position exceeds a certain threshold, which significantly reduces the number of frames that have to be processed. Furthermore, a generic list-mode-based reconstruction algorithm, called PRESTO, was proposed to eliminate the need for axial and transaxial data compression, as is typically required when sinogram-based image reconstruction algorithms are used (Ullisch et al. 2012).

15.3.4.2 NON-RIGID-BODY MOTION CORRECTION

As opposed to the rigid-body case, the displacement of each voxel in the PET FOV has to be estimated for performing non-rigid-body motion correction.

Non-rigid PET motion correction using MR-derived motion estimates was first demonstrated using a two-section phantom (Tsoumpas et al. 2010). Although the motion of the phantom did not mimic the typical motion observed in human studies, the goal of the study was to demonstrate that simultaneously acquired MR data could be used for this purpose.

Internal organ deformations related to cardiac and respiratory motion affect the PET data quality and quantification in the thorax and abdomen. Although these two sources of error have to be addressed concurrently (particularly in the thorax) before these methods can be used routinely, the first efforts in this area focused on providing solutions to each of them separately. Since respiratory motion predominates in the abdomen, various techniques (e.g., respiratory bellows and interleaved MR navigators that track the translation of the diaphragm) are currently used for respiratory gating in both PET and MRI studies. However, these techniques provide minimal information about the non-rigid-body motion of the internal organs.

Tagged-MRI has been suggested for tracking the motion in the abdomen (Guerin et al. 2011; Chun et al. 2012). In simulation, phantom, small-animal, and nonhuman primate studies, a complementary spatial modulation of magnetization (C-SPAMM) sequence (Axel and Dougherty 1989) was proposed for MRI-tagging and either a regularized HARmonic phase (r-HARP) (Osman et al. 2000) or B-spline nonrigid image registration algorithm was used for tracking the motion vector fields. This information was included in the system matrix of an iterative PET reconstruction algorithm so that all the detected coincidences can be used to generate the final image. In other words, this method allowed the "freezing" of the motion in any of the desired reference frames. As opposed to standard gating techniques, in which the majority of the detected events are actually discarded and do not contribute to the final image for a particular frame, the image variance is considerably reduced after motion correction, which leads to improvements in SNR and contrast recovery coefficients (Figure 15.7). One disadvantage of this method is that the tagged-MR images cannot be used for clinical purposes given the lack of contrast and relatively low spatial resolution.

Another challenge that has to be considered is the significant variability in breathing patterns both during the respiratory cycle (the motion paths during inspiration are different than those observed during respiration) and between respiratory cycles. A statistical model was proposed to characterize and account for the intra- and inter-cycle motion of the thorax during respiration (King et al. 2012). The model is derived from a dynamic 3D MRI dataset by estimating the motion vector fields using principal component analysis. Instead of using a one-dimensional (1D) navigator (e.g., external marker or displacement of the diaphragm), the model applied is based on two-dimensional (2D) image navigators. The navigator can be positioned in a way that maximizes the performance of the model and is continuously acquired until the similarity between the target and warped images exceeds a certain threshold. When this happens, a new set of dynamic 3D MRI data is acquired and the model is updated.

Although these methods showed promise for addressing the issue of respiratory motion in the abdomen (e.g., the liver, spleen, pancreas or kidney, and adrenal gland), one common limitation was that it is currently challenging to apply them in the thorax because of the reduced SNR of the lungs. In these early studies, either the lung tissue was masked out to avoid introducing bias in adjacent regions (Guerin et al. 2011) or the lung motion fields were interpolated from those estimated at the boundaries (King et al. 2012). It should be noted, though, that MR methods for improving lung imaging are constantly being developed, and the performance of MR-assisted PET motion (as well as attenuation) correction in this very important region will likely improve.

A similar method has been proposed for MR-assisted cardiac motion correction, and proof-of-principle studies were initially performed on the BrainPET scanner using a cardiac beating phantom (Petibon et al.

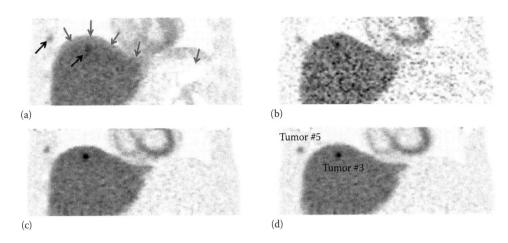

(a)

(b)

Tumor #5

(c)

Tumor #3

(d)

Figure 15.7 Simulation studies demonstrating the potential of MR-assisted PET non-rigid-body motion correction for improving the PET image quality in abdominal imaging. Simulated PET images without motion correction (a), reconstructed using only the events from one gate (b), corrected with motion estimates derived from the tagged-MRI simulations (c), and using the reference motion fields (d). (Originally published in Guerin, B., et al., *Med. Phys.*, 38(6), 3025–3038, 2011.)

2013). A SPAMM sequence was used for MR tagging, and a multislice/multiphase gradient recalled echo sequence was run to acquire multiple representative volumes during the cycle. A nonrigid B-spline registration algorithm (Ledesma-Carbayo et al. 2008) was preferred in this case for estimating the motion vector fields in all three directions from the tagged-MRI volumes, instead of the HARP method that was previously proposed for characterizing the respiratory motion. Partially sampling the k-space was proposed for reducing the acquisition time. The motion estimates were incorporated into a list-mode iterative reconstruction framework. Additionally, the point-spread function of the scanner was estimated and also included in the model so that the image degradation due to partial volume effects could also be minimized. Significantly improved contrast recovery and lesion detectability compared with the gated and no-motion-corrected cases were reported.

Proof-of-principle MR-based motion correction studies have been performed in oncological patients scanned on the Biograph mMR scanner (Wurslin et al. 2013). A multislice 2D spoiled gradient echo sequence was used to estimate the motion for the region located in the PET FOV. Multiple slices were defined in the sagittal orientation (which was chosen to maintain the largest in-plane displacements), and multiple frames were acquired for each slice over one respiratory cycle. The position of the diaphragm was also recorded before each frame using a navigator. These data were used to define the respiratory gates and the frame mean respiratory position. Four-dimensional (4D) volumes were generated from the acquired 2D data by selecting for each slice the image closest to the mean position out of all the available frames and discarding the rest. The motion fields were derived from these 4D data using a nonrigid registration algorithm. Instead of including this information in the reconstruction, the PET images reconstructed for each respiratory gate were individually reconstructed. For this purpose, attenuation maps corresponding to each gate were generated from the attenuation map generated as described in Section 15.3.3. The final PET image was generated by summing the individual PET images corresponding to each gate transformed based on the motion field and weighted according to the number of counts detected during each gate. The resulting images were superior to those uncorrected in terms of contrast, lesion delineation, estimated lesion volume, and SNR. However, the contrast and uptake quantification were better for the gated images, which is probably due to the limited number of gates and the fact that the images are combined postreconstruction. Methods that include the motion model directly into the iterative reconstruction algorithm have been shown to be superior to those applying the correction postreconstruction (Dikaios et al. 2012). Another limitation of this method is that the 2D MR images acquired for estimating the motion are not particularly useful for clinical diagnosis.

A framework for estimating both the respiratory and cardiac motion at the same time has recently been presented (Ouyang et al. 2013). A combination of MR tagging and 1D navigator sequences can be used to estimate the cardiac and respiratory motion, respectively. If the cardiac and respiratory cycles are each divided into 8 phases, a total of 64 combined phases need to be considered. One of these phases is selected as the reference, and the motion fields for the other 63 phases need to be estimated to characterize the complex displacements. The motion field can be estimated using the HARP or B-spline nonrigid image registration algorithms. The main limitation of this approach is that acquiring the data needed for accurately estimating the motion fields for all the phases would require very long acquisition times. In practical situations, many of these phases will be undersampled. The missing information could be "recovered" using compressed sensing techniques to reconstruct the MR volumes corresponding to undersampled phases. In extreme cases, when virtually no data are available for a particular phase, the motion fields for the missing volumes could be obtained through interpolation from those estimated for the adjacent phases.

More work is still required for the development and validation of MR-assisted non-rigid-body PET motion estimation and correction methods. More importantly, before any such method can be adopted for routine clinical use, the total acquisition time of the MR sequence used for characterizing the motion has to be minimized. Accelerated tagged-MRI using either parallel imaging or compressed sensing approaches has been recently suggested for this purpose, and the PET image quality was similar to that obtained from fully sampled MR data for up to four times acceleration (Huang et al. 2015). Alternatively, a generalized reconstruction by inversion of coupled systems (GRICS) approach (Odille et al. 2008) could be used with any MR sequence to obtain both the MR image and the motion model that can be retrospectively applied to the PET data (Fayad et al. 2015). Although not specifically discussed here, data-driven methods have also been suggested for deriving the motion information directly from the PET data (Dawood et al. 2013). A recent study comparing the MR- and PET-based approaches has shown that comparable results can be obtained with the latter in terms of both the respiratory signal extraction and motion vector field derivation (Furst et al. 2015). Studies comparing and cross-validating the two approaches for various applications will likely be performed in the near future. Additionally, more advanced phantoms, such as the torso phantom that mimics respiratory and cardiac motion, will be needed for generating no-motion ground truth data and for testing these methods in near-realistic situations (Fieseler et al. 2013).

An MR-based motion correction approach could also eventually be used in even more difficult situations, such as nonperiodic non-rigid-body motion (e.g., motion of the neck or spine, bowel movement, and filling of the bladder). For example, this motion could be modeled from the repeatedly acquired volumetric data using fast MR sequences.

Although many challenges still remain, MR-assisted PET motion correction could dramatically reduce the spatial blurring and artifacts associated with PET movement of solid organs. If techniques to track the motion in the background of the sequences used for acquiring standard MR data are successfully developed, this unique opportunity enabled by simultaneous PET and MRI could completely revolutionize the way PET is performed in certain body regions (e.g., brain, lung, heart, and liver).

15.3.5 Other methods for improving the PET data quantification using the MR information

15.3.5.1 PARTIAL VOLUME EFFECTS CORRECTION

Partial volume effects are caused by the PET scanner's limited spatial resolution (and tissue fraction effects) and lead to an underestimation of the radiotracer concentration in structures of interest that are smaller than two to three times the FWHM spatial resolution of the scanner, as well as an overestimation of the activity in the adjacent structures, the so-called spill-out and spill-in effects. The problem is further complicated by the spatial variability of the point-spread function across the FOV of the PET scanner. An example of partial volume effects correction for an NNC112 study performed on the BrainPET scanner is shown in Figure 15.8. A very comprehensive review of the myriad partial volume effects correction methods and examples of their use in neurology, oncology, and cardiology has recently been published (Erlandsson et al. 2012). In the context of PET/MRI, those approaches that use the anatomical information derived from MRI for performing the correction, either post- or during the image reconstruction, are particularly relevant. At this time, no one method has been accepted or is routinely used for research applications, and even less so in clinical practice. This is probably because the

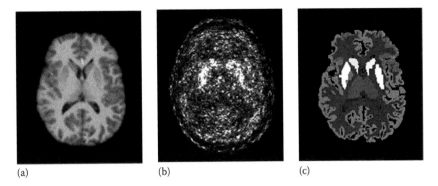

(a)   (b)   (c)

Figure 15.8 Partial volume effects correction. (a) Morphological MR data used to segment the brain structures of interest and the corresponding PET image before partial volume effects correction (b) and the map showing the mean regional uptake after PVEC (c). (Data courtesy of Dr. Joshua Roffman, Massachusetts General Hospital, Boston.)

performance of these methods is task specific and there is no optimal method that can be used in all situations. More importantly, the performance also depends on the accuracy of the anatomical segmentation procedure and the precision of the spatial coregistration of the PET and MRI volumes. Even in the case of neurological applications, the segmentation of very small brain structures is difficult and the image registration is affected by head motion during the scan. These tasks are even more challenging outside the brain, although partial volume effects correction could be very relevant for treatment monitoring in oncology or assessing myocardial perfusion, to give just two examples. The rigid- and non-rigid-body motion correction methods discussed in Section 15.3.4 would eliminate the image coregistration problem in integrated PET/MRI scanners.

15.3.5.2 IMAGE-BASED RADIOTRACER ARTERIAL INPUT FUNCTION ESTIMATION

Deriving parameters of interest after kinetic modeling of the time–activity curves derived from dynamic PET data requires knowledge of the radiotracer arterial input function. The gold standard technique involves arterial cannulation and manual (or automatic) blood sampling throughout the PET acquisition. However, this procedure is invasive, cannot be used in all patient populations, and requires specialized personnel for placing and managing the arterial line. Alternatively, image-based methods have been proposed to derive similar information directly from the PET images (e.g., see Zanotti-Fregonara et al. 2011 for an excellent review on this topic), and the anatomical and physiological information acquired simultaneously with MRI could facilitate this task.

As a first step to deriving the radiotracer arterial input function from the PET images, an arterial mask has to be defined. In the case of whole-body applications, the input function can be obtained from regions of interest defined on the heart, aorta, and even femoral arteries, which are relatively large and thus minimally affected by partial volume effects. In the case of brain studies, the vessels of interest are considerably smaller. Time-of-flight MR angiography sequences are capable of resolving both large and small arterial structures using bright-blood techniques; however, acquiring these data for extended FOVs can be quite time-consuming. The standard sequences for acquiring morphological data (e.g., MPRAGE) also exhibit a hyperintense arterial blood signal in larger vessels. A very accurate arterial mask can be obtained from these data using filtering, postprocessing operations, and clustering techniques. Preliminary studies performed using data acquired on the BrainPET prototype demonstrated good correspondence between the image-based FDG arterial input function obtained after accounting for partial volume effects in the vessels included in the arterial mask and the gold standard technique (Chonde and Catana 2012). The final validation will likely benefit from an MR-compatible blood sampler capable of high-temporal arterial sampling (Breuer et al. 2010).

Another interesting opportunity is to use the MR contrast agent input function for improving the estimation of the radiotracer input function. In a recent study comparing the two curves in a small-animal glioma model, it was shown that the Gd-DTPA input curve could be converted into the FDG curve (and vice versa) so that only one is needed for performing dual pharmacokinetic modeling (Poulin et al. 2013). At first, this might seem to benefit MRI more than PET given the challenging task of quantitatively estimating the MR contrast agent input function from the images. However, once such methods are validated, they could be used to improve the estimation of the radiotracer input function, particularly of the rapidly changing early part of the curve that is difficult to estimate from the PET data given the limited statistics in these early frames.

15.4 PROMISING RESEARCH AND CLINICAL APPLICATIONS

In this section, only a few examples of potential applications are briefly discussed. For a more detailed discussion, the interested reader is referred to several review papers published on this topic focusing on neuropsychiatry, oncology, and cardiology applications (Catana et al. 2012, 2013; Yankeelov et al. 2012; Judenhofer and Cherry 2013; Rischpler et al. 2013; Garibotto et al. 2013; Buchbender et al. 2012a, 2012b).

The improvement in PET data quantification using the MR-assisted methods discussed in the previous sections could benefit virtually all neurological applications for which quantification is important. To give just one example, motion and partial volume effects correction are particularly relevant in Alzheimer's disease patients, and more accurate corrections would allow one to address two of the most important confounding factors that bias the interpretation of PET measurements in the small and anatomically complex structures (e.g., hippocampus) that are of interest in this patient population.

Many other neuropsychiatric disorders (e.g., depression and schizophrenia) are in need of multimodal imaging biomarkers, and PET/MRI could facilitate translational investigations in these patient populations. A very interesting opportunity is to use PET/MRI to simultaneously assess changes in brain neurochemistry (PET) and brain activity (MRI) in response to pharmacological or physiological challenges. In the first study of this type, the temporal and spatial relationship between the changes in dopamine receptor occupancy and cerebral blood volume in response to the administration of pharmacological doses of a D2/D3 receptor antagonist was assessed in nonhuman primates using the BrainPET prototype (Figure 15.9) (Sander et al. 2013).

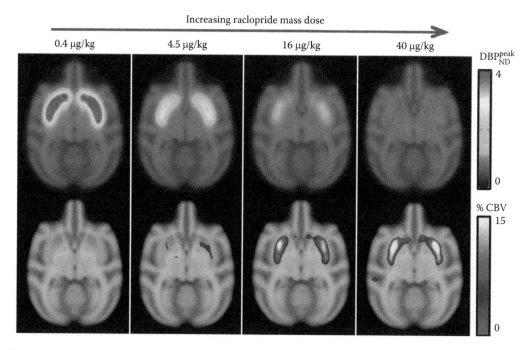

Figure 15.9 Nonhuman primate simultaneous PET and MRI study demonstrating similar spatial distribution and dose-dependent changes in raclopride PET binding and functional MRI–measured cerebral blood volume. (Originally published in Sander, C. Y., et al., *Proc. Natl. Acad. Sci. U.S.A.*, 110(27), 11169–11174, 2013.)

There are several low-hanging fruit applications in oncology in which the benefits of PET/MR over PET/CT are most obvious (Catana et al. 2013). First, replacing CT with MRI for providing anatomical correlates for PET significantly reduces the radiation exposure, which is particularly relevant in patients for which this is of concern (e.g., children, lymphoma patients that require multiple PET/CT scans, and women). Second, PET/MRI will be the modality of choice in areas of the body where CT is suboptimal because of the poor soft tissue contrast (i.e., head and neck, and pelvis). Third, PET/MRI will be preferred in areas in which MRI provides improved tissue specificity (e.g., liver, breast, and bone marrow) (Figure 15.10).

There are of course more advanced applications in which PET/MRI can go beyond what PET/CT can offer. An example is treatment monitoring in oncology in which the richer dataset collected using both modalities and the improved PET quantification might have a significant impact. The possibility of assessing simultaneously microvascular proliferation and permeability (using advanced MRI techniques) and tumor metabolism and proliferation (using various PET tracers) could help us better understand the tumor biology and mechanism of action of promising therapeutic agents.

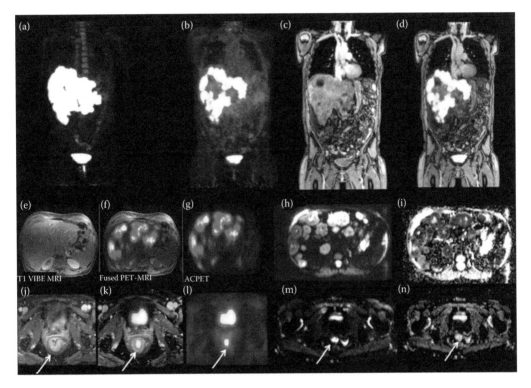

Figure 15.10 Simultaneous PET and MR exam in a colorectal cancer patient with liver metastases. (a) Maximum intensity projection and (b) coronal FDG-PET images demonstrating increased uptake in scattered innumerable liver metastases. (c) Coronal T1-weighted turbo spin echo image demonstrating multiple enhancing lesions throughout the liver. (d) Fused PET and MR images. (e) Axial T1-weighted VIBE postcontrast images demonstrating multiple enhancing lesions scattered throughout the liver parenchyma. (f) Axial FDG-PET images fused with T1-weighted VIBE postcontrast images. (g) FDG-PET images demonstrating multifocal FDG-avid lesions. (h, i) Diffusion-weighted images at the same level demonstrating hyperintense lesions with excellent correspondence to the FDG-avid and -enhancing lesions. Apparent diffusion coefficient (ADC) parametric maps demonstrating areas of low signal intensity throughout compatible with restricted diffusion. (j) T1-weighted VIBE postcontrast image demonstrating an enhancing mass within the rectum (white arrow). (k) FDG-PET images fused with T1-weighted VIBE postcontrast axial images demonstrating this mass to be FDG avid. (l) FDG-PET images demonstrating avidity of the mass without anatomic correlate. (m) Diffusion-weighted images at the same level demonstrating hyperintense lesion in the rectum with excellent correspondence to the FDG-avid lesion (white arrow). (n) ADC parametric map demonstrating low signal intensity in this lesion compatible with restricted diffusion and concordant with the FDG-avid lesion. (Data acquired on the Biograph mMR scanner, A. A. Martinos Center, Massachusetts General Hospital, Boston. Images courtesy of Alexander R. Guimaraes, A. A. Martinos Center, Massachusetts General Hospital, Boston.)

In the case of cardiovascular applications, simultaneous PET and MRI will facilitate the validation and cross-calibration of various techniques that have been proposed for the same purpose. For example, FDG-PET is considered the gold standard for assessing myocardial viability, but the late gadolinium enhancement MRI technique is also very valuable in this context. While myocardial perfusion assessed with PET is routinely used clinically, flow quantification by MRI is still challenging and requires further validation studies. Since these studies involve a pharmacological challenge to detect perfusion changes at stress, the simultaneous PET and MRI data acquisition will allow a true comparison between the performances of each of the techniques in identical conditions (Rischpler et al. 2013). In the context of molecular imaging, PET/MRI could become the modality of choice for the noninvasive assessment of stem cell therapies or for atherosclerotic plaque imaging using dual-labeled PET/MRI probes (Ciesienski et al. 2013; Uppal et al. 2011). All these applications would benefit from the improved PET quantification enabled by the advanced MR-assisted data correction techniques described earlier in this chapter.

REFERENCES

Ahmadian, A., Ay, M. R., Bidgoli, J. H., Sarkar, S., and Zaidi, H. 2008. Correction of oral contrast artifacts in CT-based attenuation correction of PET images using an automated segmentation algorithm. *European Journal of Nuclear Medicine and Molecular Imaging* no. 35 (10):1812–1823.

Ai, T., Padua, A., Goerner, F., et al. 2012. SEMAC-VAT and MSVAT-SPACE sequence strategies for metal artifact reduction in 1.5T magnetic resonance imaging. *Investigative Radiology* no. 47 (5):267–276.

Akbarzadeh, A., Ay, M. R., Ahmadian, A., Riahi Alam, N., and Zaidi, H. 2013. MRI-guided attenuation correction in whole-body PET/MR: Assessment of the effect of bone attenuation. *Annals of Nuclear Medicine* no. 27 (2):152–162.

Aklan, B., Paulus, D. H., Wenkel, E., et al. 2013. Toward simultaneous PET/MR breast imaging: Systematic evaluation and integration of a radiofrequency breast coil. *Medical Physics* no. 40 (2):024301.

Andersen, F. L., Ladefoged, C. N., Beyer, T., et al. 2014. Combined PET/MR imaging in neurology: MR-based attenuation correction implies a strong spatial bias when ignoring bone. *Neuroimage* no. 84:206–216.

Antoch, G., Freudenberg, L. S., Beyer, T., Bockisch, A., and Debatin, J. F. 2004. To enhance or not to enhance? 18F-FDG and CT contrast agents in dual-modality 18F-FDG PET/CT. *Journal of Nuclear Medicine* no. 45 (1 Suppl.):56S–65S.

Antoch, G., Jentzen, W., Freudenberg, L. S., et al. 2003. Effect of oral contrast agents on computed tomography-based positron emission tomography attenuation correction in dual-modality positron emission tomography/computed tomography imaging. *Invest Radiol.* no. 38 (12):784–789.

Arabi, H., Rager, O., Alem, A., Varoquaux, A., Becker, M., and Zaidi, H. 2015. Clinical assessment of MR-guided 3-class and 4-class attenuation correction in PET/MR. *Molecular Imaging and Biology* no. 17 (2):264–276.

Axel, L., and Dougherty, L. 1989. MR imaging of motion with spatial modulation of magnetization. *Radiology* no. 171 (3):841–845.

Aznar, M. C., Sersar, R., Saabye, J., et al. 2014. Whole-body PET/MRI: The effect of bone attenuation during MR-based attenuation correction in oncology imaging. *European Journal of Radiology* no. 83 (7):1177–1183.

Berker, Y., Franke, J., Salomon, A., et al. 2012. MRI-based attenuation correction for hybrid PET/MRI systems: A 4-class tissue segmentation technique using a combined ultrashort-echo-time/Dixon MRI sequence. *Journal of Nuclear Medicine* no. 53 (5):796–804.

Bindseil, G. A., Gilbert, K. M., Scholl, T. J., Handler, W. B., and Chronik, B. A. 2011. First image from a combined positron emission tomography and field-cycled MRI system. *Magnetic Resonance in Medicine* no. 66 (1):301–305.

Bini, J., Izquierdo-Garcia, D., Mateo, J., et al. 2013. Preclinical evaluation of MR attenuation correction versus CT attenuation correction on a sequential whole-body MR/PET scanner. *Investigative Radiology* no. 48 (5):313–322.

Borra, R., Bowen, S. L., Attenberger, U., et al. 2013. Effects of ferumoxytol on quantitative accuracy of PET in simultaneous PET/MR imaging—A validation study. Presented at the 99th Scientific Assembly and Annual Meeting of the Radiological Society of North America, Chicago.

Breuer, J., Grazioso, R., Zhang, N., Schmand, M., and Wienhard, K. 2010. Evaluation of an MR-compatible blood sampler for PET. *Physics in Medicine and Biology* no. 55 (19):5883–5893.

Buchbender, C., Heusner, T. A., Lauenstein, T. C., Bockisch, A., and Antoch, G. 2012a. Oncologic PET/MRI. Part 1. Tumors of the brain, head and neck, chest, abdomen, and pelvis. *Journal of Nuclear Medicine* no. 53 (6):928–938.

Buchbender, C., Heusner, T. A., Lauenstein, T. C., Bockisch, A., and Antoch, G. 2012b. Oncologic PET/MRI. Part 2. Bone tumors, soft-tissue tumors, melanoma, and lymphoma. *Journal of Nuclear Medicine* no. 53 (8):1244–1252.

Catana, C., Benner, T., van der Kouwe, A., et al. 2011. MRI-assisted PET motion correction for neurologic studies in an integrated MR-PET scanner. *Journal of Nuclear Medicine* no. 52 (1):154–161.

Catana, C., Drzezga, A., Heiss, W. D., and Rosen, B. R. 2012. PET/MRI for neurologic applications. *Journal of Nuclear Medicine* no. 53 (12):1916–1925.

Catana, C., Guimaraes, A. R., and Rosen, B. R. 2013. PET and MR imaging: The odd couple or a match made in heaven? *Journal of Nuclear Medicine* no. 54 (5):815–824.

Catana, C., Procissi, D., Wu, Y., et al. 2008. Simultaneous in vivo positron emission tomography and magnetic resonance imaging. *Proceedings of the National Academy of Sciences of the United States of America* no. 105 (10):3705–3710.

Catana, C., van der Kouwe, A., Benner, T., et al. 2010. Toward implementing an MRI-based PET attenuation-correction method for neurologic studies on the MR-PET brain prototype. *Journal of Nuclear Medicine* no. 51 (9):1431–1438.

Catana, C., Wu, Y., Judenhofer, M. S., Qi, J., Pichler, B. J., and Cherry, S. R. 2006. Simultaneous acquisition of multislice PET and MR images: Initial results with a MR-compatible PET scanner. *Journal of Nuclear Medicine* no. 47 (12):1968–1976.

Censor, Y., Gustafson, D. E., Lent, A., and Tuy, H. 1979. A new approach to the emission computerized tomography problem: Simultaneous calculation of attenuation and activity coefficients. *IEEE Transactions on Nuclear Science* no. 26 (2):2775–2779.

Cho, Z. H., Son, Y. D., Choi, E. J., et al. 2013. In-vivo human brain molecular imaging with a brain-dedicated PET/MRI system. *Magnetic Resonance Materials in Physics, Biology and Medicine* no. 26 (1):71–79.

Cho, Z. H., Son, Y. D., Kim, H. K., et al. 2008. A fusion PET-MRI system with a high-resolution research tomograph-PET and ultra-high field 7.0 T-MRI for the molecular-genetic imaging of the brain. *Proteomics* no. 8 (6):1302–1323.

Cho, Z. H., Son, Y. D., Kim, H. K., et al. 2011. Observation of glucose metabolism in the thalamic nuclei by fusion PET/MRI. *Journal of Nuclear Medicine* no. 52 (3):401–404.

Chonde, D. B., Abolmaali, N., Arabasz, G., Guimaraes, A. R., and Catana, C. 2013. Effect of MRI acoustic noise on cerebral fludeoxyglucose uptake in simultaneous MR-PET imaging. *Investigative Radiology* no. 48 (5):302–312.

Chonde, D., and Catana, C. 2012. MR-guided radiotracer input function estimation in simultaneous MR/PET. Presented at the 20th Annual Meeting of the International Society of Magnetic Resonance in Medicine, Melbourne, Australia.

Christensen, N. L., Hammer, B. E., Heil, B. G., and Fetterly, K. 1995. Positron emission tomography within a magnetic field using photomultiplier tubes and lightguides. *Physics in Medicine and Biology* no. 40 (4):691–697.

Chun, S. Y., Reese, T. G., Ouyang, J., et al. 2012. MRI-based nonrigid motion correction in simultaneous PET/MRI. *Journal of Nuclear Medicine* no. 53 (8):1284–1291.

Ciesienski, K. L., Yang, Y., Ay, I., et al. 2013. Fibrin-targeted PET probes for the detection of thrombi. *Molecular Pharmaceutics* no. 2013 (10):1100–1110.

Cohade, C., Osman, M., Nakamoto, Y., et al. 2003. Initial experience with oral contrast in PET/CT: Phantom and clinical studies. *Journal of Nuclear Medicine* no. 44 (3):412–416.

Conradi, J. 1974. Temperature effects in silicon avalanche photodiodes. *Solid-State Electronics* no. 17:99–106.

Dawood, M., Gigengack, F., Jiang, X. Y., and Schafers, K. P. 2013. A mass conservation-based optical flow method for cardiac motion correction in 3D-PET. *Medical Physics* no. 40 (1):9.

Delso, G., Furst, S., Jakoby, B., et al. 2011. Performance measurements of the Siemens mMR integrated whole-body PET/MR scanner. *Journal of Nuclear Medicine* no. 52 (12):1914–1922.

Delso, G., Martinez-Moller, A., Bundschuh, R. A., Nekolla, S. G., and Ziegler, S. I. 2010. The effect of limited MR field of view in MR/PET attenuation correction. *Medical Physics* no. 37 (6):2804–2812.

Dikaios, N., Izquierdo-Garcia, D., Graves, M. J., Mani, V., Fayad, Z. A., and Fryer, T. D. 2012. MRI-based motion correction of thoracic PET: Initial comparison of acquisition protocols and correction strategies suitable for simultaneous PET/MRI systems. *European Radiology* no. 22 (2):439–446.

Dizendorf, E., Hany, T. F., Buck, A., von Schulthess, G. K., and Burger, C. 2003. Cause and magnitude of the error induced by oral CT contrast agent in CT-based attenuation correction of PET emission studies. *Journal of Nuclear Medicine* no. 44 (5):732–738.

Dregely, I., Lanz, T., Metz, S., et al. 2015. A 16-channel MR coil for simultaneous PET/MR imaging in breast cancer. *European Journal of Radiology* no. 25 (4):1154–1161.

Drzezga, A., Souvatzoglou, M., Eiber, M., et al. 2012. First clinical experience with integrated whole-body PET/MR: Comparison to PET/CT in patients with oncologic diagnoses. *Journal of Nuclear Medicine* no. 53 (6):845–855.

Eldib, M., Bini, J., Calcagno, C., Robson, P. M., Mani, V., and Fayad, Z. A. 2014. Attenuation correction for flexible magnetic resonance coils in combined magnetic resonance/positron emission tomography imaging. *Investigative Radiology* no. 49 (2):63–69.

Erlandsson, K., Buvat, I., Pretorius, P. H., Thomas, B. A., and Hutton, B. F. 2012. A review of partial volume correction techniques for emission tomography and their applications in neurology, cardiology and oncology. *Physics in Medicine and Biology* no. 57 (21):R119–R159.

Fayad, H., Odille, F., Schmidt, H., et al. 2015. The use of a generalized reconstruction by inversion of coupled systems (GRICS) approach for generic respiratory motion correction in PET/MR imaging. *Physics in Medicine and Biology* no. 60 (6):2529–2546.

Fieseler, M., Kugel, H., Gigengack, F., et al. 2013. A dynamic thorax phantom for the assessment of cardiac and respiratory motion correction in PET/MRI: A preliminary evaluation. *Nuclear Instruments & Methods in Physics Research Section A* no. 702:59–63.

Frullano, L., Catana, C., Benner, T., Sherry, A. D., and Caravan, P. 2010. Bimodal MR-PET agent for quantitative pH imaging. *Angewandte Chemie—International Edition* no. 49 (13):2382–2384.

Furst, S., Grimm, R., Hong, I., et al. 2015. Motion correction strategies for integrated PET/MR. *Journal of Nuclear Medicine* no. 56 (2):261–269.

Furst, S., Souvatzoglou, M., Martinez-Moller, A., Schwaiger, M., Nekolla, S. G., and Ziegler, S. I. 2014. Impact of flexible body surface coil and patient table on PET quantification and image quality in integrated PET/MR. *Nuklearmedizin* no. 53 (3):79–87.

Garibotto, V., Heinzer, S., Vulliemoz, S., et al. 2013. Clinical applications of hybrid PET/MRI in neuroimaging. *Clinical Nuclear Medicine* no. 38 (1):E13–E18.

Garlick, P. B., Marsden, P. K., Cave, A. C., et al. 1997. PET and NMR dual acquisition (PANDA): Applications to isolated, perfused rat hearts. *NMR in Biomedicine* no. 10 (3):138–142.

Guerin, B., Cho, S., Chun, S. Y., et al. 2011. Nonrigid PET motion compensation in the lower abdomen using simultaneous tagged-MRI and PET imaging. *Medical Physics* no. 38 (6):3025–3038.

Hammer, B. E., and Christensen, N. L. 1995. Measurement of positron range in matter in strong magnetic fields. *IEEE Transactions on Nuclear Science* no. 42 (4):1371–1376.

Heusch, P., Buchbender, C., Beiderwellen, K., et al. 2013. Standardized uptake values for [18F] FDG in normal organ tissues: Comparison of whole-body PET/CT and PET/MRI. *European Journal of Radiology* no. 82 (5):870–876.

Hofmann, M., Steinke, F., Scheel, V., et al. 2008. MRI-based attenuation correction for PET/MRI: A novel approach combining pattern recognition and atlas registration. *Journal of Nuclear Medicine* no. 49 (11):1875–1883.

Hong, S. J., Kang, H. G., Ko, G. B., Song, I. C., Rhee, J. T., and Lee, J. S. 2012. SiPM-PET with a short optical fiber bundle for simultaneous PET-MR imaging. *Physics in Medicine and Biology* no. 57 (12):3869–3883.

Huang, C., Petibon, Y., Ouyang, J., et al. 2015. Accelerated acquisition of tagged MRI for cardiac motion correction in simultaneous PET-MR: Phantom and patient studies. *Medical Physics* no. 42 (2):1087–1097.

Iida, H., Kanno, I., Miura, S., Murakami, M., Takahashi, K., and Uemura, K. 1986. A simulation study of a method to reduce positron-annihilation spread distributions using a strong magnetic-field in positron emission tomography. *IEEE Transactions on Nuclear Science* no. 33 (1):597–600.

Izquierdo-Garcia, D., Chen, K., Hansen, A., et al. 2014. New SPM8-based MRAC method for simultaneous PET/MR brain images: Comparison with state-of-the-art non-rigid registration methods. *EJNMMI Physics* no. 1 (Suppl. 1):A29.

Johansson, A., Karlsson, M., and Nyholm, T. 2011. CT substitute derived from MRI sequences with ultrashort echo time. *Medical Physics* no. 38 (5):2708–2714.

Johansson, A., Karlsson, M., Yu, J., Asklund, T., and Nyholm, T. 2012. Voxel-wise uncertainty in CT substitute derived from MRI. *Medical Physics* no. 39 (6):3283–3290.

Judenhofer, M. S., Catana, C., Swann, B. K., et al. 2007. PET/MR images acquired with a compact MR-compatible PET detector in a 7-T magnet. *Radiology* no. 244 (3):807–814.

Judenhofer, M. S., and Cherry, S. R. 2013. Applications for preclinical PET/MRI. *Seminars in Nuclear Medicine* no. 43 (1):19–29.

Judenhofer, M. S., Wehrl, H. F., Newport, D. F., et al. 2008. Simultaneous PET-MRI: A new approach for functional and morphological imaging. *Nature Medicine* no. 14 (4):459–465.

Kalemis, A., Delattre, B. M. A., and Heinzer, S. 2013. Sequential whole-body PET/MR scanner: Concept, clinical use, and optimisation after two years in the clinic. The manufacturer's perspective. *Magnetic Resonance Materials in Physics, Biology and Medicine* no. 26 (1):5–23.

Kang, J., Choi, Y., Hong, K. J., et al. 2011. A small animal PET based on GAPDs and charge signal transmission approach for hybrid PET-MR imaging. *Journal of Instrumentation* no. 6(08):P08012.

Keereman, V., Vandenberghe, S., De Deene, Y., Luypaert, R., and Broux, T. 2008. MR-based attenuation correction for PET using an ultrashort echo time (UTE) sequence. In *IEEE Nuclear Science Symposium Conference Record*, 4656–4661. New York: IEEE.

Keereman, V., Van Holen, R., Mollet, P., and Vandenberghe, S. 2011. The effect of errors in segmented attenuation maps on PET quantification. *Medical Physics* no. 38 (11):6010–6019.

Kershah, S., Partovi, S., Traughber, B. J., et al. 2013. Comparison of standardized uptake values in normal structures between PET/CT and PET/MRI in an oncology patient population. *Molecular Imaging and Biology* no. 15 (6):776–785.

Kim, J. H., Lee, J. S., Song, I. C., and Lee, D. S. 2012. Comparison of segmentation-based attenuation correction methods for PET/MRI: Evaluation of bone and liver standardized uptake value with oncologic PET/CT data. *Journal of Nuclear Medicine* no. 53 (12):1878–1882.

King, A. P., Buerger, C., Tsoumpas, C., Marsden, P. K., and Schaeffter, T. 2012. Thoracic respiratory motion estimation from MRI using a statistical model and a 2-D image navigator. *Medical Image Analysis* no. 16 (1):252–264.

Kolb, A., Lorenz, E., Judenhofer, M. S., Renker, D., Lankes, K., and Pichler, B. J. 2010. Evaluation of Geiger-mode APDs for PET block detector designs. *Physics in Medicine and Biology* no. 55 (7):1815–1832.

Kolb, A., Wehrl, H. F., Hofmann, M., et al. 2012. Technical performance evaluation of a human brain PET/MRI system. *European Radiology* no. 22 (8):1776–1788.

Ladefoged, C. N., Andersen, F. L., Keller, S. H., et al. 2013. PET/MR imaging of the pelvis in the presence of endoprostheses: Reducing image artifacts and increasing accuracy through inpainting. *European Journal of Nuclear Medicine and Molecular Imaging* no. 40 (4):594–601.

Ledesma-Carbayo, M. J., Derbyshire, J. A., Sampath, S., Santos, A., Desco, M., and McVeigh, E. R. 2008. Unsupervised estimation of myocardial displacement from tagged MR sequences using nonrigid registration. *Magnetic Resonance in Medicine* no. 59 (1):181–189.

Levin, C., Glover, G., Deller, T., McDaniel, D., Peterson, W., and Maramraju, S. H. 2013. Prototype time-of-flight PET ring integrated with a 3T MRI system for simultaneous whole-body PET/MR imaging. *Journal of Nuclear Medicine* no. 54 (Suppl. 2):148.

Lois, C., Bezrukov, I., Schmidt, H., et al. 2012. Effect of MR contrast agents on quantitative accuracy of PET in combined whole-body PET/MR imaging. *European Journal of Nuclear Medicine and Molecular Imaging* no. 39 (11):1756–1766.

Lucas, A. J., Hawkes, R. C., Ansorge, R. E., et al. 2006. Development of a combined microPET((R))-MR system. *Technology in Cancer Research & Treatment* no. 5 (4):337–341.

MacDonald, L. R., Kohlmyer, S., Liu, C., Lewellen, T. K., and Kinahan, P. E. 2011. Effects of MR surface coils on PET quantification. *Medical Physics* no. 38 (6):2948–2956.

Mackewn, J. E., Halsted, P., Charles-Edwards, G., et al. 2010. Performance evaluation of an MRI-compatible pre-clinical PET system using long optical fibers. *IEEE Transactions on Nuclear Science* no. 57 (3):1052–1062.

Mackewn, J. E., Strul, D., Hallett, W. A., et al. 2005. Design and development of an MR-compatible PET scanner for imaging small animals. *IEEE Transactions on Nuclear Science* no. 52 (5):1376–1380.

Maramraju, S. H., Smith, S. D., Junnarkar, S. S., et al. 2011. Small animal simultaneous PET/MRI: Initial experiences in a 9.4 T microMRI. *Physics in Medicine and Biology* no. 56 (8):2459–2480.

Marshall, H. R., Patrick, J., Laidley, D., et al. 2013. Description and assessment of a registration-based approach to include bones for attenuation correction of whole-body PET/MRI. *Medical Physics* no. 40 (8):082509.

Marshall, H. R., Prato, F. S., Deans, L., Theberge, J., Thompson, R. T., and Stodilka, R. Z. 2012. Variable lung density consideration in attenuation correction of whole-body PET/MRI. *Journal of Nuclear Medicine* no. 53(6):977–984.

Martinez-Moller, A., Souvatzoglou, M., Delso, G., et al. 2009. Tissue classification as a potential approach for attenuation correction in whole-body PET/MRI: Evaluation with PET/CT data. *Journal of Nuclear Medicine* no. 50 (4):520–526.

Mediso. nanoPET PM PET/MRI—In vivo molecular and preclinical imager. Budapets: Mediso. Available from http://www.mediso.hu/uploaded/product_features84.pdf.

Mehranian, A., and Zaidi, H. 2015. Impact of time-of-flight PET on quantification errors in MR imaging-based attenuation correction. *Journal of Nuclear Medicine* no. 56 (4):635–641.

Mollet, P., Keereman, V., Clementel, E., and Vandenberghe, S. 2012. Simultaneous MR-compatible emission and transmission imaging for PET using time-of-flight information. *IEEE Transactions on Medical Imaging* no. 31 (9):1734–1742.

Montandon, M. L., and Zaidi, H. 2005. Atlas-guided non-uniform attenuation correction in cerebral 3D PET imaging. *Neuroimage* no. 25 (1):278–286.

Navalpakkam, B. K., Braun, H., Kuwert, T., and Quick, H. H. 2013. Magnetic resonance-based attenuation correction for PET/MR hybrid imaging using continuous valued attenuation maps. *Investigative Radiology* no. 48 (5):323–332.

Nehmeh, S. A., Erdi, Y. E., Kalaigian, H., et al. 2003. Correction for oral contrast artifacts in CT attenuation-corrected PET images obtained by combined PET/CT. *Journal of Nuclear Medicine* no. 44 (12):1940–1944.

Nuyts, J., Dupont, P., Stroobants, S., Benninck, R., Mortelmans, L., and Suetens, P. 1999. Simultaneous maximum a posteriori reconstruction of attenuation and activity distributions from emission sinograms. *IEEE Transactions on Medical Imaging* no. 18 (5):393–403.

Nuyts, J., Michel, C., Fenchel, M., Bal, G., Watson, C., and Ieee. 2010. Completion of a truncated attenuation image from the attenuated PET emission data. In *2010 IEEE Nuclear Science Symposium Conference Record*, 2123–2127. New York: IEEE.

Odille, F., Vuissoz, P. A., Marie, P. Y., and Felblinger, J. 2008. Generalized reconstruction by inversion of coupled systems (GRICS) applied to free-breathing MRI. *Magnetic Resonance in Medicine* no. 60 (1):146–157.

Osman, N. F., McVeigh, E. R., and Prince, J. L. 2000. Imaging heart motion using harmonic phase MRI. *IEEE Transactions on Medical Imaging* no. 19 (3):186–202.

Ouyang, J. S., Li, Q. Z., and El Fakhri, G. 2013. Magnetic resonance-based motion correction for positron emission tomography imaging. *Seminars in Nuclear Medicine* no. 43 (1):60–67.

Panin, V. Y., Aykac, M., and Casey, M. E. 2013. Simultaneous reconstruction of emission activity and attenuation coefficient distribution from TOF data, acquired with external transmission source. *Physics in Medicine and Biology* no. 58 (11):3649–3669.

Partovi, S., Kohan, A., Gaeta, C., et al. 2013. Image quality assessment of automatic three-segment MR attenuation correction vs. CT attenuation correction. *American Journal of Nuclear Medicine and Molecular Imaging* no. 3 (3):291–299.

Paulus, D. H., Braun, H., Aklan, B., and Quick, H. H. 2012. Simultaneous PET/MR imaging: MR-based attenuation correction of local radiofrequency surface coils. *Medical Physics* no. 39 (7):4306–4315.

Peng, H., Handler, W. B., Scholl, T. J., Simpson, P. J., and Chronik, B. A. 2010. Proof-of-principle study of a small animal PET/field-cycled MRI combined system using conventional PMT technology. *Nuclear Instruments & Methods in Physics Research Section A* no. 612 (2):412–420.

Petibon, Y., Ouyang, J., Zhu, X., et al. 2013. Cardiac motion compensation and resolution modeling in simultaneous PET-MR: A cardiac lesion detection study. *Physics in Medicine and Biology* no. 58 (7):2085.

Pichler, B., Lorenz, E., Mirzoyan, R., et al. 1997. Performance test of a LSO-APD PET module in a 9.4 Tesla magnet. Presented at 1997 IEEE Nuclear Science Symposium, Albuquerque, NM.

Pichler, B. J., Pimpl, W., Buttler, W., et al. 2001. Integrated low-noise low-power fast charge-sensitive preamplifier for avalanche photodiodes in JFET-CMOS technology. *IEEE Transactions on Nuclear Science* no. 48 (6):2370–2374.

Poulin, E., Lebel, R., Croteau, E., et al. 2013. Conversion of arterial input functions for dual pharmacokinetic modeling using Gd-DTPA/MRI and 18F-FDG/PET. *Magnetic Resonance in Medicine* no. 69 (3):781–792.

Poynton, C. B., Chen, K. T., Chonde, D. B., et al. 2014. Probabilistic atlas-based segmentation of combined T1-weighted and DUTE MRI for calculation of head attenuation maps in integrated PET/MRI scanners. *American Journal of Nuclear Medicine and Molecular Imaging* no. 4 (2):160–171.

Raylman, R. R. 1991. Reduction of positron range effects by the use of a magnetic field: For use in positron emission tomography. University of Michigan, Ann Arbor.

Raylman, R. R., Hammer, B. E., and Christensen, N. L. 1996. Combined MRI-PET scanner: A Monte Carlo evaluation of the improvements in PET resolution due to the effects of a static homogeneous magnetic field. *IEEE Transactions on Nuclear Science* no. 43 (4):2406–2412.

Raylman, R. R., Majewski, S., Lemieux, S. K., et al. 2006. Simultaneous MRI and PET imaging of a rat brain. *Physics in Medicine and Biology* no. 51 (24):6371–6379.

Raylman, R. R., Majewski, S., Velan, S. S., et al. 2007. Simultaneous acquisition of magnetic resonance spectroscopy (MRS) data and positron emission tomography (PET) images with a prototype MR-compatible, small animal PET imager. *Journal of Magnetic Resonance* no. 186 (2):305–310.

Reichert, I. L. H., Robson, M. D., Gatehouse, P. D., et al. 2005. Magnetic resonance imaging of cortical bone with ultrashort TE pulse sequences. *Magnetic Resonance Imaging* no. 23 (5):611–618.

Rezaei, A., Defrise, M., Bal, G., et al. 2012. Simultaneous reconstruction of activity and attenuation in time-of-flight PET. *IEEE Transactions on Medical Imaging* no. 31 (12):2224–2233.

Rischpler, C., Nekolla, S. G., Dregely, I., and Schwaiger, M. 2013. Hybrid PET/MR imaging of the heart: Potential, initial experiences, and future prospects. *Journal of Nuclear Medicine* no. 54 (3):402–415.

Robson, M. D., and Bydder, G. M. 2006. Clinical ultrashort echo time imaging of bone and other connective tissues. *NMR in Biomedicine* no. 19 (7):765–780.

Roncali, E., and Cherry, S. R. 2011. Application of silicon photomultipliers to positron emission tomography. *Annals of Biomedical Engineering* no. 39 (4):1358–1377.

Rota Kops, E., and Herzog, H. 2008. Template-based attenuation correction of PET in hybrid MR-PET scanners. *Society of Nuclear Medicine Annual Meeting Abstracts* no. 49 (Suppl. 1):162P-c.

Roy, S., Wang, W. T., Carass, A., Prince, J. L., Butman, J. A., and Pham, D. L. 2014. PET attenuation correction using synthetic CT from ultrashort echo-time MR imaging. *Journal of Nuclear Medicine* no. 55 (12):2071–2077.

Salomon, A., Goedicke, A., Schweizer, B., Aach, T., and Schulz, V. 2011. Simultaneous reconstruction of activity and attenuation for PET/MR. *IEEE Transactions on Medical Imaging* no. 30 (3):804–813.

Samarin, A., Burger, C., Wollenweber, S. D., et al. 2012. PET/MR imaging of bone lesions—Implications for PET quantification from imperfect attenuation correction. *European Journal of Nuclear Medicine and Molecular Imaging* no. 39 (7):1154–1160.

Sander, C. Y., Hooker, J. M., Catana, C., et al. 2013. Neurovascular coupling to D2/D3 dopamine receptor occupancy using simultaneous PET/functional MRI. *Proceedings of the National Academy of Sciences of the United States of America* no. 110 (27):11169–11174.

Sander, C. Y., Keil, B., Chonde, D. B., Rosen, B. R., Catana, C., and Wald, L. L. 2015. A 31-channel MR brain array coil compatible with positron emission tomography. *Magnetic Resonance in Medicine* no. 73 (6):2363–2375.

Schenck, J. F. 1996. The role of magnetic susceptibility in magnetic resonance imaging: MRI magnetic compatibility of the first and second kinds. *Medical Physics* no. 23 (6):815–850.

Schlemmer, H.-P. W., Pichler, B. J., Schmand, M., et al. 2008. Simultaneous MR/PET imaging of the human brain: Feasibility study. *Radiology* no. 248 (3):1028–1035.

Schmid, A., Schmitz, J., Mannheim, J. G., et al. 2013. Feasibility of sequential PET/MRI using a state-of-the-art small animal PET and a 1 T benchtop MRI. *Molecular Imaging and Biology* no. 15 (2):155–165.

Schramm, G., Langner, J., Hofheinz, F., et al. 2013. Quantitative accuracy of attenuation correction in the Philips Ingenuity TF whole-body PET/MR system: A direct comparison with transmission-based attenuation correction. *Magnetic Resonance Materials in Physics, Biology and Medicine* no. 26 (1):115–126.

Schulz, V., Torres-Espallardo, I., Renisch, S., et al. 2011. Automatic, three-segment, MR-based attenuation correction for whole-body PET/MR data. *European Journal of Nuclear Medicine and Molecular Imaging* no. 38 (1):138–152.

Seong Jong, H., In, C., Ito, M., et al. 2008. An investigation into the use of Geiger-mode solid-state photomultipliers for simultaneous PET and MRI acquisition. *IEEE Transactions on Nuclear Science* no. 55 (3):882–888.

Shao, Y., Cherry, S. R., Farahani, K., et al. 1997a. Simultaneous PET and MR imaging. *Physics in Medicine and Biology* no. 42 (10):1965–1970.

Shao, Y., Cherry, S. R., Farahani, K., et al. 1997b. Development of a PET detector system compatible with MRI/NMR systems. *IEEE Transactions on Nuclear Science* no. 44 (3):1167–1171.

Shao, Y., Cherry, S. R., Siegel, S., Silverman, R. W., and Majewski, S. 1997c. Evaluation of multi-channel PMTs for readout of scintillator arrays. *Nuclear Instruments & Methods in Physics Research Section A* no. 390 (1–2):209–218.

Sutter, R., Ulbrich, E. J., Jellus, V., Nittka, M., and Pfirrmann, C. W. A. 2012. Reduction of metal artifacts in patients with total hip arthroplasty with slice-encoding metal artifact correction and view-angle tilting MR imaging. *Radiology* no. 265 (1):204–214.

Tatsumi, M., Yamamoto, S., Imaizumi, M., et al. 2012. Simultaneous PET/MR body imaging in rats: Initial experiences with an integrated PET/MRI scanner. *Annals of Nuclear Medicine* no. 26 (5):444–449.

Tellmann, L., Quick, H. H., Bockisch, A., Herzog, H., and Beyer, T. 2011. The effect of MR surface coils on PET quantification in whole-body PET/MR: Results from a pseudo-PET/MR phantom study. *Medical Physics* no. 38 (5):2795–2805.

Townsend, D. W., Carney, J. P., Yap, J. T., and Hall, N. C. 2004. PET/CT today and tomorrow. *Journal of Nuclear Medicine* no. 45 (Suppl. 1):4S–14S.

Tsoumpas, C., Mackewn, J., Halsted, P., et al. 2010. Simultaneous PET-MR acquisition and MR-derived motion fields for correction of non-rigid motion in PET. *Annals of Nuclear Medicine* no. 24 (10):745–750.

Ullisch, M. G., Scheins, J. J., Weirich, C., et al. 2012. MR-based PET motion correction procedure for simultaneous MR-PET neuroimaging of human brain. *PLoS ONE* no. 7 (11):e48149.

Uppal, R., Catana, C., Ay, I., et al. 2011. Simultaneous MR-PET imaging of thrombus with a fibrin-targeted dual MR-PET probe: A feasibility study. *Radiology* no. 258 (3):812–820.

van der Kouwe, A. J., Benner, T., and Dale, A. M. 2006. Real-time rigid body motion correction and shimming using cloverleaf navigators. *Magnetic Resonance in Medicine* no. 56 (5):1019–1032.

Veit-Haibach, P., Kuhn, F. P., Wiesinger, F., Delso, G., and Schulthess, G. 2013. PET-MR imaging using a tri-modality PET/CT-MR system with a dedicated shuttle in clinical routine. *Magnetic Resonance Materials in Physics, Biology and Medicine* no. 26 (1):25–35.

Wirrwar, A., Vosberg, H., Herzog, H., Halling, H., Weber, S., and Muller-Gartner, H.-W. 1997. 4.5 tesla magnetic field reduces range of high-energy positrons—Potential implications for positron emission tomography. *IEEE Transactions on Nuclear Science* no. 44 (2):184–189.

Wollenweber, S. D., Delso, G., Deller, T., Goldhaber, D., Hullner, M., and Veit-Haibach, P. 2014. Characterization of the impact to PET quantification and image quality of an anterior array surface coil for PET/MR imaging. *MAGMA* no. 27 (2):149–159.

Woody, C., Schlyer, D., Vaska, P., et al. 2007. Preliminary studies of a simultaneous PET/MRI scanner based on the RatCAP small animal tomograph. *Nuclear Instruments & Methods in Physics Research Section A* no. 571 (1–2):102–105.

Wurslin, C., Schmidt, H., Martirosian, P., et al. 2013. Respiratory motion correction in oncologic PET using T1-weighted MR imaging on a simultaneous whole-body PET/MR system. *Journal of Nuclear Medicine* no. 54 (3):464–471.

Yamamoto, S., Imaizumi, M., Kanai, Y., et al. 2010. Design and performance from an integrated PET/MRI system for small animals. *Annals of Nuclear Medicine* no. 24 (2):89–98.

Yamamoto, S., Kuroda, K., and Senda, M. 2003. Scintillator selection for MR-compatible gamma detectors. *IEEE Transactions on Nuclear Science* no. 50 (5):1683–1685.

Yamamoto, S., Watabe, H., Kanai, Y., et al. 2011. Interference between PET and MRI sub-systems in a silicon-photomultiplier-based PET/MRI system. *Physics in Medicine and Biology* no. 56 (13):4147–4159.

Yamamoto, S., Watabe, T., Watabe, H., et al. 2012. Simultaneous imaging using Si-PM-based PET and MRI for development of an integrated PET/MRI system. *Physics in Medicine and Biology* no. 57 (2):N1–N13.

Yankeelov, T. E., Peterson, T. E., Abramson, R. G., et al. 2012. Simultaneous PET-MRI in oncology: A solution looking for a problem? *Magnetic Resonance Imaging* no. 30 (9):1342–1356.

Yoon, H. S., Ko, G. B., Il Kwon, S., et al. 2012. Initial results of simultaneous PET/MRI experiments with an MRI-compatible silicon photomultiplier PET scanner. *Journal of Nuclear Medicine* no. 53 (4):608–614.

Zaidi, H., Montandon, M. L., and Slosman, D. O. 2003. Magnetic resonance imaging-guided attenuation and scatter corrections in three-dimensional brain positron emission tomography. *Medical Physics* no. 30 (5):937–948.

Zaidi, H., Ojha, N., Morich, M., et al. 2011. Design and performance evaluation of a whole-body Ingenuity TF PET/MRI system. *Physics in Medicine and Biology* no. 56 (10):3091–3106.

Zanotti-Fregonara, P., Chen, K., Liow, J. S., Fujita, M., and Innis, R. B. 2011. Image-derived input function for brain PET studies: Many challenges and few opportunities. *Journal of Cerebral Blood Flow and Metabolism* no. 31 (10):1986–1998.

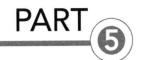
PRECLINICAL IMAGING AND CLINICAL APPLICATIONS

16 Preclinical PET and SPECT   413
    Steven R. Meikle, Andre Z. Kyme, Peter Kench, Frederic Boisson, and Arvind Parmar
17 Clinical applications of PET/CT and SPECT/CT imaging   439
    *Johannes Czernin and Ora Israel, Ken Herrmann, Martin Barrio, David Nathanson, and
    Martin Allen-Auerbach*

Preclinical PET and SPECT

STEVEN R. MEIKLE, ANDRE Z. KYME, PETER KENCH, FREDERIC
BOISSON, AND ARVIND PARMAR

16.1	Introduction	414
16.2	Instrumentation	414
	16.2.1 Overview	414
	16.2.2 Preclinical PET	415
	16.2.2.1 Scanner geometry	415
	16.2.2.2 Detector technologies	416
	16.2.3 SPECT	417
	16.2.3.1 Retrofitted clinical SPECT systems	417
	16.2.3.2 Systems based on compact high-resolution detectors	417
	16.2.3.3 Rotating versus stationary SPECT systems	417
	16.2.3.4 Detector technologies	418
	16.2.3.5 Collimation	419
	16.2.4 Multimodality systems	419
16.3	PET Performance characterization and quality control	419
	16.3.1 Spatial resolution	419
	16.3.2 Sensitivity	420
	16.3.3 Factors affecting PET performance	420
	16.3.3.1 Detector design	420
	16.3.3.2 Scanner geometry	421
	16.3.3.3 Depth of interaction	421
	16.3.3.4 Scatter, attenuation, and partial volume correction	422
	16.3.4 Performance testing	423
	16.3.4.1 Spatial resolution	423
	16.3.4.2 Scatter, count losses, and randoms measurement	423
	16.3.4.3 Sensitivity	424
	16.3.4.4 Image quality	424
	16.3.5 Current state-of-the-art in preclinical PET	424
16.4	Spect performance characterization and quality control	425
	16.4.1 Factors affecting SPECT performance	426
	16.4.1.1 Detector design	426
	16.4.1.2 Collimator profile	426

	16.4.2 Preclinical SPECT quality control	428
16.5	Practical aspects of small-animal imaging	428
	16.5.1 Anesthesia	430
	16.5.1.1 Injectable anesthetics	430
	16.5.1.2 Inhalation anesthesia	431
	16.5.2 Injection techniques	431
	16.5.3 Physiological monitoring and gating	432
	16.5.3.1 Body temperature	432
	16.5.3.2 Respiration	432
	16.5.3.3 Electrocardiograph	432
	16.5.3.4 Blood oxygenation	433
	16.5.3.5 Blood pressure	433
	16.5.3.6 Pulmonary CO_2	433
	16.5.4 Blood sampling	433
16.6	Summary	434
References		434

16.1 INTRODUCTION

Since radiation detectors were first used in the 1950s to noninvasively image the distribution of radiolabeled tracers in the body, animals have been used to test new radiopharmaceuticals and imaging methods and to better understand the pathophysiology of disease. Until relatively recently, such studies were conducted using the same instrumentation and methods as those used in human studies. This approach delivered satisfactory results when imaging large animals, such as dogs and sheep, but clinical SPECT and PET scanners have inadequate spatial resolution and sensitivity for imaging smaller animals, such as rodents.

The last two decades have witnessed rapid advances in gene technologies that dramatically increased our ability to record the entire gene sequence (genome) of a living organism and breed animals with individual genes selectively manipulated. For example, a gene of interest can be introduced into a genome where it would not normally be found (knock-in) or selectively deleted from the genome (knockout). The animal with the altered gene, referred to as a transgenic animal, can then be studied in order to understand the function of the specific gene and its potential role in disease. The laboratory mouse is particularly well suited to modeling human diseases in this way, since it has a large proportion (approximately 90%) of its genome in common with humans and other mammals, has a rapid breeding cycle, and is relatively inexpensive to breed and maintain. Thus, the ability to characterize rodent disease models and study them longitudinally has become increasingly important in medical research in the last two decades.

During this same period, advances in detector technologies were made that lent themselves to the design and development of PET and SPECT scanners suitable for imaging small animals, such as mice and rats. In this chapter, we discuss the key design principles of modern preclinical PET and SPECT systems, the factors affecting their performance, and practical considerations for their use in the biomedical research setting.

16.2 INSTRUMENTATION

16.2.1 OVERVIEW

The instruments and techniques used to acquire a small-animal imaging study are determined by the research question, the species of animal, the structure and physiology of the organ(s) of interest, and the desired spatial resolution and sensitivity. Because of the relatively long physical half-lives of single-photon emitters, SPECT is best suited to the study of macromolecules, such as antibodies and proteins, which have relatively slow rates of accrual at their target sites and slow plasma clearance (Meikle et al. 2005). Additionally, proteins and antibodies are easily labeled with one of the radioisotopes of iodine (^{125}I, ^{123}I, or ^{131}I), or else by attaching a chelating agent incorporating one of the other common single-photon emitters with suitable imaging properties, such as ^{99m}Tc or ^{111}In. Conversely, PET is best suited to the study of small molecules, such as synthetic drugs, which have relatively fast kinetics in the body, matched to the relatively short physical half-lives of common positron-emitting radioisotopes such as ^{18}F (109.8 min) and ^{11}C (20.4 min). Thus, the two techniques are highly complementary in the preclinical research environment. We note, however, that PET can also be successfully used in conjunction with longer-lived positron emitters labeled to antibody fragments (McCabe and Wu 2010). Furthermore, both PET and SPECT are inherently quantitative techniques (particularly in small-animal imaging where the magnitudes of photon attenuation and scattering are relatively small) and well suited to longitudinal study designs.

The performance requirements of preclinical imaging systems are highly object and task dependent, and the size of the smallest structure to be imaged and the activity distribution within tissue are often important considerations (Jansen and Vanderheyden 2007). For example, the brain is a complex organ requiring reasonably high spatial resolution and sensitivity in order to quantify radiopharmaceutical uptake in specific structures, such as the striatum and cerebellum (Acton et al. 2002; Pissarek et al. 2008). Imaging the rodent skeleton requires high spatial resolution, but sensitivity may be less critical depending on the research question being asked. Engrafted tumors often exhibit a heterogeneous distribution of radiopharmaceuticals due to rapid tumor growth and tissue necrosis, which requires high spatial resolution for accurate quantification, whereas high system sensitivity is required when investigating and quantifying tracer kinetics. Modern preclinical PET and SPECT systems are capable of performing all these tasks with the appropriate selection of instruments and parameters for image acquisition and analysis.

16.2.2 PRECLINICAL PET

16.2.2.1 SCANNER GEOMETRY

Compared with PET scanners designed for imaging humans, small-animal scanners are characterized by a roughly fivefold reduction in diameter and a considerably larger ratio of axial to transaxial field of view (FOV). The diameter and axial extent of several current ring-based small-animal scanners are listed in Table 16.2, where the ratio of axial to transaxial FOV is typically in the range of 0.4–1.0. By comparison, for human systems the ratio varies from approximately 0.2 to 0.4. Overall, in spite of the smaller crystal size, the reduced scanner diameter means that, even with an extended axial FOV, small-animal systems maintain a similar number of crystals (and electronic channels) as human systems.

The majority of small-animal PET scanners have a transaxial FOV large enough for imaging both mice and rats. Some are specifically designed for mice, having a ring diameter of <80 mm (Yang et al. 2013; Zhang et al. 2011), and some are large enough to image non-human primates such as baboons and monkeys, in addition to rodents (Tai et al. 2005). The RatCAP scanner (Vaska 2004) is an example of a system purpose-built for rats.

Although the majority of scanners utilize full-ring geometry similar to systems designed for humans, several unconventional geometries have also been implemented. These include the Genisys4 (aka PETbox) (Sofie Biosciences) (Zhang et al. 2011; Herrmann et al. 2013; Gu et al. 2013) comprising two or four opposing block detector panels in a box-like geometry. Rotating systems involving two or more block detectors have also been implemented (Lage et al. 2009; Ziemons et al. 2005). The ClearPET system (Ziemons et al. 2005) has the flexibility to change the number of detectors being rotated and also adjust the ring diameter. The RatCAP scanner, although utilizing a ring geometry, is unconventional in that it has very small overall dimensions (80 mm diameter, 39 mm internal diameter, 25 mm axial length), being designed for rigid attachment to a rat's head via cranial screws. The system is used in conjunction with a counterbalance mechanism to alleviate the 200 g weight on the animal's head and allow the awake animal to maneuver itself within a 40 × 40 cm enclosure during imaging (Schulz et al. 2011).

16.2.2.2 DETECTOR TECHNOLOGIES

Almost all small-animal PET systems use scintillation-based gamma ray detectors in conjunction with photodetectors. The various scintillator materials in common use are discussed in Section 16.3.3.1. Most scanners use a block detector design with arrays of pixelated crystals comprising from 8×8 to 30×30 or more elements (Figure 16.1). To obtain high efficiency and high resolution in PET implies long thin crystals (i.e., crystals that are short in the axial and transaxial directions and long in the radial direction). In commercial systems, crystal sizes vary in cross section from 1.4×1.4 mm to 2.2×2.2 mm, and in length from about 7 to 25 mm. Single-layer systems typically use crystals of 10 mm length, whereas dual-layer (phoswich) systems use two layers with a combined crystal thickness of 15–25 mm (dual-layer systems enable depth-of-interaction estimation, as discussed below). In most cases, the crystal elements are rectangular prisms; however, tapered designs for improved packing (i.e., by minimizing intercrystal gaps) have also been proposed, with a cross section at the inner face as small as 0.4×0.4 mm (Yang et al. 2013).

For the photodetector, until quite recently most PET or PET–CT systems have used single-anode or position-sensitive photomultipler tubes (PS-PMTs). Two notable exceptions are the LabPET and RatCAP scanners, both of which use position-sensitive avalanche photodiodes (PS-APDs). In the case of the RatCAP, the use of a solid-state photodetector was essential to reduce detector size and enable the scanner to be head-mounted to a rat. In general, the advantages of using solid-state photodetectors over PMTs include compactness, low cost, flexibility in the readout configuration for obtaining DOI information (see Section 16.3.3.3), and magnetic field compatibility, thereby making them suitable for use in hybrid PET/MRI systems. Silicon photomultiplier (SiPM) technology (see Sections 16.2.3.4 and 16.3.3.1) has led to very promising compact solid-state photodetectors in recent years and is already replacing APD designs due to low noise, low bias

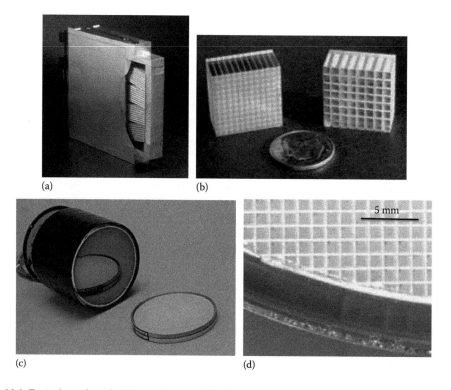

(a) (b)

(c) (d)

Figure 16.1 Typical preclinical PET (a and b) and SPECT (c and d) detectors: (a) PET detector module with optical fiber light guides partially exposed. (b) LSO crystal arrays from two different commercial systems with 1.5 mm (left) and 2.1 mm (right) crystals. (c) Hamamatsu R3292-02 PS-PMT and pixelated NaI:Tl crystal array. (d) Zoomed section of the crystal array showing individual elements separated by polytetrafluoroethylene powder.

voltage (~25–60 V), and much better thermal stability. Almost all new small-animal PET systems being developed are now using this technology.

16.2.3 SPECT

16.2.3.1 RETROFITTED CLINICAL SPECT SYSTEMS

Initial feasibility studies of small-animal SPECT imaging were performed using clinical SPECT systems retrofitted with specially designed pinhole collimators to obtain high spatial resolution and reasonable sensitivity (Jaszczak et al. 1994; Weber and Ivanovic 1999). This provided a cost-effective method for small-animal SPECT imaging. The large surface of the detector allowed for highly magnified projections, and placing the animal close to the pinhole produced reasonable sensitivity. The approach of retrofitting a clinical system however, causes some loss of spatial resolution near the edge of the detector due to parallax error from the oblique angle of incidence of gamma rays and the finite thickness of the crystal. Moreover, because clinical SPECT systems are optimized for photon energies of 140–300 keV, they are not well suited to small-animal studies using low-photon-energy radionuclides such as ^{125}I (20–35 keV), which produce low light output within the crystal (Weisenberger et al. 1997). Overall, the size and cost of a clinical SPECT system make it less than ideal for a dedicated small-animal imaging facility (Barrett and Hunter 2005).

16.2.3.2 SYSTEMS BASED ON COMPACT HIGH-RESOLUTION DETECTORS

The need for dedicated small-animal SPECT and organ-specific imaging systems resulted in the development of radiation detectors with higher intrinsic spatial resolution (Schramm et al. 2000; Wojcik et al. 1998). The array of single-anode PMTs used in a clinical system was replaced by one or more PS-PMTs, which are capable of very high intrinsic spatial resolution. These devices have multiple anodes whose outputs are used to calculate an x and y position signal for each detected scintillation event using Anger logic. The sum of the signals from all anodes is proportional to the number of light photons detected in the photocathode, and hence the energy of the gamma ray absorbed in the crystal. A limitation of PS-PMTs is their relatively poor uniformity and linearity of response, particularly near the edge of the FOV. However, their spatial response is very stable over time. A linearity correction or event position lookup map is created to ensure that all detected events are mapped to the correct crystal position.

16.2.3.3 ROTATING VERSUS STATIONARY SPECT SYSTEMS

A variety of SPECT system designs are used to acquire sufficient angular samples of the animal for tomography. The simplest small-animal SPECT system involves the vertical or horizontal rotation of the anesthetized animal in front of a stationary detector (MacDonald et al. 2001). The animal gantry needs to rotate through at least 180° in incremental steps. With this design, vertical rotation (animal in the upright position) is preferred over horizontal rotation (animal in decubitus position) to reduce the chance of organ movement during the scan, although horizontally rotating systems that address the organ motion issue have also been developed (Habraken et al. 2001). Vertical positioning should be done for short periods of time only, as it is not well suited to the rodent's physiology and has been related to an increased incidence of mortality (Stevenson 2005). The advantage of rotating the animal instead of the SPECT detector is that the weight of the animal is considerably less than that of the detector, and the rotating gantry is simpler and cheaper to design. However, this regime does make physiological monitoring and reproducible positioning of the animal for longitudinal studies more challenging.

Most clinical and some small-animal SPECT systems have the detector and collimator mounted on a gantry that rotates around the subject in precise incremental steps or continuous motion. To improve sensitivity and reduce imaging times, additional detectors may be added. Multiple detector systems reduce the need for a system to rotate over a full 180° or 360°. Each additional detector adds weight to the gantry and extra cost to the system, although multiple equally placed detectors do help to balance the gantry as it rotates.

The FOV is often limited for small-animal pinhole SPECT systems that use high magnification or small compact detectors. The FOV can be enlarged by increasing the radius of rotation (ROR), but this also reduces the spatial resolution and sensitivity of pinhole systems. Another approach is to move the animal stepwise

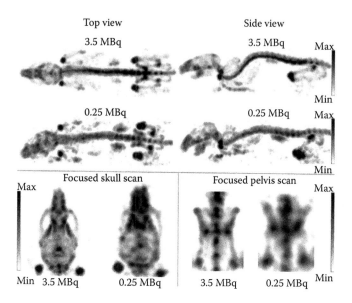

Figure 16.2 Whole-body (top) and focused (bottom) images obtained from two bone SPECT studies of a mouse. One study was acquired after administering 3.5 MBq of ^{99m}Tc-MDP to the mouse, while the other study was acquired after injecting the animal with only 0.25 MBq of ^{99m}Tc-MDP. (Reproduced from Ivashchenko, O., et al., *J. Nucl. Med.*, 56[3], 470–476 2015. With permission of the Society of Nuclear Medicine and Molecular Imaging.)

through the FOV during the SPECT acquisition, allowing a degree of projection overlap. The acquired data can be reconstructed separately and the volumes stitched together, or the entire dataset can be reconstructed as one extended volume (van der Have et al. 2009). When this approach is combined with many high-resolution pinholes focused on a small area, this method can yield submillimeter spatial resolution and greater than 1% absolute sensitivity, rivaling the performance of small-animal PET systems (Figure 16.2) (Ivashchenko et al. 2015).

Several systems have been developed with stationary detectors that surround the animal and multiple stationary or rotating pinholes (Beekman and Vastenhouw 2004; Furenlid et al. 2004; Goertzen et al. 2005; van der Have et al. 2009). Surrounding the animal with detectors and pinholes improves system sensitivity, and rotating the collimator instead of the detector reduces gantry construction costs and avoids mechanical misalignments due to gantry rotation. An important advantage of stationary SPECT systems is that all the required projections are acquired simultaneously, eliminating reconstruction errors due to redistribution of the radiopharmaceutical and enabling dynamic SPECT of tracers with fast kinetics (Furenlid et al. 2004; Fresneau et al. 2015).

16.2.3.4 DETECTOR TECHNOLOGIES

As in PET, most SPECT detectors are based on inorganic crystals coupled to one or more photodetectors via a light guide. NaI:Tl is a good choice of scintillator for SPECT due to its stopping power for 140 keV gamma rays, high light output, and the close match between its 410 nm emission wavelength and the peak efficiency of bialkali PMTs. CsI:Tl has a greater density and light output but slower decay time than NaI:Tl. They have similar refractive indexes, but CsI:Tl is only slightly hygroscopic, making it less likely to deteriorate over time. CsI:Na exhibits the best characteristics of NaI:Tl and CsI:Tl but has a longer scintillation decay time, which may be a problem for high-count-rate applications.

The most common photodetectors are PMTs (and PS-PMTs), silicon photodiodes, and charge-coupled devices (CCDs). PMTs have reasonable quantum efficiency (15%–40%) for converting light photons into photoelectrons, which is required for good spatial and energy resolution. Photodiodes are efficient at converting light into electrical current but produce very weak and noisy signals. Geiger-mode APDs (also known as silicon photomultipliers or SiPMs) show significant promise as alternatives to PS-PMTs, as they have a gain similar to that of PMTs (10^5–10^7), fast timing properties, and MR compatibility. Improvements in the performance of CCDs make these devices viable alternatives to PMTs. Modern CCDs do not suffer from dark current when modestly cooled and can achieve quantum efficiencies as high as 90%. Some CCDs are suitable for both optical (bioluminescence or fluorescence) and SPECT imaging with suitable modifications (Barrett and Hunter 2005).

Recent developments in semiconductor radiation imaging detectors make them a viable choice for small-animal SPECT in place of inorganic scintillators coupled to photodetectors. For example, cadmium-zinc-telluride (CZT) is a high-density semiconductor (6.06 g cm^{-3}) with good performance at room temperature. The probability of interaction for a 140 keV gamma ray is 83% for 5.0 mm of CZT, and the energy resolution is approximately 6%–7% for a typical array element, which is better than the energy resolution of similar-sized scintillation array detectors (Izaguirre et al. 2006; Seo et al. 2000). CZT detectors have the added advantage of being insensitive to magnetic field strengths of up to 7 T, therefore making them a suitable choice for hybrid SPECT/MR systems.

16.2.3.5 COLLIMATION

The purpose of collimation is to restrict gamma rays impinging on the detector to those traveling in certain preferred, and therefore known, directions. Collimators are constructed from gamma ray–absorbing material that has a high atomic number and electron density, such as lead, tungsten, gold, and depleted uranium. There are a wide variety of collimator designs that provide different trade-offs between spatial resolution and detection efficiency (see Section 16.4.1.2). The different types of collimation and their effect on SPECT performance are discussed in detail in Chapter 5.

16.2.4 MULTIMODALITY SYSTEMS

It is desirable to localize foci of increased or decreased radiopharmaceutical uptake in relation to surrounding anatomical structures to ensure correct interpretation of the image. It is often the case that radiopharmaceuticals with high specificity for their target site also exhibit less nonspecific uptake in surrounding organs and tissues. Paradoxically, radiopharmaceuticals with a lot of nonspecific uptake in surrounding tissues provide information that helps to localize uptake in the target tissues.

It is becoming increasingly important in research applications to accurately localize radiopharmaceutical biodistribution relative to known anatomical structures, particularly for new targeted radiopharmaceuticals with low nonspecific binding. X-ray CT and MR can provide detailed anatomical information that is highly complementary to the SPECT study. Thus, it is common in commercial systems for PET or SPECT to be one component of a dual- or trimodality imaging system. There are several possible combinations and approaches to multimodality imaging, including PET/CT, SPECT/CT, PET/MR and SPECT/MR.

16.3 PET PERFORMANCE CHARACTERIZATION AND QUALITY CONTROL

PET imaging of small animals is, in many respects, very similar to PET imaging of humans. For example, the principles of scanner operation, data acquisition, and image reconstruction, attenuation and scatter correction strategies, and the tendency toward integration of the PET component with other modalities (e.g., CT or SPECT) all remain the same or very similar. The most obvious difference is the much smaller object size, with rats and mice being two to three orders of magnitude less in weight and volume compared with humans. This introduces significant challenges with regard to spatial resolution and sensitivity.

16.3.1 SPATIAL RESOLUTION

For PET to be a useful investigative tool for small animals, high spatial resolution enabling visualization and quantification of the radiotracer distribution in structures on the order of millimeters or less (e.g., the striatum in the rat brain) is a key requirement. Spatial resolution is related to several factors, including the size of the detector elements, positron range, annihilation photon noncollinearity, depth-of-interaction (DoI), efficiency of light production and collection, intercrystal scatter, and signal multiplexing. The contribution to resolution degradation by factors other than the size of the detector elements is ~0.7 mm at the scanner center when using low-energy positrons and scanners with a small ring diameter. Therefore, for crystals of ~1.2 mm, a realistic target for the reconstructed spatial resolution of small-animal PET systems is about 1 mm (Lecomte 2004). Note that a reconstructed spatial resolution of 1 mm in rats and 0.4 mm in mice provides a volumetric imaging performance (in terms of the ability to recover signals from anatomically relevant structures) that is approximately equivalent to that of 6 mm spatial resolution in humans (Yao et al. 2012).

16.3.2 SENSITIVITY

Scanner sensitivity determines the feasibility of obtaining a measurable PET signal from small structures. Since typical tracer doses are 10–100 times less for rats and mice, respectively, compared to humans, the requirement for high-sensitivity scanners is increased significantly. For example, a dual challenge in receptor ligand–based studies is achieving a high enough specific activity of the tracer to allow the administration of tracer doses while simultaneously meeting the sensitivity requirements to reconstruct small volumes (Lecomte 2004).

Sensitivity depends on three main factors: the solid-angle coverage of the detectors, the detector material and thickness, and the choice of energy window. Sensitivity will be decreased if (1) there is a high probability that one or both 511 keV photons produced from an annihilation event fail to intersect with the active detector volume, (2) the photons intersect the detector ring but fail to deposit their energy in the detectors, or (3) the photons interact in the detector but are outside the allowable energy range. Conversely, sensitivity increases as the solid angle of detector coverage increases, as the crystal thickness (stopping power) increases, and as the energy window is widened. For a given scanner diameter and choice of scintillator, the first two of these factors represent an increase in total detector material, and therefore also in cost.

16.3.3 FACTORS AFFECTING PET PERFORMANCE

It is the requirement of high spatial resolution simultaneously with high sensitivity that determines (or limits) the range of applications for PET in small-animal imaging (Stickel and Cherry 2005). The development of small-animal PET systems over the last two decades has been characterized by considerable innovation in terms of the detector design and system geometry in order to address these dual challenges. Accordingly, small-animal PET systems exhibit much more variety in design than human systems. Below, several of the main factors affecting small-animal PET performance are outlined, together with examples of different systems from the published literature and their various design choices to meet the requirements of specific applications.

16.3.3.1 DETECTOR DESIGN

The main design factors affecting performance are the type and configuration of the scintillator material, the individual crystal size, and the type (e.g., PMT vs. solid state) and configuration (e.g., single-ended vs. dual-ended readout) of photodetectors.

Single-layer scintillation detectors usually comprise lutetium oxyorthosilicate (LSO) or lutetium-yttrium oxyorthosilicate (LYSO) because of its high stopping power and excellent light output. Dual-layer (phoswich) detectors usually combine LYSO with either lutetium-yttrium aluminum perovskite (LuYAP), germanium oxyorthosilicate (GSO), or lutetium gadolinium oxyorthosilicate (LGSO) (Goertzen et al. 2012). Several scanners make use of cheaper bismuth germanium oxide (BGO) (Zhang et al. 2011; Parnham et al. 2006), although the light output and timing properties of this scintillator are poorer than for lutetium-based scintillators. BGO does, however, have the advantage of having no intrinsic radioactivity like lutetium.

Simulations suggest that the main limiting factors for spatial resolution are the pixel size and the positron range, therefore allowing considerable flexibility in the choice of scintillator and photodetector (Stickel and Cherry 2005). Although long thin crystals go a long way to allowing high resolution and efficiency simultaneously, the parallax error is greatly increased for such crystals. Therefore, to fully benefit from this design,

DOI capability (discussed below) is essential. Solid-state photodetectors have advantages over PMTs when it comes to DOI-capable detectors, since they provide considerably greater flexibility in the design of the readout system.

Although direct detection of annihilation photons via solid-state detectors (e.g., CZT) has advantages over the traditional scintillator or photodetector module—most notably through the avoidance of light production or collection effects and in having the potential for smaller pixel sizes—the efficiency of such detectors is limited for 511 keV photons in PET due to their relatively small thickness. The detection efficiency of solid-state detectors can be improved by using a layered approach (Stickel and Cherry 2005), but this has yet to be implemented in a full system.

16.3.3.2 SCANNER GEOMETRY

The reduced diameter of preclinical PET systems compared with clinical scanners leads to improved spatial resolution by minimizing the impact of noncollinearity of the annihilation photons. Together with the increased ratio of axial to transaxial FOV, this leads to an improvement in the absolute sensitivity by increasing the solid angle of detection. In some systems, absolute sensitivity is compromised by the use of short crystals. For example, due to size and weight restrictions, the scintillator crystals of the RatPET scanner are only 5 mm long, resulting in lower sensitivity than more conventional designs where the crystals are typically at least twice this length.

Unconventional geometries, such as a departure from circular (i.e., ring) systems and the presence of nonuniform gaps between detector modules, have important implications for image reconstruction. In particular, artifacts may result when FBP is used to reconstruct images from such systems. Instead, an iterative algorithm in which the nonstandard geometry is correctly modeled in the system matrix is preferable (Goertzen et al. 2012).

16.3.3.3 DEPTH OF INTERACTION

For sources near the center of the FOV, the use of long thin crystals confines the width of the coincidence channel between any two crystals so that the DOI of a gamma ray has little impact on eventual localization. However, for annihilations nearer to the edge of the FOV, localization is strongly affected by the point of interaction of the gamma rays along the length of the crystal. This is the so-called parallax or DOI effect, which results in nonuniform spatial resolution throughout the FOV. The DOI effect is exaggerated in small-diameter detector rings such as those used in small-animal PET systems. For example, for a 6–8 cm diameter system dedicated to mouse imaging, with no DOI capability, the radial resolution can degrade by several millimeters in moving from the center to the edge of the FOV. Conversely, a DOI resolution of 2 mm will result in approximately uniform spatial resolution throughout the 3 cm FOV for a high-resolution system comprised of $0.5 \times 0.5 \times 20$ mm crystals (St. James et al. 2009).

The impact of ambiguous DOI is reduced either by using shorter crystals or by enlarging the ring diameter. However, both approaches lower the efficiency of detection. In addition, shorter crystals increase the proportion of scattered events in the measured data, while enlarging the ring diameter increases the impact of noncollinearity on spatial resolution degradation and necessitates a quadratic increase in the number of detector elements to achieve the same solid angle of detection. It is therefore preferable to have PET detectors with DOI capability so that high sensitivity and spatial resolution can be maintained simultaneously.

Numerous methods have been developed for DOI determination. Broadly, these methods are categorized according to whether they provide discrete or continuous DOI information. The most common discrete DOI approach involves the so-called phoswich detector, which uses multiple scintillator layers with different detection properties such as scintillation decay times (Seidel et al. 1999). Detected events are assigned to a particular layer based on the pulse shape characteristics. Phoswich technology provides relatively coarse DOI information, limited by the number and thickness of scintillator layers. Although many-layer implementations have been reported (Saoudi et al. 1999; Tsuda et al. 2004), only two-layer implementations have appeared commercially (e.g., Wang et al. 2006). Several variations on the phoswich concept for discrete DOI information exist, for example using a clever arrangement of reflectors around groups of crystal elements within the different scintillator layers (Tsuda et al. 2004).

Continuous DOI information can be obtained using a dual-ended photodetector readout scheme (Yang et al. 2006). Dual-ended readout is facilitated by compact solid-state photodetectors such as PS-APDs and SiPMs, both of which are largely transparent to 511 keV photons. In dual-ended readout designs, continuous DOI information is obtained based on the ratio of the signal amplitude from each photodetector. A DOI resolution of approximately 2 mm is achievable for $1 \times 1 \times 20$ mm crystals (Yang et al. 2008). The major drawback of this approach is that it doubles the number of photodetectors and the number of electronic channels for processing. The number of channels can be reduced considerably using orthogonally placed wavelength-shifting (WS) optical fibers at each end of the scintillator array (Du et al. 2007). The WS fibers contain a photofluorescent core that absorbs the scintillation light emitted from the crystal and reemits it at a longer wavelength along the fibers. The number of electronic channels is reduced to the number of fibers in the x and y directions.

Several methods exist to obtain continuous DOI information using a single-ended photodetector readout configuration. Precalibrated lookup tables can be used to relate the measured light response to various parameters correlated with DOI (van Dam et al. 2011). Another approach is to use a phosphor coating over one end of the crystal to cause a wavelength shift and time delay for a component of the scintillation light that is dependent on the DOI (Du et al. 2009). DOI estimates can then be obtained by decoding the mixture signal read out from the photodetector. Yet another approach is to estimate the photon entry point into a detector array to provide an intrinsic DOI correction. This method has the drawback of extensive precalibration using photons at many angles of incidence (Maas et al. 2009).

Although most small-animal PET systems use pixelated detector arrays, systems with monolithic crystals are also making a comeback because of the advantages in detection sensitivity, and several methods for DOI determination in such systems have been reported. These methods usually involve DOI estimation based on characterization of the light spread at the photodetector or a model of the light transport (Antich et al. 2002; Lerche et al. 2009; Li et al. 2010).

DOI capability has several important benefits for PET performance. Primarily, it improves the uniformity of spatial resolution throughout the FOV. It also enables longer crystals to be used, thus improving sensitivity. Furthermore, it enables the scanner radius to be reduced so that fewer detectors are required to achieve the same solid-angle coverage of the subject. Fewer detectors in turn means fewer electronic channels to read out and process. DOI capability has also been shown to enable improved timing resolution in TOF PET systems (Vinke et al. 2010).

16.3.3.4 SCATTER, ATTENUATION, AND PARTIAL VOLUME CORRECTION

Attenuation and scatter of the annihilation photons in PET imaging of small animals can affect quantification and degrade image quality, although to a lesser extent than in human PET due to the much smaller subject size. Typical scatter fractions are 5%–10% for mice, 15%–35% for rats, and 35%–50% for nonhuman primates. Measurement of the scatter fraction for tissue equivalent mouse, rat, and monkey-like phantoms is included as part of the National Electrical Manufacturers Association (NEMA) standardized methodology for evaluating the performance of preclinical PET scanners (NEMA 2008) (see Section 16.3.4).

In small-animal scanners, the reduced scanner diameter and smaller object size tend to make the scatter fractions more reflective of the gantry design and materials than systems designed for humans. For example, for mouse-sized objects the gantry is the dominant source of scatter (Yang and Cherry 2006). The scatter fraction tends to reduce as the ring diameter is increased or as the energy window is narrowed. However, some widening of the energy window in order to improve sensitivity is reasonable given that the scatter is considerably smaller than for a human. Dual-layer detector configurations can result in higher scatter fractions, most likely because of the use of scintillator materials with lower photofractions (Goertzen et al. 2012). It is usually safe to ignore attenuation and scatter effects for qualitative investigations, especially in mice. In cases where attenuation and scatter correction are implemented, the methods are essentially the same as for human studies (see Chapter 8 for details).

The partial volume effect (PVE) is defined as signal dilution and mixing due to spatial resolution and sampling limitations of the imaging system. The magnitude of PVE depends on the ratio of the size of the characteristic structures being imaged to the reconstructed spatial resolution, and therefore is more likely to be problematic in small-animal studies than in human studies (Dupont and Warwick 2009). The extent to which PVE affects the primary outcome measure of a PET study depends on the research question. In many cases PVE can probably be ignored, however it is likely to be an issue when estimating quantitative parameters in small structures such as mouse brain regions and also when quantifying heterogeneous radiopharmaceutical uptake in a tumor. As with attenuation and scatter correction, methods of partial volume correction are mainly based on those developed for human PET data analyses. However, because non-DOI-capable small-animal PET systems typically have more variable spatial resolution than human PET systems, more careful modeling of the spatially variant point-spread function (PSF) and voxel-based rather than region-based correction are recommended (Lehnert et al. 2012).

16.3.4 PERFORMANCE TESTING

NEMA sets out a standardized methodology for evaluating the performance of preclinical PET scanners (NEMA 2008). The methodology enables users to establish a baseline of system performance for typical imaging conditions. Importantly, it is applicable across a wide range of tomograph designs, including circular ring and planar (panel) detector designs, segmented or continuous scintillator crystals, gas avalanche detectors, tomographs with fixed or movable detector elements, and tomographs with or without time-of-flight capability. To perform all standard NEMA measurements, the transverse FOV must be able to accommodate a 33.5 mm diameter image-quality phantom.

The main tests specified by NEMA are outlined below. All measurements should be performed with critical parameters (e.g., coincidence timing window, choice of angular or axial mashing, reconstruction algorithm, and associated parameters) kept constant, unless the parameters are reported together with the relevant measurement. Following the NEMA definition, the axial FOV is the maximum length parallel to the long axis of the tomograph along which transaxial tomographic images can be generated. The transverse FOV is the diameter of the maximal circular region, centered on the long axis of the tomograph and perpendicular to it, in which an object could be imaged.

16.3.4.1 SPATIAL RESOLUTION

Spatial resolution according to the NEMA standardized methodology is specified as the width (full width at half maximum and full width at tenth maximum) of a reconstructed ^{22}Na point source (≤ 0.3 mm in all directions) imaged in a scattering medium (10 mm^3 acrylic cube), where the dead-time losses and randoms rates during data acquisition are $\leq 5\%$. The standard specifies repetition of the measurement at several radial positions for each of two axial positions, each time reporting the width of the PSF in all three directions.

16.3.4.2 SCATTER, COUNT LOSSES, AND RANDOMS MEASUREMENT

For scatter and count rate measurements NEMA specifies three phantoms in line with the animals most commonly imaged preclinically: the mouse, rat, and monkey. All three phantoms constitute solid right circular cylinders composed of high-density polyethylene ($\rho = 0.96$ g cm^{-3}) with a hole drilled parallel to the central axis in which a line source can be inserted. The lengths and diameters of the mouse, rat, and monkey phantoms are summarized in Table 16.1.

The raw data needed to estimate true, scatter, and randoms rates as a function of activity are obtained by scanning the relevant phantom repeatedly over several half-lives of the isotope (either ^{18}F or ^{11}C), beginning with a line source of activity that produces appreciable dead time. Scans should be repeated until the count rate loss and randoms rate are <1% of the trues rate. Sinograms containing true, randoms and scattered

Table 16.1 NEMA animal phantom dimensions

Phantom	Length (mm)	Diameter (mm)
Mouse	70	25
Rat	150	50
Monkey	400	100

coincidences are then processed to determine the true, random, and scatter event rates for the system, the noise-equivalent count rate (NECR) (see Section 1.6.9), and the total event rate, each as a function of activity. The relative sensitivity of a system to scattered radiation, characterized by the scatter fraction (see Section 8.2.2), is determined from the acquisitions in which count rate losses and random event rates are less than 1% of the true event rate, since it is assumed that the randoms are negligible by this stage. Scanner performance characterizations in the literature typically report values such as the scatter fraction for the phantom (mouse, rat, or monkey), the peak true count rate or peak NECR, and the activity concentration corresponding to the peak NECR.

16.3.4.3 SENSITIVITY

Sensitivity is the rate of true coincidences per Becquerel of source activity, measured when count rate losses and the random coincidence rate are negligible. The absolute sensitivity describes how this value compares to the branching fraction of the radionuclide. For sensitivity measurements, data are collected by acquiring a fixed-duration scan each time a ^{22}Na source is stepped along the axis in increments of one slice thickness. The background-corrected sensitivities for slices in the central 70 and 150 mm are summed to obtain the overall sensitivity for mouse and rat scans, respectively. Total sensitivity is obtained by summing the sensitivities for all slices.

16.3.4.4 IMAGE QUALITY

A multicompartment image-quality phantom is used to obtain a measure of the spatial resolution, signal-to-noise ratio, and scatter and attenuation correction performance in a representative small-animal imaging scenario. The 30 mm diameter, 50 mm long cylindrical phantom consists of a main fillable chamber, five fillable rods ranging from 1 to 5 mm in diameter, and two cold compartments (one containing nonradioactive water and one containing air). The main chamber and rods are filled with a known concentration of ^{18}F such that the total activity falls within the range of a typical mouse study. The phantom is imaged for 20 min, and transaxial images are reconstructed with all available corrections. Uniformity is calculated from a volume of interest (VOI) drawn within the main fillable chamber. This provides a measure of the accuracy of the corrections for attenuation and scatter, as does the spillover ratio for each of the cold regions. The standard deviation within the main hot VOI is indicative of the SNR of the system. The recovery coefficient for each rod size provides a measure of spatial resolution performance.

16.3.5 CURRENT STATE-OF-THE-ART IN PRECLINICAL PET

Table 16.2 summarizes the design and performance of commercial and research preclinical PET scanners. The current state-of-the-art is characterized by an approximately 1 mm³ volumetric spatial resolution, peak sensitivity of >10%, energy resolution of approximately 12%–15%, and DOI resolution of <2 mm (Mizuta et al. 2008; Wang et al. 2006; Constantinescu and Mukherjee 2009; Jeavons et al. 1999; Tai et al. 2005). For mouse imaging, the peak NECR occurs at >3.2 MBq in the FOV for all scanners and in most cases is >20 MBq. For rat imaging, peak NECR occurs at >5.6 MBq for all scanners and in most cases is >30 MBq.

In general, using finely pixelated gamma ray detectors with DOI encoding provides a means of simultaneously improving sensitivity, spatial resolution, and uniformity of resolution throughout the FOV, and these features have come to characterize the latest generation of small-animal PET scanners (e.g., Yang et al. 2013). However, it should be noted that the performance variation seen between scanners is often due in large part to differences in design specification and the intended application. For example, the sensitivity of the RatCAP, where miniaturization is the primary design goal, is not expected to be as high as that of the long-axial-FOV Quad HIDAC.

In terms of equivalent volumetric imaging performance compared with human systems, this has been achieved for rat imaging but not yet for mouse imaging. Analysis of the components affecting intrinsic spatial resolution indicates that the physical limit for PET is ~0.5 mm and may be achieved using 0.25 mm crystal elements (Stickel and Cherry 2005). This assumes unambiguous positioning of the energy centroid for all elements. In practice, there may be some ambiguity in resolving the energy centroid for discrete elements

Table 16.2 Design and performance of preclinical PET scanners[a]

Characteristic	Range
Ring diameter (mm)	38–261
Axial FOV (mm)[b]	7–280
Crystal size—cross section (mm)	0.43–2.32
Crystal size—length (mm)	5–13 (14–25.2[c])
Spatial resolution	
Radial (mm)	0.6–2.32
Tangential (mm)	0.6–2.32
Axial (mm)	0.61–3.24
Peak sensitivity (%)[d]	0.7–14
Scatter fraction (%)	
Mouse	5–37
Rat	12–35
Monkey	35–50
Recovery coefficient	
1 mm rod	0.1–0.27
5 mm rod	0.75–1.0
Peak NECR (peak activity)	
Mouse	20 kcps (3.2 MBq)–1670 kcps (131 MBq)
Rat	31 kcps (34 MBq)–592 kcps (110 MBq)

[a] Based on 17 research and commercial systems (Goertzen et al. 2012; Jeavons et al. 1999; Parnham et al. 2006; Yang et al. 2013; Szanda et al. 2011; Mizuta et al. 2008; Zhang et al. 2011).
[b] Fixed axial FOV only (i.e., does not include systems with motorized bed to move subject axially).
[c] Values in parentheses are for dual-layer phoswich systems.
[d] Energy window 150–650 keV.

due to cross talk and multiplexing in the photodetection. However, the impact of this on spatial resolution is usually small (Stickel and Cherry 2005). The recently achieved 0.6 mm spatial resolution demonstrated in a single-ring prototype scanner (Yang et al. 2013) suggests that the limits of PET performance may be on the horizon. Such improvements in PET performance make it suitable for applications such as early detection of metastatic disease and studies of disease progression, and assessing treatment response in mouse models of human cancer and brain diseases. In the future, it is also likely that we will see the use of solid-state photodetector technology become standard in preclinical PET systems, as well as the mature integration of PET and MRI components.

16.4 SPECT PERFORMANCE CHARACTERIZATION AND QUALITY CONTROL

The performance of preclinical SPECT systems is primarily determined by the geometrical relationship between the target organ and the detectors, the detector specifications, and the collimator profile. As with preclinical PET, spatial resolution and sensitivity are the key performance parameters for most applications, although energy resolution can also be very important, especially in multi-isotope studies. The performance of three commercial preclinical SPECT systems with typical collimator profiles is shown in Figure 16.3 as a resolution versus sensitivity plot.

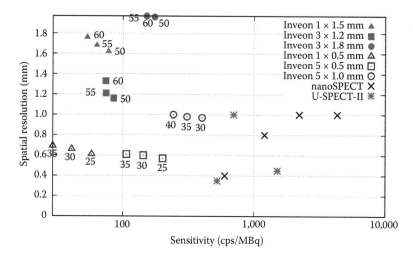

Figure 16.3 Tomographic spatial resolution as a function of sensitivity measured for three commercial small-animal SPECT scanners: Inveon SPECT, U-SPECT-II, and nanoSPECT. Results for a range of collimator profiles designed for mouse and rat studies are shown. For the Inveon scanner, the number and diameter of pinholes are indicated in the legend and the ROR is indicated next to the data points. NanoSPECT results are for 36 pinhole arrays with 0.6 and 1.0 mm diameter, U-SPECT-II results are for 75 pinhole arrays with 0.35 and 0.6 mm diameter. (Reproduced from Boisson, F., et al., *J. Nucl. Med.*, 54[10], 1833–1840, 2013. With permission of the Society of Nuclear Medicine and Molecular Imaging.)

16.4.1 FACTORS AFFECTING SPECT PERFORMANCE

16.4.1.1 DETECTOR DESIGN

While NaI:Tl is virtually ubiquitous in clinical SPECT imaging systems, several other inorganic scintillators are also used in preclinical systems. Typically, the scintillation wavelengths are in the range of 350–600 nm. Table 16.3 presents the different properties of scintillating crystals commonly used in single-photon imaging.

A pixelated crystal array comprising small (typically 1 mm wide), tightly packed, and optically isolated crystals is commonly used in preclinical systems to ensure high intrinsic spatial resolution. The intrinsic spatial resolution of the detector is approximately the same as the crystal pitch, provided it is coupled to a high-resolution detector capable of resolving individual crystal elements, such as a PS-PMT (Figure 16.1c and d). While a small crystal pitch is desirable for high spatial resolution, the thickness must be sufficient to absorb most photons for good detection efficiency. However, as the crystal length-to-width ratio increases, light output decreases due to internal reflections, resulting in a loss of energy resolution (Wirrwar et al. 1999, 2000; Barrett and Hunter 2005).

16.4.1.2 COLLIMATOR PROFILE

Small-animal SPECT systems typically use pinhole collimation, which presents a conical geometry leading to high magnification and high spatial resolution (Franc et al. 2008; Schramm et al. 2003; Weber and Ivanovic 1999). Higher detection efficiency can be obtained using multipinhole collimation (Meikle et al. 2002; Vunckx et al. 2009) without, in theory, trading away spatial resolution. These collimators are normally designed to rotate at a specific ROR. The combination of the collimator geometrical design (number and placement of the pinholes, collimator length, aperture, and degree of multiplexing) and the ROR fixes many characteristics, such as the active FOV and the performance of the system in terms of spatial resolution and sensitivity. It is therefore important to understand the performance trade-offs obtained with each type of collimation profile before applying them to biological studies. These trade-offs are discussed in detail in Chapter 5. Here, we focus on collimator profiles that are most commonly employed in small-animal SPECT, such as pinhole and multipinhole configurations, and their effects on small-animal imaging performance parameters.

Table 16.3 Properties of scintillating crystals commonly used in single-photon imaging

Scintillation crystal	NaI:Tl	CsI:Tl	YAP:Ce	LaBr$_3$	GSO:Ce	LaCl$_3$
Density (g cm^{-1})	3.67	4.51	5.55	5.29	6.71	3.79
Index of refraction	1.85	1.79	1.94	1.9	1.85	1.9
Luminescence (ph keV^{-1})	38	54	18	63	9	49
Peak emission wavelength (nm)	415	550	350	380	430	350
Emission decay time (ns)	250	1000	27	26	60	28
Attenuation length at 140 keV (cm)	0.41	0.28	0.58	0.29	0.17	0.37
Hygroscopicity	Yes	Poor	No	Yes	No	Yes

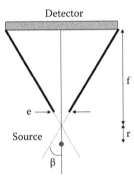

Figure 16.4 Pinhole collimator geometry showing key parameters affecting SPECT performance.

The pinhole collimator is well suited to imaging small objects such as mice and rats. Its conical geometry (Figure 16.4) leads to high magnification, and therefore excellent spatial resolution, when the subject is positioned close to the pinhole aperture. However, it also reduces the size of the FOV, and the potentially excellent spatial resolution is accompanied by very poor detection efficiency, as shown in the following equations:

$$R_c = e\left(1 + \frac{r}{f}\right)$$

$$S_c = e^2\left(\frac{\cos^3 \beta}{16r^2}\right)$$

where R_c and S_c are the collimator resolution and sensitivity, respectively; e is the effective hole diameter (taking edge penetration into account); f is the focal length; r is the distance between the source and the hole; and β is the opening angle of the collimator. Note that the r/f term can be written as $1/M$, where M is the magnification factor.

The magnification factor and the diameter of the hole are the parameters that control the pinhole collimator resolution. However, the magnification factor has an upper limit that is determined by the detector FOV and the required size of the reconstructed FOV. The low detection efficiency of the pinhole collimator can be compensated for by increasing the number of holes (Beekman et al. 2005; Meikle et al. 2002, 2003; Vanhove et al. 2008; DiFilippo 2008). In general, the use of multiple-pinhole collimation increases sensitivity without significantly affecting spatial resolution. However, it can also lead to truncation of the object being imaged or overlapping projections, which may introduce artifacts in the reconstructed image unless the collimator is carefully designed and properly modeled (Kench et al. 2011; Lin 2013; Vunckx et al. 2008).

The slit-slat collimator proposed by Metzler et al. (2006) is also well suited to small-animal imaging. As the name implies, it consists of a slit perpendicular to a parallel array of slats, as shown in Figure 16.5. It can

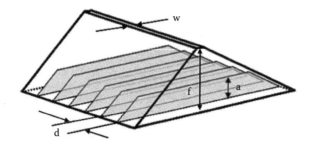

Figure 16.5 Slit-slat collimator geometry showing key parameters affecting SPECT performance.

be considered the combination of a pinhole collimator in one direction and a parallel-hole collimator in the other direction. The dependence of the spatial resolution perpendicular to the slit, R_{trans}, and in the direction of the slit, R_{axial}, on the slit-slat parameters is given by the following equations:

$$R_{\text{trans}} = \sqrt{w^2\left(\frac{h+f}{f}\right)^2 + \left(\frac{hR_i}{f}\right)^2}$$

$$R_{\text{axial}} = \sqrt{d^2\left(\frac{h+f}{a}\right)^2 + R_i^2}$$

where R_i is the intrinsic spatial resolution of the detector, w is the width of the slit, f is the focal length, a is the slat height, d is the space between two consecutive slats, and h is the distance between the emission point and the collimator entrance face.

The detection efficiency of a slit-slat collimator is given by

$$S_c = \frac{d^2}{\left(4\pi ah(d+t)\right)}$$

where t is the thickness of the slats. This collimator profile has superior detection efficiency compared with a single-pinhole collimator. However, the compromise between resolution and detection efficiency remains and is more complicated in this case due to the large number of fixed parameters. The performance of the slit-slat collimator is compared with that of typical collimator profiles in Figure 16.6.

16.4.2 PRECLINICAL SPECT QUALITY CONTROL

Unlike preclinical PET systems, for which NEMA has defined the NU 4 2008 standard (NEMA 2008), pre-clinical SPECT systems are, to date, subject to no standards. A task force has recently been assigned to establish such standards, including a new phantom adapted to small-animal SPECT systems, and to define the image-quality parameters. In anticipation of this possible NEMA NU 5, the image-quality phantom defined by the NU 4 2008 standard was used in previous studies to characterize the performance of small-animal SPECT scanners (Harteveld et al. 2011).

16.5 PRACTICAL ASPECTS OF SMALL-ANIMAL IMAGING

In addition to the instrumentation-related factors that make small-animal imaging with PET and SPECT a significant challenge, there are several practical issues arising from the biology and physiology of rodents that

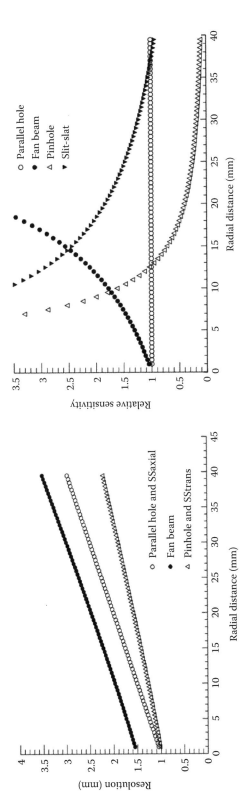

Figure 16.6 Comparative performance of collimators used in preclinical SPECT with typical collimator parameters (collimator height = 20 mm, septal thickness = 0.2 mm, hole diameter = 1 mm, focal length = 40 mm, pinhole angle = 45°, slit width = 1 mm, slat gap = 1.5 mm). SSaxial, slit-slat axial; SStrans, slit-slat transaxial.

can affect the reliability of imaging results, and therefore require careful attention. These include the need for anesthesia, injection techniques, physiological monitoring, and blood sampling.

16.5.1 ANESTHESIA

Artifacts due to biological motion remain a major challenge for obtaining image data in serial *in vivo* imaging studies (Nicholson and Klaunberg 2008; Hildebrandt et al. 2008). In principle, the motion problem can be overcome by restraining the animal (Mizuma et al. 2010), fixing the PET detectors rigidly to the skull (Vaska 2004), or implementing accurate motion tracking and correction (Kyme et al. 2008). However, for routine applications in most laboratories, anesthesia is required to minimize gross physical motion. Anesthesia has a profound depressant effect on the autonomic nervous system, which also depresses the cardiovascular system, respiration rate, and thermoregulation. In addition, repeated anesthesia, as well as radiation exposure and contrast agent administration, affect the homeostasis of the animal, which may adversely affect image quality (Tremoleda et al. 2012). Therefore, it is important to ensure that the animal remains in a stable physiological state while undergoing an imaging study and to be aware of the physiological effects of different anesthetic regimens. In addition, the response to anesthesia may vary among animals; therefore, it is important to monitor and adjust the anesthesia protocol throughout the study. The depth of anesthesia can be monitored by assessing muscle tone, response to painful stimulus, rate and depth of respiration, and loss of righting and palpebral reflexes.

The anesthetic regimen may be of two types: injectable and inhaled. Both are used in rodents. Inhalation anesthesia is most suitable for long procedures, such as imaging studies, because it is safer, has rapid onset and recovery, and provides greater control of the dose of anesthetic agent and better maintenance of anesthetic depth than injectable anesthetics. Moreover, inhaled agents are quickly eliminated via the lungs, and produce less cardiovascular depression and less effect on liver and kidney function. However, inhalation anesthetic agents produce respiratory depression, myocardial depression, and hypotension and are weak analgesics (Tremoleda et al. 2012). In addition, expensive equipment and a greater level of expertise are needed for using inhalation anesthesia.

Injectable agents are usually metabolized in the liver and eliminated by the kidneys. Specific reversal agents are available for some of the newer injectable agents, which hastens the recovery. Use of injectable agents for a longer duration increases the risk of hypoxia, and oxygen supplementation is needed to prevent respiratory depression, hypercapnia, and acidosis (Tremoleda et al. 2012).

16.5.1.1 INJECTABLE ANESTHETICS

Injectable anesthetic agents can be administered via various routes: intraperitoneal, intramuscular, subcutaneous, or intravenous. They offer the advantages of convenience and familiarity, and no special equipment is required, which justifies their use for short procedures. However, problems may arise when longer anesthesia is required. A dose of drug that achieves stable anesthesia in some animals may be insufficient in others or, conversely, may lead to overdose, toxicity, or death in others. Repeated doses may also have these adverse effects. This is especially true while using drugs with narrow margins of safety, such as pentobarbital. Increasing the length of anesthesia may require further injections, which can also change the depth of anesthesia. This may be overcome by using continuous infusion to maintain a steady plasma concentration. Some drugs like propofol and alpha-chlorolose may be used in continuous infusion to adjust the length and depth of anesthesia as needed. Although this method offers better control over the planes of anesthesia, it has limitations. Alpha-chlorolose can be administered via an intraperitoneal line; the success of this drug depends on the hydration status, cardiac output, and systemic blood pressure of the animal, in addition to its absorption from the peritoneal cavity. Propofol is an ultra-short-acting intravenous anesthetic agent for which anesthetic levels are easy to adjust; however, venous access is a requirement. Apart from the technical challenges in placing an intravenous catheter in rodents, it is also difficult to maintain patency. Metabolism and elimination of these drugs are dependent on hepatic and renal pathways, and because of the time taken to remove these drugs, recovery time is often prolonged. The investigator must allow enough time for proper recovery of the animals and provide adequate postprocedural care. If animals are sent back to their housing room without full recovery, they may suffer hypothermia overnight. This can be partially overcome by using anesthetic drugs that are reversible (Gargiulo et al. 2012). Many factors, including the species used, age, sex, strain, health condition, environment, experimental setup, administration route, and previous drug treatments, can affect an animal's response to a drug (Tremoleda et al. 2012). In addition, anesthetic outcomes are affected by subclinical infections of rodent pathogens. It therefore may be wise to expose several animals to the proposed anesthetic regime before commencing the actual experiment.

16.5.1.2 INHALATION ANESTHESIA

The adverse effects of injectable anesthesia are usually better controlled with inhalation anesthesia due to its rapid onset and short recovery time. For long procedures (1 h or more), it is safer to use inhalation anesthesia, as it can be adjusted more rapidly than injectables and recovery is shorter. In addition, it is usually not possible to manipulate the animal for maintenance anesthesia once positioned for imaging. With the use of a precision vaporizer, the delivery of anesthesia can be adjusted remotely without manipulating the animal. For these reasons, the use of inhalation anesthesia is generally preferred for animal imaging.

There are three methods for delivering inhalation anesthesia: endotracheal tube (ET), face mask, or anesthesia chamber. An ET tube has the advantage that in the case of cardiac or respiratory arrest, artificial ventilation can be started immediately. Anesthetizing the animal with a face mask is simple but precludes ventilation. Anesthetizing the animal using a chamber is the simplest method; however, the animal cannot be repositioned once anesthetized, and this method has the same limitation on ventilation as the face mask approach. While using these methods, proper scavenging of exhaled anesthetic gases must be ensured to prevent occupational exposure to potentially harmful gases.

When an ET tube is used, the largest tube that fits the trachea without causing trauma is used. Oral insertion of an ET tube is a difficult task, especially in the mouse. Even in experienced hands, there is a risk of trauma to the oropharynx, larynx, trachea, or esophagus. To avoid complications, monitoring of vital signs and physiological parameters is important during this procedure. While using an ET tube in rodents, the use of positive-pressure ventilation is strongly recommended. Ventilating physiologically stable rats is quite robust, but such reliable methods are yet to be developed for the mouse.

The risk of adverse outcomes due to prolonged anesthesia is increased in old or sick animals. Moreover, genetically engineered mice are usually smaller in size and have greater risk of adverse outcomes from anesthesia, which increases the technical challenges involved in imaging these valuable animals. Although it is advisable to monitor as many physiological parameters as possible, this may not be feasible in all imaging studies.

16.5.2 INJECTION TECHNIQUES

There are three main methods used for radiotracer administration in mice: intraperitoneal, retro-orbital, and intravenous. Each has its own advantages and disadvantages. Intraperitoneal injections are easy and quick to administer, but erroneous injection into the bowel may distort results. The major limitation of this method is the wide variability in radiotracer pharmacokinetics arising from intraperitoneal administration due to radiotracer-dependent variability in peritoneal absorption. Retro-orbital injections are also easy and quick to perform, but the mouse must be anesthetized for this procedure. At many institutions, this method is not approved by the animal care committee (Vines et al. 2011). Thus, neither of these methods is used frequently, and therefore intravenous injection remains the most commonly used method for radiotracer administration. It offers the advantage over other methods of providing 100% bioavailability of the radiotracer, resulting in more consistent pharmacokinetics, and it can be performed on both awake and anesthetized animals.

Intravenous injections are usually given via the lateral veins of the tail. These veins serve the purpose of thermal regulation of the animal, and thus will dilate for heat dissemination when body temperature rises. Applying heat to the torso or locally to the tail will cause vasodilation, making the vein easily accessible.

The tail should be held taut with the lateral tail vein facing the injector. The needle should be inserted into the vein at a minimal angle and advanced about 2 mm into the vein, taking care not to perforate it. Blood should be drawn back into the needle hub before making an injection to confirm that the needle is in the vein. Now the plunger can be pushed to deliver the radiopharmaceutical into the vein. There should be no resistance or swelling at the injection site, and the radiopharmaceutical should be detectable in the tissues of the animal within 10 s; otherwise, the injection has failed and needs to be repeated. An ethanol swab should be applied at the injection site to stop any bleeding.

A tail vein cannula is used when continuous infusion of radiopharmaceutical is required. This method also simplifies the procedure when multiple bolus injections are required or when the radiotracer must be administered at a specified rate.

16.5.3 PHYSIOLOGICAL MONITORING AND GATING

All anesthetic drugs affect the respiratory system, cardiovascular system, and thermoregulation to varying extents. These physiologic parameters can be used to determine the level of anesthesia, as well as to maintain homeostasis of the anesthetized animal during the imaging procedure. Thus, monitoring of physiological parameters of animals is vital during imaging procedures. Although there are no clearly defined parameters, cardiovascular and respiratory functions are usually monitored continuously throughout the study. Basic parameters include heart rate, blood pressure, respiratory rate, blood oxygenation, body temperature, and arterial blood gas (Tremoleda et al. 2012).

The selection of appropriate equipment, as well as technical expertise, is important, as the small size of rodents, along with their high heart rate and small respiratory volume, presents unique challenges and may require monitoring equipment that is different than that used in larger species. While selecting appropriate equipment for physiological monitoring, the type and duration of imaging procedures, previous procedures the animal has undergone, and capabilities of the available equipment all need to be considered.

16.5.3.1 BODY TEMPERATURE

Most anesthetic agents have a depressant effect on the thermoregulatory centers of the brain, and risk of hypothermia increases with the duration of anesthesia (Tremoleda et al. 2012). Hypothermia is a major concern in laboratory rodents due to their small size, high metabolic rate, and high ratio of surface area to body weight. Thus, monitoring the core body temperature of the anesthetized animal is crucial to avoid hypothermia and risk of mortality in the postprocedural period. The animal must recover completely before it is returned to its home cage.

Several systems are available for use with all imaging modalities, but the rectal temperature probe is the most common. Rectal temperature may be 1°C lower than the core body temperature. Several methods are available for treating hypothermia, such as hot water blanket, air-blowing system, electric heating pad, bubble wrap, and infrared lamps. The method used depends mainly on compatibility with the imaging device.

16.5.3.2 RESPIRATION

In a spontaneously breathing animal, the level of anesthesia and adequate ventilation can be assessed by respiratory rate. During homeostasis, the blood levels of O_2 and CO_2 are controlled by sensors present in the brain that change the rate of respiration to adjust blood gas levels. If the level of CO_2 in the blood rises, the respiratory rate increases to exhale more CO_2. However, careful monitoring is needed, as increased respiratory rate may also indicate insufficient level of anesthesia. In deeply anesthetized animals, this reflex may be suppressed. The respiratory rate can be counted by breaths visually or with a monitoring device. Some devices may translate the respiratory movement into a signal and display the respiratory waveform on a monitor.

16.5.3.3 ELECTROCARDIOGRAPH

Electrical activity of the heart is monitored by electrocardiograph (ECG). With each cardiac beat, an electrical signal is generated that is picked up by electrodes, amplified, and displayed on a screen. The ECG is useful for diagnosing and treating arrhythmias and may help in critical situations, such as loss of blood pressure, resulting in peripheral pulses being so low that they cannot be palpated. The ECG is also useful for cardiac gated imaging studies where the cardiac signal is synchronized with data acquired by the scanner (Hildebrandt et al. 2008).

16.5.3.4 BLOOD OXYGENATION

Arterial blood oxygenation is measured using a device called a pulse oximeter. Hypoxia is a common and serious problem in anesthetized animals, and the pulse oximeter is able to detect it before the animal develops cyanosis. It consists of a probe, a light-emitting diode, and a photodetector. It can be applied on a superficial vessel. This device gives information about both the circulatory and respiratory system, as it measures both pulse rate and oxygen saturation in the blood. The device provides continuous measurement of arterial oxygen saturation, pulse strength, blood flow, and heart rate (Tremoleda et al. 2012). Thus, it is a valuable tool for monitoring anesthetized animals. The sensor can be applied over the thigh, foot, neck, or tail of rodents, depending on their body size. An arterial oxygen saturation of >95% is good. If it falls to less than 90%, the anesthetist should be watchful. If it falls to less than 80%, action is required to improve oxygen saturation.

16.5.3.5 BLOOD PRESSURE

Systemic blood pressure is affected by all anesthetic agents. Blood pressure monitoring helps in maintaining the appropriate level of anesthesia and adequate tissue perfusion. Two basic methods are used for measurement of arterial blood pressure: direct and indirect. In the indirect method, a pulse transducer and inflatable tail pressure cuff specially configured for rodents can be used. The cuff pressure and pulse transducer signals are recorded from the tail artery. However, anesthetized rodents may undergo hypothermia, leading to peripheral vasoconstriction, which may interfere with pulse detection by the indirect method. The direct method consists of placing an arterial catheter and connecting it to a pressure transducer or optical sensor that is able to convert pressure changes into electrical impulses for display. With the development of fiber-optic technology, newer devices have become available to invasively monitor blood pressure in rodents. However, technical challenges are involved in placing an arterial catheter in rodents, and signals from other equipment may interfere with amplification of the blood pressure signal.

Some anesthetic agents decrease arterial blood pressure, while others may produce coronary vasodilatation, leading to changes in flow parameters. Thus, blood pressure monitoring is very important while assessing the perfusion of a radiotracer through specific tissues during PET/SPECT imaging (Tremoleda et al. 2012).

16.5.3.6 PULMONARY CO_2

Capnography consists of a highly sensitive infrared spectroscopy sensor that provides continuous measurement of the CO_2 level in respiratory circuits. Samples are taken from the respiratory circuit and CO_2 is analyzed in both inhaled and exhaled gas. The capnograph is a very good indicator of pulmonary function. In exhaled air, the level of CO_2 rapidly rises initially and then plateaus off. In situations of compromised lung function or poor lung perfusion, this plateau phase disappears. The level of CO_2 in the exhaled gas at the end of expiration (end-tidal CO_2) is very useful in evaluating ventilator sufficiency in spontaneous as well as artificial ventilation.

The end-tidal CO_2 provides information about physiological status of the animal, as well as problems in the respiratory circuits, such as leaks or an incorrectly placed ET tube. The respiratory rate and end-tidal CO_2 are useful in assessing depth of anesthesia, as well as ventilation status. In cases of improper ventilation or a problem in the respiratory circuit, end-tidal CO_2 rises. In cases of excessive ventilation or death of the animal, end-tidal CO_2 is low. With an increase in the CO_2 level in blood, pH decreases and acidosis develops. If this condition persists, metabolic compensatory mechanisms may become activated to rectify this, but respiratory intervention is the fastest method of correcting this imbalance (Larach et al. 1988).

16.5.4 BLOOD SAMPLING

Various methods are available for measuring the time course of radiotracer activity concentration in arterial plasma (the input function) for application in kinetic models (Kim et al. 2006). Arterial blood sampling is the most appropriate and direct method for measuring the input function (Shimoji et al. 2004). Although manual sampling is considered the gold standard (Convert et al. 2007), it is technically challenging, and implementation of this method in small-animal imaging is complicated and labor-intensive.

The technique provides blood input function measurements with high accuracy, but it is limited by the number of samples that can be withdrawn and logistics. First, to accurately characterize the peak of the radio-activity concentration curve, samples must be collected very rapidly, as circulation in small animals is very rapid. Second, the number of samples that can be withdrawn is limited by the small blood volume available in small animals. Additionally, methods need to be developed for rapid analysis of small sample volumes. Despite these challenges and limitations, manual sampling has been used for small-animal PET imaging (Shimoji et al. 2004).

A number of methods have been developed for online blood sampling, such as the automatic blood sampling system (Ingvar et al. 1991) and the beta microprobe (Warnock et al. 2011). Measurement of the input function in mice is even more difficult than in rats, and thus image-based methods have been developed to obviate the need for cannulas and intravital detectors. The newly developed CD-Well technology (Kimura et al. 2013) permits serial small-volume blood collections for measurement of radioactivity concentrations in plasma and whole blood separately. This technology allows the measurement of arterial whole blood and plasma using 2–3 μL per sample which is ideal for studying mice.

16.6 SUMMARY

The performance of dedicated preclinical PET and SPECT systems has improved markedly over the last 20 years, largely as a result of improvements in detector technology, collimator design (in the case of SPECT), and image reconstruction algorithms, as well as an improved understanding of animal handling and homeo-stasis during imaging studies. Indeed, the ability to spatially and temporally resolve important organs, such as the rapidly beating heart, is now approximately equivalent in the mouse and the human. Furthermore, the sensitivity of preclinical imaging systems is sufficient, particularly in the case of PET, to perform types of kinetic analyses of dynamic tracer studies similar to those typically performed in human research studies. The development of hybrid imaging systems, such as PET/CT and PET/MRI, has mirrored developments in clinical hybrid imaging, enabling multiparametric studies of animal models in one imaging session. There are several practical considerations when performing PET and SPECT studies on small animals, such as choice of anesthetic protocol, blood sampling regime, and temperature and heart rate monitoring, to name a few. When careful attention is paid to these factors and quality control of the imaging systems, preclinical PET and SPECT technologies are capable of producing high-quality research data and making a valuable contribution to a wide variety of fields in the biological sciences.

REFERENCES

Acton, PD, SR Choi, K Plossl, and HF Kung. 2002. Quantification of Dopamine Transporters in the Mouse Brain Using Ultra-High Resolution Single-Photon Emission Tomography. *Eur J Nucl Med Mol Imaging* 29 (5): 691–98.

Antich, P, N Malakhov, R Parkey, N Slavin, and E Tsyganov. 2002. 3D Position Readout from Thick Scintillators. *Nucl Instrum Methods Phys Res A* 480 (2–3): 782–87.

Barrett, HH, and WCJ Hunter. 2005. Detectors for Small-Animal SPECT I. Overview of Technologies. In *Small Animal SPECT Imaging*, ed. MA Kupinski and HH Barrett, 9–48. New York: Springer.

Beekman, FJ, F van der Have, B Vastenhouw, AJ van der Linden, PP van Rijk, JP Burbach, and MP Smidt. 2005. U-SPECT-I: A Novel System for Submillimeter-Resolution Tomography with Radiolabelled Molecules in Mice. *J Nucl Med* 46: 1194–200.

Beekman, FJ, and B Vastenhouw. 2004. Design and Simulation of a High-Resolution Stationary SPECT System for Small Animals. *Phys Med Biol* 49 (19): 4579–92.

Boisson, F, D Zahra, A Parmar, M-C Gregoire, SR Meikle, H Hamse, and A Reilhac. 2013. Imaging Capabilities of the Inveon SPECT System Using Single-and Multipinhole Collimators. *J Nucl Med* 54 (10): 1833–40.

Constantinescu, CC, and J Mukherjee. 2009. Performance Evaluation of an Inveon PET Preclinical Scanner. *Phys Med Biol* 54 (9): 2885–99.

Convert, L, G Morin-Brassard, J Cadorette, M Archambault, M Bentourkia, and R Lecomte. 2007. A New Tool for Molecular Imaging: The Microvolumetric Beta Blood Counter. *J Nucl Med* 48 (7): 1197–206.

DiFilippo, FP. 2008. Design and Performance of a Multi-Pinhole Collimation Device for Small Animal Imaging with Clinical SPECT and SPECT-CT Scanners. *Phys Med Biol* 53 (15): 4185–201.

Du, HN, YF Yang, and SR Cherry. 2007. Measurements of Wavelength Shifting (WLS) Fibre Readout for a Highly Multiplexed, Depth-Encoding PET Detector. *Phys Med Biol* 52 (9): 2499–514.

Du, HN, YF Yang, J Glodo, YB Wu, K Shah, and SR Cherry. 2009. Continuous Depth-of-Interaction Encoding Using Phosphor-Coated Scintillators. *Phys Med Biol* 54 (6): 1757–71.

Dupont, P, and J Warwick. 2009. Kinetic Modelling in Small Animal Imaging with PET. *Methods* 48 (2): 98–103.

Franc BL Mari C, Hasegawa BH, Acton PD. 2008. Small-Animal SPECT and SPECT/CT: Important Tools for Preclinical Investigation. *J Nucl Med* 49: 1651–63.

Fresneau, N, N Dumas, BB Tournier, C Fossey, C Ballandonne, A Lesnard, P Millet, et al. 2015. Design of a Serotonin 4 Receptor Radiotracer with Decreased Lipophilicity for Single Photon Emission Computed Tomography. *Eur J Med Chem* 94: 386–96.

Furenlid, LR, DW Wilson, C Yi-chun, K Hyunki, PJ Pietraski, MJ Crawford, and HH Barrett. 2004. FastSPECT II: A Second-Generation High-Resolution Dynamic SPECT Imager. *IEEE Trans Nucl Sci* 51: 631–35.

Gargiulo, S, A Greco, M Gramanzini, S Esposito, A Affuso, A Brunetti, and G Vesce. 2012. Mice Anesthesia, Analgesia, and Care. Part II. Special Considerations for Preclinical Imaging Studies. *Ilar J* 53 (1): E70–81.

Goertzen, AL, QN Bao, M Bergeron, E Blankemeyer, S Blinder, M Canadas, AF Chatziioannou, et al. 2012. NEMA NU 4-2008 Comparison of Preclinical PET Imaging Systems. *J Nucl Med* 53 (8): 1300–9.

Goertzen, AL, J Seidel, K Li, MV Green, and DW Jones. 2005. First Results from the High-Resolution mouse-eSPECT Annular Scintillation Camera. *IEEE Trans Med Imaging* 24 (7): 863–67.

Gu, Z, R Taschereau, NT Vu, H Wang, DL Prout, RW Silverman, B Bai, DB Stout, ME Phelps, and AF Chatziioannou. 2013. NEMA NU-4 Performance Evaluation of PETbox4, a High Sensitivity Dedicated PET Preclinical Tomograph. *Phys Med Biol* 58 (11): 3791–814.

Habraken, JBA, K de Bruin, M Shehata, J Booij, R Bennink, B LF van Eck Smit, and EB Sokole. 2001. Evaluation of High-Resolution Pinhole SPECT Using a Small Rotating Animal. *J Nucl Med* 42 (12): 1863–69.

Harteveld, AA, APW Meeuwis, JA Disselhorst, CH Slump, WJG Oyen, OC Boerman, and EP Visser. 2011. Using the NEMA NU 4 PET Image Quality Phantom in Multipinhole Small-Animal SPECT. *J Nucl Med* 52: 1646–53.

Herrmann, K, M Dahlbom, D Nathanson, L Wei, C Radu, A Chatziioannou, and J Czernin. 2013. Evaluation of the Genisys4, a Bench-Top Preclinical PET Scanner. *J Nucl Med* 54 (7): 1162–67.

Hildebrandt, IJ, H Su, and WA Weber. 2008. Anesthesia and Other Considerations for In Vivo Imaging of Small Animals. *ILAR J* 49 (1): 17–26.

Ingvar, M, L Eriksson, GA Rogers, S Stone-Elander, and L Widén. 1991. Rapid Feasibility Studies of Tracers for Positron Emission Tomography: High-Resolution PET in Small Animals with Kinetic Analysis. *J Cereb Blood Flow Metab* 11 (6): 926–31.

Ivashchenko, O, F van der Have, M Goorden, R Ramakers, and FJ Beekman. 2015. Ultra-High-Sensitivity Sub-mm Mouse SPECT. *J Nucl Med* 56 (3): 470–76.

Izaguirre, EW, S Mingshan, T Vandehei, P Despres, H Yong, T Funk, L Junqiang, K Parnham, BE Pratt, and BH Hasegawa. 2006. Evaluation of a Large Pixellated Cadmium Zinc Telluride Detector for Small Animal Radionuclide Imaging. In *2006 IEEE Nuclear Science Symposium Conference Record*, vol. 6, pp. 3817–20. Piscataway, NJ: IEEE.

Jansen, FP, and J-L Vanderheyden. 2007. The Future of SPECT in a Time of PET. *Nucl Med Biol* 34 (7): 733–35.

Jaszczak, RJ, J Li, H Wang, MR Zalutsky, and RE Coleman. 1994. Pinhole Collimation for Ultra-High-Resolution, Small-Field-of-View SPECT. *Phys Med Biol* 39: 425–37.

Jeavons, AP, RA Chandler, and CAR Dettmar. 1999. A 3D HIDAC-PET Camera with Sub-Millimetre Resolution for Imaging Small Animals. *IEEE Trans Nucl Sci* 46 (3): 468–73.

Kench, PL, J Lin, MC Gregoire, and SR Meikle. 2011. An Investigation of Inconsistent Projections and Artefacts in Multi-Pinhole SPECT with Axially Aligned Pinholes. *Phys Med Biol* 56 (23): 7487–503.

Kim, J, P Herrero, T Sharp, R Laforest, DJ Rowland, Y-C Tai, JS Lewis, and MJ Welch. 2006. Minimally Invasive Method of Determining Blood Input Function from PET Images in Rodents. *J Nucl Med* 47 (2): 330–36.

Kimura, Y, C Seki, N Hashizume, T Yamada, H Wakizaka, T Nishimoto, K Hatano, K Kitamura, H Toyama, and I Kanno. 2013. Novel System Using Microliter Order Sample Volume for Measuring Arterial Radioactivity Concentrations in Whole Blood and Plasma for Mouse PET Dynamic Study. *Phys Med Biol* 58 (22): 7889–903.

Kyme, AZ, VW Zhou, SR Meikle, and RR Fulton. 2008. Real-Time 3D Motion Tracking for Small Animal Brain PET. *Phys Med Biol* 53: 2651–66.

Lage, E, JJ Vaquero, A Sisniega, S Espana, G Tapias, M Abella, A Rodriguez-Ruano, JE Ortuno, A Udias, and M Desco. 2009. Design and Performance Evaluation of a Coplanar Multimodality Scanner for Rodent Imaging. *Phys Med Biol* 54 (18): 5427–41.

Larach, DR, G Schuler, TM Skeehan, and JA Derr. 1988. Mass Spectrometry for Monitoring Respiratory and Anaesthetic Gas Waveforms in Rats. *J Appl Physiol* 65: 955–63.

Lecomte, R. 2004. Technology Challenges in Small Animal PET Imaging. *Nucl Instrum Methods Phys Res A* 527 (1–2): 157–65.

Lehnert, W, M-C Gregoire, A Reilhac, and SR Meikle. 2012. Characterisation of Partial Volume Effect and Region-Based Correction in Small Animal Positron Emission Tomography (PET) of the Rat Brain. *Neuroimage* 60 (4): 2144–57.

Lerche, CW, M Doring, A Ros, V Herrero, R Gadea, RJ Aliaga, R Colom, et al. 2009. Depth of Interaction Detection for Gamma-Ray Imaging. *Nucl Instrum Methods Phys Res A* 600 (3): 624–34.

Li, Z, M Wedrowski, P Bruyndonckx, and G Vandersteen. 2010. Nonlinear Least-Squares Modeling of 3D Interaction Position in a Monolithic Scintillator Block. *Phys Med Biol* 55 (21): 6515–32.

Lin, J. 2013. On Artifact-Free Projection Overlaps in Multi-Pinhole Tomographic Imaging. *IEEE Trans Med Imaging* 32 (12): 2215–29.

Maas, MC, DR Schaart, DJ van der Laan, P Bruyndonckx, C Lemaitre, FJ Beekman, and CW E van Eijk. 2009. Monolithic Scintillator PET Detectors with Intrinsic Depth-of-Interaction Correction. *Phys Med Biol* 54 (7): 1893–908.

MacDonald, LR, BE Patt, JS Iwanczyk, BMW Tsui, Y Wang, EC Frey, DE Wessell, PD Acton, and HF Kung. 2001. Pinhole SPECT of Mice Using the LumaGEM Gamma Camera. *IEEE Trans Nucl Sci* 48 (3): 830–36.

McCabe, KE, and AM Wu. 2010. Positive Progress in immunoPET—Not Just a Coincidence. *Cancer Biother Radiopharm* 25 (3): 253–61.

Meikle, SR, P Kench, M Kassiou, and RB Banati. 2005. Small Animal SPECT and Its Place in the Matrix of Molecular Imaging Technologies. *Phys Med Biol* 50: R45–61.

Meikle, SR, P Kench, AG Weisenberger, R Wojcik, MF Smith, S Majewski, S Eberl, RR Fulton, AB Rosenfeld, and MJ Fulham. 2002. A Prototype Coded Aperture Detector for Small Animal SPECT. *IEEE Trans Nucl Sci* 49 (5): 2167–71.

Meikle, SR, P Kench, R Wojcik, MF Smith, AG Weisenberger, S Majewski, M Lerch, and AB Rosenfeld. 2003. Performance Evaluation of a Multipinhole Small Animal SPECT System. In *2003 IEEE Nuclear Science Symposium and Medical Imaging Conference Record*, vol. 3, 1988–92. Portland, OR: IEEE.

Metzler, SD, R Accorsi, J Novak, AS Ayan, and RJ Jaszczak. 2006. On-Axis Sensitivity and Resolution of a Slit-Slat Collimator. *J Nucl Med* 47: 1884–90.

Mizuma, H, M Shukuri, T Hayashi, Y Watanabe, and H Onoe. 2010. Establishment of In Vivo Brain Imaging Method in Conscious Mice. *J Nucl Med* 51 (7): 1068–75.

Mizuta, T, K Kitamura, H Iwata, Y Yamagishi, A Ohtani, K Tanaka, and Y Inoue. 2008. Performance Evaluation of a High-Sensitivity Large-Aperture Small-Animal PET Scanner: ClairvivoPET. *Ann Nucl Med* 22 (5): 447–55.

NEMA [National Electrical Manufacturers Association]. 2008. NEMA Standard Publication NU 4-2008: Performance Measurements of Small Animal Positron Emission Tomographs. Rosslyn, VA: NEMA.

Nicholson, A, and B Klaunberg. 2008. Anesthetic Considerations for *In Vivo* Imaging Studies. In: RE Fish, MJ Brown, PJ Danneman, and AZ Karas (eds) *Anesthesia and Analgesia for Laboratory Animals*, 2nd edn, Boston, MA: Elsevier Academic Press, pp. 629–39.

Parnham, KB, S Chowdhury, J Li, DJ Wagenaar, and BE Patt. 2006. Second-Generation, Tri-Modality Pre-Clinical Imaging System. In *2006 IEEE Nuclear Science Symposium Conference Record*, vol. 1–6, pp. 1802–5. Piscataway, NJ: IEEE.

Pissarek, MB, AM Oros-Peusquens, and NU Schramm. 2008. Challenge by the Murine Brain: Multi-Pinhole SPECT of 123I-Labelled Pharmaceuticals. *J Neurosci Methods* 168 (2): 282–92.

Saoudi, A, CM Pepin, F Dion, M Bentourkia, R Lecomte, M Andreaco, M Casey, R Nutt, and H Dautet. 1999. Investigation of Depth-of-Interaction by Pulse Shape Discrimination in Multicrystal Detectors Read Out by Avalanche Photodiodes. *IEEE Trans Nucl Sci* 46 (3): 462–67.

Schramm, NU, G Ebel, U Engeland, T Schurrat, M Behe, and TM Behr. 2003. High-Resolution SPECT Using Multipinhole Collimation. *IEEE Trans Nucl Sci* 50 (3): 315–20.

Schramm, N, A Wirrwar, F Sonnenberg, and H Halling. 2000. Compact High Resolution Detector for Small Animal SPECT. *IEEE Trans Nucl Sci* 47 (3): 1163–67.

Schulz, S, S Southekal, SS Junnarkar, J-F Pratte, ML Purschke, SP Stoll, B Ravindranath, et al. 2011. Simultaneous Assessment of Rodent Behavior and Neurochemistry Using a Miniature Positron Emission Tomograph. *Nat Methods* 8: 347–52.

Seidel, J, JJ Vaquero, S Siegel, WR Gandler, and MV Green. 1999. Depth Identification Accuracy of a Three Layer Phoswich PET Detector Module. *IEEE Trans Nucl Sci* 46 (3): 485–90.

Seo, HK, Y Choi, JH Kim, KC Im, SK Woo, YS Choe, KH Lee, SE Kim, YI Choi, and BT Kim. 2000. Performance Evaluation of the Plate and Array Types of NaI(Tl), CsI(Tl) and CsI(Na) for Small Gamma Camera Using PSPMT. In *2000 IEEE Nuclear Science Symposium Conference Record*, vol. 3, pp. 21/94–21/97. Piscataway, NJ: IEEE.

Stevenson, G. 2005. In ed MA Kupinski and HH Barrett (eds), Small-Animal SPECT Imaging. New York: Springer, pp 87–100.

Shimoji, K, L Ravasi, K Schmidt, ML Soto-Montenegro, T Esaki, J Seidel, E Jagoda, L Sokoloff, MV Green, and WC Eckelman. 2004. Measurement of Cerebral Glucose Metabolic Rates in the Anesthetized Rat by Dynamic Scanning with 18F-FDG, the ATLAS Small Animal PET Scanner, and Arterial Blood Sampling. *J Nucl Med* 45 (4): 665–72.

Stickel, JR, and SR Cherry. 2005. High-Resolution PET Detector Design: Modelling Components of Intrinsic Spatial Resolution. *Phys Med Biol* 50 (2): 179–95.

St James, S, YF Yang, YB Wu, R Farrell, P Dokhale, KS Shah, and SR Cherry. 2009. Experimental Characterization and System Simulations of Depth of Interaction PET Detectors Using 0.5 mm and 0.7 mm LSO Arrays. *Phys Med Biol* 54 (14): 4605–19.

Szanda, I, J Mackewn, G Patay, P Major, K Sunassee, GE Mullen, G Nemeth, Y Haemisch, PJ Blower, and PK Marsden. 2011. National Electrical Manufacturers Association NU-4 Performance Evaluation of the PET Component of the NanoPET/CT Preclinical PET/CT Scanner. *J Nucl Med* 52 (11): 1741–47.

Tai, YC, A Ruangma, D Rowland, S Siegel, DF Newport, PL Chow, and R Laforest. 2005. Performance Evaluation of the microPET Focus: A Third-Generation microPET Scanner Dedicated to Animal Imaging. *J Nucl Med* 46 (3): 455–63.

Tremoleda, JL, A Kerton, and W Gsell. 2012. Anaesthesia and Physiological Monitoring during In Vivo Imaging of Laboratory Rodents: Considerations on Experimental Outcomes and Animal Welfare. *EJNMMI Res* 2 (1): 44.

Tsuda, T, H Murayama, K Kitamura, T Yamaya, E Yoshida, T Omura, H Kawai, N Inadama, and N Orita. 2004. A Four-Layer Depth of Interaction Detector Block for Small Animal PET. *IEEE Trans Nucl Sci* 51 (5): 2537–42.

van Dam, HT, S Seifert, R Vinke, P Dendooven, H Lohner, FJ Beekman, and DR Schaart. 2011. A Practical Method for Depth of Interaction Determination in Monolithic Scintillator PET Detectors. *Phys Med Biol* 56 (13): 4135–45.

van der Have, F, B Vastenhouw, RM Ramakers, W Branderhorst, JO Krah, C Ji, SG Staelens, and FJ Beekman. 2009. U-SPECT-II: An Ultra-High-Resolution Device for Molecular Small-Animal Imaging. *J Nucl Med* 50: 599–605.

Vanhove, C, M Defrise, T Lahoutte, and A Bossuyt. 2008. Three-Pinhole Collimator to Improve Axial Spatial Resolution and Sensitivity in Pinhole SPECT. *Eur J Nucl Med Mol Imaging* 35: 407–15.

Vaska, P. 2004. RatCAP: Miniaturized Head-Mounted PET for Conscious Rodent Brain Imaging. *IEEE Trans Nucl Sci* 51: 2718–22.

Vines, DC, DE Green, G Kudo, and H Keller. 2011. Evaluation of Mouse Tail-Vein Injections Both Qualitatively and Quantitatively on Small-Animal PET Tail Scans. *J Nucl Med Technol* 39 (4): 264–70.

Vinke, R, H Lohner, DR Schaart, HT van Dam, S Seifert, FJ Beekman, and P Dendooven. 2010. Time Walk Correction for TOF-PET Detectors Based on a Monolithic Scintillation Crystal Coupled to a Photosensor Array. *Nucl Instrum Methods Phys Res A* 621 (1–3): 595–604.

Vunckx, K, J Nuyts, B Vanbilloen, M De Saint-Hubert, D Vanderghinste, D Rattat, FM Mottaghy, and M Defrise. 2009. Optimized Multipinhole Design for Mouse Imaging. *IEEE Trans Nucl Sci* 56 (5): 2696–705.

Vunckx, K, P Sutens, and J Nuyts. 2008. Effect of Overlapping Projections on Reconstruction Image Quality in Multipinhole SPECT. *IEEE Trans Med Imaging* 27 (7): 972–83.

Wang, YC, J Seidel, BM W Tsui, JJ Vaquero, and MG Pomper. 2006. Performance Evaluation of the GE Healthcare eXplore VISTA Dual-Ring Small-Animal PET Scanner. *J Nucl Med* 47 (11): 1891–900.

Warnock, G, M-A Bahri, D Goblet, F Giacomelli, C Lemaire, J Aerts, A Seret, X Langlois, A Luxen, and A Plenevaux. 2011. Use of a Beta Microprobe System to Measure Arterial Input Function in PET via an Arteriovenous Shunt in Rats. *EJNMMI Res* 1 (1): 13.

Weber, DA, and M Ivanovic. 1999. Ultra-High-Resolution Imaging of Small Animals: Implications for Preclinical and Research Studies. *J Nucl Cardiol* 6 (3): 332–44.

Weisenberger, AG, S Majewski, M Saha, and E Bradley. 1997. Coincident Radiation Imaging of Iodine 125 for In Vivo Gene Imaging in Small Animals. *Nucl Instrum Methods Phys Res A* 392: 299–303.

Wirrwar, A, N Schramm, H Halling, and HW Muller-Gartner. 2000. The Optimal Crystal Geometry for Small-Field-of-View Gamma Cameras: Arrays or Disks? In *2000 IEEE Nuclear Science Symposium Conference Record*, vol. 3, pp. 21/91–21/93. Piscataway, NJ: IEEE.

Wirrwar, A, N Schramm, H Vosberg, and HW Muller-Gartner. 1999. Influence of Crystal Geometry and Wall Reflectivity on Scintillation Photon Yield and Energy Resolution. In *1999 IEEE Nuclear Science Symposium*, vol. 3, pp. 1443–45. Piscataway, NJ: IEEE.

Wojcik, R, S Majewski, B Kross, D Steinbach, and AG Weisenberger. 1998. High Spatial Resolution Gamma Imaging Detector Based on a 5" Diameter R3292 Hamamatsu PSPMT. *IEEE Trans Nucl Sci* 45 (3): 487–91.

Yang, Y, J Bec, J Zhou, M Zhang, M Judenhofer, X Bai, K Di, et al. 2013. A High Spatial Resolution PET Scanner Designed for Neuroimaging in Mice. In *2013 World Molecular Imaging Congress*, Savannah, Georgia, p. SS83.

Yang, Y, Y Wu, J Qi, S St James, H Du, PA Dokhale, KS Shah, R Farrell, and SR Cherry. 2008. A Prototype PET Scanner with DOI-Encoding Detectors. *J Nucl Med* 49 (7): 1132–40.

Yang, YF, and SR Cherry. 2006. Observations Regarding Scatter Fraction and NEC Measurements for Small Animal PET. *IEEE Trans Nucl Sci* 53 (1): 127–32.

Yang, YF, PA Dokhale, RW Silverman, KS Shah, MA McClish, R Farrell, G Entine, and SR Cherry. 2006. Depth of Interaction Resolution Measurements for a High Resolution PET Detector Using Position Sensitive Avalanche Photodiodes. *Phys Med Biol* 51 (9): 2131–42.

Yao, R, R Lecomte, and E Crawford. 2012. Small-Animal PET: What Is It, and Why Do We Need It? *J Nucl Med Technol* 40 (3): 157–65.

Zhang, H, QA Bao, NT Vu, RW Silverman, R Taschereau, BN Berry-Pusey, A Douraghy, FR Rannou, DB Stout, and AF Chatziioannou. 2011. Performance Evaluation of PETbox: A Low Cost Bench Top Preclinical PET Scanner. *Mol Imaging Biol* 13 (5): 949–61.

Ziemons, K, E Auffray, R Barbier, G Brandenburg, P Bruyndonckx, Y Choi, D Christ, et al. 2005. The ClearPET (TM) Project: Development of a 2nd Generation High-Performance Small Animal PET Scanner. *Nucl Instrum Methods Phys Res A* 537 (1–2): 307–11.

Clinical applications of PET/CT and SPECT/CT imaging

JOHANNES CZERNIN AND ORA ISRAEL, KEN HERRMANN, MARTIN
BARRIO, DAVID NATHANSON, AND MARTIN ALLEN-AUERBACH

17.1	Introduction		439
	17.1.1	Brief history of PET/CT and SPECT/CT imaging	440
17.2	State-of-the-art PET/CT and SPECT/CT systems and protocols		441
	17.2.1	PET/CT	441
	17.2.2	State-of-the-art SPECT/CT systems and protocols	441
17.3	Advantages of PET/CT and SPECT/CT imaging		442
17.4	Reading molecular and metabolic disease signatures with PET and SPECT		444
	17.4.1	PET: molecular imaging modalities enable the phenotyping of cancer	444
	17.4.2	SPECT	448
17.5	Specific applications of PET/CT and SPECT/CT in oncology		451
	17.5.1	PET/CT in oncology	451
	17.5.2	SPECT/CT in oncology	453
	17.5.3	SPECT/CT and PET/CT imaging of metastatic bone disease	453
17.6	Probing functional and molecular signatures of the heart with PET and SPECT		454
	17.6.1	Cardiac PET/CT	454
	17.6.2	Cardiac SPECT/CT imaging	455
17.7	Insights into brain function and metabolism with PET and SPECT		456
	17.7.1	PET applications in neurology	456
	17.7.2	SPECT applications in neurology	459
17.8	Impact of PET/CT on patient management and outcome		459
17.9	Impact of SPECT/CT on patient management and outcome		459
17.10	Summary		460
References			460

17.1 INTRODUCTION

PET–computed tomography (CT) and SPECT/CT have been successfully integrated and translated into the clinical practice of oncology, cardiology, and neurology. They have also emerged as valuable tools for managing many other disorders, including degenerative, endocrine, and infectious or inflammatory diseases. This chapter includes a brief review of the history of PET/CT and SPECT/CT, followed by a discussion of current state-of-the-art instrumentation and a presentation of their major clinical applications. PET/MRI is not addressed in this chapter since its clinical value has not yet been established [1].

17.1.1 BRIEF HISTORY OF PET/CT AND SPECT/CT IMAGING

PET imaging became a reality when Phelps and his coworkers invented and developed the first true tomographic PET system [2,3]. The increased glucose utilization of cancer cells was discovered almost 100 years ago, when Otto Warburg observed that cancer cells metabolize glucose to lactate even in the presence of oxygen (Warburg effect) [4,5]. The use of ^{14}C-deoxyglucose (^{14}C-DG) autoradiography for mapping neuroanatomical pathways *ex vivo* [6,7] subsequently led to the introduction of the fluorinated glucose analog ^{18}F-fluorodeoxyglucose (FDG) [8]. Later, FDG and the blood flow marker ^{13}N-ammonia were used to investigate regional cerebral blood flow and glucose metabolism in patients with epilepsy [9], stroke [9], cancer [10,11], and neurodegenerative [12] and cardiovascular diseases [13,14]. Further pivotal events in the translation of PET included the development of whole-body PET image acquisition protocols [15], and of small electronic generators to facilitate the distribution of PET isotopes.

While stand-alone PET provided accurate assessments of cancer and other disorders, its relatively poor anatomical resolution limited widespread clinical adoption. To overcome this limitation, Beyer et al. designed, developed, and implemented the first integrated PET/CT system in 1998 to provide anatomical and molecular diagnostic capabilities in a single device that enabled near-ideal alignment between PET and CT images [16]. The introduction of PET/CT led to the rapid and widespread adoption of glucose metabolic cancer imaging, facilitated also by its relatively broad insurance coverage.

The integrated PET/CT systems were designed to permit exact localization of metabolic abnormalities, but also allowed implementation of CT-based photon attenuation correction [17]. For the initial proof-of-principle device, a low-end, single-detector CT was merged with a rotating, partial-ring PET scanner. This simple device already demonstrated improved diagnostic accuracy and reader confidence over PET and CT alone [18]. Subsequently, multislice CT devices equipped with up to 64 or even 128 detector rows have been merged with state-of-the-art PET systems to provide whole-body anatomic images of high diagnostic quality in a one-stop-shop solution. Image resolution was also improved by the use of fast scintillator crystals with high detection efficiency, such as cerium-doped lutetium oxyorthosilicate (LSO) and cerium-doped lutetium-yttrium oxyorthosilicate (LYSO), which has made time-of-flight PET a clinical reality [19,20]. Further improvements in resolution were achieved by the use of smaller PET detector elements and novel image reconstruction methods, such as ordered subset expectation maximization (OSEM) [21]. PET/CT imaging is now accepted worldwide as a critically important diagnostic tool for the improved management of cancer patients. PET/CT is cost-effective [22] and does not significantly contribute to health care costs [23].

Imaging following administration of single-photon-emitting radiotracers traditionally includes planar scintigraphy and SPECT. SPECT requires relatively long scanning times, and photon statistics are relatively poor. The limited spatial resolution, together with photon attenuation and scatter, further reduce image quality [24–30]. Methods designed to correlate information from x-ray transmission and SPECT data [16,31–41] to overcome some of these limitations and correlate anatomical and physiological information have been developed [42–44]. CT data have further been used to generate patient-specific maps of attenuation coefficients, which can correct SPECT images for photon attenuation or scatter errors [17,31–36,45].

SPECT/CT offers several clinically significant advantages when compared with stand-alone SPECT, conventional anatomical imaging alone, or with coregistration of separately performed SPECT and CT [46]. These advantages were recognized several decades ago. In the 1980s and early 1990s, the late Bruce Hasegawa and his team at the University of California, San Francisco, pioneered the development of dedicated imaging systems that could coregister radionuclide SPECT and x-ray data [34,37]. They designed the first SPECT/CT scanner as a CT in tandem with a SPECT device, a configuration in which the patient remained on a common table for imaging with two separate subsystems. They tested this machine on phantoms, animals, and patients and demonstrated that the use of combined imaging improved the visual quality, as well as the quantitative accuracy of SPECT [31,32]. Starting in the mid-1990s, independent pioneering work on SPECT/CT was performed by scientists and engineers in the medical imaging industry. The first commercially available SPECT/

CT system, known as the Hawkeye, consisted of a dual-headed sodium iodide (^{131}I) crystal gamma camera with a gantry incorporating an x-ray tube with fan-beam technology that enabled low-dose CT at a maximum current of 2.5 mA [47,48]. It included a single gantry and patient table, as well as an integrated computer system and software for reconstruction, display, and analysis. The first prototype units of this system were placed for evaluation and further development at the nuclear medicine departments at Vanderbilt University (Nashville, Tennessee) and the Rambam Medical Center (Haifa, Israel), with the first clinical images being acquired in 1999. Although PET/CT initially gained more publicity and acceptance, SPECT/CT is now considered the state of the art in single-photon emission imaging.

17.2 STATE-OF-THE-ART PET/CT AND SPECT/CT SYSTEMS AND PROTOCOLS

17.2.1 PET/CT

PET/CT provides a one-stop-shop solution in diagnostics, mainly of cancer, but also of cardiovascular diseases and infection. High-resolution PET images as a result of the use of fast scintillator crystals that enable time-of-flight PET studies have become the standard [49]. High-count-rate capabilities and detection efficiency have resulted in short PET image acquisitions of as low as 1 minute/bed position in patients with a low body weight [50]. The availability of multidetector CT components as part of the PET/CT system enables the implementation of fully diagnostic intravenous contrast protocols [51,52], currently the standard of care in cancer imaging. They should be implemented for clinical oncology PET/CT studies whenever feasible and not contraindicated. At University of California, Los Angeles, the scan commences with a breath-hold chest CT to identify small lung nodules that may be missed during shallow breathing [53]. Subsequently, intravenous contrast is administered. Performing contrast-enhanced CT adds only a few minutes to the duration of PET/CT studies and results in improved diagnostic accuracy in a variety of cancers [54–56]. PET/CT imaging protocols are tailored to specific clinical problems; for instance, multi-phase-contrast protocols are used for assessing the liver and the pancreas [57,58].

Whole-body PET/CT acquisition times of as short as 20–30 minutes, even when performed with intravenous and oral contrast, provide a true one-stop-shop diagnostic imaging approach in cancer [59].

FDG-PET scan results are reproducible [60]. Nevertheless, one of the current limitations of clinical PET imaging is its lack of standardization. Recent surveys found a substantial variability in image acquisition, reconstruction, and analysis, emphasizing the need for standardization [51,52]. Initial attempts for standardization have been spearheaded by various groups [61–63]. However, no international consensus has been reached, a critically important shortcoming that needs to be addressed in the near future.

17.2.2 STATE-OF-THE-ART SPECT/CT SYSTEMS AND PROTOCOLS

A range of dual-modality SPECT/CT devices incorporating multidetector CT technology are now commercially available, and a large number of nuclear medicine and radiology departments are equipped with at least one SPECT/CT device. In contrast to PET/CT, the performance of whole-body CT as part of the SPECT/CT study is at present not justified. A limited field of view (FOV) SPECT—mainly CT—is performed based on one of the following criteria: (1) the specific clinical referral indication, (2) the specific symptomatology of the patient or results of previous imaging studies, and (3) the presence of suspicious or unclear findings observed on planar scintigraphy.

Acquisition of SPECT and CT is performed sequentially. Acquisition protocols of the SPECT component of the study are the same as for stand-alone SPECT, adapted to the physical characteristics of the radioisotope used, the anatomical region that has to be imaged, and the clinical question at hand. As a rule, dual-headed, variable-angle ^{131}I scintillation cameras are used. SPECT images are reconstructed using iterative methods such as the OSEM algorithm incorporating photon attenuation correction and scatter correction. Newly developed reconstruction algorithms also allow for reduced SPECT acquisition times, up to less than 50% of previous routine protocols [64].

For first-generation devices equipped with a low-end CT component, CT data are typically acquired with the x-ray tube operated at 140 kV and 2.5 mA rotating 220° around the patient. The scan time of approximately 16 seconds per slice results in a total study duration of 10 minutes for the entire set of CT data. Systems equipped with a higher-end CT are characterized by higher spatial resolution and a faster scanning time of approximately 30 seconds for the whole FOV, but also accompanied by higher radiation doses.

17.3 ADVANTAGES OF PET/CT AND SPECT/CT IMAGING

Diagnostic approaches that are based solely on anatomical image information have well-known limitations. For instance, in cancer, tissue composition cannot be discerned reliably based on morphological features and benign tissue cannot be discriminated consistently from cancer. These distinctions can be made using molecular imaging. FDG imaging can be used, for example, for improved target definition and dose painting in radiation therapy [65] or for better targeting of tissue biopsies [66,67] (Figure 17.1). Furthermore, while changes in tumor size are still most frequently used to assess tumor responses to treatment [68], they have considerable limitations, including a time delay in detecting anatomical changes, as well as the inability to define the composition of residual masses [69,70]. The contribution of molecular imaging to therapy response assessment has been firmly established [71] (Figure 17.2). Integrating metabolic with anatomic information by measuring total lesion glycolysis [72] or metabolic tumor volume [73,74] is expected to further improve treatment response assessments.

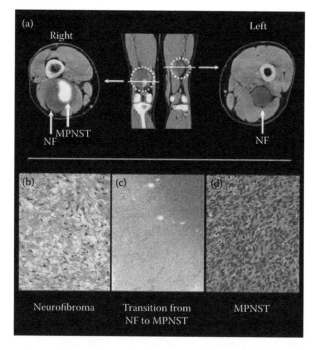

Figure 17.1 (a) A PET/CT study in a patient with neurofibromatosis (NF) type 1–associated malignant peripheral nerve sheath tumor (MPNST). The MPNST is located in the right distal thigh and arises from a benign neurofibroma (NFib). A neurofibroma with low FDG uptake is located in the left medial thigh. (b) A region of benign neurofibroma shows the usual low cellularity and slender spindled cells with interspersed pink collagen fibers. (c) A low-power view shows transition from neurofibroma (lower left corner) to high-grade MPNST (upper right corner). Note the increase in cellularity from the benign to the malignant area. (d) A high-power view (original magnification, ×20) of the high-grade MPNST is shown. Note the marked increase in cellularity, obvious mitoses, and nuclear pleomorphism. (Reprinted from Benz, M. R., et al., *Cancer*, 116, 451–458, 2010. With permission.)

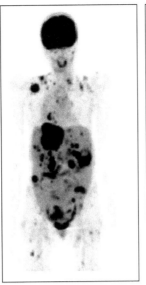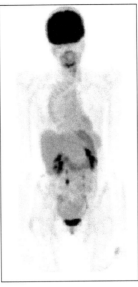

Figure 17.2 A patient with widespread metastatic melanoma is imaged with ¹⁸F-FDG PET before and 2 weeks after treatment with a BRAF inhibitor. Note the complete resolution of hypermetabolic malignant disease.

On the other hand, anatomic information is indispensable for localization of metabolic abnormalities, as well as for the planning of biopsy, surgery, or radiation therapy. Also, well-differentiated tumors can exhibit a low glycolytic rate, rendering them undetectable with PET alone. Integrated imaging has become critically important whenever exact lesion localization is important or when anatomical imaging can add to the specificity of molecular imaging. Since background tracer activity is frequently significant, exact anatomical coregistration of focally increased tracer uptake is highly relevant for PET and SPECT imaging. One such example is the routine utilization of SPECT/CT for detecting and localizing parathyroid adenomas (Figure 17.3).

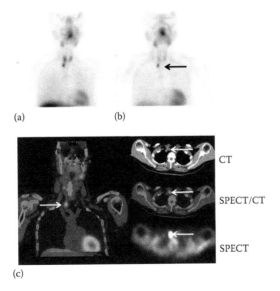

Figure 17.3 A 58-year-old patient is referred for a ⁹⁹ᵐTc-SestaMIBI SPECT/CT scan to evaluate for parathyroid adenoma. (a) An immediate anterior planar image demonstrates bilateral thyroid uptake. (b) A 1.5-hour-delayed anterior planar image demonstrates complete tracer washout from thyroid tissue and tracer retention in the parathyroid adenoma (arrow). (c) Corresponding coronal and axial SPECT/CT images localize the parathyroid adenoma (white arrow) inferior to the lower pole of the right thyroid lobe.

While not frequently utilized, integrated cardiac PET/CT and SPECT/CT imaging can provide comprehensive cardiac evaluations, including coronary anatomy, calcifications, left ventricular function, and myocardial perfusion. In contrast, the addition of CT to SPECT or PET imaging of the brain appears to be less relevant. The brain is a rigid organ, and SPECT and PET images can be readily fused with MRI data, the most important anatomical imaging modality in neurology.

17.4 READING MOLECULAR AND METABOLIC DISEASE SIGNATURES WITH PET AND SPECT

17.4.1 PET: MOLECULAR IMAGING MODALITIES ENABLE THE PHENOTYPING OF CANCER

The metabolic switch to glucose that can be imaged with FDG PET is governed by changes in gene expression that in turn affect signaling pathways involved in cell proliferation, neoangiogenesis, evasion of apoptosis, and metastatic potential. Mutations of the proto-oncogene KRAS in colorectal cancer are associated with increased GLUT1 and Hk-2 expression when compared with wild-type tumors, which results in higher tumor FDG uptake [75]. FDG tumor uptake also correlates with p53 expression [76] and with hormone receptor expression in breast cancer. Triple-negative breast cancers exhibit significantly higher FDG uptake than estrogen or progesterone receptor–positive tumors [77]. Thus, the tumor uptake of FDG represents the net effect of the complex interplay among gene expression, translation, and various signal transduction pathways in cancer (reviewed by [78]). The information extracted from these images relates to the tumor proliferative activity and aggressiveness and provides useful readouts of therapeutic interventions targeting one or several of these altered gene expression or signal transduction pathways.

Glucose is not the only relevant substrate for anabolic and catabolic processes in cancer cells. Upregulation of alternate pathways such as amino acid metabolism may represent a different strategy to meet the anabolic and catabolic needs of cancer cells [79,80] in tumors such as glioblastoma [81] (Figure 17.4), lung [82], and pancreatic cancer [83]. PET tracers of amino acid transport such as ^{11}C-methionine (CMET), ^{18}F-DOPA

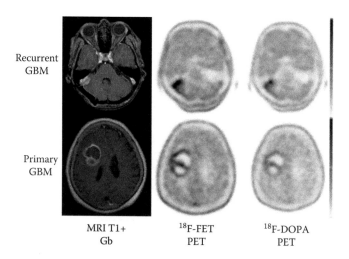

Recurrent
GBM

Primary
GBM

MRI T1+ ^{18}F-FET ^{18}F-DOPA
Gb   PET   PET

Figure 17.4 Display of axial contrast-enhanced T1-weighted MRI (left), FET (middle), and FDOPA PET/CT scans (right) of patient with recurrent and primary glioblastoma (GBM). In both patients, ^{18}F-FET uptake was higher than that of FDOPA. However, diagnostic information was identical. (Reprinted from Lapa, C., et al., *J. Nucl. Med.*, 55, 1611–1616, 2014. With permission.)

(FDOPA), or ^{18}F-tyrosine (FET) have been used to diagnose these and neuroendocrine tumors, including paraganglioma, pheochromocytoma (Figure 17.5), neuroblastoma, and dedifferentiated carcinoids [84–88]. ^{11}C-choline and ^{11}C-acetate target choline kinase and fatty acid synthesis, respectively. They have therefore been used to image mainly prostate (Figure 17.6) [89,90] and hepatocellular carcinoma [91].

The activity of the DNA salvage pathway can be imaged with ^{18}F-fluorothymidine (FLT), a thymidine analog that serves as a marker of tumor cell proliferation [92]. FLT uptake correlated with the expression of Ki-67 in tumors such as lung or colorectal cancer [93,94] (Figure 17.7).

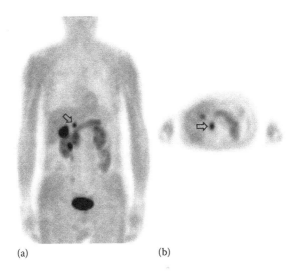

(a) (b)

Figure 17.5 (a) Anterior view of maximum intensity projection image demonstrates right adrenal pheochromocytoma (open arrow) and adjacent pancreas, gallbladder, kidneys, and liver. (b) Transverse cross section through tumor. (Reprinted from Imani, F., et al., *J. Nucl. Med.*, 50, 513–519, 2009. With permission.)

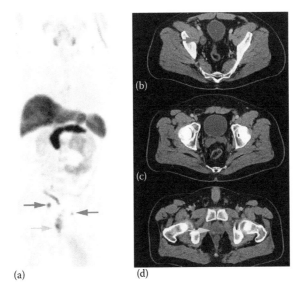

(a) (d)

Figure 17.6 A 55-year-old male diagnosed with prostate cancer is referred for a ^{11}C-acetate PET/CT scan for staging of disease. Maximum intensity projection (a) and selected fused axial images (b–d) demonstrate lymph nodes with increased acetate uptake (red arrows, a–c) consistent with local metastatic disease, and focal intense prostatic uptake (cyan arrows, a, d) consistent with the primary site of disease.

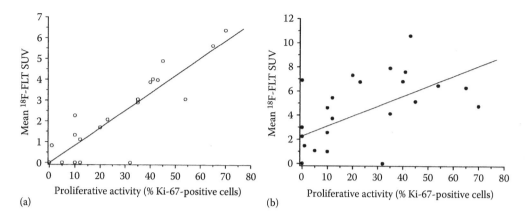

Figure 17.7 Relationship between mean tumor ^{18}F-FLT (left) and ^{18}F-FDG (right) SUV and proliferation rate (% of Ki-67-positive tumor cells). $p < 0.0001$ for ^{18}F-FLT ($r = 0.92$); $p < 0.001$ for ^{18}F-FDG ($r = 0.59$). (Reprinted from Buck, A. K., et al., *J. Nucl. Med.*, 44, 1426–1431, 2003. With permission.)

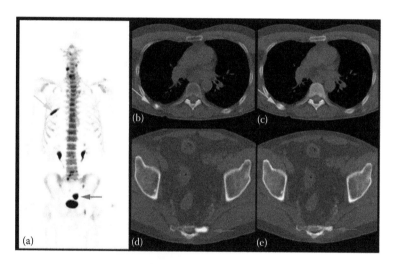

Figure 17.8 A 72-year-old patient with prostate cancer who presented with rising prostate-specific antigen (PSA). Maximum intensity projection (a) and selected axial fused (b, c) and CT (d, e) images demonstrated benign tracer ^{18}F-NaF in a healing rib fracture (cyan arrows, a–c) and intense ^{18}F-NaF uptake due to a sclerotic metastasis in the sacrum (red arrows, a, d, e).

^{18}F-sodium fluoride (NaF) is a PET probe to target hydroxyapatite in areas of increased bone turnover [95] (Figure 17.8). The area of "exposed" bone surface is larger in various benign or malignant bone disorders, resulting in abnormal uptake patterns.

Cell surface receptor and antigen imaging approaches include small molecules and labeled peptides. Estrogen receptor expression measured with ^{18}F-fluoroestradiol (FES) permits response predictions to hormonal therapy in breast cancer [96]. Androgen receptor expression measured with ^{18}F-fluorodehydrotestosteron (FDHT) may allow for response predictions to hormonal therapy in prostate cancer [97]. Imaging prostate cell membrane antigen using a radiolabeled antibody to the prostate-specific membrane antigen (PSMA) that is overexpressed in castrate-resistant prostate cancer has been introduced [98,99]. ^{68}Ga-labeled somatostatin receptor ligands are used successfully for imaging neuroendocrine tumors [100] (Figure 17.9). When labeled with ^{177}Lu or ^{90}Y, these probes serve as successful therapeutics.

The cell surface receptor avb3 integrin involved in tumor neoangiogenesis can be imaged with ^{68}Ga- or ^{18}F-labeled galacto-arginine-glycineaspartate (RGD) peptides, thus enabling response prediction to

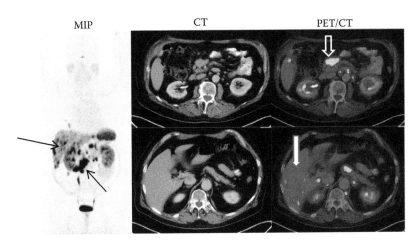

Figure 17.9 ^{68}Ga-DOTATATE PET/CT images acquired in a 60-year-old male patient with a neuroendocrine tumor of the ileum and multiple lymph node and liver metastases (black arrows on maximum intensity projection [MIP]). Left: MIP images. Corresponding axial CT and PET/CT images display the primary tumor (open white arrow) and multiple lymph node and liver metastases (solid white arrow).

Table 17.1 Clinical applications and mechanisms of action of frequently used PET probes

Probe	Target	Process	Application
[18]F-fluorodeoxyglucose	GLUT1, GLUT3, hexokinase	Glycolysis	Cancer, cerebral cortical function, myocardial viability, inflammation/infection
[18]F-tyrosine, ^{11}C-methionine	LAT	Amino acid transport	Cancer
^{18}F-DOPA	LAT	Amino acid transport	Cancer
	DOPA decarboxylase	Presynaptic dopaminergic function	NET
			Movement disorders
^{68}Ga-DOTATATE/TOC	SSR2	SSR expression	NET
[13]N-ammonia	Glutamine synthase	Myocardial blood flow	Coronary artery disease
[82]Rb	Na/K pump	Myocardial blood flow	Coronary artery disease
[18]F-florbetapir	Beta-amyloid	Amyloid accumulation	Progressive neurodegenerative diseases
[18]F-sodium fluoride	Hydroxyapatite	Bone metabolism	Cancer, degenerative bone disease, trauma

Note: GLUT, glucose transporter; LAT, L-amino acid transporter; SSR2, somatostatin receptor 2; NET, neuroendocrine tumor.

antiangiogenic therapy [101]. Antibodies targeting cell surface antigen can be labeled with diagnostic or therapeutic radioisotope pairs, such as ^{64}Cu/[67]Cu, [86]Y/^{90}Y, and [124]I/[131]I (reviewed in [102]). Thus, theranostic approaches have become feasible, and radiopeptide and immune therapy, respectively, will emerge as critically important cancer therapeutics.

In summary, a large and diverse portfolio of molecular PET imaging probes can be used as diagnostic and phenotypic imaging biomarkers (Tables 17.1 through 17.3).

Table 17.2 Clinical applications and mechanisms of action of frequently used SPECT probes

Radiopharmaceutical	Clinical application	Mechanism
^{99m}Tc-MIBI	Myocardial perfusion	Active transport
	Breast	Enhanced uptake
		Active transport
	Parathyroid adenoma	Mitochondrial uptake and delayed washout
^{99m}Tc leukocytes	Infection and inflammation	Cellular sequestration
^{99m}Tc-HMPAO	Cerebral perfusion imaging	Active transport
^{99m}Tc-DMSA	Renal imaging	Active transport
^{99m}Tc-MDP	Bone imaging	Chemical adsorption
^{131}I	Thyroid disease imaging	Active transport
^{99m}Tc-RBC	Spleen imaging	Compartmental localization
	Liver hemangioma	
	Intestinal bleeding	
^{67}Ga-citrate	Tumor and inflammation	Active transport
^{99m}Tc sulfur colloid	Imaging of liver/spleen	
	Bone marrow	
	Gastric emptying	Compartmental localization
	GI bleeds	Compartmental localization
^{123}I-MIBG	Neuroendocrine tumors	Active transport
^{111}In-zevalin	Lymphoma imaging	Antigen–antibody
^{99m}Tc-MAA	Lung scan	Capillary blockage
^{111}In-octreotide	Neuroendocrine system	Receptor binding

Note: MIBI, methoxyisobutylisonitrile; HMPAO, hexamethylpropyleneamine oxime; MDP, methylene diphosphonate; RBC, red blood cells; MAA, macroaggregated albumin; GI, gastrointestinal.

Table 17.3 PET and SPECT probes of the dopaminergic system

Probe	Target	Location
^{18}F-DOPA	AADC	Presynaptic
^{11}C-dihydrotetrabenazine	VMAT2	Presynaptic
^{11}C-nomifensine	DAT	Presynaptic
^{11}C-CFT	DAT	Presynaptic
^{18}F-CFT	DAT	Presynaptic
^{11}C-raclopride	D2	Postsynaptic
^{11}C-SCH23390	D1	Postsynaptic

Note: DAT, dopamine transporter; D2, dopamine D2 receptor; D1, dopamine D1 receptor.

17.4.2 SPECT

For nuclear medicine procedures using single-photon-emitting radiotracers, technetium-99 (^{99m}Tc) is the most commonly used radionuclide. In spite of periods of intermittent shortage, ^{99m}Tc is widely available. It has favorable physical characteristics for imaging, good dosimetry, and a physical half-life of 6 hours that allows for efficient labeling and, when needed, performing serial studies that will assess the dynamics of the tracer as part of characterizing a pathophysiologic process. ^{99m}Tc-labeled products account for nearly 80% of radiopharmaceuticals used in clinical nuclear medicine. Additional single-photon-emitting radionuclides

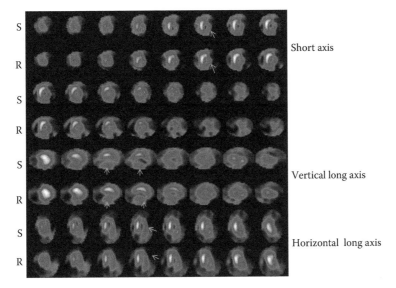

Figure 17.10 Stress–rest myocardial perfusion study using ^{99m}Tc-tetrofosmin in a female patient with fixed perfusion defects in the inferior and lateral wall extending into the inferior aspect of the apex (arrows). This is consistent with infarcts in the RCA and LCX territories. S, stress; R, rest; RCA, right coronary artery; LCX, left circumflex coronary artery.

used in the clinical routine include radioiodine (^{131}I and ^{123}I), ^{111}In, ^{67}Ga, and ^{201}TI. These tracers assess a variety of pathophysiological processes, including flow, function, metabolism, and receptor status [103].

Myocardial blood flow is assessed mainly by ^{99m}Tc-SestaMIBI or ^{99m}Tc-tetrofosmin (Figure 17.10). ^{201}TI uptake by the heart muscle is mediated by the Na$^+$-K$^+$ pump. It is taken up by myocytes as well as by malignant cells. It has a high extraction fraction in the heart and is therefore a marker of myocardial blood flow. In tumors, it indicates the presence of viable cancer tissue and can be used, among other clinical indications, in the differential diagnosis of radiation necrosis versus recurrence of brain tumors [104,105].

Radiotracers assessing function are physiologic components of various organs or similar compounds, and thus take active part in the functional characterization of pathophysiological processes in various diseases. ^{131}I and ^{123}I, administered orally, are taken up, similarly to nonradioactive iodine, via the ^{131}I symporter in the thyroid gland and are therefore useful for assessing the functional status of the thyroid gland and for diagnosing diseases such as toxic nodular goiter and cancer (Figure 17.11). In large doses, ^{131}I is used for therapeutic purposes in both benign and malignant thyroid disorders.

Following its intravenous administration, ^{67}Ga-citrate is chelated by transferrin. This radioisotope has been used for more than four decades for diagnosis and follow-up of tumors, mainly lymphoma, and for assessment of infection. Recently, its use has diminished because of the availability of PET agents that provide more specific, high-quality images. ^{111}In, as indium chloride, is also injected intravenously and chelated by transferrin, similar to ^{67}Ga-citrate. ^{111}In-labeled white blood cells are used successfully for imaging of infectious processes.

Radiotracers used for imaging of metabolism are, as a rule, small molecules rapidly taken up into cells by transporters and subsequently metabolized in the cytoplasm. They can be analogs of small native molecules. They are retained within the cells by metabolic trapping. For example, the above-mentioned myocardial perfusion tracers show increased uptake in parathyroid adenomas due to both increased blood flow to the lesion, as well as increased mitochondrial metabolism. ^{123}I-metaiodobenzylguanidine (MIBG), an analog of norepinephrine, is an index of the sympathetic cardiac innervation and can provide quantitative data on the uptake in and washout from the heart [106].

Uptake of ^{131}I-iodocholesterol is a marker of adrenal cortical metabolism, a region where gluco- and mineralocorticoids are synthesized. Increased uptake is seen in cortisol- and aldosterone-producing adenomas and in Cushing's disease [107].

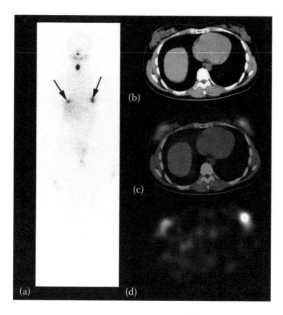

Figure 17.11 A 34-year-old female patient with papillary thyroid cancer status postresection and treatment with 153 mCi of ^{131}I. The posttreatment anterior planar image (a) demonstrates focal tracer uptake in the chest (black arrows), potentially indicating metastatic disease. SPECT/CT images helped localize the tracer uptake to the bilateral breast tissue, consistent with a normal physiologic variant: (b) CT, (c) SPECT/CT, and (d) SPECT.

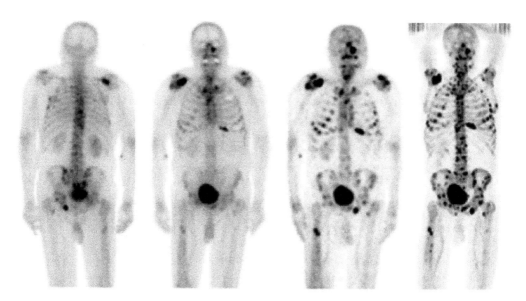

Figure 17.12 An 82-year-old patient with numerous bone metastases. From left to right: Posterior and anterior planar BS, multi-FOV SPECT, and ^{18}F-fluoride PET images. More lesions are detected on SPECT compared with planar images and on ^{18}F-fluoride PET compared with SPECT images. (Reprinted from Even-Sapir, E., et al., *J. Nucl. Med.*, 47, 287–297, 2006. With permission.)

Radionuclide imaging of bone metabolism identifies areas of increased new bone formation associated with higher osteoblastic activity. The radiotracers at hand are various phosphonates labeled with ^{99m}Tc (Figure 17.12). Clinical indications for imaging of bone metabolism include diagnosis of skeletal metastases, fracture, or osteomyelitis, diseases characterized by an increased osteoblastic activity necessary to repair injured bone [108].

Liver metabolism can be assessed with ^{99m}Tc-iminodiacetic acid analogs that are taken up by hepatocytes and further undergo a pathway similar to bilirubin. A second aspect of liver metabolism, phagocytosis performed by reticuloendothelial cells, is assessed using ^{99m}Tc-labeled colloid particles [109].

Functional imaging of the kidneys is done with ^{99m}Tc-mercaptoacetyltriglycine (MAG-3), which is taken up and excreted through the proximal tubules and provides data on renal blood flow and the status of the proximal tubules; ^{99m}Tc-dimercaptosuccinic acid (DMSA), a renal cortex imaging agent, is used primarily for imaging of renal scarring. An additional, commonly used renal tracer, ^{99m}Tc-diethylenetriaminepentaacetic acid (DTPA), is a passively filtered glomerular agent [110].

Agents used for receptor imaging are, as a rule, antibodies (or their fragments), small peptides, or molecules characterized by specific binding. Ideally, these agents should have a high receptor specificity with no or only minimal nonspecific uptake and affinity, low metabolism, and rapid clearance from the blood. One such example relates to integrins, cell adhesion receptors involved in the regulation of endothelial cell growth. The V-3 integrin receptor, overexpressed during neoangiogenesis, can be targeted with ^{123}I-RGD, an agent used mainly in experimental models to assess the effect of angiogenesis therapy with vascular endothelial growth factor [111].

Octreotide, an ^{111}In-labeled oligopeptide, targets somatostatin receptors and has been used for imaging various neuroendocrine malignancies, such as pituitary and pancreatic tumors, carcinoid, paraganglioma, medullary thyroid carcinoma, and Merkel cell tumors [112].

[111]In-capromab-pendetide (Prostascint) an antibody directed against PSMA, has been developed for assessment of cancer of the prostate but provides images of poor quality because of its rather low target-to-background ratio [113].

[123]I-ioflupane (DaTscan™, GE Healthcare) has a high binding affinity for presynaptic dopamine transporters. DaTscan imaging is used for diagnosis and follow-up of patients with various movement disorders, in particular Parkinson's disease characterized by, mostly asymmetrically, a decrease in uptake in the caudate and putamen [114].

17.5 SPECIFIC APPLICATIONS OF PET/CT AND SPECT/CT IN ONCOLOGY

17.5.1 PET/CT IN ONCOLOGY

More than 2 million PET/CT studies have been performed in the United States in 2012, and more than 95% of these studies were conducted using FDG for oncological indications. The combined anatomical and molecular information obtained with FDG PET/CT is superior to that derived from PET or CT alone for establishing initial and subsequent treatment strategies in cancer [115]. This is because anatomical lesions can represent numerous benign or malignant entities, including inflammation scar necrosis and fibrosis. Metabolic phenotyping of these lesions with PET permits more accurate assessments of the nature of such lesions. A high staging accuracy of FDG PET/CT in malignancies of the lung [116], breast [117], esophagus [118], colon [55], cervix [119], and head and neck [118], as well as in lymphoma [120], melanoma [121], sarcoma [122], and myeloma [123], has been demonstrated.

The accuracy of FDG PET/CT imaging for detecting distant metastases or synchronous second cancers is high, as reported in an analysis that was based on more than 4300 patients from 41 published studies, including those with primary or recurrent cancers. Using histopathology as the reference standard in a subset of 800 patients, the patient-based sensitivity and specificity of PET/CT averaged 93% and 96%, respectively, comparing favorably to those of conventional imaging [124].

Tumor responses to treatment can be assessed reliably as early as after a single cycle, at midtherapy, or after completion of chemotherapy [125,126]. For instance, in 260 patients with Hodgkin's lymphoma, positive PET scans after two cycles of chemotherapy were associated with a 2-year progression-free survival of only 13%, compared with 95% of patients with negative PET studies [127]. Treatment response assessment is accurate in both Hodgkin's [128] and non-Hodgkin's lymphoma [129] and in a variety of solid tumors, including cervical cancer, soft tissue sarcoma, non–small cell lung cancer, esophageal cancer, breast cancer, and gastric cancer [130]. Changes in tumor FDG uptake early during treatment are frequently predictive of histopathologic response to neoadjuvant therapy and of long-term outcome (Figure 17.13). As a limitation, microscopic residual disease cannot be detected by PET. FDG PET has also been used successfully to assess tumor responses to targeted therapies such as imatinib [131], gefitinib [132], or erlotinib [133].

Combining anatomical and functional tumor response assessments may further improve treatment response assessments. Standardized uptake values (SUVs) or glucose metabolic rates (μmol/g/min) describe metabolic activity per gram of tissue, but not within the entire tumor volume [134]. This limitation can be overcome with PET/CT by deriving the total lesion glycolysis (i.e., SUV × volume) [73]. There is still a need for prospective studies to define the value of this integrated approach for tumor treatment response

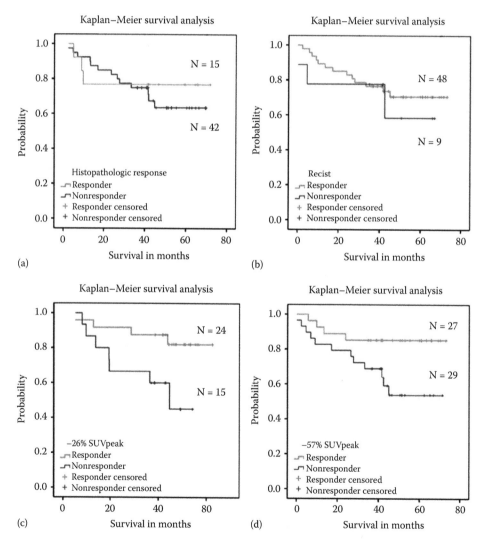

Figure 17.13 Kaplan–Meier survival curves in patients with soft tissue sarcoma stratified by (a) histopathologic response, (b) response evaluation criteria in solid tumors (RECIST), (c) early PET response and (d) late metabolic response. Only early and late reductions in tumor FDG uptake in response to therapy were predictive of long-term survival. (Reprinted from Herrmann, K., et al., *Clin. Cancer Res.*, 18, 2024–2031, 2012. With permission.)

assessments [135]. FDG PET–based response criteria in solid tumors (PERCIST) have been proposed [126] and are increasingly used in clinical management of patients with cancer. In addition, the harmonization criteria for response assessments in lymphoma have gained widespread acceptance [136,137]. While in need for future refinements, these criteria nevertheless provide a solid initial framework to standardize molecular PET imaging–based treatment response criteria.

17.5.2 SPECT/CT IN ONCOLOGY

SPECT/CT imaging has also found widespread clinical utilization in oncology. ^{123}I/^{131}I is sensitive for detecting well-differentiated thyroid cancer metastases [138], with lesion location being greatly improved by SPECT/CT [139]. Other frequently used clinical SPECT/CT studies include the detection and localization of parathyroid adenoma [140], neuroendocrine tumors [141], and sentinel lymph nodes in breast cancer and melanoma patients [142].

17.5.3 SPECT/CT AND PET/CT IMAGING OF METASTATIC BONE DISEASE

Imaging methods for detecting bone metastases include planar whole-body, SPECT, SPECT/CT, and PET/CT imaging; plain film x-rays; CT; and MRI. Integrated SPECT/CT and PET/CT have improved the capabilities to characterize bone lesions as malignant or benign [143,144]. Bone scintigraphy using ^{99m}Tc-labeled phosphonates is a widely available imaging modality in patients with cancer, as well as in orthopedic indications. The reported sensitivity for detection of bone metastases or benign lesions ranges between 62% and 100%. However, the specificity of bone scintigraphy is lower, with a large number of equivocal studies that require further anatomic imaging or invasive diagnostic procedures for final diagnosis. SPECT as an add-on to planar scans has improved lesion detectability through higher contrast and resolution, and has, to some extent, improved localization of suspicious foci of increased radiotracer uptake, mainly in the skull, spine, and pelvis, but with no significant increase in the diagnostic accuracy of bone scintigraphy [145]. SPECT/CT has an incremental diagnostic value in patients with equivocal findings on bone scintigraphy, increasing the specificity through accurate anatomic localization and by assessment of the morphologic CT patterns of specific suspicious sites, thereby obviating the need for further, more sophisticated investigations [145,146]. CT contributes by determining typical patterns of benign versus malignant lesions, thereby improving the specificity of the study for detection of bone metastases. SPECT/CT provided a correct diagnosis in the majority (85%–92%) of indeterminate bone lesions in patients with malignancy, with a significant increase in specificity to 81%, being particularly useful in the spine, thoracic cage, and ribs [145,146]. Further improvements in accuracy have been accomplished with the use of SPECT/CT and ^{18}F-NaF PET/CT [147]. While the utilization of conventional bone scintigraphy for bone metastases detection has decreased in recent years due to increased utilization of FDG PET/CT and MRI, it is remerging now with SPECT/CT as an important diagnostic tool. Following the recent emergence of ^{223}Ra (Xofigo), a therapeutic radionuclide that reduces skeletal-related events and improves overall survival in castrate-resistant prostate cancer, bone scintigraphy has regained an important role, allowing the precise localization of regionally increased bone turnover, resulting in improved treatment tailoring and identification of patients who might benefit from this novel therapeutic approach [148].

^{99m}Tc-MDP and ^{18}F-NaF accumulate in regions of bone growth or trauma, and in response to neoplastic and inflammatory processes [149]. Thus, increased tracer uptake is specific for osteoblastic activity. In general, osteoblastic lesions are well detected with planar or SPECT bone scintigraphy and ^{18}F-NaF PET/CT, while osteolytic lesions that are prevalent in breast, lung, thyroid, and renal cancer patients are well assessed with FDG PET/CT [117,150–153]. Sclerotic bone lesions show lower or no FDG uptake [154]. After treatment, progressive sclerotic lesions became increasingly FDG positive, while responding lytic lesions showed increased sclerosis on CT and diminishing FDG uptake on PET. Thus, both metabolic and anatomic changes can provide important insights into treatment responses of bone metastases.

17.6 PROBING FUNCTIONAL AND MOLECULAR SIGNATURES OF THE HEART WITH PET AND SPECT

Coronary function can be evaluated with a variety of SPECT and PET probes. While clinical imaging of coronary function is the strength of SPECT/(CT) imaging, metabolic imaging is the domain of PET/(CT). The short half-life of currently used perfusion PET probes requires the availability of on-site cyclotrons or generators for PET imaging. SPECT or SPECT/CT myocardial perfusion imaging is more frequently used in clinical practice, a situation that may change with the advance of fluorinated PET myocardial perfusion imaging probes [155]. As an advantage of PET, tracer kinetic models can be used to quantify myocardial blood flow in units of milliliters per gram per minute at rest and during various interventions [156].

17.6.1 Cardiac PET/CT

Imaging of the glucose metabolism of the heart was introduced decades ago. Its key clinical application is the detection of hibernating myocardium, defined as maintained glucose metabolism in the presence of resting blood flow reductions and potentially reversible myocardial contractile dysfunction [157]. Other cardiac metabolic pathways evaluated with PET include using ^{11}C-acetate as an index of oxidative metabolism and myocardial oxygen consumption and assessment of fatty acid metabolism with ^{11}C-palmitate [157].

Several attempts have been made to use established or develop new probes for identifying vulnerable atherosclerotic plaques with PET. Inflammatory cells such as macrophages and activated lymphocytes consume considerable amounts of glucose [158]. Since inflammation is a hallmark of the vulnerable plaque, FDG-PET imaging may detect high-risk atherosclerotic lesions. Coronary FDG uptake was four times more frequently found in patients with than in those without coronary artery disease [158]. ^{18}F-NaF has been used for detecting calcified coronary artery plaques, and a correlation between its vascular uptake and CT-measured calcium score and risk factor profiles has been found [159]. On the other hand, 41% of patients with high calcium scores had no significant probe uptake, suggesting that information derived from CT and PET may be complementary. Other recently developed PET probes target fibrin, an important component of atherosclerotic plaques [160]. The potential to characterize coronary artery plaques at high or low risk would greatly benefit risk stratification and aid in developing and monitoring therapeutic approaches in cardiac diseases.

While used relatively infrequently, PET/CT could play an important role in managing patients with ischemic and nonischemic heart disease. Key applications include diagnosis and risk stratification of coronary artery disease patients and the assessment of myocardial viability in patients with ischemic heart disease and impaired left ventricular contractile function. PET probes of myocardial perfusion include ^{13}N-ammonia [161] (Figure 17.14), ^{82}Rb, ^{15}O-H$_2$O, and several emerging fluorinated probes [155,162]. The accuracy of PET stress–rest perfusion imaging for detecting coronary disease is high and can be further improved by PET/CT angiography [163,164]. Measurements of myocardial glucose metabolism with ^{18}F-FDG in conjunction with perfusion imaging are considered the gold standard for the assessment of myocardial viability [157]. It beneficially affects patient outcome [165] because viable yet hypoperfused myocardium can regain function following revascularization [157].

Using appropriate tracer kinetic models, myocardial blood flow and glucose metabolism can be quantified in units of milliliters per gram per minute or micromoles per gram per minute, respectively [156]. Such quantitative measurements can assist in detecting mild vasomotor dysfunction in patients at risk for coronary artery disease [166]. Relatively low-grade coronary artery stenosis [167] and triple-vessel disease can be identified with PET [168]. Impaired myocardial flow reserve correlated with the degree of coronary stenosis, with a higher accuracy of PET than of SPECT perfusion imaging [169].

Quantitative measurements of myocardial glucose metabolism have been used to characterize acutely infarcted or ischemic myocardium [170] and shown to provide prognostic information [171]. Importantly, PET perfusion imaging is cost-effective and has a significant impact on patient management [172,173].

The high sensitivity of PET, combined with the high negative predictive value of CT angiography, suggests that PET/CT could replace, in some instances, invasive assessments of coronary artery disease. Moreover, CT

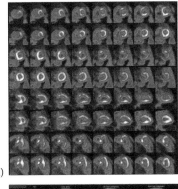

(a)

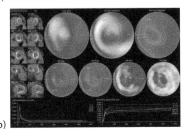

(b)

Table

	Str Flow	Rest Flow	CFR	Str SF	Rest SF
LAD	2.27	0.58	2.66	0.54	0.42
LCX	1.22	0.78	1.63	0.47	0.28
RCA	1.24	0.54	2.33	0.61	0.34
TOT	1.24	0.57	2.31	0.55	0.37

Figure 17.14 A 77-year-old male with a mild to moderate reversible perfusion defect in the proximal to midanterolateral wall, as well as a small fixed perfusion defect in the inferoseptal wall, suggestive of a prior infarct as seen on (a) corresponding perfusion images and (b) abnormal flow reserve in the LCX territory (Table). Str, stress; FR, coronary flow reserve; LCX, left circumflex coronary artery; LAD, left anterior descending coronary artery; RCA, right coronary artery, SF, spillover fraction; TOT: total.

measurements of coronary calcification and left ventricular function may also aid in diagnosis and prognostication [174]. CT data can also be used for photon attenuation correction [17]. Thus, cardiac PET/CT imaging can provide a one-stop-shop solution for the quantitative diagnostic evaluation of patients with ischemic and nonischemic heart disease.

17.6.2 Cardiac SPECT/CT Imaging

Several myocardial perfusion probes have been used for SPECT imaging, including ^{201}Tl-chloride, ^{99m}Tc-SestaMIBI, and ^{99m}Tc-tetrofosmin. Myocardial perfusion SPECT (MPS) is a well-established method for the diagnosis and localization of areas of ischemic or persistent myocardial damage and provides objective measurements of cardiac perfusion and function, as well as accurate risk assessment. Appropriate use of SPECT stress–rest perfusion imaging includes diagnosis and risk assessment in intermediate- and high-risk patients with coronary artery disease, while testing in low-risk patients, routine repeat testing, and general screening are discouraged [175].

Through the CT component, SPECT/CT of the heart can provide valuable additional information that will enhance the performance indices of myocardial perfusion imaging by (1) optimized attenuation correction (see Chapter 14), (2) providing coronary calcium score measurements in addition to estimates of perfusion, and (3) assessing coronary anatomy when CT coronary angiography (CTA) is performed.

Cardiac SPECT images are susceptible to attenuation artifacts from the breast and diaphragm, which can be misinterpreted, mainly by less experienced readers, as perfusion defects. Efforts are made to reduce the number of inconclusive SPECT studies, and it has been shown that attenuation correction increases the specificity of MPS from 60%–70% to 80%–90% [176]. Transmission source attenuation correction was developed a few decades ago, but it has not gained widespread clinical acceptance. However, in recent years cardiac CT from SPECT/CT has been used routinely for attenuation correction of SPECT perfusion studies. CT also allows for accurate and early detection of coronary calcifications. The coronary calcium score is a useful prognostic risk stratification tool. For SPECT/CT devices equipped with a diagnostic CT component, calcium scoring and perfusion studies can be performed sequentially during a single imaging session. The combined information increases the diagnostic accuracy, provides a tool to select patients that may need aggressive risk factor modification, and can assist in optimization of treatment strategies in patients with suspected or known coronary artery disease [177]. Cardiac CT angiography is limited, as it cannot determine the hemodynamic significance of stenosis. On the other hand, SPECT perfusion imaging has a high success rate in stratifying patients who are likely to benefit from revascularization or angioplasty; however, it cannot detect early atherosclerosis and has a tendency to underestimate the extent of coronary artery disease. The combined information from cardiac SPECT/CT angiography provides more specific diagnostic anatomic and functional data in cases where perfusion abnormalities are detected on SPECT and CTA will reveal the underlying cause and its location [178,179]. High-end CT devices provide gating capabilities in which x-rays are transmitted only during the required phase of the cardiac cycle, further reducing patient exposure. The patient must have the ability to tolerate IV contrast, to remain motionless on the table, to perform a breath-hold of at least 15 seconds, and to have a stable heart rate lower than 70 beats per minute. Beta-blockers may be needed to reduce the heart rate. The need for simultaneous anatomic and hemodynamic assessment of coronary artery disease using either SPECT/CT or PET/CT has not been demonstrated in large-scale studies. Preliminary results show an increased positive predictive value and specificity of both perfusion imaging and CT angiography by hybrid images. SPECT/CT angiography can potentially eliminate or at least reduce pitfalls in patients with advanced ischemic heart disease and balanced reduction of blood flow, as well as in patients with early atherosclerosis where the extent of coronary artery disease can be underestimated. When considering the best clinical algorithm for assessment of patients with known or suspected coronary artery disease, it is also important to appreciate the relative radiation burden to which the patient is exposed during each of the imaging modalities, and with hybrid imaging in particular [180].

17.7 INSIGHTS INTO BRAIN FUNCTION AND METABOLISM WITH PET AND SPECT

More PET probes have been developed for targeted brain imaging than for any other organ system. These include probes for beta-amyloid and tau protein, pre- and postsynaptic receptor expression, and transporter systems. PET imaging has also been described for assessing various neurotransmitter systems and receptors involved in progressive neurodegeneration and movement disorders [181–184]. Neurotransmitter and receptor systems are frequently impaired in Alzheimer's disease, as well as in dementias associated with Parkinson's disease and other movement disorders. PET probes may serve as diagnostic and predictive biomarkers and may help in individualizing patient treatments. SPECT probes are most frequently used to evaluate cerebral blood flow in a variety of neurological disorders. Additional SPECT probes have been introduced for imaging the dopaminergic neurotransmitter system [185].

17.7.1 PET APPLICATIONS IN NEUROLOGY

Cross-sectional MR is the imaging modality of choice for brain tumors, with some limitations related to the ability to differentiate tumor infiltration from surrounding edema or, after treatment, to differentiate recurrent tumor from radiation necrosis. The breakdown of the blood brain barrier provides the physiological rationale for using contrast-enhanced MRI. However, the value of MRI for metabolic phenotyping of brain tumors is not well established; moreover, the breakdown of the blood brain barrier is a nonspecific finding [186]. PET probes of glucose metabolism, amino acid transport, lipid metabolism, and tumor cell proliferation have enriched the diagnostic portfolio in brain tumor imaging [187].

Glucose metabolism is increased in malignant brain tumors [188]. However, the normal brain tissue high-background glucose metabolic activity renders tumor assessments with FDG PET difficult. Nevertheless, the degree of FDG uptake is correlated with tumor grade [189], and high-grade recurrent tumors can be differentiated from radiation necrosis, which in turn provides important prognostic information [190,191].

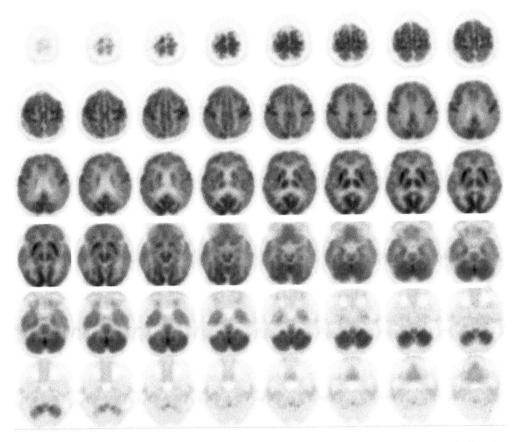

Figure 17.15 Axial ^{18}F-FDG-PET images in a 92-year-old female patient with severe cognitive decline demonstrating severely decreased metabolism of the posterior cingulate cortex, as well as the parietal, frontal, and temporal lobes, consistent with an advanced progressive neurodegenerative disorder, likely Alzheimer's disease.

Some of the limitations of FDG PET for brain tumor imaging have been overcome by the use of various fluorinated PET probes of amino acid transport. The increased utilization of amino acids in brain tumor cells meets anabolic (nucleic acid protein and protein synthesis) and catabolic (via the Krebs cycle) needs of rapidly growing tissue and is in many instances governed by upregulated c-myc [79]. The metabolic fate of various labeled amino acids and analogs is incompletely understood. However, after transport into tumor cells via L-amino acid transporters that are upregulated in brain cancer, CMET, but not FET, is incorporated into intracellular protein pools. FDOPA is metabolized peripherally by aromatic amino acid decarboxylase (AADC) to dopamine. Due to low normal brain background activity, low-grade and high-grade tumors can be detected equally well regardless of blood brain barrier integrity. FET, CMET, and FDOPA have thus been used successfully to detect and grade primary and recurrent brain tumors [192,193], to provide prognostic information, and to monitor therapeutic responses [194].

Cerebral glucose metabolic imaging can be used for detection of and differentiation between progressive and nonprogressive neurodegenerative diseases (Figure 17.15) [195–198] since brain physiology and function can be mapped with FDG PET [188]. FDG PET discriminates robustly among various disease entities, including Alzheimer's, frontotemporal dementias, and Lewy body disease [199]. ^{11}C- and ^{18}F-labeled probes for measuring cortical amyloid plaque and tau burden have been developed [200,201]. Three amyloid imaging compounds (florbetapir [Amyvid], flutemetamol [Vizamyl], and florbetaben [Neuraceq]) have been approved by the U.S. Food and Drug Administration (FDA) for brain imaging of beta-amyloid plaque burden in patients with cognitive impairment who are being evaluated for Alzheimer's disease and other causes of cognitive decline (Figure 17.16). At present, potential incremental benefits of these new probes over FDG

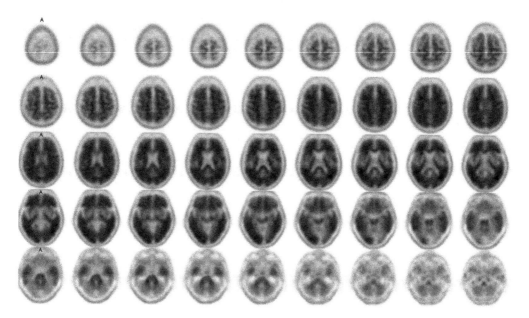

Figure 17.16 ¹⁸F-florbetapir study in an 88-year-old patient with mild cognitive decline demonstrates diffuse global moderate tracer activity in the cortical cerebral gray matter with a loss of the gray–white matter contrast. Findings are consistent with the presence of moderate to frequent amyloid neuritic plaques.

PET, especially for diagnosing and specifying neurodegenerative diseases, have not yet been demonstrated. If shown in future studies, the molecular imaging approach may significantly impact the diagnostic workup of patients with cognitive decline and be useful to determine the initiation of therapy early and for monitoring the effect of targeted therapies on the cerebral amyloid and tau burden. Given the widespread attempts to develop therapies, the role of diagnosing progressive neurodegenerative diseases early is gaining importance. This cannot be accomplished with anatomical imaging modalities, and PET will, in the future, play a critically important role in managing patients with these diseases.

Various neurotransmitter systems involved in progressive neurodegeneration with resulting movement disorders have also been targeted for PET imaging. These include acetylcholine esterase activity [183], and nicotinic [184], 5-hydroxytryptamine (5-HT) [181], and dopamine receptors [182]. These neurotransmitter systems are frequently impaired in dementias associated with Parkinson's disease. This clinical entity is characterized clinically by tremor, rigidity, and bradykinesia, symptoms caused by loss of dopaminergic neurons in the caudate nuclei and putamen. Other disorders, including essential tremor, cannot be readily distinguished from Parkinson's disease. Noninvasive diagnostic tools that permit such differentiation and that allow for monitoring the progression of disease are therefore needed. FDOPA PET imaging targets presynaptic AADC activity in terminal nerve endings. Striatal FDOPA uptake correlates inversely with the severity of motor dysfunction, bradykinesia, and rigidity, but not with tremor severity [202]. PET imaging can also be used to monitor the course of the disease, and studies have revealed that the degenerative process progresses faster in the putamen than in the caudate nuclei [203]. Presynaptic dopamine transport can be imaged using probes of the vesicular monoamine transporter 2 (VMAT2) [204] or those that target presynaptic dopamine transporters. Postsynaptic D1 and D2 dopamine receptor expression and function have also been imaged with PET. This approach has been used to assess the effects of oral levodopa therapy [205].

However, while a portfolio of metabolic and receptor-based imaging approaches has been developed, with some probes even deployed in the clinic, therapeutic advances, unfortunately, have not kept pace with the progress of diagnostics. Therefore, the impact of these PET imaging approaches on patient outcome frequently remains limited at the current time.

17.7.2 SPECT APPLICATIONS IN NEUROLOGY

SPECT studies have also been used in patients with known brain tumors to differentiate residual or recurrent malignant tissue infiltration from surrounding edema or posttreatment changes seen on CT or MRI following surgery or radiotherapy. Furthermore, CT and MRI cannot accurately distinguish primary brain lymphoma from cerebral toxoplasmosis in patients with acquired immunodeficiency syndrome [206,207]. SPECT imaging of the brain using radiotracers such as ^{201}Tl-chloride, ^{99m}Tc-SestaMIBI, or ^{99m}Tc-tetrofosmin has the potential to solve some of these clinical dilemmas [208]. The usefulness of SPECT for accurate preoperative detection and localization of brain tumors, as well as for radiotherapy planning and treatment monitoring, has been reported, with a proven clinical impact on the management of almost half of the investigated patient population. Specifically, SPECT with ^{201}Tl-chloride has been integrated into surgical planning and as a guide for directing biopsy to the target, with the highest uptake within the brain mass [209]. SPECT/CT, in particular, can achieve a more precise anatomical localization of viable malignant cerebral lesions and separate them from adjacent sites of physiological tracer uptake, such as the ventricles, choroid plexus, and venous sinuses [210]. Brain SPECT following the administration of tracers such as ^{99m}Tc-HMPAO has also been used for the assessment of cognitive disorders, particularly in the diagnosis of brain disorders such as dementia or to determine brain death. In these cases, no specific incremental value has been demonstrated so far.

17.8 IMPACT OF PET/CT ON PATIENT MANAGEMENT AND OUTCOME

Diagnostic tests need to be accurate and should improve patient management and outcome. The National Oncology PET Registry (NOPR) [211,212] has provided evidence for a substantial impact of FDG-PET imaging on patient management across a wide variety of cancers and indications, including initial and subsequent management strategies. Patient management was affected in 30%–40% of all patients, regardless of the study indication. As a limitation, NOPR did not include PET studies of patients with cancers already covered by the U.S. Center for Medicare and Medicaid Services (CMS). However, the impact of PET on managing patients with previously covered malignancies, such as lung, colon, and cervix cancers, as well as lymphoma, is consistent with the NOPR data [213–215].

Several studies have investigated the potential impact of FDG-PET imaging on patient outcome. The risk-adaptive PETAL trial [216] demonstrated a beneficial impact of interim PET imaging on the outcome of lymphoma patients. Another risk-adaptive trial, the Municon study [217], demonstrated that esophageal cancer patients who responded to neoadjuvant therapy had improved long-term survival, while nonresponders experienced no detrimental effects from earlier surgery. Lung cancer patients were randomized to presurgical staging with or without FDG PET/(CT) [116,218]. A significant reduction in the number of futile surgeries was reported in the group when FDG PET was included in the staging process. Similar beneficial effects were observed when PET was included in the presurgical staging of patients with liver metastases from colorectal cancer [219]. Finally, colorectal cancer patients were randomized to either conventional or FDG-PET follow-up [220]. Tumor recurrence was detected significantly earlier in the PET group, and these recurrences were more frequently cured by surgery. These observations strongly suggest that FDG-PET/CT staging can beneficially affect patient outcome and that PET early after the start of therapy can be used to change the management of cancer patients effectively.

17.9 IMPACT OF SPECT/CT ON PATIENT MANAGEMENT AND OUTCOME

Several studies have addressed the impact of SPECT/CT imaging on the management of patients with breast cancer [62,221–223], melanoma [222,224], head and neck cancer [224,225], thyroid cancer [226,227], parathyroid adenoma [228,229], and neuroendocrine tumors [230–232]. Patient management was affected in one-third to one-half of patients undergoing sentinel node imaging for head and neck and breast cancers, respectively. Management was similarly affected in up to 40% of patients scanned with ^{131}I for thyroid cancer and of those who had ^{99m}Tc-SestaMIBI studies for parathyroid adenoma. Finally, integrated SPECT/CT affected the management of up to one-third of patients with neuroendocrine tumors.

17.10 SUMMARY

In summary, PET/CT and SPECT/CT have emerged as indispensable imaging tools to better characterize and manage oncologic, cardiologic, neurologic, endocrine, and other diseases. The technologies are safe, mature, and robust, and their appropriate application can result in improved patient outcomes. The clinical role of PET/MRI has yet to be determined, but it appears possible that it will find its place in the management of pediatric patients and those with neurological diseases, and in other selected applications.

REFERENCES

1. Spick, C., K. Herrmann, and J. Czernin. 2016. 18F-FDG PET/CT and PET/MRI perform equally well in cancer: Evidence from studies on more than 2,300 patients. *J Nucl Med* 7(3):420–430.
2. Ter-Pogossian, M. M., M. E. Phelps, E. J. Hoffman, and N. A. Mullani. 1975. A positron-emission transaxial tomograph for nuclear imaging (PETT). *Radiology* 114:89–98.
3. Phelps, M., E. Hoffman, N. Mullani, and M. Ter-Pogossian. 1975. Application of annihilation coincidence detection to transaxial reconstruction tomography. *J Nucl Med* 16:210–224.
4. Warburg, O., K. Posener, and E. Negelein. 1924. The metabolism of cancer cells. *Biochem Zeitschr* 152:129–169.
5. Warburg, O., F. Wind, and E. Negelein. 1927. The metabolism of tumors in the body. *J Gen Physiol* 8:519–530.
6. Sokoloff, L. 1996. *The History of Neuroscience in Autobiography*. Washington, DC: Society of Neuroscience.
7. Sokoloff, L., M. Reivich, C. Kennedy, M. Des Rosiers, C. Patlak, K. Pettigrew, O. Sakurada, and M. Shinohara. 1977. The [14C]deoxyglucose method for the measurement of local cerebral glucose utilization: Theory, procedure, and normal values in the conscious and anesthetized albino rat. *J Neurochem* 28:897–916.
8. Gallagher, B. M., J. S. Fowler, N. I. Gutterson, R. R. MacGregor, C. N. Wan, and A. P. Wolf. 1978. Metabolic trapping as a principle of oradiopharmaceutical design: Some factors responsible for the biodistribution of [18F] 2-deoxy-2-fluoro-D-glucose. *J Nucl Med* 19:1154–1161.
9. Kuhl, D. E., M. E. Phelps, A. P. Kowell, E. J. Metter, C. Selin, and J. Winter. 1980. Effects of stroke on local cerebral metabolism and perfusion: Mapping by emission computed tomography of 18FDG and 13NH3. *Ann Neurol* 8:47–60.
10. Phelps, M. E., E. J. Hoffman, R. E. Coleman, M. J. Welch, M. E. Raichle, E. S. Weiss, B. E. Sobel, and M. M. Ter-Pogossian. 1976. Tomographic images of blood pool and perfusion in brain and heart. *J Nucl Med* 17:603–612.
11. Yen, C.-K., Y. Yano, T. F. Budinger, R. P. Friedland, S. E. Derenzo, R. H. Huesman, and H. A. O'Brien. 1982. Brain tumor evaluation using Rb-82 and positron emission tomography. *J Nucl Med* 23:532–537.
12. Benson, D., D. Kuhl, M. Phelps, J. Cummings, and S. Tsai. 1981. Positron emission computed tomography in the diagnosis of dementia. *Trans Am Neurol Assoc* 106:68–71.
13. Schelbert, H. 1989. Myocardial ischemia and clinical applications of positron emission tomography. *Am J Cardiol* 64:46E–53E.
14. Bax, J. J., R. S. Beanlands, F. J. Klocke, J. Knuuti, A. A. Lammertsma, M. A. Schaefers, H. R. Schelbert, G. K. Von Schulthess, L. J. Shaw, G. Z. Yang, and P. G. Camici. 2007. Diagnostic and clinical perspectives of fusion imaging in cardiology: Is the total greater than the sum of its parts? *Heart* 93:16–22.

15. Dahlbom, M., E. J. Hoffman, C. K. Hoh, C. Schiepers, G. Rosenqvist, R. A. Hawkins, and M. E. Phelps. 1992. Whole-body positron emission tomography. Part I. Methods and performance characteristics. *J Nucl Med* 33:1191–1199.

16. Beyer, T., D. Townsend, T. Brun, P. Kinahan, M. Charron, R. Roddy, J. Jerin, J. Young, L. Byars, and R. Nutt. 2000. A combined PET/CT scanner for clinical oncology. *J Nucl Med* 41:1369–1379.

17. Kinahan, P. E., D. W. Townsend, T. Beyer, and D. Sashin. 1998. Attenuation correction for a combined 3D PET/CT scanner. *Med Phys* 25:2046–2053.

18. Martinelli, M., D. Townsend, C. Meltzer, and V. Villemagne. 2000. 7. Survey of results of whole body imaging using the PET/CT at the University of Pittsburgh Medical Center PET facility. *Clin Positron Imaging* 3:161.

19. Mullani, N., J. Markham, and M. Ter-Pogossian. 1980. Feasibility of time-of-flight reconstruction in positron emission tomography. *J Nucl Med* 21:1095–1097.

20. Budinger, T. 1983. Time-of-flight positron emission tomography: Status relative to conventional PET. *J Nucl Med* 24:73–78.

21. Hudson, H., and R. Larkin. 1994. Accelerated image reconstruction using ordered subsets of projection data. *IEEE Trans Med Imaging* 13:601–609.

22. Gambhir, S. S., J. E. Shepherd, B. D. Shah, E. Hart, C. K. Hoh, P. E. Valk, T. Emi, and M. E. Phelps. 1998. Analytical decision model for the cost-effective management of solitary pulmonary nodules. *J Clin Oncol* 16:2113–2125.

23. Yang, Y., and J. Czernin. 2011. Contribution of imaging to cancer care costs. *J Nucl Med* 52:86S–92S.

24. Hoffman, E. J., S. C. Huang, and M. E. Phelps. 1979. Quantitation in positron emission computed tomography. 1. Effect of object size. *J Comput Assist Tomogr* 3:299–308.

25. Huang, S. C., E. J. Hoffman, M. E. Phelps, and D. E. Kuhl. 1979. Quantitation in positron emission computed tomography. 2. Effects of inaccurate attenuation correction. *J Comput Assist Tomogr* 3:804–814.

26. Larsson, A., L. Johansson, T. Sundstrom, and K. R. Ahlstrom. 2003. A method for attenuation and scatter correction of brain SPECT based on computed tomography images. *Nucl Med Commun* 24:411–420.

27. Rosenthal, M. S., J. Cullom, W. Hawkins, S. C. Moore, B. M. Tsui, and M. Yester. 1995. Quantitative SPECT imaging: A review and recommendations by the Focus Committee of the Society of Nuclear Medicine Computer and Instrumentation Council. *J Nucl Med* 36:1489–1513.

28. Tsui, B. M., E. C. Frey, X. Zhao, D. S. Lalush, R. E. Johnston, and W. H. McCartney. 1994. The importance and implementation of accurate 3D compensation methods for quantitative SPECT. *Phys Med Biol* 39:509–530.

29. Zaidi, H., and B. Hasegawa. 2003. Determination of the attenuation map in emission tomography. *J Nucl Med* 44:291–315.

30. Tsui, B. M., X. Zhao, E. C. Frey, and W. H. McCartney. 1994. Quantitative single-photon emission computed tomography: Basics and clinical considerations. *Semin Nucl Med* 24:38–65.

31. Blankespoor, S., X. Wu, and J. Kalki. 1996. Attenuation correction of SPECT using x-ray CT on an emission–transmission CT system: Myocardial perfusion assessment. *IEEE Trans Nucl Sci* 43:2263–2274.

32. Da Silva, A. J., H. R. Tang, K. H. Wong, M. C. Wu, M. W. Dae, and B. H. Hasegawa. 2001. Absolute quantification of regional myocardial uptake of 99mTc-sestamibi with SPECT: Experimental validation in a porcine model. *J Nucl Med* 42:772–779.

33. Hasegawa, B., H. R. Tang, A. J. Silva, K. H. Wong, K. Iwata, and M. C. Wu. 2000. Dual-modality imaging. *Nucl Instrum Methods Phys Res* A471:140–144.

34. Hasegawa, B., E. Gingold, and S. Reilly. 1990. Description of a simultaneous emission-transmission CT system. *Proc SPIE* 1231:50–60.

35. Hasegawa, B., K. Iwata, K. Wong, M. Wu, A. Da Silva, H. Tang, W. Barber, A. Hwang, and A. Sakdinawat. 2002. Dual-modality imaging of function and physiology. *Acad Radiol* 9:1305–1321.

36. Hasegawa, B., K. Wong, K. Iwata, W. Barber, A. Hwang, A. Sakdinawat, M. Ramaswamy, D. Price, and R. Hawkins. 2002. Dual-modality imaging of cancer with SPECT/CT. *Technol Cancer Res Treat* 6:449–458.

37. Lang, T. F., B. H. Hasegawa, S. C. Liew, J. K. Brown, S. C. Blankespoor, S. M. Reilly, E. L. Gingold, and C. E. Cann. 1992. Description of a prototype emission transmission computed tomography imaging system. *J Nucl Med* 33:1881–1887.

38. Townsend, D., T. Beyer, and T. Blodgett. 2003. PET/CT scanners: A hardware approach to image fusion. *Semin Nucl Med* 33:193–199.

39. Townsend, D., J. Carney, J. Yap, and N. Hall. 2004. PET/CT today and tomorrow. *J Nucl Med* 45(Suppl. 1):4S–12S.

40. Townsend, D., and S. Cherry. 2001. Combining anatomy and function: The path to true image fusion. *Eur Radiol* 11:1968–1974.

41. Townsend, D. W. 2001. A combined PET/CT scanner: The choices. *J Nucl Med* 42:533–534.

42. Hutton, B., and M. Braun. 2003. Software for image registration: Algorithms, accuracy, efficacy. *Semin Nucl Med* 33:180–192.

43. Maintz, J., and M. Viergever. 1998. A survey of medical image registration. *Med Image Anal* 2:1–36.

44. Slomka, P. 2004. Software approach to merging molecular with anatomic information. *J Nucl Med* 45:36S–45S.

45. Kinahan, P. E., B. H. Hasegawa, and T. Beyer. 2003. X-ray-based attenuation correction for positron emission tomography/computed tomography scanners. *Semin Nucl Med* 33:166–179.

46. Israel, O., Z. Keidar, G. Iosilevsky, L. Bettman, J. Sachs, and A. Frenkel. 2001. The fusion of anatomic and physiologic imaging in the management of patients with cancer. *Semin Nucl Med* 31:191–205.

47. Bocher, M., A. Balan, Y. Krausz, Y. Shrem, A. Lonn, M. Wilk, and R. Chisin. 2000. Gamma camera-mounted anatomical x-ray tomography: Technology, system characteristics and first images. *Eur J Nucl Med* 27:619–627.

48. Even-Sapir, E., Z. Keidar, J. Sachs, A. Engel, L. Bettman, D. Gaitini, L. Guralnik, N. Werbin, G. Iosilevsky, and O. Israel. 2001. The new technology of combined transmission and emission tomography in evaluation of endocrine neoplasms. *J Nucl Med* 42:998–1004.

49. Lois, C., B. Jakoby, M. Long, K. Hubner, D. Barker, M. Casey, M. Conti, V. Panin, D. Kadrmas, and D. Townsend. 2010. An assessment of the impact of incorporating time-of-flight information into clinical PET/CT imaging. *J Nucl Med* 51:237–245.

50. Halpern, B., M. Dahlbom, A. Quon, C. Schiepers, C. Waldherr, D. Silverman, O. Ratib, and J. Czernin. 2004. Impact of patient weight and emission scan duration on PET/CT image quality and lesion detectability. *J Nucl Med* 45:797–801.

51. Beyer, T., J. Czernin, and L. S. Freudenberg. 2011. Variations in clinical PET/CT operations: Results of an international survey of active PET/CT users. *J Nucl Med* 52:303–310.

52. Graham, M. M., R. D. Badawi, and R. L. Wahl. 2011. Variations in PET/CT methodology for oncologic imaging at U.S. academic medical centers: An imaging response assessment team survey. *J Nucl Med* 52:311–317.

53. Allen-Auerbach, M., K. Yeom, J. Park, M. Phelps, and J. Czernin. 2006. Standard PET/CT of the chest during shallow breathing is inadequate for comprehensive staging of lung cancer. *J Nucl Med* 47:298–301.

54. Pfannenberg, A. C., P. Aschoff, K. Brechtel, M. Müller, M. Klein, R. Bares, C. D. Claussen, and S. M. Eschmann. 2007. Value of contrast-enhanced multiphase CT in combined PET/CT protocols for oncological imaging. *Br J Radiol* 80:437–445.

55. Soyka, J. D., P. Veit-Haibach, K. Strobel, S. Breitenstein, A. Tschopp, K. A. Mende, M. P. Lago, and T. F. Hany. 2008. Staging pathways in recurrent colorectal carcinoma: Is contrast-enhanced 18F-FDG PET/CT the diagnostic tool of choice? *J Nucl Med* 49:354–361.

56. Tateishi, U., T. Maeda, T. Morimoto, M. Miyake, Y. Arai, and E. E. Kim. 2007. Non-enhanced CT versus contrast-enhanced CT in integrated PET/CT studies for nodal staging of rectal cancer. *Eur J Nucl Med Mol Imaging* 34:1627–1634.

57. Aschoff, P., C. Plathow, T. Beyer, M. Lichy, G. Erb, M. Öksüz, C. Claussen, and C. Pfannenberg. 2012. Multiphase contrast-enhanced CT with highly concentrated contrast agent can be used for PET attenuation correction in integrated PET/CT imaging. *Eur J Nucl Med Mol Imaging* 39:316–325.

58. Ippolito, D., C. Capraro, L. Guerra, E. Ponti, C. Messa, and S. Sironi. 2013. Feasibility of perfusion CT technique integrated into conventional 18FDG/PET-CT studies in lung cancer patients: Clinical staging and functional information in a single study. *Eur J Nucl Med Mol Imaging* 40:156–165.

59. Czernin, J., M. Benz, and M. Allen-Auerbach. 2010. PET/CT imaging: The incremental value of assessing the glucose metabolic phenotype and the structure of cancers in a single examination. *Eur J Radiol* 73:470–480.

60. de Langen, A. J., A. Vincent, L. M. Velasquez, H. van Tinteren, R. Boellaard, L. K. Shankar, M. Boers, E. F. Smit, S. Stroobants, W. A. Weber, and O. S. Hoekstra. 2012. Repeatability of 18F-FDG uptake measurements in tumors: A metaanalysis. *J Nucl Med* 53:701–708.

61. Boellaard, R. 2011. Need for standardization of 18F-FDG PET/CT for treatment response assessments. *J Nucl Med* 52:93S–100S.

62. Delbeke, D., H. Schöder, W. H. Martin, and R. L. Wahl. 2009. Hybrid imaging (SPECT/CT and PET/CT): Improving therapeutic decisions. *Semin Nucl Med* 39:308–340.

63. Young, H., R. Baum, U. Cremerius, K. Herholz, O. Hoekstra, A. Lammertsma, J. Pruim, and P. Price. 1999. Measurement of clinical and subclinical tumour response using [[18F]-fluorodeoxyglucose and positron emission tomography: Review and 1999 EORTC recommendations. *Eur J Cancer* 35:1773–1782.

64. Bar, R., K. Przewloka, R. Karry, A. Frenkel, A. Golz, and Z. Keidar. 2012. Half-time SPECT acquisition with resolution recovery for Tc-MIBI SPECT imaging in the assessment of hyperparathyroidism. *Mol Imaging Biol* 14:647–651.

65. Wahl, R. L., J. M. Herman, and E. Ford. 2011. The promise and pitfalls of positron emission tomography and single-photon emission computed tomography molecular imaging–guided radiation therapy. *Semin Radiat Oncol* 21:88–100.

66. Tatli, S., V. H. Gerbaudo, C. M. Feeley, P. B. Shyn, K. Tuncali, and S. G. Silverman. 2011. PET/CT-guided percutaneous biopsy of abdominal masses: Initial experience. *J Vasc Interv Radiol* 22:507–514.

67. Benz, M. R., J. Czernin, S. M. Dry, W. D. Tap, M. S. Allen-Auerbach, D. Elashoff, M. E. Phelps, W. A. Weber, and F. C. Eilber. 2010. Quantitative F18-fluorodeoxyglucose positron emission tomography accurately characterizes peripheral nerve sheath tumors as malignant or benign. *Cancer* 116:451–458.

68. Eisenhauer, E., P. Therasse, and J. Bogaerts. 2009. New response evaluation criteria in solid tumours: Revised RECIST guideline (version 1.1). *Eur J Cancer* 45:228–247.

69. Evilevitch, V., W. A. Weber, W. D. Tap, M. Allen-Auerbach, K. Chow, S. D. Nelson, F. R. Eilber, et al. 2008. Reduction of glucose metabolic activity is more accurate than change in size at predicting histopathologic response to neoadjuvant therapy in high-grade soft-tissue sarcomas. *Clin Cancer Res* 14:715–720.

70. Benz, M. R., J. Czernin, M. S. Allen-Auerbach, W. D. Tap, S. M. Dry, D. Elashoff, K. Chow, et al. 2009. FDG-PET/CT imaging predicts histopathologic treatment responses after the initial cycle of neoadjuvant chemotherapy in high-grade soft-tissue sarcomas. *Clin Cancer Res* 15:2856–2863.

71. Weber, W. 2009. Assessing tumor response to therapy. *J Nucl Med* 50:1S–10S.

72. Larson, S. M., Y. Erdi, T. Akhurst, M. Mazumdar, H. A. Macapinlac, R. D. Finn, C. Casilla, et al. 1999. Tumor treatment response based on visual and quantitative changes in global tumor glycolysis using PET-FDG imaging: The visual response score and the change in total lesion glycolysis. *Clin Positron Imaging* 2:159–171.

73. Francis, R. J., M. J. Byrne, A. A. van der Schaaf, J. A. Boucek, A. K. Nowak, M. Phillips, R. Price, A. P. Patrikeos, A. W. Musk, and M. J. Millward. 2007. Early prediction of response to chemotherapy and survival in malignant pleural mesothelioma using a novel semiautomated 3-dimensional volume-based analysis of serial 18F-FDG PET scans. *J Nucl Med* 48:1449–1458.

74. Lee, P., D. K. Weerasuriya, P. W. Lavori, A. Quon, W. Hara, P. G. Maxim, Q.-T. Le, H. A. Wakelee, J. S. Donington, E. E. Graves, and B. W. Loo Jr. 2007. Metabolic tumor burden predicts for disease progression and death in lung cancer. *Int J Radiat Oncol Biol Phys* 69:328–333.

75. Kawada, K., Y. Nakamoto, M. Kawada, K. Hida, T. Matsumoto, T. Murakami, S. Hasegawa, K. Togashi, and Y. Sakai. 2012. Relationship between 18F-fluorodeoxyglucose accumulation and KRAS/BRAF mutations in colorectal cancer. *Clin Cancer Res* 18:1696–1703.

76. Riedl, C. C., T. Akhurst, S. Larson, S. F. Stanziale, S. Tuorto, A. Bhargava, H. Hricak, D. Klimstra, and Y. Fong. 2007. 18F-FDG PET scanning correlates with tissue markers of poor prognosis and predicts mortality for patients after liver resection for colorectal metastases. *J Nucl Med* 48:771–775.

77. Koolen, B., M. Vrancken Peeters, T. Aukema, W. Vogel, H. Oldenburg, J. Hage, C. Hoefnagel, et al. 2012. 18F-FDG PET/CT as a staging procedure in primary stage II and III breast cancer: Comparison with conventional imaging techniques. *Breast Cancer Res Treat* 131:117–126.

78. Kelloff, G. J., J. M. Hoffman, B. Johnson, H. I. Scher, B. A. Siegel, E. Y. Cheng, B. D. Cheson, et al. 2005. Progress and promise of FDG-PET imaging for cancer patient management and oncologic drug development. *Clin Cancer Res* 11:2785–2808.

79. Lieberman, B. P., K. Ploessl, L. Wang, W. Qu, Z. Zha, D. R. Wise, L. A. Chodosh, G. Belka, C. B. Thompson, and H. F. Kung. 2011. PET imaging of glutaminolysis in tumors by 18F-(2S,4R)4-fluoroglutamine. *J Nucl Med* 52:1947–1955.

80. Vander Heiden, M., S. Lunt, T. Dayton, B. Fiske, W. Israelsen, K. Mattaini, N. Vokes, G. Stephanopoulos, L. Cantley, C. Metallo, and J. Locasale. 2011. Metabolic pathway alterations that support cell proliferation. *Cold Spring Harb Symp Quant Biol* 76:325–334.

81. Okubo, S., H.-N. Zhen, N. Kawai, Y. Nishiyama, R. Haba, and T. Tamiya. 2010. Correlation of L-methyl-11C-methionine (MET) uptake with L-type amino acid transporter 1 in human gliomas. *J Neurooncol* 99:217–225.

82. Kaira, K., N. Oriuchi, H. Imai, K. Shimizu, N. Yanagitani, N. Sunaga, T. Hisada, T. Ishizuka, Y. Kanai, T. Nakajima, and M. Mori. 2009. Prognostic significance of L-type amino acid transporter 1 (LAT1) and 4F2 heavy chain (CD98) expression in stage I pulmonary adenocarcinoma. *Lung Cancer* 66:120–126.

83. Yanagisawa, N., M. Ichinoe, T. Mikami, N. Nakada, K. Hana, W. Koizumi, H. Endou, and I. Okayasu. 2012. High expression of L-type amino acid transporter 1 (LAT1) predicts poor prognosis in pancreatic ductal adenocarcinomas. *J Clin Pathol* 65:1019–1023.

84. Fottner, C., A. Helisch, M. Anlauf, H. Rossmann, T. J. Musholt, A. Kreft, S. Schadmand-Fischer, et al. 2010. 6-18F-fluoro-L-dihydroxyphenylalanine positron emission tomography is superior to 123I-metaiodobenzyl-guanidine scintigraphy in the detection of extraadrenal and hereditary pheochromocytomas and paragangliomas: Correlation with vesicular monoamine transporter expression. *J Clin Endocrinol Metab* 95:2800–2810.

85. Imani, F., V. G. Agopian, M. S. Auerbach, M. A. Walter, F. Imani, M. R. Benz, R. A. Dumont, C. K. Lai, J. G. Czernin, and M. W. Yeh. 2009. 18F-FDOPA PET and PET/CT accurately localize pheochromocytomas. *J Nucl Med* 50:513–519.

86. Lu, M.-Y., Y.-L. Liu, H.-H. Chang, S.-T. Jou, Y.-L. Yang, K.-H. Lin, D.-T. Lin, et al. 2013. Characterization of neuroblastic tumors using 18F-FDOPA PET. *J Nucl Med* 54:42–49.

87. Montravers, F., K. Kerrou, V. Nataf, V. Huchet, J.-P. Lotz, P. Ruszniewski, P. Rougier, et al. 2009. Impact of fluorodihydroxyphenylalanine-(18F) positron emission tomography on management of adult patients with documented or occult digestive endocrine tumors. *J Clin Endocrinol Metab* 94:1295–1301.

88. Piccardo, A., E. Lopci, M. Conte, A. Garaventa, L. Foppiani, V. Altrinetti, C. Nanni, et al. 2012. Comparison of 18F-dopa PET/CT and 123I-MIBG scintigraphy in stage 3 and 4 neuroblastoma: A pilot study. *Eur J Nucl Med Mol Imaging* 39:57–71.

89. Czernin, J., M. Benz, and M. Allen-Auerbach. 2009. PET imaging of prostate cancer using C-acetate. *PET Clin* 4:163–172.

90. Langsteger, W., M. Heinisch, and I. Fogelman. 2006. The role of fluorodeoxyglucose, 18F-dihydroxyphenylalanine, 18F-choline, and 18F-fluoride in bone imaging with emphasis on prostate and breast. *Semin Nucl Med* 36:73–92.

91. Ho, C.-L., S. C. H. Yu, and D. W. C. Yeung. 2003. 11C-acetate PET imaging in hepatocellular carcinoma and other liver masses. *J Nucl Med* 44:213–221.

92. Shields, A., J. Grierson, B. Dohmen, H. Machulla, J. Stayanoff, J. Lawhorn-Crews, J. Obradovich, O. Muzik, and T. Mangner. 1998. Imaging proliferation in vivo with [F-18]FLT and positron emission tomography. *Nat Med* 4:13343–11336.

93. Francis, D. L., A. Freeman, D. Visvikis, D. C. Costa, S. K. Luthra, M. Novelli, I. Taylor, and P. J. Ell. 2003. In vivo imaging of cellular proliferation in colorectal cancer using positron emission tomography. *Gut* 52:1602–1606.

94. Vesselle, H., J. Grierson, M. Muzi, J. M. Pugsley, R. A. Schmidt, P. Rabinowitz, L. M. Peterson, E. Vallières, and D. E. Wood. 2002. In vivo validation of 3′deoxy-3′-[18F]fluorothymidine ([18F]FLT) as a proliferation imaging tracer in humans: Correlation of [18F]FLT uptake by positron emission tomography with Ki-67 immunohistochemistry and flow cytometry in human lung tumors. *Clin Cancer Res* 8:3315–3323.

95. Blau, M., R. Ganatra, and M. Bender. 1972. 18 F-fluoride for bone imaging. *Semin Nucl Med* 2:31–37.

96. Linden, H. M., S. A. Stekhova, J. M. Link, J. R. Gralow, R. B. Livingston, G. K. Ellis, P. H. Petra, et al. 2006. Quantitative fluoroestradiol positron emission tomography imaging predicts response to endocrine treatment in breast cancer. *J Clin Oncol* 24:2793–2799.

97. Liu, A., C. S. Dence, M. J. Welch, and J. A. Katzenellenbogen. 1992. Fluorine-18-labeled androgens: Radiochemical synthesis and tissue distribution studies on six fluorine-substituted androgens, potential imaging agents for prostatic cancer. *J Nucl Med* 33:724–734.

98. Eder, M., M. Eisenhut, J. Babich, and U. Haberkorn. 2013. PSMA as a target for radiolabelled small molecules. *Eur J Nucl Med Mol Imaging* 40:819–823.

99. Evans, M. J., P. M. Smith-Jones, J. Wongvipat, V. Navarro, S. Kim, N. H. Bander, S. M. Larson, and C. L. Sawyers. 2011. Noninvasive measurement of androgen receptor signaling with a positron-emitting radiopharmaceutical that targets prostate-specific membrane antigen. *Proc Natl Acad Sci USA* 108:9578–9582.

100. Reubi, J. C., and H. R. Maecke. 2008. Peptide-based probes for cancer imaging. *J Nucl Med* 49:1735–1738.

101. Gaertner, F. C., H. Kessler, H. J. Wester, M. Schwaiger, and A. J. Beer. 2012. Radiolabelled RGD peptides for imaging and therapy. *Eur J Nucl Med Mol Imaging* 39:126–138.

102. Wu, A. M. 2009. Antibodies and antimatter: The resurgence of immuno-PET. *J Nucl Med* 50:2–5.

103. Graham, M. 2012. Clinical molecular imaging with radiotracers: Current status. *Med Princ Pract* 21:197–208.

104. Nishiyama, H., V. J. Sodd, R. J. Adolph, E. L. Saenger, J. T. Lewis, and M. Gabel. 1976. Intercomparison of myocardial imaging agents: 201Ti, 129Cs, 43K, and 81Rb. *J Nucl Med* 17:880–889.

105. Gómez-Río, M., A. Rodríguez-Fernández, C. Ramos-Font, E. López-Ramírez, and J. Llamas-Elvira. 2008. Diagnostic accuracy of 201Thallium-SPECT and 18F-FDG-PET in the clinical assessment of glioma recurrence. *Eur J Nucl Med Mol Imaging* 35:966–975.

106. Ji, S., and M. Travin. 2010. Radionuclide imaging of cardiac autonomic innervation. *J Nucl Cardiol* 17:655–666.

107. Freitas, J. E., R. J. Grekin, J. H. Thrall, M. D. Gross, D. P. Swanson, and W. H. Beierwaltes. 1979. Adrenal imaging with iodomethyl-norcholesterol (I-131) in primary aldosteronism. *J Nucl Med* 20:7–10.

108. Jones, A., M. Francis, and M. Davis. 1976. Bone scanning: Radionuclidic reaction mechanisms. *Semin Nucl Med* 6:3–18.

109. de Graaf, W., R. J. Bennink, R. Veteläinen, and T. M. van Gulik. 2010. Nuclear imaging techniques for the assessment of hepatic function in liver surgery and transplantation. *J Nucl Med* 51:742–752.

110. Moran, J. 1999. Technetium-99m-EC and other potential new agents in renal nuclear medicine. *Semin Nucl Med* 29:91–101.

111. Sinusas, A. 2008. Targeted imaging offers advantages over physiological imaging for evaluation of angiogenic therapy. *JACC Cardiovasc Imaging* 1:511–514.

112. Kaltsas, G., A. Rockall, D. Papadogias, R. Reznek, and A. Grossman. 2004. Recent advances in radiological and radionuclide imaging and therapy of neuroendocrine tumours. *Eur J Endocrinol* 151:15–27.

113. Haseman, M., S. Rosenthal, and T. Polascik. 2000. Capromab pendetide imaging of prostate cancer. *Cancer Biother Radiopharm* 15:131–140.

114. Vlaar, A., T. de Nijs, A. Kessels, F. Vreeling, A. Winogrodzka, W. Mess, S. Tromp, M. van Kroonenburgh, and W. Weber. 2008. Diagnostic value of 123I-ioflupane and 123I-iodobenzamide SPECT scans in 248 patients with parkinsonian syndromes. *Eur Neurol* 59:258–266.

115. Czernin, J., M. Allen-Auerbach, and H. Schelbert. 2007. Improvements in cancer staging with PET/CT: Literature-based evidence as of September 2006. *J Nucl Med* 48:78S–88S.

116. Fischer, B. M., U. Lassen, and L. Højgaard. 2011. PET-CT in preoperative staging of lung cancer. *N Engl J Med* 364:980–981.

117. Riegger, C., J. Herrmann, J. Nagarajah, J. Hecktor, S. Kuemmel, F. Otterbach, S. Hahn, A. Bockisch, T. Lauenstein, G. Antoch, and T. A. Heusner. 2012. Whole-body FDG PET/CT is more accurate than conventional imaging for staging primary breast cancer patients. *Eur J Nucl Med Mol Imaging* 39:852–863.

118. Barber, T. W., C. P. Duong, T. Leong, M. Bressel, E. G. Drummond, and R. J. Hicks. 2012. 18F-FDG PET/CT has a high impact on patient management and provides powerful prognostic stratification in the primary staging of esophageal cancer: A prospective study with mature survival data. *J Nucl Med* 53:864–871.

119. Choi, H. J., J. W. Roh, S.-S. Seo, S. Lee, J.-Y. Kim, S.-K. Kim, K. W. Kang, J. S. Lee, J. Y. Jeong, and S.-Y. Park. 2006. Comparison of the accuracy of magnetic resonance imaging and positron emission tomography/computed tomography in the presurgical detection of lymph node metastases in patients with uterine cervical carcinoma. *Cancer* 106:914–922.

120. El-Galaly, T. C., F. d'Amore, K. J. Mylam, P. de Nully Brown, M. Bøgsted, A. Bukh, L. Specht, et al. 2012. Routine bone marrow biopsy has little or no therapeutic consequence for positron emission tomography/computed tomography—Staged treatment-naive patients with Hodgkin lymphoma. *J Clin Oncol* 30:4508–4514.

121. Reinhardt, M. J., A. Y. Joe, U. Jaeger, A. Huber, A. Matthies, J. Bucerius, R. Roedel, H. Strunk, T. Bieber, H.-J. Biersack, and T. Tüting. 2006. Diagnostic performance of whole body dual modality 18F-FDG PET/CT imaging for N- and M-staging of malignant melanoma: Experience with 250 consecutive patients. *J Clin Oncol* 24:1178–1187.

122. Benz, M. R., S. M. Dry, F. C. Eilber, M. S. Allen-Auerbach, W. D. Tap, D. Elashoff, M. E. Phelps, and J. Czernin. 2010. Correlation between glycolytic phenotype and tumor grade in soft-tissue sarcomas by 18F-FDG PET. *J Nucl Med* 51:1174–1181.

123. van Lammeren-Venema, D., J. Regelink, I. I. Riphagen, S. Zweegman, O. Hoekstra, and J. Zijlstra. 2012. 18F-fluoro-deoxyglucose positron emission tomography in assessment of myeloma-related bone disease: A systematic review. *Cancer* 118:1971–1981.

124. Xu, G., L. Zhao, and Z. He. 2012. Performance of whole-body PET/CT for the detection of distant malignancies in various cancers: A systematic review and meta-analysis. *J Nucl Med* 53:1847–1854.

125. Plathow, C., and W. A. Weber. 2008. Tumor cell metabolism imaging. *J Nucl Med* 49:43S–63S.

126. Wahl, R. L., H. Jacene, Y. Kasamon, and M. A. Lodge. 2009. From RECIST to PERCIST: Evolving considerations for PET response criteria in solid tumors. *J Nucl Med* 50:122S–150S.

127. Gallamini, A., M. Hutchings, L. Rigacci, L. Specht, F. Merli, M. Hansen, C. Patti, et al. 2007. Early interim 2-[18F]fluoro-2-deoxy-D-glucose positron emission tomography is prognostically superior to international prognostic score in advanced-stage Hodgkin's lymphoma: A report from a joint Italian-Danish study. *J Clin Oncol* 25:3746–3752.

128. Dann, E. 2012. PET/CT adapted therapy in Hodgkin disease: Current state of the art and future directions. *Curr Oncol Rep* 14:403–410.

129. Casasnovas, R.-O., M. Meignan, A. Berriolo-Riedinger, E. Itti, D. Huglo, C. Haioun, and F. Morschhauser. 2012. Early interim PET scans in diffuse large B-cell lymphoma: Can there be consensus about standardized reporting, and can PET scans guide therapy choices? *Curr Hematol Malig Rep* 7:193–199.

130. Weber, W. A. 2006. Positron emission tomography as an imaging biomarker. *J Clin Oncol* 24:3282–3292.

131. Van den Abbeele, A., and R. Badawi. 2002. Use of positron emission tomography in oncology and its potential role to assess response to imatinib mesylate therapy in gastrointestinal stromal tumors (GISTs). *Eur J Cancer* 38(Suppl. 5):S60–S65.

132. Sunaga, N., N. Oriuchi, K. Kaira, N. Yanagitani, Y. Tomizawa, T. Hisada, T. Ishizuka, K. Endo, and M. Mori. 2008. Usefulness of FDG-PET for early prediction of the response to gefitinib in non-small cell lung cancer. *Lung Cancer* 59:203–210.

133. Benz, M. R., K. Herrmann, F. Walter, E. B. Garon, K. L. Reckamp, R. Figlin, M. E. Phelps, W. A. Weber, J. Czernin, and M. S. Allen-Auerbach. 2011. 18F-FDG PET/CT for monitoring treatment responses to the epidermal growth factor receptor inhibitor erlotinib. *J Nucl Med* 52:1684–1689.

134. Weber, W. A., and R. Figlin. 2007. Monitoring cancer treatment with PET/CT: Does it make a difference? *J Nucl Med* 48:36S–44S.

135. Wiele, C., V. Kruse, P. Smeets, M. Sathekge, and A. Maes. 2013. Predictive and prognostic value of metabolic tumour volume and total lesion glycolysis in solid tumours. *Eur J Nucl Med Mol Imaging* 40:290–301.

136. Cheson, B. D., B. Pfistner, M. E. Juweid, R. D. Gascoyne, L. Specht, S. J. Horning, B. Coiffier, et al. 2007. Revised response criteria for malignant lymphoma. *J Clin Oncol* 25:579–586.

137. Barrington, S. F., N. G. Mikhaeel, L. Kostakoglu, M. Meignan, M. Hutchings, S. P. Mueller, L. H. Schwartz, et al. 2014. Role of imaging in the staging and response assessment of lymphoma: Consensus of the International Conference on Malignant Lymphomas Imaging Working Group. *J Clin Oncol* 32:3048–3058.

138. de Geus-Oei, L., H. Oei, G. Hennemann, and E. Krenning. 2002. Sensitivity of 123I whole-body scan and thyroglobulin in the detection of metastases or recurrent differentiated thyroid cancer. *Eur J Nucl Med Mol Imaging* 29:768–774.

139. Xue, Y.-L., Z.-L. Qiu, H.-J. Song, and Q.-Y. Luo. 2013. Value of 131I SPECT/CT for the evaluation of differentiated thyroid cancer: A systematic review of the literature. *Eur J Nucl Med Mol Imaging* 40:768–778.

140. Eslamy, H. K., and H. A. Ziessman. 2008. Parathyroid scintigraphy in patients with primary hyperparathyroidism: 99mTc sestamibi SPECT and SPECT/CT1. *Radiographics* 28:1461–1476.

141. Lu, S., G. Gnanasegaran, J. Buscombe, and S. Navalkissoor. 2013. Single photon emission computed tomography/computed tomography in the evaluation of neuroendocrine tumours: A review of the literature. *Nucl Med Commun* 34:98–107.

142. Brandon, D., A. Alazraki, R. K. Halkar, and N. P. Alazraki. 2011. The role of single-photon emission computed tomography and SPECT/computed tomography in oncologic imaging. *Semin Oncol* 38:87–108.

143. Horger, M., S. Eschmann, C. Pfannneberg, R. Vonthein, H. Besenfelder, C. Claussen, and R. Bares. 2004. Evaluation of combined transmission and emission tomography for classification of skeletal lesions. *Am J Roentgenol* 183:655–661.

144. Römer, W., A. Nömayr, M. Uder, W. Bautz, and T. Kuwert. 2006. SPECT-guided CT for evaluating foci of increased bone metabolism classified as indeterminate on SPECT in cancer patients. *J Nucl Med* 47:1102–1106.

145. Utsunomiya, D., S. Shiraishi, M. Imuta, S. Tomiguchi, K. Kawanaka, S. Morishita, K. Awai, and Y. Yamashita. 2006. Added value of SPECT/CT fusion in assessing suspected bone metastasis: Comparison with scintigraphy alone and nonfused scintigraphy and CT. *Radiology* 238:264–271.

146. Even-Sapir, E., G. Flusser, H. Lerman, G. Lievshitz, and U. Metser. 2007. SPECT/multislice low-dose CT: A clinically relevant constituent in the imaging algorithm of nononcologic patients referred for bone scintigraphy. *J Nucl Med* 48:319–324.

147. Even-Sapir, E., U. Metser, E. Mishani, G. Lievshitz, H. Lerman, and I. Leibovitch. 2006. The detection of bone metastases in patients with high-risk prostate cancer: 99mTc-MDP planar bone scintigraphy, single- and multi-field-of-view SPECT, 18F-fluoride PET, and 18F-fluoride PET/CT. *J Nucl Med* 47:287–297.

148. Parker, C., S. Nilsson, D. Heinrich, S. I. Helle, J. M. O'Sullivan, S. D. Fosså, A. Chodacki, et al. 2013. Alpha emitter radium-223 and survival in metastatic prostate cancer. *N Engl J Med* 369:213–223.

149. Czernin, J., N. Satyamurthy, and C. Schiepers. 2010. Molecular mechanisms of bone 18F-NaF deposition. *J Nucl Med* 51:1826–1829.

150. Cheran, S., J. Herndon II, and E. Patz Jr. 2004. Comparison of whole-body FDG-PET to bone scan for detection of bone metastases in patients with a new diagnosis of lung cancer. *Lung Cancer* 44:317–325.

151. Iwata, M., K. Kasagi, T. Misaki, K. Matsumoto, Y. Iida, T. Ishimori, Y. Nakamoto, T. Higashi, T. Saga, and J. Konishi. 2004. Comparison of whole-body 18F-FDG PET, 99mTc-MIBI SPET, and post-therapeutic 131I-Na scintigraphy in the detection of metastatic thyroid cancer. *Eur J Nucl Med Mol Imaging* 31:491–498.

152. Nakatani, K., Y. Nakamoto, T. Saga, T. Higashi, and K. Togashi. 2011. The potential clinical value of FDG-PET for recurrent renal cell carcinoma. *Eur J Radiol* 79:29–35.

153. Riegger, C., J. Herrmann, J. Nagarajah, J. Hecktor, S. Kuemmel, F. Otterbach, S. Hahn, A. Bockisch, T. Lauenstein, G. Antoch, and T. Heusner. 2012. Whole-body FDG PET/CT is more accurate than conventional imaging for staging primary breast cancer patients. *Eur J Nucl Med Mol Imaging* 39:852–863.

154. Du, Y., I. Cullum, T. Illidge, and P. Ell. 2007. Fusion of metabolic function and morphology: Sequential [18F]fluorodeoxyglucose positron-emission tomography/computed tomography studies yield new insights into the natural history of bone metastases in breast cancer. *J Clin Oncol* 25:3440–3447.

155. Berman, D. S., J. Maddahi, B. K. Tamarappoo, J. Czernin, R. Taillefer, J. E. Udelson, C. M. Gibson, M. Devine, J. Lazewatsky, G. Bhat, and D. Washburn. 2013. Phase II safety and clinical comparison with single-photon emission computed tomography myocardial perfusion imaging for detection of coronary artery disease: Flurpiridaz F 18 positron emission tomography. *J Am Coll Cardiol* 61:469–477.

156. Kuhle, W., G. Porenta, S. Huang, D. Buxton, S. Gambhir, H. Hansen, M. Phelps, and H. Schelbert. 1992. Quantification of regional myocardial blood flow using 13N-ammonia and reoriented dynamic positron emission tomographic imaging. *Circulation* 86:1004–1017.

157. Schelbert, H. R. 2002. 18F-deoxyglucose and the assessment of myocardial viability. *Semin Nucl Med* 32:60–69.

158. Dunphy, M. P. S., A. Freiman, S. M. Larson, and H. W. Strauss. 2005. Association of vascular 18F-FDG uptake with vascular calcification. *J Nucl Med* 46:1278–1284.

159. Dweck, M. R., M. W. L. Chow, N. V. Joshi, M. C. Williams, C. Jones, A. M. Fletcher, H. Richardson, et al. 2012. Coronary arterial 18F-sodium fluoride uptake: A novel marker of plaque biology. *J Am Coll Cardiol* 59:1539–1548.

160. Uppal, R., C. Catana, I. Ay, T. Benner, A. G. Sorensen, and P. Caravan. 2011. Bimodal thrombus imaging: Simultaneous PET/MR imaging with a fibrin-targeted dual PET/MR probe—Feasibility study in rat model. *Radiology* 258:812–820.

161. Schelbert, H., G. Wisenberg, M. Phelps, K. Gould, E. Henze, E. Hoffman, A. Gomes, and D. Kuhl. 1982. Noninvasive assessment of coronary stenoses by myocardial imaging during pharmacologic coronary vasodilation. VI. Detection of coronary artery disease in human beings with intravenous N-13 ammonia and positron computed tomography. *Am J Cardiol* 49:1197–1207.

162. Maddahi, J. 2012. Properties of an ideal PET perfusion tracer: New PET tracer cases and data. *J Nucl Cardiol* 19:9491–9498.

163. Danad, I., P. G. Raijmakers, Y. E. Appelman, H. J. Harms, S. de Haan, M. L. P. van den Oever, M. W. Heymans, et al. 2013. Hybrid imaging using quantitative H215O PET and CT-based coronary angiography for the detection of coronary artery disease. *J Nucl Med* 54:55–63.

164. Kajander, S., E. Joutsiniemi, M. Saraste, M. Pietilä, H. Ukkonen, A. Saraste, H. T. Sipilä, et al. 2010. Cardiac positron emission tomography/computed tomography imaging accurately detects anatomically and functionally significant coronary artery disease. *Circulation* 122:603–613.

165. Beanlands, R. S. B., G. Nichol, E. Huszti, D. Humen, N. Racine, M. Freeman, K. Y. Gulenchyn, et al. 2007. F-18-fluorodeoxyglucose positron emission tomography imaging-assisted management of patients with severe left ventricular dysfunction and suspected coronary disease: A randomized, controlled trial (PARR-2). *J Am Coll Cardiol* 50:2002–2012.

166. Schindler, T. H., H. R. Schelbert, A. Quercioli, and V. Dilsizian. 2010. Cardiac PET imaging for the detection and monitoring of coronary artery disease and microvascular health. *JACC Cardiovascular Imaging* 3:623–640.

167. Alexánderson Rosas, E., P. J. Slomka, L. García-Rojas, R. Calleja, R. Jácome, M. Jiménez-Santos, E. Romero, A. Meave, and D. S. Berman. 2010. Functional impact of coronary stenosis observed on coronary computed tomography angiography: Comparison with 13N-ammonia PET. *Arch Med Res* 41:642–648.

168. Sampson, U. K., S. Dorbala, A. Limaye, R. Kwong, and M. F. Di Carli. 2007. Diagnostic accuracy of rubidium-82 myocardial perfusion imaging with hybrid positron emission tomography/computed tomography in the detection of coronary artery disease. *J Am Coll Cardiol* 49:1052–1058.

169. Bateman, T., G. Heller, A. McGhie, J. Friedman, J. Case, J. Bryngelson, G. Hertenstein, K. Moutray, K. Reid, and S. Cullom. 2006. Diagnostic accuracy of rest/stress ECG-gated Rb-82 myocardial perfusion PET: Comparison with ECG-gated Tc-99m sestamibi SPECT. *J Nucl Cardiol* 13:24–33.

170. Czernin, J., G. Porenta, R. Brunken, J. Krivokapich, K. Chen, R. Bennett, A. Hage, C. Fung, J. Tillisch, M. Phelps, and H. Schelbert. 1993. Regional blood flow, oxidative metabolism, and glucose utilization in patients with recent myocardial infarction. *Circulation* 88:884–895.

171. Slart, R. H. J. A., C. J. Zeebregts, H. L. Hillege, J. de Sutter, R. A. J. O. Dierckx, D. J. van Veldhuisen, F. Zijlstra, and R. A. Tio. 2011. Myocardial perfusion reserve after a PET-driven revascularization procedure: A strong prognostic factor. *J Nucl Med* 52:873–879.

172. Patterson, R. E., R. L. Eisner, and S. F. Horowitz. 1995. Comparison of cost-effectiveness and utility of exercise ECG, single photon emission computed tomography, positron emission tomography, and coronary angiography for diagnosis of coronary artery disease. *Circulation* 91:54–65.

173. Siegrist, P., L. Husmann, M. Knabenhans, O. Gaemperli, I. Valenta, T. Hoefflinghaus, H. Scheffel, P. Stolzmann, H. Alkadhi, and P. Kaufmann. 2008. 13N-ammonia myocardial perfusion imaging with a PET/CT scanner: Impact on clinical decision making and cost-effectiveness. *Eur J Nucl Med Mol Imaging* 35:889–895.

174. Berman, D. S., R. Hachamovitch, L. J. Shaw, J. D. Friedman, S. W. Hayes, L. E. J. Thomson, D. S. Fieno, et al. 2006. Roles of nuclear cardiology, cardiac computed tomography, and cardiac magnetic resonance: Assessment of patients with suspected coronary artery disease. *J Nucl Med* 47:74–82.

175. R. C. Hendel, D. S. Berman, M. F. Di Carli, P. A. Heidenreich, R. E. Henkin, P. A. Pellikka, G. M. Pohost, and K. A. Williams. 2009. ACCF/ASNC/ACR/AHA/ASE/SCCT/SCMR/SNM 2009 appropriate use criteria for cardiac radionuclide imaging: A report of the American College of Cardiology Foundation Appropriate Use Criteria Task Force, the American Society of Nuclear Cardiology, the American College of Radiology, the American Heart Association, the American Society of Echocardiography, the Society of Cardiovascular Computed Tomography, the Society for Cardiovascular Magnetic Resonance, and the Society of Nuclear Medicine: Endorsed by the American College of Emergency Physicians. *Circulation* 119:e561–e587.

176. Masood, Y., Y. Liu, G. Depuey, R. Taillefer, L. Araujo, S. Allen, D. Delbeke, et al. 2005. Clinical validation of SPECT attenuation correction using x-ray computed tomography-derived attenuation maps: Multicenter clinical trial with angiographic correlation. *J Nucl Cardiol* 12:676–686.

177. Rana, J., A. Rozanski, and D. Berman. 2011. Combination of myocardial perfusion imaging and coronary artery calcium scanning: Potential synergies for improving risk assessment in subjects with suspected coronary artery disease. *Curr Atheroscler Rep* 13:381–389.

178. Rispler, S., Z. Keidar, E. Ghersin, A. Roguin, A. Soil, R. Dragu, D. Litmanovich, et al. 2007. Integrated single-photon emission computed tomography and computed tomography coronary angiography for the assessment of hemodynamically significant coronary artery lesions. *J Am Coll Cardiol* 49:1059–1067.

179. Rispler, S., D. Aronson, S. Abadi, A. Roguin, A. Engel, R. Beyar, O. Israel, and Z. Keidar. 2011. Integrated SPECT/CT for assessment of haemodynamically significant coronary artery lesions in patients with acute coronary syndrome. *Eur J Nucl Med Mol Imaging* 38:1917–1925.

180. Slart, R. J. A., R. Tio, F. Zijlstra, and R. Dierckx. 2009. Diagnostic pathway of integrated SPECT/CT for coronary artery disease. *Eur J Nucl Med Mol Imaging* 36:1829–1834.

181. Drevets, W. C., M. E. Thase, E. L. Moses-Kolko, J. Price, E. Frank, D. J. Kupfer, and C. Mathis. 2007. Serotonin-1A receptor imaging in recurrent depression: Replication and literature review. *Nucl Med Biol* 34:865–877.

182. Kaasinen, V., and J. O. Rinne. 2002. Functional imaging studies of dopamine system and cognition in normal aging and Parkinson's disease. *Neurosci Biobehav Rev* 26:785–793.

183. Kuhl, D., R. Koeppe, S. Minoshima, S. Snyder, E. Ficaro, N. Foster, K. Frey, and M. Kilbourn. 1999. In vivo mapping of cerebral acetylcholinesterase activity in aging and Alzheimer's disease. *Neurology* 52:691–699.

184. Nordberg, A., H. Lundqvist, P. Hartvig, A. Lilja, and B. Långström. 1995. Kinetic analysis of regional (S)(-)11C-nicotine binding in normal and Alzheimer brains—In vivo assessment using positron emission tomography. *Alzheimer Dis Assoc Disord* 9:21–27.

185. Brooks, D. J. 2010. Imaging dopamine transporters in Parkinson's disease. *Biomark Med* 4:651–660.

186. Taal, W., D. Brandsma, H. G. de Bruin, J. E. Bromberg, A. T. Swaak-Kragten, P. A. E. Sillevis Smitt, C. A. van Es, and M. J. van den Bent. 2008. Incidence of early pseudo-progression in a cohort of malignant glioma patients treated with chemoirradiation with temozolomide. *Cancer* 113:405–410.

187. Herholz, K., K.-J. Langen, C. Schiepers, and J. M. Mountz. 2012. Brain tumors. *Semin Nucl Med* 42:356–370.

188. Reivich, M., D. Kuhl, A. Wolf, J. Greenberg, M. Phelps, T. Ido, V. Casella, J. Fowler, E. Hoffman, A. Alavi, P. Son, and L. Sokoloff. 1979. The (18F) fluorodeoxyglucose method for the measurement of local cerebral glucose utilization in man. *Circ Res* 44:127–137.

189. Di Chiro, G., R. DeLaPaz, R. Brooks, L. Sokoloff, P. Kornblith, B. Smith, N. Patronas, et al. 1982. Glucose utilization of cerebral gliomas measured by [18F] fluorodeoxyglucose and positron emission tomography. *Neurology* 32:1323–1329.

190. Alavi, J., A. Alavi, J. Chawluk, M. Kushner, J. Powe, W. Hickey, and M. Reivich. 1988. Positron emission tomography in patients with glioma. A predictor of prognosis. *Cancer* 62:1074–1078.

191. Patronas, N. J., G. Di Chiro, R. A. Brooks, R. L. DeLaPaz, P. L. Kornblith, B. H. Smith, H. V. Rizzoli, et al. 1982. Work in progress: [18F] fluorodeoxyglucose and positron emission tomography in the evaluation of radiation necrosis of the brain. *Radiology* 144:885–889.

192. Herrmann, K., J. Czernin, T. Cloughesy, A. Lai, K. L. Pomykala, M. R. Benz, A. K. Buck, M. E. Phelps, and W. Chen. 2014. Comparison of visual and semiquantitative analysis of 18F-FDOPA-PET/CT for recurrence detection in glioblastoma patients. *Neuro Oncol* 16:603–609.

193. Chen, W., D. H. S. Silverman, S. Delaloye, J. Czernin, N. Kamdar, W. Pope, N. Satyamurthy, C. Schiepers, and T. Cloughesy. 2006. 18F-FDOPA PET imaging of brain tumors: Comparison study with 18F-FDG PET and evaluation of diagnostic accuracy. *J Nucl Med* 47:904–911.

194. Piroth, M. D., M. Pinkawa, R. Holy, J. Klotz, S. Nussen, G. Stoffels, H. H. Coenen, H. J. Kaiser, K. J. Langen, and M. J. Eble. 2011. Prognostic value of early [18F]fluoroethyltyrosine positron emission tomography after radiochemotherapy in glioblastoma multiforme. *Int J Radiat Oncol Biol Phys* 80:176–184.

195. Bohnen, N. I., D. S. W. Djang, K. Herholz, Y. Anzai, and S. Minoshima. 2012. Effectiveness and safety of 18F-FDG PET in the evaluation of dementia: A review of the recent literature. *J Nucl Med* 53:59–71.

196. Heiss, W., J. Kessler, B. Szelies, M. Grond, G. Fink, and K. Herholz. 1991. Positron emission tomography in the differential diagnosis of organic dementias. *J Neural Transm Suppl* 33:13–19.

197. Small, G. W., P. Siddarth, V. Kepe, L. M. Ercoli, A. C. Burggren, S. Y. Bookheimer, K. J. Miller, J. Kim, H. Lavretsky, S. C. Huang, and J. R. Barrio. 2012. Prediction of cognitive decline by positron emission tomography of brain amyloid and tau. *Arch Neurol* 69:215–222.

198. Silverman, D., G. Small, and C. Chang. 2001. Positron emission tomography in evaluation of dementia: Regional brain metabolism and long-term outcome. *JAMA* 286:2120–2127.

199. Herholz, K., S. F. Carter, and M. Jones. 2007. Positron emission tomography imaging in dementia. *Br J Radiol* 80:S160–S167.

200. Agdeppa, E. D., V. Kepe, J. Liu, S. Flores-Torres, N. Satyamurthy, A. Petric, G. M. Cole, G. W. Small, S.-C. Huang, and J. R. Barrio. 2001. Binding characteristics of radiofluorinated 6-dialkylamino-2-naphthylethylidene derivatives as positron emission tomography imaging probes for β-amyloid plaques in Alzheimer's disease. *J Neurosci* 21:RC189.

201. Mathis, C. A., Y. Wang, D. P. Holt, G.-F. Huang, M. L. Debnath, and W. E. Klunk. 2003. Synthesis and evaluation of 11C-labeled 6-substituted 2-arylbenzothiazoles as amyloid imaging agents. *J Med Chem* 46:2740–2754.

202. Otsuka, M., Y. Ichiya, Y. Kuwabara, S. Hosokawa, M. Sasaki, T. Yoshida, T. Fukumura, K. Masuda, and M. Kato. 1996. Differences in the reduced 18F-Dopa uptakes of the caudate and the putamen in Parkinson's disease: Correlations with the three main symptoms. *J Neurol Sci* 136:169–173.

203. Brück, A., S. Aalto, E. Rauhala, J. Bergman, R. Marttila, and J. O. Rinne. 2009. A follow-up study on 6-[18F]fluoro-L-dopa uptake in early Parkinson's disease shows nonlinear progression in the putamen. *Mov Disord* 24:1009–1015.

204. Stoessl, A. J. 2007. Positron emission tomography in premotor Parkinson's disease. *Parkinsonism Relat Disord* 13(Suppl. 3):S421–S424.

205. Pavese, N., A. Evans, Y. Tai, G. Hotton, D. Brooks, A. Lees, and P. Piccini. 2006. Clinical correlates of levodopa-induced dopamine release in Parkinson disease: A PET study. *Neurology* 67:1612–1617.

206. Brandes, A. A., A. Tosoni, F. Spagnolli, G. Frezza, M. Leonardi, F. Calbucci, and E. Franceschi. 2008. Disease progression or pseudoprogression after concomitant radiochemotherapy treatment: Pitfalls in neurooncology. *Neuro Oncol* 10:361–367.

207. Chinn, R. J., I. D. Wilkinson, M. A. Hall-Craggs, M. N. Paley, R. F. Miller, B. E. Kendall, S. P. Newman, and M. J. Harrison. 1995. Toxoplasmosis and primary central nervous system lymphoma in HIV infection: Diagnosis with MR spectroscopy. *Radiology* 197:649–654.

208. Schillaci, O., L. Filippi, C. Manni, and R. Santoni. 2007. Single-photon emission computed tomography/computed tomography in brain tumors. *Semin Nucl Med* 37:34–47.

209. Hemm, S., N. Vayssiere, M. Zanca, P. Ravel, and P. Coubes. 2004. Thallium SPECT-based stereotactic targeting for brain tumor biopsies. A technical note. *Stereotact Funct Neurosurg* 82:70–76.

210. Filippi, L., O. Schillaci, R. Santoni, C. Manni, R. Danieli, and G. Simonetti 2006. Usefulness of SPECT/CT with a hybrid camera for the functional anatomical mapping of primary brain tumors by [Tc99m] tetrofosmin. *Cancer Biother Radiopharm* 21:41–48.

211. Hillner, B. E., B. A. Siegel, D. Liu, A. F. Shields, I. F. Gareen, L. Hanna, S. H. Stine, and R. E. Coleman. 2008. Impact of positron emission tomography/computed tomography and positron emission tomography (PET) alone on expected management of patients with cancer: Initial results from the National Oncologic PET Registry. *J Clin Oncol* 26:2155–2161.

212. Hillner, B. E., B. A. Siegel, A. F. Shields, D. Liu, I. F. Gareen, E. Hunt, and R. E. Coleman. 2008. Relationship between cancer type and impact of PET and PET/CT on intended management: Findings of the National Oncologic PET Registry. *J Nucl Med* 49:1928–1935.

213. Yap, C. S., M. A. Seltzer, C. Schiepers, S. S. Gambhir, J. Rao, M. E. Phelps, P. E. Valk, and J. Czernin. 2001. Impact of whole-body 18F-FDG PET on staging and managing patients with breast cancer: The referring physician's perspective. *J Nucl Med* 42:1334–1337.

214. Seltzer, M. A., C. S. Yap, D. H. Silverman, J. Meta, C. Schiepers, M. E. Phelps, S. S. Gambhir, J. Rao, P. E. Valk, and J. Czernin. 2002. The impact of PET on the management of lung cancer: The referring physician's perspective. *J Nucl Med* 43:752–756.

215. Schöder, H., J. Meta, C. Yap, M. Ariannejad, J. Rao, M. E. Phelps, P. E. Valk, J. Sayre, and J. Czernin. 2001. Effect of whole-body 18F-FDG PET imaging on clinical staging and management of patients with malignant lymphoma. *J Nucl Med* 42:1139–1143.

216. Dührsen, U., A. Hüttmann, K.-H. Jöckel, and S. Müller. 2009. Positron emission tomography guided therapy of aggressive non-Hodgkin lymphomas—The PETAL trial. *Leuk Lymphoma* 50:1757–1760.

217. Lordick, F., K. Ott, B.-J. Krause, W. A. Weber, K. Becker, H. J. Stein, S. Lorenzen, et al. 2007. PET to assess early metabolic response and to guide treatment of adenocarcinoma of the oesophagogastric junction: The MUNICON phase II trial. *Lancet Oncol* 8:797–805.

218. van Tinteren, H., O. S. Hoekstra, E. F. Smit, J. H. A. M. van den Bergh, A. J. M. Schreurs, R. A. L. M. Stallaert, P. C. M. van Velthoven, et al. 2002. Effectiveness of positron emission tomography in the preoperative assessment of patients with suspected non-small-cell lung cancer: The PLUS multicentre randomised trial. *Lancet* 359:1388–1392.

219. Ruers, T. J. M., B. Wiering, J. R. M. van der Sijp, R. M. Roumen, K. P. de Jong, E. F. I. Comans, J. Pruim, H. M. Dekker, P. F. M. Krabbe, and W. J. G. Oyen. 2009. Improved selection of patients for hepatic surgery of colorectal liver metastases with 18F-FDG PET: A randomized study. *J Nucl Med* 50:1036–1041.

220. Sobhani, I., E. Tiret, R. Lebtahi, T. Aparicio, E. Itti, F. Montravers, C. Vaylet, et al. 2008. Early detection of recurrence by 18FDG-PET in the follow-up of patients with colorectal cancer. *Br J Cancer* 98:875–880.

221. Lerman, H., U. Metser, G. Lievshitz, F. Sperber, S. Shneebaum, and E. Even-Sapir. 2006. Lymphoscintigraphic sentinel node identification in patients with breast cancer: The role of SPECT-CT. *Eur J Nucl Med Mol Imaging* 33:329–337.

222. van der Ploeg, I. M. C., R. A. Valdés Olmos, O. E. Nieweg, E. J. T. Rutgers, B. B. R. Kroon, and C. A. Hoefnagel. 2007. The additional value of SPECT/CT in lymphatic mapping in breast cancer and melanoma. *J Nucl Med* 48:1756–1760.

223. Lerman, H., G. Lievshitz, O. Zak, U. Metser, S. Schneebaum, and E. Even-Sapir. 2007. Improved sentinel node identification by SPECT/CT in overweight patients with breast cancer. *J Nucl Med* 48:201–206.

224. Even-Sapir, E., H. Lerman, G. Lievshitz, A. Khafif, D. M. Fliss, A. Schwartz, E. Gur, Y. Skornick, and S. Schneebaum. 2003. Lymphoscintigraphy for sentinel node mapping using a hybrid SPECT/CT system. *J Nucl Med* 44:1413–1420.

225. Khafif, A., S. Schneebaum, D. M. Fliss, H. Lerman, U. Metser, R. Ben-Yosef, Z. Gil, L. Reider-Trejo, L. Genadi, and E. Even-Sapir. 2006. Lymphoscintigraphy for sentinel node mapping using a hybrid single photon emission CT (SPECT)/CT system in oral cavity squamous cell carcinoma. *Head Neck* 28:874–879.

226. Tharp, K., O. Israel, J. Hausmann, L. Bettman, W. H. Martin, M. Daitzchman, M. P. Sandler, and D. Delbeke. 2004. Impact of 131I-SPECT/CT images obtained with an integrated system in the follow-up of patients with thyroid carcinoma. *Eur J Nucl Med Mol Imaging* 31:1435–1442.

227. Ruf, J., L. Lehmkuhl, H. Bertram, D. Sandrock, H. Amthauer, B. Humplik, L. Munz, and D. Felix. 2004. Impact of SPECT and integrated low-dose CT after radioiodine therapy on the management of patients with thyroid carcinoma. *Nucl Med Commun* 25:1177–1182.

228. Serra, A., P. Bolasco, L. Satta, A. Nicolosi, A. Uccheddu, and M. Piga. 2006. Role of SPECT/CT in the preoperative assessment of hyperparathyroid patients. *Radiol Med* 111:999–1008.

229. Krausz, Y., L. Bettman, L. Guralnik, G. Yosilevsky, Z. Keidar, R. Bar-Shalom, E. Even-Sapir, R. Chisin, and O. Israel. 2006. Technetium-99m-MIBI SPECT/CT in primary hyperparathyroidism. *World J Surg* 30:76–83.

230. Krausz, Y., Z. Keidar, I. Kogan, E. Even-Sapir, R. Bar-Shalom, A. Engel, R. Rubinstein, J. Sachs, M. Bocher, S. Agranovicz, R. Chisin, and O. Israel. 2003. SPECT/CT hybrid imaging with 111In-pentetreotide in assessment of neuroendocrine tumours. *Clin Endocrinol* 59:565–573.

231. Pfannenberg, A., S. Eschmann, M. Horger, R. Lamberts, R. Vonthein, C. Claussen, and R. Bares. 2003. Benefit of anatomical-functional image fusion in the diagnostic work-up of neuroendocrine neoplasms. *Eur J Nucl Med Mol Imaging* 30:835–843.

232. Hillel, P. G., E. J. R. van Beek, C. Taylor, E. Lorenz, N. D. S. Bax, V. Prakash, and W. B. Tindale. 2006. The clinical impact of a combined gamma camera/CT imaging system on somatostatin receptor imaging of neuroendocrine tumours. *Clin Radiol* 61:579–587.

233. Lapa, C., T. Linsenmann, C. M. Monoranu, S. Samnick, A. K. Buck, C. Bluemel, J. Czernin, et al. 2014. Comparison of the amino acid tracers 18F-FET and 18F-DOPA in high-grade glioma patients. *J Nucl Med* 55:1611–1616.

234. Buck, A. K., G. Halter, H. Schirrmeister, J. Kotzerke, I. Wurziger, G. Glatting, T. Mattfeldt, B. Neumaier, S. N. Reske, and M. Hetzel. 2003. Imaging proliferation in lung tumors with PET: 18F-FLT versus 18F-FDG. *J Nucl Med* 44:1426–1431.

235. Herrmann, K., M. R. Benz, J. Czernin, M. S. Allen-Auerbach, W. D. Tap, S. M. Dry, T. Schuster, J. J. Eckardt, M. E. Phelps, W. A. Weber, and F. C. Eilber. 2012. 18F-FDG-PET/CT imaging as an early survival predictor in patients with primary high-grade soft tissue sarcomas undergoing neoadjuvant therapy. *Clin Cancer Res* 18:2024–2031.

Index

A

AC. *see* Attenuation correction (AC)
Adaptive imaging, 154
Analytic 2D image reconstruction, 239–241
Anatometabolic PET/CT imaging, 340–341
Anatomical priors, 250–251
Anesthesia
    inhalation, 431
    injectable, 430–431
APD-based systems, 383–385
Attenuation
    and PET imaging, 33–34
    and quantitative SPECT imaging, 196–199
Attenuation correction (AC)
    artifacts and bias from, 356–359
    basics, 352–353
    contrast agents, 358
    effect of the various parameters, 356
    metal implants, 356–358
    models for calculation, 353–355
    patient motion, 358–359
    and PET imaging, 214–219
Attenuation maps, 136
Avalanche photodiodes (APDs), 77–80
    applications of, 80
    gain, 78–79
    noise, 79–80

B

Back- and forward projection, using CUDA,
    278–279
Backprojection
    filtered, 35–36
    and image reconstruction, 263–264
    using texture mapping, 277–278
Basic signal multiplexing, 94–97
Basis function selection, 244–245
Bias affect, and quantitative SPECT imaging, 196
Block detector design, 174–176
Block effect, 167–168
Blood oxygenation, 433

Blood pressure, 433
Blood sampling, 433–434
Body temperature, 432
Bone scans, SPECT/CT imaging in, 375
Brain SPECT imaging, 138–140
    consideration for, 139
    single-purpose systems, 139–140
    using general-purpose systems, 139

C

Cardiac SPECT imaging systems, 140–153
    general considerations for, 140–141
    general-purpose dual-head systems, 141–142
    single-purpose, 142–153
        cardio-centric geometry, 142–143
        Cardius series from Digirad, 144–145
        Discovery 530c, 150–152
        D-SPECT, 149–150
        high normalized system sensitivity, 142
        IQ-SPECT, 146–149
        mini-dual-head systems, 144
        motion-free imaging operation, 143
        MP-SPECT, 145–146
        scout imaging and patient
            positioning, 143
Cardio-centric geometry, 142–143
Cardiology
    PET/CT imaging in, 454–455
    SPECT/CT imaging in, 374–375, 455–456
Clinical single-photon dynamic studies, 286–287
Clinical SPECT imaging, 138
Coincidence detection, 31
Collimator systems, 154, 419, 426–428
    converging, 128
    diverging, 128
    parallel-hole, 127–128
    pinhole, 126–127
    slit-slat, 128–129
    and x-ray contamination, 129
Compact high-resolution SPECT detectors, 417
Continuous table motion, 361–362
Converging collimator systems, 128

Coprocessor, GPU as, 270–272
Cost, and SPECT instrumentation, 125–126

D

Dark current, 70
  and noise, 84–85
Data acquisition
  and dynamic SPECT imaging
    fast camera rotation methods, 289–290
    mixed planar-SPECT acquisitions, 290
    slow camera rotation methods, 288–289
    and stationary systems, 290–291
  goals of, 91–94
  and PET instrumentation
    coincidence identification methods, 182–183
    overview, 180–181
    singles event acquisition, 181–182
  pulse integration and basic signal multiplexing,
    94–97
  sequential, 386–387
  simultaneous, 382–386
    APD-based systems, 383–385
    PMT-based systems, 382–383
    SIPM-based systems, 385–386
  and SPECT instrumentation, 134
  supporting software, 103–112
  system topologies, 97–103
Data normalization, and PET imaging, 228–231
Data-parallel algorithms, 261–262
Decoding error/block effect, 167–168
Delayed coincidence identification, 182–183
Detection geometry
  and PET instrumentation, 170–172
  SPECT instrumentation, 119
Detector design, PET instrumentation, 420–421
  block detector, 174–176
  panel-type, 176
  for preclinical and high-resolution systems,
    176–180
  requirements for performance, 173–174
Detector efficiency, 172
Detector response, and quantitative SPECT
    imaging, 203–204
Detector technologies, for SPECT, 154, 416–419
  monolithic scintillator-based detector, 131–132
  pixelated CZT-based detector, 133–134
  pixelated scintillator-based detector, 132–133
Digital silicon photomultiplier, 85–86
Diverging collimator systems, 128
Dual-modality PET/CT imaging, 341–343

Dynamic PET imaging
  framing rate, 324
  image reconstruction, 325
  injected dose, 324
  issues of concern, 330–332
  movement correction, 325–326
  overview, 321–323
  scan time of, 323–324
  tracer kinetic modeling
    application of, 328–330
    parametric imaging, 330
    validation of, 327–328
  volume of interest (VOI)/ROI, 326–327
    and time–activity curve extraction, 327
Dynamic SPECT imaging, 154–155
  challenges of, 286
  classification based on data acquisition
    methods
    fast camera rotation methods, 289–290
    mixed planar-SPECT acquisitions, 290
    slow camera rotation methods, 288–289
    and stationary systems, 290–291
  classification based on data processing
    methods
    image-based approaches, 291–292
    projection-based approaches, 292
  clinical single-photon dynamic studies,
    286–287
  factor analysis of, 306–309
    algorithms for, 308–309
    clinical example of, 309
    mathematical formulation and
      nonuniqueness, 307–308
  and image reconstruction, 293–298
    spatiotemporal basis functions, 304–306
  overview, 286
  spatiotemporal modeling of, 298–300
    using splines, 300–304
  with stationary systems
    with Discovery NM530C, 311–314
    myocardial blood flow, 309–311

E

ECG. *see* Electrocardiograph (ECG)
Electrocardiograph (ECG), 432
Electromagnetic interference, 380–381
Electron multiplication, 68–69
Energy calibration, and PET imaging, 211–212
Energy resolution, and SPECT instrumentation,
    124–125

F

Factor analysis, of dynamic SPECT imaging, 306–309
    algorithms for, 308–309
    clinical example of, 309
    mathematical formulation and nonuniqueness, 307–308
Fast camera rotation methods, 289–290
Fast Fourier transform (FFT), 262–263
FFT. *see* Fast Fourier transform (FFT)
Framing rate, of dynamic PET imaging, 324

G

Gantry system, 135
General-purpose dual-head systems, 141–142
Geometric efficiency, 170–171
Graphics pipeline, 267–270
Graphics processing unit (GPU)
    advanced concepts, 277
    back- and forward projection using CUDA, 278–279
    backprojection using texture mapping, 277–278
    as coprocessor, 270–272
    graphics pipeline, 267–270
    history of, 266–267
    list-mode projection operations, 279–280
    memory operations, 275–277
    multi-GPU reconstruction, 279
    resource allocation, 274–275
    and streaming multiprocessor (SM), 272–274

H

Hardware attenuation correction, 393–394
High normalized system sensitivity, 142
Hybrid PMT (HPMT), 73–75

I

Image-based approaches, and dynamic SPECT imaging, 291–292
Image-based radiotracer arterial input function estimation, 399–400
Image quality, 424
Image reconstruction
    analytic 2D methods, 239–241
    analytic 3D methods
        parallel-beam methods for PET, 241–243
        SPECT reconstruction, 243

    of dynamic PET imaging, 325
    and dynamic SPECT imaging, 293–298
        spatiotemporal basis functions, 304–306
    model-based
        anatomical priors, 250–251
        basis function selection, 244–245
        noise modeling, 246–247
        numerical optimization, 251–253
        objective functions, 247–251
        overview, 243–244
        prior functions, 248–250
        statistical, 244–253
        system modeling, 245–246
    overview, 235–236
    PET data formation, 237–238
    and PET imaging
        backprojection, 263–264
        fast Fourier transform (FFT), 262–263
        filtered backprojection, 35–36
        iterative reconstruction, 264–265
        list-mode reconstruction, 265
    and PET instrumentation, 169
    radon and x-ray transforms, 236–237
    SPECT data formation, 238–239
Imaging volume, and SPECT instrumentation, 119
Inhalation anesthesia, 431
Injectable anesthetics, 430–431
Injected dose, of dynamic PET imaging, 324
Injection techniques, and small-animal imaging, 431–432
Instrumentation
    multimodality systems, 419
    overview, 414–415
    PET
        current state-of-the-art in, 424–425
        depth of interaction, 421–422
        detector design, 420–421
        detector technologies, 416–417
        image quality, 424
        performance testing, 423–424
        scanner geometry, 415, 421
        scanner sensitivity, 420, 424
        scatter, attenuation, and partial volume correction, 422–423
        scatter, count losses, and randoms measurement, 423–424
        spatial resolution, 419–420, 423
    small-animal imaging, 428–434
        anesthesia, 430–431
        blood oxygenation, 433
        blood pressure, 433

blood sampling, 433–434
body temperature, 432
electrocardiograph (ECG), 432
inhalation anesthesia, 431
injectable anesthetics, 430–431
injection techniques, 431–432
pulmonary CO_2, 433
respiration, 432
SPECT
collimation, 419
compact high-resolution detectors, 417
detector technologies, 418–419
retrofitted clinical systems, 417
rotating *versus* stationary systems, 417–418
Iterative reconstruction, 264–265
and PET, 36
and PSF, 364

L

Light yield, 22
List-mode projection operations, 279–280
List-mode reconstruction, 265
Location of interaction, 181

M

Magnetic fields, 70
sensitivity of PET photon detectors, 380
Measurement, and quantitative SPECT imaging,
207–208
Memory operations, and GPU, 275–277
Metastatic bone disease, 453
Microchannel plate, 75
Mini-multi-dual-head cardiac SPECT systems,
144–145
Mixed planar-SPECT acquisitions, 290
Model-based image reconstruction
anatomical priors, 250–251
basis function selection, 244–245
noise modeling, 246–247
numerical optimization, 251–253
objective functions, 247–251
overview, 243–244
prior functions, 248–250
statistical, 244–253
system modeling, 245–246
Molecular and metabolic disease signatures,
448–451
Monolithic scintillator-based detector, 131–132
Monte Carlo methods, 265–266, 280–281

Motion system, 135
correction and gating, 364–365
-free imaging operation, 143
and quantitative SPECT imaging, 206–207
Movement correction, and dynamic PET imaging,
325–326
MR-based photon attenuation correction,
387–388
Multi-GPU reconstruction, 279
Multimodality systems, 419
Myocardial blood flow, 309–311

N

NECR. *see* Noise equivalent count rate (NECR)
Neurology
PET/CT imaging in, 456–458
SPECT/CT imaging in, 459
Noise
avalanche photodiodes (APDs), 79–80
and dark current, 84–85
modeling, 246–247
PIN photodiodes, 76–77
Noise equivalent count rate (NECR), 34–35
Non-rigid-body motion correction, 396–398
Numerical optimization, 251–253

O

Objective functions, 247–251
Objective metrics, and SPECT instrumentation,
122–124
Oncology
PET/CT imaging in, 451–453
SPECT/CT imaging in, 375, 453

P

Panel-type detector design, 176
Parallel-beam analytic 3D methods, 241–243
Parallel-hole collimator systems, 127–128
Partial volume effect, 204–206
correction of, 398–399
Photocathode, 66–67
Photodetection efficiency, 83–84
Photodetectors
overview, 64–65
photomultipler tube (PMT), 22–23
dark current, 70
electron multiplication, 68–69
hybrid PMT (HPMT), 73–75

magnetic fields, 70
microchannel plate, 75
photocathode, 66–67
position-sensitive, 72–73
spatial uniformity, 69–70
time response, 70–71
voltage divider, 71–72
semiconductor detectors
avalanche photodiodes (APDs), 77–80
noise, 76–77
PIN photodiodes, 76–77
silicon photomultiplier, 80–86
solid-state detectors, 24–25
solid-state photodetectors, 23–24
Photomultiplier tube (PMT), 21
-based detectors, 51–52
dark current, 70
electron multiplication, 68–69
hybrid PMT (HPMT), 73–75
magnetic fields, 70
microchannel plate, 75
photocathode, 66–67
position-sensitive, 72–73
spatial uniformity, 69–70
time response, 70–71
voltage divider, 71–72
Photon noncollinearity, 167
Pinhole collimator systems, 126–127
Pixelated CZT-based detector, 133–134
Pixelated scintillator-based detector, 132–133
PMT. see Photomultiplier tube (PMT)
PMT-based systems, 382–383
Position-sensitive PMT, 72–73
Positron emission process, 165–167
Positron emission tomography (PET)–computed
tomography (CT) imaging
advantages of, 442–444
anatometabolic imaging, 340–341
applications, 343–345
attenuation correction
artifacts and bias from, 356–359
basics, 352–353
contrast agents, 358
effect of the various parameters, 356
metal implants, 356–358
models for calculation, 353–355
patient motion, 358–359
cardiac, 454–455
dual-modality, 341–343
history of, 440–441
of metastatic bone disease, 453

molecular and metabolic disease signatures,
444–448
in neurology, 456–458
in oncology, 451–453
patient management and outcome, 459
quality assurance, 350–352
system architecture/models, 345–348
system characteristic performance, 348–350
systems and protocols, 441–442
technical advances in, 359–365
axial FOV, 360
continuous table motion, 361–362
iterative reconstruction and PSF, 364
motion correction and gating, 364–365
TOF, 362–364
transverse FOV, truncation, and wide gantry,
360–361
Positron emission tomography (PET) imaging
and attenuation, 33–34
correction, 214–219
basic principle, 28–30
coincidence detection, 31
and data normalization, 228–231
and data-parallel algorithms, 261–262
and energy calibration, 211–212
exponential attenuation of beam of photons,
16–18
and graphics processing unit (GPU)
advanced concepts, 277
back- and forward projection using CUDA,
278–279
backprojection using texture mapping,
277–278
as coprocessor, 270–272
graphics pipeline, 267–270
history of, 266–267
list-mode projection operations, 279–280
memory operations, 275–277
multi-GPU reconstruction, 279
resource allocation, 274–275
and streaming multiprocessor (SM), 272–274
image analysis and evaluation, 36–37
and image reconstruction
backprojection, 263–264
emission activity level, 231
fast Fourier transform (FFT), 262–263
filtered backprojection, 35–36
iterative reconstruction, 36, 264–265
list-mode reconstruction, 265
interactions of photons with matter, 14–16
Monte Carlo methods, 265–266, 280–281

multiple events, 33
noise equivalent count rate (NECR), 34–35
photodetectors
    photomultiplier tube, 22–23
    solid-state detectors, 24–25
    solid-state photodetectors, 23–24
photon detection
    detection systems, 21
    pulse height analysis, 19–21
    scintillation detection, 21–22
and radioactive decay, 7–12
    mathematics of, 12–13
random coincidences, 32–33
and randoms correction, 224–226
and read-time correction, 226–228
and scatter correction, 219–224
and scattering, 33–34
and sinogram correction, 262
stable and radioactive nuclides, 5–7
time-of-flight, 35
and time resolution, 31–32
and timing calibration, 212–214
true coincidences, 32
units for mass and energy, 4–5
used in scintillators, 48
    properties of, 48–51
Positron emission tomography (PET)
        instrumentation
    basic design, 30–31
    current state-of -the-art in, 424–425
    and data acquisition
        coincidence identification methods, 182–183
        overview, 180–181
        singles event acquisition, 181–182
    decoding error or block effect, 167–168
    delayed coincidence identification, 182–183
    depth of interaction, 165, 421–422
    and detection efficiency, 170–172
        detector efficiency, 172
        geometric efficiency, 170–171
    detector design, 420–421
        block detector, 174–176
        panel-type, 176
        for preclinical and high-resolution systems,
            176–180
        requirements for performance, 173–174
    detector technologies, 165, 416–417
    general 2D sinogram organization, 184–185
    goal of, 164
    image quality, 424
    image reconstruction, 169

overview, 163–164
performance testing, 423–424
photon noncollinearity, 167
positron emission process, 165–167
and sampling, 169
scanner geometry, 415, 421
scanner sensitivity, 420, 424
scatter, attenuation, and partial volume
        correction, 422–423
scatter, count losses, and randoms measurement,
        423–424
sinogram data organization, 183
spatial resolution, 164–169, 419–420, 423
3D sinograms, 185–188
and timing performance, 172–173
total spatial resolution, 169
2D sinogram organization, 183–185
Positron emission tomography (PET)/MRI
    electromagnetic interference, 380–381
    hardware attenuation correction, 393–394
    image-based radiotracer arterial input function
        estimation, 399–400
    magnetic field sensitivity of photon detectors,
        380
    main magnetic field homogeneity, 381
    MR-based photon attenuation correction,
        387–388
    non-rigid-body motion correction, 396–398
    overview, 380
    partial volume effects correction, 398–399
    research and clinical applications, 400–402
    RF coils' PET compatibility, 381–382
    rigid-body motion correction, 394–396
    sequential data acquisition, 386–387
    simultaneous data acquisition, 382–386
        APD-based systems, 383–385
        PMT-based systems, 382–383
        SIPM-based systems, 385–386
    space limitations inside MR bore, 382
    and temperature effects, 381
    tissue attenuation correction, 388–393
Prior functions, 248–250
Projection-based approaches, and dynamic SPECT
        imaging, 292
Pulmonary CO_2, 433
Pulse integration, 94–97

Q

Quantitative SPECT imaging
    attenuation, 196–199

and bias affect, 196
CT imaging, 374
detector response, 203–204
and measurement, 207–208
and motion, 206–207
overall accuracy, 208–209
overview, 195
and partial volume effect, 204–206
and scattering, 199–203
Quenching, 83

R

Radioactive decay, 7–12
    mathematics of, 12–13
Radioactive nuclides, 5–7
Radon and x-ray transforms, 236–237
Randoms correction, and PET imaging, 224–226
Read-time correction, and PET imaging, 226–228
Resource allocation, 274–275
Respiration, and small-animal imaging, 432
Retrofitted SPECT clinical systems, 417
RF coils' PET compatibility, 381–382
Rigid-body motion correction, 394–396
Rotating *versus* stationary SPECT systems,
        417–418

S

Sampling
    and PET instrumentation, 169
    and SPECT instrumentation, 124
Scanner geometry, 415
Scanner sensitivity, 420, 424
Scan time, of dynamic PET imaging, 323–324
Scatter correction, and PET imaging, 219–224
Scattering
    and PET imaging, 33–34
    and quantitative SPECT imaging, 199–203
Scintillators/scintillation
    current SPECT systems, 57
    description, 44–46
    instrumentation choice, 55–56
    overview, 43–44
    photomultiplier tube–based detectors, 51–52
    properties of commercial, 46–47
    silicon photomultiplier–based detectors, 53
    small-animal SPECT, 57
    and SPECT, 55
    time resolution data of PMTs and SiPMs, 54
    used in PET, 48

properties of, 48–51
Scout imaging and patient positioning, 143
Semiconductor detectors
    avalanche photodiodes (APDs), 77–80
        applications of, 80
        gain, 78–79
        noise, 79–80
    PIN photodiodes, 76–77
        noise, 76–77
    silicon photomultiplier, 80–86
        applications, 86
        basic operation, 80–83
        digital silicon photomultiplier, 85–86
        linearity, 84
        noise and dark current, 84–85
        photodetection efficiency, 83–84
        quenching, 83
        time resolution, 85
Septal penetration, 129
Sequential data acquisition, 386–387
Signal-to-noise ratio (SNR), 23
Silicon photomultiplier (SiPM), 80–86
    applications, 86
    basic operation, 80–83
    digital silicon photomultiplier, 85–86
    linearity, 84
    noise and dark current, 84–85
    photodetection efficiency, 83–84
    quenching, 83
    time resolution, 85
Silicon photomultiplier-based detectors, 53
Simultaneous data acquisition, 382–386
    APD-based systems, 383–385
    PMT-based systems, 382–383
    SIPM-based systems, 385–386
Single-photon emission computed tomography
        (SPECT) imaging
    advantages of, 442–444
    analytic 3D methods for image reconstruction,
        243
    attenuation correction, 371–373
    in bone scans, 375
    in cardiology, 374–375, 455–456
    CT reconstruction, 371
    and data-parallel algorithms, 261–262
    future developments and applications of,
        375–376
    and graphics processing unit (GPU)
        advanced concepts, 277
        back- and forward projection using CUDA,
            278–279

backprojection using texture mapping, 277–278
  as coprocessor, 270–272
  graphics pipeline, 267–270
  history of, 266–267
  list-mode projection operations, 279–280
  memory operations, 275–277
  multi-GPU reconstruction, 279
  resource allocation, 274–275
  and streaming multiprocessor (SM), 272–274
history of, 440–441
and image reconstruction
  backprojection, 263–264
  fast Fourier transform (FFT), 262–263
  iterative reconstruction, 264–265
  list-mode reconstruction, 265
of metastatic bone disease, 453
molecular and metabolic disease signatures, 448–451
Monte Carlo methods, 265–266, 280–281
in neurology, 459
in oncology, 375, 453
overview, 25–27, 369–370
patient management and outcome, 459–460
quantitative, 374
  attenuation, 196–199
  and bias affect, 196
  detector response, 203–204
  and measurement, 207–208
  and motion, 206–207
  overall accuracy, 208–209
  overview, 195
  and partial volume effect, 204–206
  and scattering, 199–203
scatter correction, 373–374
and scintillators/scintillation, 55
  new trends in, 57–58
and sinogram correction, 262
systems and protocols, 441–442
Single-photon emission computed tomography (SPECT) instrumentation
adaptive imaging, 154
basic issues, 117–118
collimator systems, 154, 419, 426–428
  converging, 128
  diverging, 128
  parallel-hole, 127–128
  pinhole, 126–127
  slit-slat, 128–129
  and x-ray contamination, 129
compact high-resolution detectors, 417

and cost, 125–126
count rate capability and dead time, 125
CT component, 370–371
CT reconstruction, 371
data acquisition system, 134
detection geometry, 119
detector design, 426
detector technologies, 154, 418–419
  monolithic scintillator-based detector, 131–132
  pixelated CZT-based detector, 133–134
  pixelated scintillator-based detector, 132–133
dynamic imaging, 154–155
and energy resolution, 124–125
gantry system, 135
and geometry, 153
hardware and software of, 117
hole pattern, 129–130
imaging considerations, 118
imaging systems
  brain, 138–140
  cardiac, 140–153
  clinical, 138
  overview, 137–138
and imaging volume, 119
motion system, 135
objective metrics, 122–124
objective of, 117
overview, 116–117
quality control, 428
quality of manufacturing, 130
retrofitted clinical systems, 417
rotating *versus* stationary systems, 417–418
and sampling, 124
sensitivity and spatial resolution, 119–122
septal penetration, 129
and system geometry, 119
transmission CT, 135–136
  attenuation maps, 136
  types of, 136–137
Single-purpose brain SPECT imaging, 139–140
Single-purpose cardiac SPECT imaging, 142–153
  cardio-centric geometry, 142–143
  Cardius series from Digirad, 144–145
  Discovery 530c, 150–152
  D-SPECT, 149–150
  high normalized system sensitivity, 142
  IQ-SPECT, 146–149
  mini-dual-head systems, 144
  motion-free imaging operation, 143
  MP-SPECT, 145–146

scout imaging and patient positioning, 143
Sinograms
    correction and PET imaging, 262
    data organization, 183
    2D organization, 183–185
SiPM. *see* Silicon photomultiplier (SiPM)
SIPM-based systems, 385–386
Slit-slat collimator systems, 128–129
Slow camera rotation methods, 288–289
SM. *see* Streaming multiprocessor (SM)
Small-animal imaging, 428–434
    anesthesia, 430–431
    blood oxygenation, 433
    blood pressure, 433
    blood sampling, 433–434
    body temperature, 432
    electrocardiograph (ECG), 432
    inhalation anesthesia, 431
    injectable anesthetics, 430–431
    injection techniques, 431–432
    pulmonary CO_2, 433
    respiration, 432
    and scintillators/scintillation, 57
SNR. *see* Signal-to-noise ratio (SNR)
Software, for data acquisition, 103–112
Solid-state detectors, 24–25
Solid-state photodetectors, 23–24
Spatial resolution, 119–122, 164–169, 419–420, 423
Spatial uniformity, 69–70
Spatiotemporal modeling
    of dynamic SPECT imaging, 298–300
        using splines, 300–304
Stationary systems
    and dynamic SPECT imaging, 290–291
    dynamic SPECT imaging with
        with Discovery NM530C, 311–314
        myocardial blood flow, 309–311
    rotating *versus,* 417–418
Statistical image reconstruction, 244–253
    basis function selection, 244–245
    noise modeling, 246–247
    numerical optimization, 251–253
    objective functions, 247–251

anatomical priors, 250–251
prior functions, 248–250
system modeling, 245–246
Streaming multiprocessor (SM), 272–274
System geometry, and SPECT instrumentation, 119
System modeling, 245–246
System topologies, 97–103

T

TCT. *see* Transmission CT (tCT)
Texture mapping, and backprojection, 277–278
3D sinograms, 185–188
Time of event, 182
Time-of-flight (TOF) PET, 35, 362–364
Time resolution
    and PET imaging, 31–32
    and SiPM, 85
Time response, 70–71
Timing performance, and PET instrumentation, 172–173
Tissue attenuation correction, 388–393
Tracer kinetic modeling
    application of, 328–330
    parametric imaging, 330
    validation of, 327–328
Transmission CT (tCT), 135–136
    attenuation maps, 136
    types of, 136–137
2D sinogram organization, 183–185

V

Voltage divider, 71–72
Volume of interest (VOI)/ROI, 326–327
    and time–activity curve extraction, 327

X

X-ray
    contamination and collimator systems, 129
    and radon transforms, 236–237